SPEECH PRODUCTION: MOTOR CONTROL, BRAIN RESEARCH AND FLUENCY DISORDERS

SPEECH PRODUCTION: MOTOR CONTROL, BRAIN RESEARCH AND FLUENCY DISORDERS

Editors:

Wouter Hulstijn, Ph.D.
University of Nijmegen
Nijmegen Institute for Cognition Research and Information Technology
Nijmegen, The Netherlands

Herman F.M. Peters, Ph.D.
University Hospital Nijmegen
Department of Voice and Speech Pathology
Nijmegen, The Netherlands

and

Pascal H.H.M. van Lieshout, Ph.D.
University Hospital Nijmegen
Department of Voice and Speech Pathology
Nijmegen, The Netherlands

 1997

ELSEVIER
Amsterdam – Lausanne – New York – Oxford – Shannon – Tokyo

International Congress Series No. 1146
ISBN 0-444-82460-x

This book is printed on acid-free paper.

Published by:
Elsevier Science B.V.
P.O. Box 211
1000 AE Amsterdam
The Netherlands

Printed in the Netherlands

CONTENTS

PART C

Brain research in speech production and fluency disorders

PART E

Developmental aspects of speech production and fluency disorders

LIST OF CONTRIBUTORS

Peter J.Alfonso, *University of Illinois, Speech and Hearing Science, 901 South Sixth Street, Champaign, IL 61820, USA*

James Au-Yeung, *University College London, Dept. of Psychology, Gower Street, London, WC 1 E 6BT, United Kingdom*

Klaas Bakker, *Southwest State University, Department of Communication Disorders, 901 S. National, Springfield, Miss. 65804, USA*

Steven M.Barlow, *Indiana University, Department of Speech and Hearing Science, Bloomingdale IN 47405, USA*

Anne Bauer, *Heinrich-Heine-University Düsseldorf, Institute of General Psychology, Universitätsstr. 1, D-40225 Düsseldorf, Deutschland*

Nan Bernstein Ratner, *University of Maryland, Department of Hearing & Speech Sciences, 0100 Lefrak Hall, College Park, MD 20142, USA*

Francesca Bettini, *Centro di Studio Ricerche di Fonetica, Universita di Padova, Via G. Anghinoni 10, 35121 Padova, Italy*

Renée van Bezooijen, *University of Nijmegen, General linguistics, 6500 HD Nijmegen, the Netherlands*

Meir Bloch, *National Institute of Health-NIDCD, 10 Center Drive MSC 1416, Room 5D38, Bethesda, MD 20892-14, USA*

Inge Boers, *University Hospital Nijmegen, IKNC-354, P.O.Box 9101, 6500 HB Nijmegen, the Netherlands*

Hans-Georg Bosshardt, *Ruhr-University Bochum, Department of Psychology, Postfach 102148, D-44780 Bochum, Deutschland*

Frank R.Boutsen, *University of South Alabama, Department of Speech and Hearing, 2000 UCOM, Mobile, AL 36688-0002, USA*

Louis Boves, *University of Nijmegen, Department of Speech and Language, 6500 HD Nijmegen, The Netherlands*

Allen R. Braun, *National Institute of Health-NIDCD, 10 Center Drive MSC 1416, Room 5D38, Bethesda, MD 20892, USA*

Catherine P.Browman, *Haskins Laboratories, 270 Crown Street, New Haven, CT 06511, USA*

Emanuela M.Caldognetto, *Universita di Padova, Centro di Studio Ricerche di Fonetica, Via G. Anghinoni 10, 35121 Padova, Italy*

Karim Calis, *National Institute of Health-NIDCD, 10 Center Drive MSC 1416, Room 5D38, Bethesda, MD 20892, USA*

Edda M.Capodaglio, *Fondazione Salvatore Maugeri, Bioengeneering, Via Revislate, 13, Veruno (NO), 28010 Veruno, Italy*

R.E. Carson, *National Institute of Health-NIDCD, 10 Center Drive MSC 1416, Room 5D38, Bethesda, MD 20892, USA*

Anthony J.Caruso, *Kent State University, Speech Pathology and Audiology, P.O.Box 5190, Kent, Ohio 44240, USA*

Roberto Colombo, *Fondazione Salvatore Maugeri, Bioengeneering, Via Revislate, 13, Veruno (NO), 28010 Veruno, Italy*

Roberto Conti, *Fondazione Salvatore Maugeri, Bioengeneering, Via Revislate, 13, Veruno (NO), 28010 Veruno, Italy*

Anne K.Cordes, *University of Georgia, Department of Communication Science and Disorders, 556 Aderhold Hall, Athens, GA 30602, USA*

Luc De Nil, *University of Toronto, Clark Institute of Psychiatry, 250 College Street, Toronto, Ontario M5T 1R8, USA*

Janis van Doorn, *University of Sydney, Australian Stuttering Research Center, Cumberland Campus, P.O.Box 170, Lidcombe, NSW 2141, Australia NSW*

Giancarlo Ferrigno, *Universita di Padova, Centro di Studio Ricerche di Fonetica, Via G. Anghinoni 10, 35121 Padova, Italy*

Peter T. Fox, *University of Texas at San Antonio, Brain Imaging Center, 7703 Floyd Curl Drive, San Antonio TX 78284, USA*

Marie-Christine Franken, *AZR-Sophia Kinderziekenhuis, KNO-Gehoor en Spraakcentrum, Dr. Molewaterplein 60, 3015 GJ Rotterdam, the Netherlands*

David L.Franklin, *University of California, Irvine Medical Center, Department of Psychiatry, Rt 88-101 City Drive, Orange, CA 92668, USA*

Frances J.Freeman, *University of Texas at Dallas, Callier Center for Communication Disorders, Dallas, TX 75235, USA*

Gerard P.van Galen, *University of Nijmegen, Nijmegen Institute for Cognition and Information, P.O. Box 9104, 6500 HE Nijmegen, The Netherlands*

Helen Glover, *East Carolina University, Department of Communication Sciences and Disorders, Belk Annex, East Carolina University, Greenville, NC 27858, USA*

Louis Goldstein, *Haskins Laboratories, 270 Crown Street, New Haven, CT 06511-6695, USA*

Barry Gordon, *John Hopkins University, Department of Neurology, 600 North Wolfe Street, Baltimore, MD 21287, USA*

Vincent R.Gracco, *Haskins Laboratories, 270 Crown Street, New Haven, CT 06511-6695, USA*

Marc Grosjean, *University of Nijmegen, Nijmegen Institute for Cognition and Information, P.O. Box 9104, 6500 HE Nijmegen, The Netherlands*

Dale Grothe, *National Institute of Health-NIDCD, 10 Center Drive MSC 1416, Room 5D38, Bethesda, MD 20892-14, USA*

Andrea Häge, *Universitäts Klinikum HNO, Sektion Phoniatrie/Pädaudiologie, Schillerstrasse 15, D-89070 Ulm, Deutschland*

Peter Hagoort, *Max Planck Institute for Psycholinguistics, Wundtlaan 1, 6525 XC Nijmegen, the Netherlands*

Kelly D.Hall, *Northern Illinois University, Department of Communicative Disorders, 332 Adams Hall, Dekalb, IL 60115, USA*

Stephen B.Hood, *University of South Alabama, Department of Speech and Hearing, 2000 UCOM, Mobile, AL 36688-0002, USA*

Philip Hoole, *ENK-Entwicklungsgruppe, Dachauerstrasse 164, 80992 München, Germany*

Susan K.Horton, *The University of Queensland, Department of Speech Pathology, Queensland 4072, Australia*

S.Houle, *University of Toronto, Clark Institute of Psychiatry, 250 College Street, Toronto, Ontario M5T 1R8, USA*

Peter Howell, *University College London, Dept. of Psychology, Gower Street, London, WC 1 E 6BT, United Kingdom*

Wouter Hulstijn, *University of Nijmegen, Nijmegen Institute for Cognition Research and Information technology, P.O. Box 9104, 6500 HE Nijmegen, the Netherlands*

Marcello Imbriani, *Fondazione Salvatore Maugeri, Bioengeneering, Via Revislate, 13, Veruno (NO), 28010 Veruno, Italy*

Peter Indefrey, *Max Planck Institute for Psycholinguistics, Wundtlaan 1, 6525 XD Nijmegen, the Netherlands*

Roger J.Ingham, *University of California at Santa Barbara, Department of Speech Hearing Science, 93106 CA, USA*

Janis Costello Ingham, *University of California at Santa Barbara, Department of Speech Hearing Science, 93106 CA, USA*

Lutz Jäncke, *Heinrich-Heine-University Düsseldorf, Institute of General Psychology, Universitätsstr. 1, D-40225 Düsseldorf, Deutschland*

Peggy Janssen, *Academic Hospital Utrecht, ENT clinic, Phoniatric Department, Postbus 85500, 3508 GA Utrecht, the Netherlands*

Helge S.Johannsen, *Universitäts Klinikum HNO, Sektion Phoniatrie/Pädaudiologie, Schillerstrasse 15, D-89070 Ulm, Deutschland*

Peter de Jong, *University of Nijmegen, Nijmegen Institute for Cognition and Information, P.O. Box 9104, 6500 HE Nijmegen, The Netherlands*

Joseph Kalinowski, *East Carolina University, Department of Communication Sciences and Disorders, Belk Annex, East Carolina University, Greenville, NC 27858, USA*

Karl-Theodor Kalveram, *Heinrich Heine Universität, Institute für Algemeine Psychologie, Universitätsstrasse 1, 40225 Düsseldorf, Germany*

S. Kapur, *University of Toronto, Clark Institute of Psychiatry, 250 College Street, Toronto, Ontario M5T 1R8, USA*

Raymond D.Kent, *University of Wisconsin, Waisman Center, 1500 Highland Avenue, Madison, WI 53705, USA*

Robert M.Kroll, *University of Toronto, Clark Institute of Psychiatry, 250 College Street, Toronto, Ontario M5T 1R8, USA*

Judith L.Lauter, *University of Oklahoma, Health Science Center, Department of Communication Science and Disorders, 825 N.E. 14th, P.O.Box 26901, Oklahoma City, OK 73190, USA*

Christy L.Ludlow, *National Institute of Health-NIDCD, 10 Center Drive MSC 1416, Room 5D38, Bethesda, MD 20892, USA*

Ben Maassen, *University Hospital Nijmegen, IKNC-354, P.O.Box 9101, 6500 HB Nijmegen, The Netherlands*

J.M. Maisog, *National Institute of Health-NIDCD, 10 Center Drive MSC 1416, Room 5D38, Bethesda, MD 20892, USA*

Gerald Maguire, *University of California, Irvine Medical Center, Department of Psychiatry, Rt 88-101 City Drive, Orange, CA 92668, USA*

Ludo Max, *Kent State University, Speech Pathology and Audiology, P.O.Box 5190, Kent, Ohio 44240, USA*

Rachel I.Mayberry, *McGill University, School of Communication Sciences & Disorders, 1266 Pine Avenue West, Montreal, Quebec H3G 1AB, Canada*

Michael D.McClean, *Walter Reed Army Medical Center, Audiology and Speech Center Washington, DC 20307-5001, USA*

Antje S.Meyer, *Max Planck Institute for Psycholinguistics, Wundtlaan 1, 6525 XD Nijmegen*

Giuseppe Minuco, *Fondazione Salvatore Maugeri, Bioengeneering, Via Revislate, 13, Veruno (NO), 28010 Veruno, Italy*

Lawrence F.Molt, *Auburn University, Neuroprocesses Research Laboratory, 1199 Haley Center, Auburn, AL 36849-5232, USA*

Jerald B.Moon, *University of Iowa, Department of Speech Pathology and Audiology, 127 A-SHC, Iowa city, Iowa 52242, USA*

Bruce E.Murdoch, *University of Queensland, Department of Speech Pathology, Queensland 4072, Australia*

Ulrich Natke, *Heinrich Heine Universität, Institute für Algemeine Psychologie, Universitätsstrasse 1, 40225 Düsseldorf, Germany*

Ron Netsell, *Southwest State University, Department of Communication Disorders, 901 S. National, Springfield, Miss. 65804, USA*

Mark Onslow, *University of Sydney, Australian Stuttering Research Center, Cumberland Campus, P.O.Box 170, Lidcombe, NSW 2141, Australia NSW*

Ann Packman, *University of Sydney, Australian Stuttering Research Center, Cumberland Campus, P.O.Box 170, Lidcombe, NSW 2141, Australia NSW*

Carlo Pasetti, *Fondazione Salvatore Maugeri, Bioengeneering, Via Revislate, 13, Veruno (NO), 28010 Veruno, Italy*

Herman F.M. Peters, *University Hospital Nijmegen, Department of Voice and Speech Pathology. P.O. Box 9101, 6500 HB Nijmegen, the Netherlands*

Paolo Pinelli, *Fondazione Salvatore Maugeri, Via Revislate, 13, Veruno (NO), 28010 Veruno, Italy*

Albert Postma, *University of Utrecht, Department of Psychonomics, P.O.Box 80140, 3508 TC Utrecht, the Netherlands*

Steven G.Potkin, *University of California, Irvine Medical Center, Department of Psychiatry, Rt 88-101 City Drive, Orange, CA 92668, USA*

Michael Rastatter, *East Carolina University, Department of Communication Sciences and Disorders, Belk Annex, East Carolina University, Greenville, NC 27858, USA*

Glyndon Riley, *365 Heather Place, Laguna, CA 92651, USA*

Donald A. Robin, *University of Iowa, Department of Speech Pathology and Audiology, 127 A-SHC, Iowa city, Iowa 52242, USA*

Dieter Rommel, *Universitäts Klinikum HNO, Sektion Phoniatrie/Pädaudiologie, Schillerstrasse 15, D-89070 Ulm, Deutschland*

David B.Rosenfield, *Baylor College of Medicine, Stuttering Center, 6550 Fannin, Suite 1801, Houston, Texas 77030, USA*

Lena Rustin, *University College London, Dept. of Psychology, Gower Street, London, WC 1 E 6BT, United Kingdom*

G. Schulz, *National Institute of Health-NIDCD, 10 Center Drive MSC 1416, Room 5D38, Bethesda, MD 20892-14, USA*

Hartmut Schulze, *Universitäts Klinikum HNO, Sektion Phoniatrie/Pädaudiologie, Schillerstrasse 15, D-89070 Ulm, Deutschland*

S. Selbie, *National Institute of Health-NIDCD, 10 Center Drive MSC 1416, Room 5D38, Bethesda, MD 20892, USA*

Rosalee C.Shenker, *McGill University, School of Communication Sciences & Disorders, 1266 Pine Avenue West, Montreal, Quebec H3G 1AB, Canada*

Kathleen Siren, *National Institute of Health-NIDCD, 10 Center Drive MSC 1416, Room 5D38, Bethesda, MD 20892, USA*

Anne Smith, *Purdue University, Department of Audiology and Speech Science, Heavilon Hall, West Lafayette, IN 47906, USA*

Gianluca Spinatonda, *Fondazione Salvatore Maugeri, Bioengeneering, Via Revislate, 13, Veruno (NO), 28010 Veruno, Italy*

Sheila Stager, *National Institute of Health-NIDCD, 10 Center Drive MSC 1416, Room 5D38, Bethesda, MD 20892, USA*

Andrew Stuart, *East Carolina University, Department of Communication Sciences and Disorders, Belk Annex, East Carolina University, Greenville, NC 27858, USA*

Debora G.Theodoros, *University of Queensland, Department of Speech Pathology, Queensland 4072, Australia*

Elizabeth C.Thompson, *University of Queensland, Department of Speech Pathology, Queensland 4072, Australia*

Geert Thoonen, *University Hospital Nijmegen, IKNC-354, P.O.Box 9101, 6500 HB Nijmegen, The Netherlands*

Naunette Turcasso, *National Institute of Health-NIDCD, 10 Center Drive MSC 1416, Room 5D38, Bethesda, MD 20892, USA*

Pascal H.H.M. Van Lieshout, *University of Nijmegen, NICI, P.O.Box 9401, 6500 HE Nijmegen, The Netherlands*

M.Varga, *National Institute of Health-NIDCD, 10 Center Drive MSC 1416, Room 5D38, Bethesda, MD 20892, USA*

Nagalapura S.Viswanath, *Baylor College of Medicine, Stuttering Center, 6550 Fannin, Suite 1801, Houston, TX 77030, USA*

David Ward, *University of Reading, Department of Linguistic Science, Whiteknights Reading RG6 2AA, United Kingdom*

Ben C.Watson, *New York Medical College, Department of Otorhinolaryngology, Munger Pavillion Room 170, Valhalla, New York 10595, USA*

William G.Webster, *Brock University, Department of Psychology, St. Catherines, Ontario, L2S 3A1 Canada*

George Wieneke, *Academic Hospital Utrecht, ENT clinic, Phoniatric Department, Postbus 85500, 3508 GA Utrecht, the Netherlands*

Joseph C.Wu, *365 Heather Place, Laguna, CA 92651, USA*

Ehud Yairi, *University of Illinois, Speech of Hearing sciences, 901 South Sixth Street, Champaign, IL 61820, USA*

J. Scott Yaruss, *Northwestern University, Speech and Language Pathology, 2299 North Campus Drive, Evanston, IL 60208, USA*

Patricia M.Zebrowski, *University of Iowa, Department of Speech Pathology and Audiology, 127 A-SHC, Iowa city, Iowa 52242, USA*

Wolfram Ziegler, *ENK-Entwicklungsgruppe, Dachauerstrasse 164, 80992 München, Germany*

Mary Zikria, *National Institute of Health-NIDCD, 10 Center Drive MSC 1416, Room 5D38, Bethesda, MD 20892, USA*

Claudio Zmarich, *Universita di Padova, Centro di Studio Ricerche di Fonetica, Via G. Anghinoni 10, 35121 Padova, Italy*

PREFACE

This volume consists of a selection of reviewed papers presented at the third International Conference on 'Speech Motor Production and Fluency Disorders', which was held in Nijmegen, The Netherlands, June 5-8, 1996. The conference was the third in a series of Nijmegen Conferences on Speech Motor Control and Stuttering. The first two conferences were held in 1985 and 1990. During the preparation of the third conference the foundations for the present edited volume were already being laid.

The present volume intends to serve three purposes. First of all, the book is meant to be an authoritative text on the basic science of motor control in speech production. Secondly, it provides a thorough introduction into the various new brain imaging techniques, with special emphasis on the ways in which these techniques are and can be put to use in the study of speech production. Thirdly, it gives a broad outline, as well as a detailed account of the current studies on fluency disorders.

To achieve these goals as many as twelve keynote speakers were invited to discuss specific topics on speech motor control and on brain research of speech production. These keynote addresses cover about one third of this book. In addition, the representatives of well-known speech and language laboratories were asked to present the results of their most recent research. They were explicitly asked not simply to report on their latest experiments, but to provide arguments that prove the relevance of their work for new, promising and lasting lines of research. These papers constitute a further third of this book. The final third of this extensive volume is occupied by a variety of, often preliminary, but nevertheless new and challenging findings, reflecting the state of the art in the research on speech motor control and fluency disorders.

Inspired by the "Decade of the Brain", this volume focuses on brain research. Contributions involving recent brain research techniques (e.g. brain imaging, electrical stimulation and ERPs), were selected only if they had the potential to add to the understanding of the motor system in both fluent and dysfluent speech production. This book provides the first, almost full account of recent brain imaging research on stuttering. The authors were requested to exclude technical details from their papers, since these can be found in other publications by the same authors. This allows an easy comparison of the many interesting and sometimes quite conflicting results.

In addition to this special topic, the book also covers themes that were prominent in the two earlier Nijmegen conferences, namely speech motor control in stuttering, and the assessment and developmental aspects of speech production in pathological speech. Key issues in the study of speech motor control in stuttering concern dynamic, kinematic and sensory aspects of speech motor production. Furthermore, special attention is paid to the influence of cognitive and linguistic processes on dysfluency.

About one half of all submitted abstracts were selected for presentation at the conference based on their relevance and quality. All subsequently submitted manuscripts were reviewed by the editors and, if necessary, by external reviewers. A small number of the papers or posters presented at the conference were not accepted for publication. A few others were withdrawn by the authors themselves for various reasons. However, it should be noted that the final responsibility for the contents of the articles lies with the authors, and not with the editors of this book.

The main goal of the first Nijmegen Conference on Speech Motor Control and Stuttering was to present and promote a motor approach through which a deeper insight into the nature of dysfluency might be gained. The emphasis of the second conference was on fundamental speech production research and not specifically on stuttering. At the third conference the research on basic speech production played an even more prominent role. Hopefully, this is a growing trend, leading to closer links between applied and fundamental research. We think that, if those who work and conduct research within the clinic draw inspiration from basic science more, this will open up new perspectives; we also hope that more fundamental research is shifted from the laboratory to the clinic. Clinically applied research does not only put basic science to the test, it may also raise important new questions that might lead to innovations in the laboratories. The editors hope that this book will provide a powerful impetus for both developments.

ACKNOWLEDGMENTS

The conference that lies at the heart of this book was organized by the Department of Voice and Speech Pathology of the Institute of Otorhinolaryngology of the University Hospital Nijmegen in close co-operation with the NICI (Nijmegen Institute for Cognition and Information), the Interfaculty Research Unit for Language and Speech of the University of Nijmegen, and the Institute of Medical Psychology of the University Hospital Nijmegen with executive assistance of the University Congress Office.

The conference and this volume could not have been realized without the help of a large number of people. We would particularly like to thank Paula Wijkamp, Elsbeth Buunk and Hans Cornelisse. Special thanks are also due to Diny Helsper for the camera-ready preparation of this book.

We are grateful for a substantial grant from the Royal Netherlands Academy of Arts and Sciences (KNAW). We also very much appreciate the considerable contributions from the Clinic of Otorhinolaryngology and the Department of Speech Pathology, both at the University Hospital of Nijmegen. Additional support was given by the Department of Medical Psychology, the Interfaculty Research Unit for Language and Speech, and the Nijmegen Institute for Cognition and Information (NICI), all of the University of Nijmegen, The Netherlands.

The Editors,
Wouter Hulstijn
Herman F.M. Peters
Pascal H.H.M. van Lieshout

Speech Production: Motor Control, Brain Research and Fluency Disorders
W. Hulstijn, H.F.M. Peters and P.H.H.M. Van Lieshout, editors

Chapter 1

SPEECH PRODUCTION: MOTOR CONTROL, BRAIN RESEARCH AND FLUENCY DISORDERS. AN INTRODUCTION.

Wouter Hulstijn, Pascal Van Lieshout, Herman F.M. Peters

In this chapter the five parts of the present book are introduced, and the rationale for the special topic of this book on brain research in speech motor production is given. Themes that will be addressed concern the rise of the dynamical approach, recent findings in brain imaging studies, the interaction between linguistic and motor processes, in particular during speech development, and ways to assess speech disfluency.

GENERAL INTRODUCTION

The present book is the third in line of a small series of books that arose from conferences on speech motor control and stuttering. The first book (Peters and Hulstijn, 1987) appeared at a time in which a motor approach to stuttering still had to find its place among the already established lines of research. Then, it was mainly characterized by a search for conspicuous events in the speech production of stutterers, and hardly driven by theory. Therefore, in the second book (Peters, Hulstijn and Starkweather, 1991), a much larger part was dedicated to models of normal speech production. It was hoped that these theoretical contributions would stimulate scientists in this area to adopt a more hypothesis testing type of research. It is our impression that the great majority of research on stuttering that has been published the last few years is better grounded in general theoretical frameworks, and we are certain that this holds for the great majority of the chapters in this book.

These considerations have provided the rationale for the ordering of the parts of this book. The first section deals with models in speech production. It is, both in chapters and in pages, more than twice as long as the model section in the previous book. By their differences in discipline and viewpoint these theoretical chapters set the stage and provide the necessary background to evaluate the research presented in the section that follows. The third and middle part is devoted to brain research, which is the central and special theme of this book. Tutorials on techniques lead research reviews on applications of these techniques in the study of fluency disorders. Part four, the section with the greatest number of chapters, is dedicated to kinematic, physiological, acoustical and perceptual methods in speech research and measurement of dysfluency. In addition, this part contains theoretical papers on the importance of prosodic and linguistic processes in explaining stuttering. The final section is devoted to developmental aspects. It begins with a theoretical chapter and is followed by research reviews as well as research data on salient aspects of children's speech, i.e., speech rate, motor control and linguistic aspects.

The special theme of this book is the imaging of brain activities during speech production and in some cases speech perception. This decade of the brain has provided us with techniques which, as described by Lauter (in chapter 20 of this volume), can open new windows to the brain. Recently these neuro-imaging techniques have also been used to investigate speech production and to study fluency disorders. It is one of the aims of this book to introduce these techniques and to survey the speech production research in which they were used.

What are "the specific areas in the human brain which subserve language production" (to quote Indefrye from chapter 22 of this volume)? The study of speech production in itself already offers many clues about how the brain works. But imagine how wonderful it would be if one could look inside the brain of a person while he is actually speaking. Would we actually 'see' the brain speaking? Or are windows opened but do curtains remain closed? What are the methodological pitfalls? Do we get a better understanding of dysfluent speech in studying the brain during stuttering?

These are some of the questions that are addressed in the chapters that together form the special theme of this book. Given the central location within the book, it thus emphasizes the importance of this type of research, but it also expresses our belief that it can only be of value if it is guided by explicit hypotheses derived from models and research on speech production. Brain imaging should help in understanding and highlighting the processes and mechanisms of speech motor control, but it will only do so if we know where to look at and in what way.

In the following sections of this chapter each of the five parts of this book will be briefly sketched. Since the abstracts of the chapters provide detailed information about chapter content, only the order of the chapters will be explained here, and common themes will be pointed at, as well as apparent controversies.

MODELS IN SPEECH PRODUCTION

The real introduction to the themes of this book is formed by the second chapter of this book, written by Kent, who gives a comprehensive and inspiring overview of the motor models and the neurophysiology of speech. This chapter not only lists the many theories on speech production and perception, but it tabulates them according to their 'fundamental strategy' and their 'primary neural structures'. A very helpful introduction to the brain imaging studies presented in Part C of this book forms Kent's simplified representations of cortical and subcortical structures involved in the production of spoken language, and the listing of their primary functions in speech. Kent describes the current status of theorizing in speech production, and in doing so introduces the concept of the "gesture" This concept, according to Kent, "needs refinement", which is done in "a conceptual model of goal-governed, trajectory-based speech motor control", that Kent pictures and describes later. An extra topic that is treated extensively in Kent's chapter is speech development. Again, Kent promotes the concept of the gesture: "A goal-based gestural account of speech production seems capable of accommodating anatomical development while preserving the essence of phonetic intention and skilled motor control."

General views on speech production. The next three chapters by Gracco, Browman and Goldstein, and Meyer present models on speech production from perspectives that can be ordered from low to high. Gracco presents a neuromotor perspective, Browman and Goldstein focus on 'higher' units, called 'gestures', which should bridge the gap between the traditionally separated physical and cognitive structures, while Meyer mainly addresses word forms.

Gracco develops a conceptual model of speech production that is grounded in neurobiology. Starting from phonological encoding, two distinct systems play a role: a SMA/basal ganglia system, responsible for preparatory and supra segmental adjustments, and a cerebellar/PM system involved in syllable-level timing and spatial adjustment. Damages to these two systems in various neurological disorders, will result in two different patterns of symptoms. On-line modification of the motor commands by sensory information is an important element of this model. It preserves a notion of loosely specified spatial goals, while still achieving accuracy. At an even lower level, i.e., that of muscle mechanics and jaw dynamics, many patterns of intra-articulator coarticulation can be explained without taking recourse to control by central movement planning. The units of speech production in Gracco's model are 'coordinative structures' or "something on the order of gestural constellations or vocal tract configurations".

The units in the model presented by Browman and Goldstein in chapter 4 of this volume are clearly more abstract. A 'gesture' is simultaneously a unit of action, or 'coordinative structure', and a unit of information that can function as a phonological primitive. The most recent version of this model is presented very intelligibly, with many elucidating examples. Terms that may cause confusion (e.g., effector, coordinative structure, gesture, gestural score, phonological unit and syllable) are clearly defined. Kent's statement that the concept of a gesture "needs refinement" has been answered adequately. The authors' conclusions are worth repeating. If the model is adopted then the measurement of articulatory kinematics might reveal much about the underlying organization of the units in speech. Additionally, it might help to discover possible overlap between gestures, which will shed a new light on so called sound errors and on dysfluent speech in general.

In the chapter by Meyer (chapter 5 of this volume) on word form generation, sound errors form the basic data for the evaluation of the existing models of word production, which are taken together in what Meyer calls the 'Standard Model'. After a clear and eloquent review of the many objections that can be made against the Standard Model, Meyer concludes that the psycholinguistic evidence for the distinction between a phonological and a phonetic level of encoding "is not compelling". Some findings, e.g. sound anticipations that span several intervening sounds, provide arguments for a theory in which speakers form a "fairly abstract form representation".

It is probably save to say that future experimental work will have to focus on the interplay between cognitive/linguistic constraints and motor demands to make clear whether this "abstract form representation" is really a representation in an abstract static sound-based code, as proposed in the traditional approach described by Meyer, or an abstract dynamic, gesture-based code as proposed by Browman and Goldstein.

Approaches to understanding speech dysfluency. The authors of the previous three chapters were not very explicit about stuttering, as in contrast to the next three chapters where a view on the origin of stuttering will be presented.

In chapter 6, Kalveram and Natke, similar to Kent, stress the problems that young children must encounter in learning speech. Stutterers in their view have failed in learning to automatize their utterances, which they cannot make independently from auditory feedback. They come to these suggestions by studying how stutterers deal with stressed and unstressed syllables, but their most interesting arguments come from trying to model a network that learns by auto-imitation. The large problems they had in deducing information on inertia, stiffness, and damping of an articulator, highlighted the problems that a normal learning network (or child that learns to speak) must have, and suggests that this may easily go wrong.

McClean, in chapter 7, also discusses 'aberrant learned motor programs' as a possible explanation for disfluency. But for him it is only one of many possibilities. He describes a functional model of the motor system in which a number of functions can give rise to stuttering behavior if disturbed. These functions include pattern selection, sensory processing, regulation of speech rate, regulation of muscle stiffness, and mediation of emotional-motivational responses. The neural systems that subserve these functions all project to a pattern generating circuitry (PGC), which is a central component in McClean's model. The PGC involves the primary motor cortex, Broca's area, and the supplementary motor area (SMA). The major contribution of the cerebellum is extensively described. Disfluent speech, according to McClean, mainly results from the ineffective interactions of all the inputs to the PGC, particularly during speech movement preparation and initiation.

Webster, in chapter 8, presents a totally different view on stuttering. His evidence comes from an impressive number of neuropsychological experiments on the lateralization and hemispheric specialization of speech control. Webster concludes this review by proposing a two factor interference model, in which people who stutter are supposed to have a normal left hemisphere lateralization of speech, but their left hemisphere mechanisms are inefficient or "fragile" and, secondly, do not show the left hemispheric activation bias that is characteristic of fluent speakers. The critical area for stuttering, according to Webster, is the supplementary motor area (SMA) because it is associated with the planning of complex sequential (speech) movements.

The issue of laterality will return in discussing the results of PET research on stuttering in Part C of this book. There we can also 'see' to what extent stuttering can be 'localized' to the SMA or whether other structures are involved too. But first, the next section will introduce the many studies on motor control that are combined in Part B of this book.

MOTOR CONTROL IN SPEECH PRODUCTION AND FLUENCY DISORDERS

In search for a dynamic measure of stability. In the first chapter of part B of this book Smith opens with a compelling plea for a dynamic multifactorial model to account for the many diverse phenomena of stuttering. Like McClean, she stresses that stuttering can not be attributed to a "single, core, causal factor". Small changes in one of the factors may produce large changes in the output of a system, resulting in disfluency, due to the nonlinearity of dynamic systems. In order to investigate the combined effects of these diverse linguistic and motor factors Smith developed a new index of speech motor variability, the spatiotemporal index or STI. In the second part of her chapter a number of experiments are reviewed that demonstrate the effects of rate and linguistic complexity on this measure. A remarkable feature of this spatiotemporal index is that it can be calculated by tracing the movements of only one lip (lower lip).

The following two chapters, in contrast, focus on the coordination of two lips (and the jaw). Chapter 10, by Alfonso and Van Lieshout, provides a thorough search for the best way to quantify the difference in coordination between persons who stutter and control subjects. Using different kinematic measures for spatial and temporal stability it seems evident that with a possible exception for the measure of motor equivalence, none is really appropriate for the task of distinghuising normal from abnormal variability. The importance of this research lies in its thorough exploration of many traditional kinematic measures offered by a dynamical approach.

However, the novel approach presented by Van Lieshout et al. in the following chapter, might prove to be more fruitful. In their experiment, the coordination of the upper and lower lip in lip-closing gestures, clearly expressed itself in the relative phasing between these articulators. The calculation of a continuous relative phase signal has not been applied to speech research earlier, and the finding that its variability clearly differentiates speech from non-speech tasks, suggests its usefulness in the study of motor coordination in fluent and disfluent speech.

Phase analysis is also used by Ward in a study described in chapter 12. He employs the discrete phase angle analysis that was put forward by Kelso and others about ten years ago (see chapter 12 for references). Measurement of phase angles was contrasted with an extrinsic timing measure, i.e., articulator sequencing as determined by peak velocities. Stuttering persons were found to be more variable in both analyses, but this seemed to hold only for a condition in which the speakers had to reverse their normal stress patterns.

Lip and jaw velocities were also investigated by Zmarich and Caldognetto. As in the studies by Alfonso et al., and by Ward, speech rate was varied. In the fast rate condition most utterances had a bell-shaped velocity profile, but in the preferred rate condition the number of multi-peaked velocity profiles was higher, particularly for stutterers.

In sum, it seems that the dynamic approach offers a valuable new approach towards the understanding of motor control in normal and disordered speech production. How valuable this contribution will turn out to be, however, remains to be seen as new experiments will have to put the model to more rigorous tests.

Coordination. Coordination was an implicit issue in the preceding chapters, that dealt with the search for the optimal measure for coordination and discoordination. In the following chapters several aspects of coordination are treated more explicitly. Mayberry and Shenker describe (in chapter 14) an interesting series of studies, trying to answer the question how spontaneous speech is related to the manual gestures that often accompany it. Their studies reveal that speech and manual gestures are tightly linked in a single integrated system, such that disfluencies are not compensated by extra gestures but interrupt or attenuate manual gesture production. The perturbation study, presented by Bauer et al. in chapter 15, followed a more classical approach. They unexpectedly loaded the jaw during the opening of the mouth for the utterance of the testword /sasasar/. However, no marked general differences between persons who stutter and nonstuttering controls were found. The next two chapters may be treated under the heading of coordination although the aim of the studies was quite different. In the study presented by Grosjean et al., in chapter 16, upper and lower lip coordination was required in a nonspeech task in which the lips had to generate an isometric force under several conditions. The authors convincingly argue that persons who stutter have a less efficient and more noisy force control than non-stuttering subjects. Hoole and Ziegler (chapter 17) study the coordination of respiratory activity and the linguistic-phonetic demands of sentences, while varying length and loudness, in normal and aphasic subjects. Their results indicate that this paradigm could be of great value for the study of a wide range of speech disorders.

Learning. The final two studies in this section deal with learning. Caruso and Max, in chapter 18, show that the decrease in stuttering frequency during repeated reading of the same text (adaptation effect) may be considered a result of motor learning. Ludlow et al. argue, in chapter 19, that developmental stuttering may be related to the ability to learn new phonological patterns. Their study showed that adults who stutter have great difficulty in learning complex novel pseudowords. Together both studies make it very clear that motor learning may prove to be a valuable research topic in the study of disfluency.

BRAIN RESEARCH IN SPEECH PRODUCTION AND FLUENCY DISORDERS

Overview of methods. The first chapter in this section, by Lauter is an excellent overview of methods in brain imaging and speech. Many different techniques are described and compared in a brief and clear manner. Moreover, the chapter provides a brief review of studies where each of these methods was used in speech research. However, more than just being an overview of methods, Lauter stresses individuality and the effect of individual differences on experimental design and on the interpretation of brain-imaging data.

The following chapter (21) reviews techniques that nicely supplement the noninvasive techniques described in the previous chapter. Gordon et al. present a study in which direct electrical cortical interference is complemented with direct electrical cortical recording. The description of this research not only serves as a good example of a very important method in the study of the neural processes involved in speech production. It also focusses on the theoretical issue of the relation between speech perception and speech production.

PET research. The subsection on PET research starts with a careful designed study by Indefrey on the generation of verbs. Although this study is interesting in its own light, it is used to illustrate methodological difficulties in PET (and fMRI) research in speech production. According to Indefrey "it does not seem to be a good idea to simply scanning ... subjects while they speak". Yet, this has been done in many previous PET studies. Speech involves different levels and different kinds of processes, therefore a subtraction paradigm only provides interpretable information if conditions are not mixed with respect to these levels and processes.

The five chapters that follow each contain one or more PET studies on persons who stutter. It is difficult to summarize these chapters, not only because they provide a wealth of data, but also because different scanning methods and speech paradigms have been used. An extensive review of earlier findings is given in chapter 25, written by Kroll et al., and a theoretical perspective is outlined by Riley et al. (chapter 26). Most of these studies can be characterized as still rather exploratory in trying to find differences between persons who stutter and control subjects, either in a resting condition or in conditions that differ in the percentage of stuttering. Ingham et al. (in chapter 24) and Wu et al. (chapter 27) manipulated stuttering frequency by comparing solo reading and chorus reading. Kroll et al. (chapter 25) used oral reading versus silent reading and Braun et al. (chapter 23) compared narrative speech and a sentence construction task with a motor control task in which subjects were asked to produce laryngeal and oral articulatory movements and associated sounds, typical for speech but devoid of linguistic content. All of the studies found group differences related to stuttering, but since so many many brain areas lighted up, it is difficult to extract one common pattern. Interestingly, most studies seem to suggest that for stutterers during dysfluent speech production, there is more right hemisphere involvement than in fluent speech of stutterers and controls. However, a decision between several explanations for this finding awaits further experiments.

The chapter by Watson et al. (chapter 28) reviews a large number of their MRI, qEEG and SPECT studies on stuttering. Their neurologically based model predicts that cognitive, linguistic or speech motor processes, or their integration might lead to dysfluencies.

ERP studies. Hagoort and Van Turenhout's chapter (29) on the possibilities of the method of recording Event Related Potentials (ERPs) more or less parallels the chapter by Indefrey. A well designed experiment (using the Lateralized Readiness Potential) is presented that nicely shows the power of ERP recording, which does not lie in precise localization of brain areas but in a high temporal resolution. An interesting experimental paradigm is offered for the study of the time course of the processes involved in lexical access during speaking, and for the study of disfluency. Molt (chapter 30) uses the readiness potential in a more simple paradigm with interesting results.

Pharmacologic studies. The final two chapters in this part of the book describe effects on fluency of pharmacologic treatment by a dopamine antagonist. Stager et al. used pimozide, which was compared with a highly selective serotonin reuptake inhibitor (paroxetine) and placebo. Maguire et al. tested risperidone. In both studies some positive effects on fluency were found.

METHODS AND MEASUREMENTS IN PATHOLOGICAL SPEECH

Measurement of disfluencies. In the first chapter, Cordes and Ingham treat a controversial issue: subperceptual stuttering. The chapter clearly reviews the concept and presents two studies with a wealth of data. The next chapter, by Howel et al., contains a promising method and software to automatically count stuttering. The third, by Bakker et al., is concerned with voice onset abruptness. Its physiologic and acoustic correlates and its measurement and feedback in a clinical context are studied and discussed. The next two chapters (36 and 37) address *voicing.* Wieneke and Janssen could not confirm the hypothesis that stuttering persons tend to avoid on-off voicing adjustments. Viswanath and Rosenfield tried to locate the terminations of part-word repetitions with respect to voicing.

EGG and EPG analysis. Natke et al. (chapter 38) present an easy and inexpensive two-channel recording technique and software for EGG and acoustic analysis, which might be useful for research and therapy. Caldognetto et al. (chapter 39) describe a system for recording and analysis of lip and jaw movements (called ELITE) that can be smoothly integrated with an electropalatograph (EPG).

Chronometric study of verbal reactions. Pinelli, in chapter 40, introduces the rationale for varying the foreperiod duration in this method and presents data of a great many neurological and psychiatric patients. Colombo et al. (chapter 41) demonstrate clear effects of age on this measure, and Spinatonda et al. (chapter 42) report dramatic effects of an neurotoxic organic solvent on laundry workers. Verbal reaction times have also been used by Van Lieshout et al. (chapter 43). In two reaction paradigms they varied word size, syllable frequency, stress location and syllable onset complexity. They did not found major differences between stuttering individuals and controls, but suggest that glottographic, myographic and respiratory measures may offer better possibilities to characterize speech motor skills.

Prosodic aspects. Packman et al. (chapter 44) tested the hypothesis that rhythmic speech reduces the variability of syllabic stress and thereby may decrease stuttering.

Jäncke et al. (chapter 45) describe two interesting studies, which clearly show that a shift in stress pattern increases disfluency, and Glover et al. (chapter 46) demonstrated that singing leads to a marked reduction in stuttering frequency even if speech rate is not lowered.

It has been claimed that speech *monitoring* is an important factor in stuttering. Postma, (chapter 47) proposes that monitoring is not only perception based but argues that multiple distributed production based monitors must exist. One might say that an extra task reduces the capacity to monitor one's speech output. The interference of cognitive processes on speech production in a dual-task paradigm is demonstrated by Bosshardt in a nice study (chapter 48).

Perceptual judgements of speech and the proper evaluation of stuttering are the subjects of the final two chapter in this methodological part of the book. Howell et al. contrast a formal and a casual interview style, Franken et al. asked raters to judge how suitable the recorded speech is for ten situations ranging in speech demands.

DEVELOPMENTAL ASPECTS OF SPEECH PRODUCTION AND FLUENCY DISORDERS

The last part of the book is devoted to the onset of speech production in early life. This part opens with an impressive theoretical introduction by Barlow in the work and ideas presented by 'dynamic' theorists as Edelman, Merzenich and Thelen. These theories are put in a clear perspective that offers the beginnings of a theory on speech development. Not many of these ideas have found their way in actual speech research yet. However, exciting research on orofacial motor activity has started recently. The experimental set up for this research and examples of recordings are described.

Speech rate. Hall and Yairi (in chapter 52) provide a thorough and comprehensive review of studies on speech rate and of the models behind them, and present initial findings of a longitudinal study of speech rate. Boutsen and Hood (chapter 53) describe a large study on normally fluent children, showing a clear distinction between fast and slow speaking children in the amount of normal disfluencies. Scott Yaruss focusses on diadochokinetic (DDK) rates (in chapter 54). The advantages, disadvantages and possible improvements of the DDK technique are very clearly described.

Visuo-motor tracking. In the studies presented in the following chapters, movement signals from lips and jaw were recorded while tracking a sinusoidally moving visual signal on a screen. A decomposition of the movements in motor and clock variance by Howell et al. (chapter 55) suggested that it is not a timing deficit but a failure in motor control that characterizes stuttering children. A similar experiment by Zebrowski et al. (chapter 56) compared predictable and nonpredictable signal tracking. Interestingly, stuttering children showed a poorer performance only on the predictable signals.

Linguistic aspects. It is an interesting question whether the linguistic demands of a speech task promote disfluency. Bernstein Ratner (chapter 57) describe the results of a pilot study on children at an age near stuttering, which suggests that language factors indeed play a role. Häge et al. (chapter 58) present the results of a large scale investigation of the cognitive and linguistic abilities of stuttering (n=94) and nonstuttering children. They found no evidence whatsoever that children who stutter suffer from a deficit or retardation in cognitive and language development. Rommel et al. (chapter 59) extended this study to other linguistic and paralinguistic aspects showing that disfluencies in the non-initial parts of words were unexpectedly high.

Dysarthria. The book ends with two studies on neurologically impaired children. In chapter 60, Maassen describes two studies comparing children with developmental apraxia of speech (DAS), children with spastic dysarthria, and children with speech language delay. Children were tested with picture naming, imitation and maximum performance tasks. This assessment procedure clearly indicated that "children with defective articulatory development show individual degrees of dysarthric and dyspraxic involvement". In the chapter by Murdoch the relevance of physiological measurements in speech motor disorders in addition to perceptual techniques is beautifully illustrated. The implications for treatment underscore the significance of this approach.

CONCLUDING REMARKS

The purpose of this book was to present a review of the current theories and research in speech production and dysfluency. Despite existing controversies, there seems to be a convergence towards the idea that the traditional separation between linguistic and motor aspects of speech production is no longer valid. Many authors in this book have emphasized the dynamic nature of speech. It offers a theoretical framework in which higher order (cognitive/linguistic) demands can be related to lower order (motor) variability. Thus, fluent speech requires the learning of a high level of verbal motor skill, which may be impeded in developmental stuttering.

The brain research presented in this book, generally showed clear differences between persons who do and who do not stutter. The interpretation of these results remains unclear, and needs to be reconciled with theoretical developments in speech motor production models. We hope that this book contributes to this integration, and will promote a further understanding of speech motor control in normal and speech disordered populations.

REFERENCES

Peters, H.F.M., & Hulstijn, W. (Eds.). (1987). *Speech motor dynamics in stuttering.* Wien: Springer Verlag.
Peters, H.F.M., Hulstijn, W., & Starkweather (Eds.). (1991). *Speech motor control and stuttering.* Amsterdam: Elsevier Science.

PART A

Models in Speech Production

Speech Production: Motor Control, Brain Research and Fluency Disorders
W. Hulstijn, H.F.M. Peters and P.H.H.M. Van Lieshout, editors

Chapter 2

SPEECH MOTOR MODELS AND DEVELOPMENTS IN NEURO-PHYSIOLOGICAL SCIENCE: NEW PERSPECTIVES

Raymond D. Kent

The theoretical understanding of speech production is fractionated. A number of theories have been proposed for various aspects of speech, such as phonological representation (e.g., articulatory phonology and various nonlinear phonologies), speech motor control (e.g., dynamic systems theory, motor programming theory), vocal tract configuration (e.g., quantal theory and related proposals). Therefore, the theoretical understanding of speech is essentially a mosaic of separate theories, each of which has a limited focus. But the real power of speech becomes evident only through a broader view of its physiologic-acoustic-perceptual domain and the versatility of its output. The different aspects of speech ultimately may be integrated through a consideration of the neural representations and neural regulatory processes that serve speech. Until recently, knowledge in this area was too limited to undergird such a synthesis. But new information from neurophysiology and brain imaging has accumulated to the point that attempts at synthesis are warranted. The promise of synthesis is contained in concepts relating to the motor regulation of a complex multiarticulate system; the conditional, adaptive use of the plurimodal afference generated during speech; and the neural control of language encoded as movement sequences. This paper explores the relations between current concepts in speech motor control and emerging information on the neural regulation of complex behavior. A major objective is to discuss the neural framework for the representation of the multidimensional properties of speech. Implications for speech developmental processes and neurogenic speech disorders are included.

INTRODUCTION

This paper discusses the following five propositions:

1. The current understanding of speech behavior is represented by a mosaic of theories, most of which pertain to only certain levels of observation or conceptualization. These theories were developed primarily or exclusively to account for speech behavior in the competent adult. Their application to the understanding of speech development in the child or of speech disorders in talkers of any age often is often uncertain.

2. A major divide exists between theories of speech production and speech perception, which have had largely separate theoretical developments. A renewed effort is underway for their unification, but controversy reigns over consensus.

3. Certain theories pertaining to the production of speech have the potential to fit together in a more comprehensive account of how movements are controlled to produce auditory-phonetic patterns. The linkage of these theories into a composite super-theory depends on a global perspective of speech as a sensorimotor behavior.

4. The gesture is a common denominator of one major direction of current thinking in both speech production and speech perception. However, the concept of gesture needs refinement if it is to offer useful and accurate descriptions of speech motor control.

5. Speech in all of its aspects develops as the human develops. Developmental phenomena may offer important insights and constraints relating to theoretical formulations about speech. Competence in speech perception is precocious: It appears that infants adapt their auditory perceptual processing to the phonetic properties of the ambient language by the end of the first year of life (Lalonde & Werker, 1995; Werker & Tees, 1984). The development of speech production is much slower and is played out against a significant anatomical restructuring as well as the maturation of neuromotor systems. As noted in #1, some of the theories and models that have been developed for the adult systems of speech production have dubious relevance to the child's systems. What is needed, then, is a view of speech production that accommodates developmental change.

A SMORGASBORD OF THEORIES

Looking across the broad sweep of speech science, one encounters a theoretical landscape of notable diversity. Because the study of speech encompasses a range of phenomena, it is not surprising that a broad view of speech behavior takes in theories pertaining to physics, physiology, psychology, linguistics, and the neurosciences, not to mention their hybrid offspring, e.g., biophysics, psycholinguistics, and neurolinguistics. Each of these basic fields of science has a rich theoretical storehouse from which theories applicable to speech might be drawn. Of course, speech has spawned its own theories to account for phenomena that are unique to, or at least most particular to, the behaviors and events of speaking.

THE GOAL OF A UNIFIED THEORY

The grail of any science is a unified theory -- a theory that grasps the foundational understanding of the field and is broad enough to embrace the major arenas of investigation. The scientific literature on speech has two prominent facets, one pertaining to speech production and the other to speech perception. These two facets seem to be separated by a theoretical divide in the sense that theories of speech production and speech perception have a largely separate development. Table 1 shows a few selected theories in the domains of production and perception. The listing is not exhaustive but it serves to make the point that theoretical alternatives exist in both domains (for further discussion, see Kent, forthcoming). Time does not permit a discussion of the substance of individual theories, but it is possible to take a quick look at their global character. This character is, if nothing else, diverse.

Table 1. Part a. Theories of speech production; listed by name of theory and a brief statement of fundamental strategy.

Theory	Strategy
Dynamic systems theory	Action responses in speech depend on task-determined synergies that operate with few degrees of freedom and well-defined control parameters. Movements are task specific and account for initial conditions.
Adaptive model theory	Planned sensory trajectories are transformed to motor commands. Performance is monitored to allow necessary revision of movement through adaptive feedback.
Connectionist theories	System "learns" by establishing weighted connections in a large network of interconnected units. Also called a Parallel Distributed Processing Model.
Feedback/feedforward	Peripheral feedback or feedforward information is used either to generate a correction signal to insure that goals are accomplished or to prepare effectors for a task-appropriate response.
Gestural Patterning	Speech goals are accomplished by the regulation of families of equivalent movement patterns (vocal tract variables are expressed as model articulator variables). This theory is compatible with dynamic systems theory and also with Articulatory (Gestural) Phonology.
Motor Program or Central Pattern theories	A plan of motor action is constructed from knowledge of speech goals and a repertoire of experience. Several theories or models of this type have been proposed.
Quantal theory	Regulation of the vocal tract reflects inherent nonlinearities between articulatory movement and acoustic output.
Schema theory	Motor plans are developed from a consideration of desired outcome, initial conditions, and previous experience with similar motor objectives.

Table 1. part b. Theories of speech perception; listed by name of theory, decision unit, and a brief statement of fundamental strategy.

Theory	Decision Unit and Fundamental Strategy
LAFS (Lexical Access from allophonic Spectra)	Short term spectra. Passive matching of short-term spectra to templates. A phonetic stage is bypassed for familiar words.
Auditory-Perceptual	Sensory responses to spectra. Makes phonemic decisions based on a perceptual-space representation that is formed from the logarithms of ratios of fundamental and formant frequencies.
Phonetic Refinement	Phones and allophones. Relies on an activation of phonetic sequences in networks to form a phonetic transcription.
ERIS	Context-sensitive allophones. Assumes that allophonic demons recognize the characteristics of sound sequences.
FLMP (Fuzzy Logical Perception)	Features and segments. Proposes that features and segments Model of are recognized by a combination of feature evaluation, feature integration and pattern classification.
Autonomous Search	Phonetic segments. Involves a mediated bottom-up processing to identify words.
Vector Analysis (Direct Realism)	Motor/ gestures. Employs natural lines of coarticulation to determine vectors from which segments are identified.
Revised Motor Theory	Syllables. Modular detection of motor gestures within syllable units to enable segment recognition.
Cohort Theory	Word-initial sound sequences. Selects a word choice from a word-initial cohort that is activated by the beginning sounds of a word.
Logogen Model	Words. Uses passive threshold devices to recognize words.
Interactive Activation	Several possible units. Active threshold devices in a connectionist net recognize features, phonemes and words.
LAME (Lateral Access Multiple Engrams)	Several possible units. assumes that units of various types are recognized using an adaptive simultaneous pattern perception representation.

Theories of speech perception differ across fundamental issues, such as: (1) Is the primaryflow of information bottom-up (data driven) or top-down (hypothesis driven)? (2) Is the processing autonomous or interactive? (3) Is the the strategy active or passive? (4) What is the basic unit of perceptual decision-making, if one is proposed? (5) If two or more units are involved, what are the privileges and limitations of their interaction? (6) What is the processing strategy? A similar diversity exists among the theories of speech production, which differ across issues such as these: (1) Does a motor program or preplanning of some kind regulate the movement patterns? (2) Is afference used in motor control, and, if so, how? (3) What is the basic unit of production, if one is proposed? (4) If two or more units are involved, how do they interact? (5) What is the strategy for motor control?

Suffice it to say that the theories in each domain pose a considerable divergence in thinking. Furthermore, in the main, theories that account for production say relatively little about speech perception, and vice versa. There are some important exceptions, beginning with the motor theory of speech production (Liberman et al., 1967), which survives today as a revised motor theory (Liberman & Mattingly, 1985). Another exception is direct realism, as described by Fowler (1984, 1986, 1996). This approach is basically compatible with system dynamics theory or its intellectual sibling, gestural patterning theory, but is not necessarily required by either of them. However, the major conclusion is that one can study theories in one domain, either perception or production, quite diligently and not have much appreciation of the theories in the other domain.

This theoretical divide is an obvious barrier to any hope for a unified theory of speech behavior. Despite the dramatic advances in the speech sciences within this century, we have only a clouded view of what such a unified theory might be. The divergence in thinking is readily apparent from a series of papers recently published in the *Journal of the Acoustical Society of America* (Vol. 99, No. 2, 1996). The papers addressed the general topic, "speech recognition and perception from an articulatory point of view." The formulation of a unified theory is not simply a matter of academic satisfaction. The perceptual and productive domains of speech must be understood in relation to each other to account for the development and maintenance of phonetic systems, and to explain various speech disorders in both children and adults.

A THEORETICAL OVERVIEW OF SPEECH PRODUCTION

Figure 1 is a view of part of the theoretical mosaic that defines the understanding of speech. The terms on the left side identify various levels at which speech is investigated and understood. The items on the right side are selected theoretical formulations associated with the levels of understanding. This is by no means the only way to conceptualize the theoretical infrastructure of speech, but it offers the advantage of showing some possible complementarities. Although some of the theories could well be associated with more than one level, the illustration simplifies things by recognizing one primary level for each theory. A major objective is to identify major arenas of theoretical contribution.

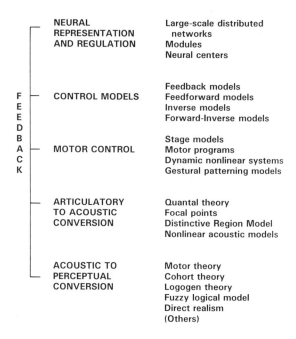

Figure 1. Levels of understanding or observation in speech (terms listed on the left) and associated theories or models (listed on the right).

The first level of understanding, neural representation and regulation, is concerned with the neural correlates of speech production and perception. Brain imaging techniques such as PET, fMRI, and qEEG have given us a rapidly spiraling database, much of which pertains to cortical activity in relation to language processing. But there is also abundant evidence on the role of the subcortical structures that support both speech production and speech perception. The importance of subcortical structures in speech production is evidenced generally by the fact that many dysarthrias (neurogenic speech disorders) are associated with damage to subcortical structures, e.g., the basal nuclei, cerebellum, brainstem, or lower motor neuron (Duffy, 1995). This is not to discount the potential role of the cerebral cortex in even the simple act of phonation. Unlike most if not all nonhuman primates, humans produce vocalizations in response to stimulation of the cortical face area (Ploog, 1992), which is evidence of the corticalization of phonatory control in humans.

Speech in its full sensorimotor array commands a vast neural territory, as shown in an admittedly understated way in Figure 2. The purpose of this simplified illustration is to show some of the primary cortical and subcortical structures that appear to be involved in speaking. The areas identified in this illustration understate the neural activation that occurs. One limitation is that this figure pertains only to the dominant hemisphere and neglects the synchronous but largely complementary activity in the nondominant hemisphere. Various attempts have been made to associate neural structures with the various processes involved

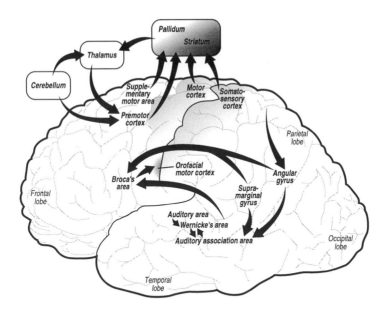

Figure 2. Simplified representation of pathways involving major cortical and subcortical structures that regulate spoken language production. This "flow chart" emphasizes neural structures involved in language formulation and speech motor assembly. Sensory components are not included because they would greatly complicate the diagram.

in spoken language. Figure 3 lists some of the associations that appear to be commonly recognized in the literature (Kent & Tjaden, forthcoming; Square & Martin, 1994; van der Merwe, forthcoming). These putative responsibilities of different neural structures are inferred from a variety of sources of data, but some of the inferences are rather weak. Perhaps the major thing to be said about Figure 3 is that some structures appear to have at least dual, if not manifold, responsibilities in the regulation of speech production.

Speech perception also seems to rely to a considerable degree on subcortical structures. Unlike the neural pathways of vision, olfaction, gustation, and somatosensation, the pathway for audition is replete with subcortical nuclei. More than 50 subcortical neuronal groups appear to be quite capable in themselves of fundamental sensory analyses including quasi-Fourier analysis, pattern recognition, localization, and an exquisite analysis of brief or transient sounds (Masterton, 1992). Furthermore, studies on the squirrel monkey have shown that subcortical structures respond differentially to self-produced calls and playbacks of the same vocalizations (Mueller-Preuss & Ploog, 1981; Ploog, 1981). Neurons in the inferior colliculus responded to both self-produced and playback calls, whereas many neurons in the medial geniculate body responded strongly to playback calls but either weakly or not at all to the self-produced vocalizations. A similar phenomenon has been observed for vocalization in the bat (Schuller, 1979; Suga & Schlegel, 1972).

Function	Primary Neural Structures
Intention	Fronto-limbic formations of the forebrain
Linguistic-symbolic processing	Cortico-cortical connections
Motor speech programming or planning	Wernicke's area, Broca's area, premotor cortex, supplementary motor area, inferior parietal lobule, inferior dorsolateral cortex, cerebellum, basal nuclei
Coordination	Basal nuclei, cerebellum, motor cortex
Execution	Pyramidal and extrapyramidal motor pathways

Figure 3. Primary functions in the production of spoken language (terms listed on the left) and neural structures hypothesized to be involved with each function (listed on the right).

Possibly, the subcortical auditory pathway is designed to afford a source-separation processing in which some neurons respond to all vocalizations (self-produced or other-produced) while other neurons respond only to externally produced sounds.

This functional segregation of the auditory pathway would support early vocal learning: first, because it should have a relatively early maturation compared to the cortical level, and second, because it would enable comparison of self-produced and other-produced sounds. This arrangement also would have obvious benefit to the purposes of self-monitoring versus sensory analysis of externally produced sounds. As Masterton (1992) observed, some auditory nuclei may be concerned more with the characteristics of sound sources than with the characteristics of sounds. The subcortical auditory processing interacts with a cortical processing that also can be widely distributed, depending on the nature of the stimulus and the listening task. Speech sounds in particular may activate regions of both left and right cerebral hemispheres (Zatorre et al., 1992) and bilateral processing seems to be the rule. This is not to suggest that the neural connections are far flung or haphazard. There is reason to believe that neural connections are designed according to the principle of "save wire," i.e., minimize the total length of the individual fibers in sensory and motor tracts (Cherniak, 1995). One simple example of conformity to this principle is the adajency of primary and association cortices for the sensory modalities.

The design of the brain, then, seems to point to a general lesson about the integration of perception and production. These two facets of communicative behavior have their neural fusion even at subcortical levels. As Huffman and Hanson (1990) commented, "The interface between auditory and vocalization centers is distributed to all levels of the brain" (p. 314). One example of such an interface is the set of direct and indirect connections between the inferior colliculus of the auditory pathway and the vocalization centers of the periaqueductal gray. The sensorimotor interface may be common to species that are highly dependent on vocalization (Schuller, 1979; Williams, 1989).

Historic formulations of speech motor control emphasized feedback models such as servosystems. More recent models include feedforward signals and/or the establishment of a forward model, inverse model, or a forward-inverse model for motor control. An important approach in modelling assumes that the control system builds an internal model of the speech production system (Wilhelms-Tricarico, 1996; Honda, 1996). The concept of forward or inverse modeling has been proposed for many motor systems. A good example is the proposal for a cerebellar-based forward-inverse model for the control of eye movements (Kawato & Gomi, 1992). This work is an example of developing a control model and placing it within a suitable part of the nervous system for its implementation. It also reflects a general belief that "internal models are essential for normal motor coordination" (Kawato & Gomi, 1992, p. 445).

The yin and yang of speech production models is the dichotomy between motor (pre)programming theories and alternatives such as nonlinear dynamic systems theory. Motor programming has been called upon especially to explain long-term dependencies across phonetic or syllabic sequences, whereas nonlinear dynamic systems theory has emphasized the biomechanical properties of the periphery in relation to goals such as compressing the degrees of freedom in system control (Kent et al., 1995). Despite vigorous counterarguments by some advocates of nonlinear dynamic systems theory, the notion of preprogramming survives to account for various aspects of speech control. Specifically, the internal model described above is used in the preprogramming of movements. The forward model is an emulation of the controller signals and the sensory information that results from responses to those signals.

Speech is known largely by, and is fundamentally directed toward, an acoustic signal that suffices for linguistic comprehension. Accordingly, a major effort in the history of speech science has been to work out the conversion from articulatory configuration to acoustic signal. In this sense, speech is like music, given that both speech and music employ skilled movements to create a highly structured acoustic signal that is readily apprehended and appreciated by listeners. Although several difficult questions remain to be answered about this articulatory to acoustic conversion, progress has been made in modeling nonlinearities and other properties that characterize the relation between articulation and acoustic product. Quantal theory (Stevens, 1989), Focal Points (Badin et L., 1990), and the Distinctive Region Model (Carre & Mrayati, 1995) are important contributions. If the acoustic product guides the speaker's motor control, then models of speech production should incorporate the nonlinearities that define the signal consequences of movement. Nonlinearities in the articulatory to acoustic conversion imply that vocal tract information is implicit in the acoustic signal. The intent of these comments is not to argue for direct realism, but simply to note that speech as an acoustic signal is governed by the physical laws that relate articulation to acoustics. The articulatory to acoustic conversion is part of the competence held by speaker and listener and it gives form to the auditory trajectory of speech.

Theories of speech perception have been developed largely to account for how other listeners understand the speech of a given talker. But talkers also listen to themselves. A complete theory of speech perception should account not only for how we understand others, but how we use self-monitoring to maintain requisite articulatory precision and to make suitable adjustments in prosody and other components of speech and voice quality. As mentioned earlier, some of the responsible neural mechanisms are likely found at several subcortical levels.

THE GESTURE IN CONTEMPORARY THEORIES OF SPEECH

Theories are built on concepts, and a powerful contemporary concept that runs through many of the subfields of speech is the gesture. Although the concept itself is not completely new or revolutionary, the gesture appears to be a kind of rallying point for much current thinking about speech production, speech perception, and even phonology. In some contemporary theories of speech production, speech control is conceptualized in terms of *gestures*, or bundles of gestures that define a motor sequence. The term *gesture* in these models refers to a family of functionally equivalent movement patterns that are actively regulated to achieve a goal of speech production. Individual gestures can be blended together to form a motoric sequence. Gestural patterning has been proposed by several investigators, including Browman and Goldstein (1986, 1988, 1992), Lofqvist (1990), and Saltzman and Munhall (1989). In speech perception, the concept of gesture is fundamental to the direct realism approach (Fowler, 1984, 1986, 1996). Finally, in phonology, Browman and Goldstein (1986, 1988, 1990, 1992) and Kroger and colleagues (Kroger, 1973; Kroger et al., 1995) have developed a theory of gestural or articulatory phonology that is based on the use of gestures as the primitives in a phonological system.

Unlike the traditional concepts of linguistics, which are static, even crystallized, the gesture is inherently dynamic. Its definition is spatiotemporal. It is not a segment, not a feature, not a steady state, but a trajectory that unfolds in time and has its essential character in movement, change, and adaptation. The two words gesture and trajectory have similar connotations in respect to speech. These closely related concepts capture a basic property of speech production and speech perception. Part of their common understanding may be found in the neural representation and organization of speech behavior.

It may be well to avoid an excessively strict spatiotemporal specification of the gesture. However attractive it may be for parsimony and other reasons to endow the gesture with a fundamental dynamic invariance, several reports question the legitimacy of such an assumption (Byrd, 1995; Gracco, 1994; Kent, 1986; Kohler, 1995; Tatham, 1995). Speech production does not appear to be constructed from dynamic structures that are rigidly determined. Instead, these structures appear to be highly adaptive in themselves, which is, after all, not surprising for an overpracticed motor skill that must blend several types of information into its composition.

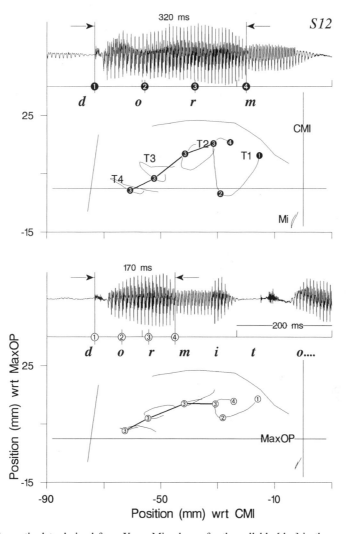

Figure 4. Kinematic data derived from X-ray Microbeam for the syllable [dor] in the words *dorm* (upper part of illustration) and *dormitory* (lower part of illustration). Trajectories are shown for four tongue points labeled as T1, T2, T3, and T4. Major segmentation events are labeled 1, 2, 3, and 4, as shown on the acoustic waveform. The solid line connecting the tongue points for event #3 represents the lingual contour for the rhotic [r]. MaxOP and CMI are reference lines, and Mi is the movement path of the lower central incisor.

Figure 4 shows kinematic data obtained with the X-ray Microbeam facility at the University of Wisconsin. -This is a sample of data from work in progress by Westbury and Flipsen. Trajectories are shown for four tongue points in two words. The upper part of the figure shows the data for the syllable [dor] from the monosyllable *dorm*, and the lower part of the figure shows the data for same syllable from the trisyllable *dormitory*. The speaker uses quite different lingual movements for the two syllables. Although there is a general similarity in mandibular excursion (Mi), the tongue point trajectories in the upper illustration have a markedly larger vertical displacement than those in the lower illustration. In addition, the tongue configuration assumed during the rhotic [r] (thick line connecting the points labeled 3) is rather different for the two syllables. This is a sample showing the flexibility of speech articulation.

DYNAMIC STRUCTURE IN SPEECH PRODUCTION

Traunmuller (1994) offers a useful perspective on the various information sources combined in the speech signal. He describes four sources as follows:

1. *Phonetic quality* refers to the linguistic content of the speech message; this information is specific to humans and is defined in terms of the conventions of a particular language.

2. *Affective quality* (or emotional quality) is paralinguistic, meaning that it accompanies the linguistic message of speech and may contribute to the interpretation of that message.

3. *Personal quality* is extralinguistic, i.e., it is outside the ordinary linguistic aspects of speech. Personal quality is informative about the talker, but not the message.

4. *Transmittal quality* gives perspectival information about the talker's location, including the distance between talker and listener, orientation in space, presence of background noise, and influence of environmental acoustics that may introduce effects such as reverberation.

These four sources of information are woven together in production and perception, and their disentanglement is a fundamental objective of longstanding efforts in speech science. By way of showing how these sources are integrated in speech, Traunmuller proposed a modulation theory of speech in which phonetic information is impressed onto speech signals by modulating a personal carrier signal. He further speculated that the carrier should be understood as a neutral schwa-like vowel with a relatively low fundamental frequency. Such a carrier is essentially stationary, as it involves a static vocal tract posture and a fixed frequency of source excitation.

An advantage that accrues to Traunmuller's proposal for a stationary carrier is that the formant and fundamental frequency information could serve the purpose of talker normalization. But a more dynamic carrier could assist in time normalization and also could supply the temporal substrate for motor regulation. One candidate for a dynamic carrier is syllabic tempo. With syllabic tempo as a carrier, the carrier frequency would be variable over a certain range, as it would have to be to account for changes in speaking rate. However, a preferred or modal frequency might be demonstrated across large ensembles of speech behavior. The frequency of 4 Hz seems to represent a typical syllabic rate of speech and also corresponds quite nicely with the ear's optimal sensitivity to amplitude modulation (Lauter & Hirsh, 1986) and therefore an awareness of the syllabic modulation of the energy envelope of speech. It may be possible to place the control of syllable rate within the nervous system. One candidate is the ventrolateral nucleus of the thalamus, stimulation of which accelerates the rate of speaking or counting (Hassler, 1966).

Another indication of an average constancy of speech rate is the observation of Voss and Clarke (1975) that the loudness fluctuations of speech have a 1/f-like power spectrum, i.e., a power spectrum that varies approximately as the inverse of frequency over many decades of frequency. Voss and Clarke determined that the average duration of a speech sound, over a long term, is about 100 ms, which is equivalent to 10 sounds per second.

Long-term temporal averages of syllable and sound-segment rate are important in defining the optimal modulation of the speech signal by information sources closely related to speech production variables. That is, both perception and production are based on syllable-timed processing. The syllable is central to the temporal regulation of speech, for it is the structure by which the major temporal regularities of speech can be determined. These regularities are defined at the molar level for syllabic sequences and at the molecular level for intrasyllabic timing relations.

THE GOAL, GESTURE, AND TRAJECTORY IN SPEECH PRODUCTION

A conceptual model of goal-governed, trajectory-based speech motor control is shown in Figure 5. The full expression of this model might represent speech as a multi-variable nonlinear dynamic system. Gestures and trajectories of various kinds are related according to the following definitions.

A *goal* or movement intention is assumed as the highest level of control. The goal is abstract, fulfilling the phonetic requirements of the utterance but not detailing muscular implementation. The goals must maintain the competence for intelligible speech across a variety of circumstances and articulatory implementations.

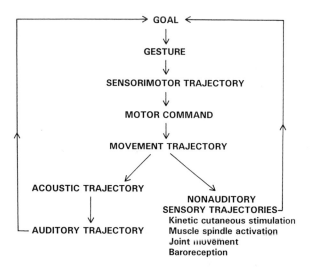

Figure 5. A depiction of a goal-gesture-trajectory model of speech production.

If goals are adjusted to speaking rate and speaking style, then goal modification can reduce some of the complexities that otherwise must be assigned to other aspects of the production model.

A *gesture* is a relatively abstract prescription for movement, derived from the goal defined above. Whereas goals pertain to a global movement objective, the gestural description introduces a level of articulatory specificity, i.e., an interpretation of the goal in terms of articulatory movements of the lips, tongue, and so on.

Gestures are redefined as *sensorimotor trajectories*, which constitute the basic plan of movement. It is assumed that speech includes both motor and sensory components which can be represented as trajectories in various parts of the nervous system. Sensory trajectories are a partial basis for the /preparation of motor trajectories, and the basal nuclei could play a major role in this operation (Lidsky, Manetto, & Schneider, 1985). The comparison of motor and sensory trajectories for a movement is a means to accurate performance of skilled behavior. Following Georgopoulos (1995), it might be expected that specific cells serve the purpose of representing memorized trajectories. It is in the formulation of sensorimotor trajectories that some differences between nonstuttering and stuttering subjects may become evident. For example, the higher EMG levels reported by van Lieshout et al. (1993) for labial gestures of stutterers compared to nonstutterers may reflect a difference in sensorimotor trajectories or the consequent motor commmands, as discussed in the following.

The trajectories are the basis for the formulation of *motor commands*. Execution of the motor commands yields movement trajectories, which, in turn, produce the acoustic trajectories of speech. Speech movements generate a dynamic afference in the form of auditory and other sensory trajectories. The auditory signal is unique among these afferent products because it is shared with other listeners. But tactile, kinesthetic, joint, and baroreceptive information is the private afference used by the talker to adjust and update sensorimotor trajectories that accomplish phonetic goals within the boundaries of prosodic and paralinguistic variation. The plurimodal afference generated by speech enables a highly flexible and adaptive regulation of speech movements.

It may be expected that the highly practiced nature of speech and the highly predictable context of speech movements would enable the articulatory execution even if one or more afferent channels is interrupted or distorted (see review by Kent, Martin, & Sufit, 1990). Trajectories are well suited to this purpose, and it is noteworthy that experiments on monkey visual cortex have shown that some neurons that respond to a moving target are active during both actual and inferred motion (Assad & Maunsell, 1995). The fact that neurons respond to such inferred motion demonstrates the powerful role of context and expectation in sensory processing. This capability permits the organism to deal with intermittencies in the distal stimulus.

The role of afferent information in the regulation of speech remains uncertain. Clinical studies may force renewed attention on the way in which sensory feedback contributes to speech motor control. For examples, evidence of impaired afferent processing has been presented for subjects with Parkinson's disease (Schneider, Diamond, & Markham, 1986) and stutterers (De Nil & Abbs, 1991; Howell et al., 1995). Interestingly, other authors (Lieshout et al., 1996) have concluded that stutterers use a motor control strategy that has an exceptional reliance on the monitoring function of proprioceptive feedback.

SPEECH DEVELOPMENT

The child's speech production system is not simply a miniaturized version of the adult's system. Recognizing the differences between the infant and the adult in vocal tract anatomy, Bosma (1976) proposed two stages of speech production, an early stage based on the infant's vocal tract anatomy and a later stage based on the vocal tract anatomy of the older child or the adult. Stathopoulos and Sapienza (1993) emphasized the functional differences between children and adults in speech production and expressed the need for models of speech production that are age specific. To be sure, a variety of changes occur during the juvenile development of the respiratory, laryngeal, and upper airway systems of sound production. Some of these changes are profound in the sense that they may indeed require quite different models than those that suffice for adults. These changes have implications for an account of the development of the motor control of speech. In addition, some of these changes are coincident with the clinical emergence of speech disorders such as stuttering (Adams, 1982; Yairi & Ambrose, 1992a, 1992b). As Williams and Bishop (1992) pointed out, a motor control deficiency may have different manifestations, depending on age or maturity of the motor control system.

Table 2. Major developmental milestones in the respiratory system.

BIRTH	Diaphragm of newborn has bellows-like displacement, unlike the piston-like effect in adults. Rest breathing rate is 30-80 breaths/min. Frequent paradoxing occurs in early infancy.
3 YRS	Respiratory function not closely geared to linguistic requirements until this age. Rest breathing rate is 20-30 breaths/min. Functional maturation is especially evident during the period of 3 to 7 yrs.
7 YRS	Essential convergence on adult-like patterns, but children use greater subglottal air pressures than adults for speaking.
10 YRS	Refinement of respiratory patterns; functional maturation achieved. Rest breathing rate is 17-22 breaths/min.
12-18 YRS	Increase in lung capacity, especially in boys.

Table 3. Major developmental milestones in the laryngeal system.

BIRTH	Laryngeal position is high in neck, similar to nonhuman primate anatomy. Vocal folds are 5 to 7 mm long. Entire lamina propria is uniform, i.e., there is no lamination corresponding to adult histology. About one-half of the infant glottal length is cartilaginous.
4 YRS	Vocal ligament appears between 1 to 4 yrs.
6 YRS	Vocal fold length is about 8 mm in both sexes. The two layers of vocal ligament become differentiated between 6 to 15 yrs.
8 YRS	Sex differences begin to emerge in laryngeal tissues.
12 YRS	Differentiation of lamina propria nearly complete.Adolescent voice change begins in males between 12.5 to 14.5 yrs. Length of vocal folds is about 12-17 mm in pubescent girls and about 15-25 mm in pubescent boys.
16 YRS	Adult morphology of vocal folds achieved.
ADULT	Vocal length is about 21 mm in women and about 29 mm in men. About one-third of vocal fold length is cartilaginous.

Table 4. Major developmental milestones in mandibular control.

BIRTH 1 YR	First primary molars achieve occlusal contact at about 16 months. Stability of jaw closing pattern follows this occlusal event.
4 YRS	Vowel system complete; this phonetic milestone may reflect mastery of tongue-jaw coordination.
7 YRS	Growth spurt in structures of lower face begins at about this time.
8 YRS	Adult-like precision of jaw movement achieved. Comparable precision for lips and tongue comes later.
12-16 YRS	Growth spurt in mandible in boys.

If speech scientists feel compelled to construct different models to account for speech production by talkers of different ages, then we may well ask if the talker's brain itself constructs new models of speech as the peripheral mechanisms of speech pass through developmental milestones. To seek an answer to this question, we need to begin with an appreciation of how the peripheral structures of speech develop in the child.

A comprehensive develomental review cannot be undertaken here, but a few examples of developmental change will be considered, as summarized in Table 2 (the respiratory system), Table 3 (the laryngeal system), and Table 4 (the mandibular system, taken as a representative of the craniofacial complex). (A review of the development of craniofacial, oral, and laryngeal structures is available in Kent and Vorperian, 1995). It is particularly important to note that development goes beyond a simple increase of structural size. Rather, development represents basic changes in configuration, histology, and sensorimotor organization.

The respiratory system

The diaphragm of the neonate has a bellows-like displacement, unlike the piston-like displacement in adults (Devlieger et al., 1991). The rest breathing rate of the neonate is in the range of 30-80 breaths/min, which is two to four times the rate in adults. As a consequence, prolonged vocalization on egressive air is a larger departure from the basic respiratory rhythm in infants. Infants also differ from adults in respiratory kinematics (Boliek et al., forthcoming). During infancy, the respiratory system shows frequent episodes of paradoxing, i.e., simultaneous inspiratory and expiratory displacements of the rib cage and diaphragm. Before the age of 3 years, regulation of the respiratory system is relatively insensitive to the linguistic requirements of the utterance. A progressive functional maturation of the respiratory system is especially evident during the period of 3 to 7 years. By the age of 7 or 8 years, the child has converged on an essentially adult-like regulation of respiration (Hoit et al., 1990). Nonetheless, it has been reported that the child generates 50-100% greater subglottal air pressures than adults for a similar phonatory task (Stathopoulos & Sapienza, 1993). Respiratory control continues to be refined until the age of about 12 years. After that age, the primary change is in the volume of the lungs, which increases with height.

The laryngeal system

Only selected developmental changes will be mentioned here; for more detailed descriptions, see Kent and Vorperian (1995). As is well known, the neonate has a high laryngeal position, rather like that seen in nonhuman primates generally. The epiglottis is sufficiently cephalad that it touches, or at least comes close to, the velum. Laryngeal descent occurs largely during the first half-year of life. However, major differences in vocal fold microanatomy continue to unfold until the child is 12 to 15 years old. The vocal ligament itself takes form only by the age of about 6 years, and the adult-like lamination of the folds is not developed until the child is about 12 to 15 years old (Hirano et al., 1981; Hirano & Sato, 1993). Therefore, the cover-body model of phonation developed for adults has limited application to the juvenile vocal folds. The differentiated visco-elastic layers of the vocal fold are a developmental phenomenon, and it appears that models of vocal fold vibration in the adult are of limited value to the child younger than 12 years.

Craniofacial and oral systems

The skull reaches nearly adult size by the age of 6 years, but the facial skeleton is still immature. Therefore, the head develops according to two calendars of skeletal maturation, one fitting the neural growth curve and the other fitting the general musculoskeletal growth curve (Scammon, 1930). The lower face has an overall growth spurt between 7 to 10 years of age. A complete discussion of the growth of the craniofacial and oral complex is beyond the scope of this paper, but it suffices for present purposes to take two systems as examples of developmental change during childhood. Let us take a brief look at the mandible and the velopharynx.

Mandibular gestures have an early spatial regularity determined by the occlusal contact of the first primary molars at about 16 mos. (Widmer, 1992). After this occlusal contact is established, the jaw returns essentially to the same position. Phonologic inventories show that the vowel system is essentially mastered by the age of 4 years. Among the last entries are the front vowels, which may require that the child solve the tongue-jaw and lip-jaw synergy problem. Spatiotemporal control of the jaw continues to mature, reaching a relatively high degree of precision at about 7 or 8 years (Nittrouer, 1993; Sharkey & Folkins, 1985; Smith, 1995). Interestingly, the age of 7 years also has been suggested as a period of transition for the cutaneous oral-motor reflex (Smith et al., 1991). Apparently, the jaw achieves a nearly adult-like precision earlier than other articulators such as the tongue or lips. Jaw regulation is indeed quite precise: the error in jaw positioning in adults is about 1° of angular variation (Broekhuijsen & van Willigen, 1983), which rivals the precision of the eye or hand in the dark (Merton, 1961). Because the gestures of the tongue and lip are to some degree predicated on jaw position, the earlier maturation of jaw regulation may be regarded as a preliminary step in the development of tongue and lip gestures.

A sequence of developmental events can be described for velopharyngeal valving. In very young children, velopharyngeal valving is predominantly velar-adenoidal, owing to the typical hypertrophy of the nasopharyngeal tonsil (Croft et al., 1981; Skolnick et al., 1975). With atrophy of this tonsil, velar-adenoidal valving gives way to another pattern. But this pattern also may be transient in most children. Siegel-Sadewitz and Shprintzen (1986) noted changes in velopharyngeal valving in more than half of normal subjects in a prepubertal-postpubertal comparison. Hence, velopharyngeal closure is not an invariant motor pattern across development. Furthermore, at least four distinct patterns of velopharyngeal closure are evident in adults.

What we might conclude from this admittedly cursory look at a complex phenomenon is that speech production occurs against a backdrop of considerable anatomical change. Individual structures and systems follow their own developmental schedules. The motor product of the composite system therefore reflects at any given point in development a complex interaction of the component movement trajectories and their relative states of maturation. In this view, it is appropriate to view the speech motor system as a multivariable nonlinear dynamic system and to consider the development of speech motor skill in terms of the emergence of various trajectories (or gestures) that are defined in terms of the anatomy and biomechanics that obtain for a given point in development. Thelen (1991) proposed a system dynamic theory of speech development to account for the role of anatomic restructuring in the emergence of attractor states, that is, stable patterns of motor control. See Stathopoulos (1995) for further arguments along this line.

A goal-based gestural account of speech production seems capable of accommodating anatomical development while preserving the essence of phonetic intention and skilled motor control. The sensorimotor trajectories that implement the goals would be subject to adaptation to reflect the changing anatomy and biomechanics. It is expected that the neural organization of speech would similarly change as the mapping between goals and trajectories is altered during development. The nervous system appears well equipped for this flexibility, given that "a single neuron can intermittently participate in different computations by rapidly changing its coupling to other neurons, without associated changes in firing rate" (Vaadia et al., 1995, p. 517). Edelman's theory of neuronal group selection (Edelman, 1993; Friston et al., 1994; Montague et al., 1991) is one way of accounting for developmental change in sensory and motor representation. Speech in its various forms of sensory and motor information could be represented as a number of neuronal "maps" that combine the different kinds of information, perhaps relying on a rhythmic substrate for their coordination.

The objective of developmental studies is not simply to add a footnote to our knowledge of adult competence. The objective is far more profound and was expressed as follows by Logan (1992) with respect to the study of bird song development: "The literature on bird song illustrates that developmental analysis is essential to understanding the origins of adult function and the processes guiding it. Development is not just what comes before; it is the historical basis for the explanation of adult function and the processes underlying it" (p. 111). The study of the young child talker is a pursuit of explanations for adult function. The conjoint study of anatomy, behavior, and neural control is the means to understanding. Sporns and Edelman state the general perspective: "There is overwhelming evidence that the emergence of coordinated movements is intimately tied both to the growth of the musculoskeletal system and to the development of the brain" (p. 966). Speech, then, is a mirror to development of the body and the brain.

CONCLUSION

Marr (1982) outlined three basic levels for understanding the brain: computational theory (to define the goal of computation), representation and algorithm (to explain how the computation can be implemented), and hardware implementation (to assign the computation to specific brain structures). Speech may well be understood at the same three levels, and we stand at an unprecedented opportunity to make a cross-level comparison of progress. It is therefore a good time for a review of the theories that capture understanding and guide research. Although some degree of theoretical competition is vital to science, there is also value to occasional attempts to evaluate the merits of individual theories and weigh their similarities and differences.

ACKNOWLEDGMENTS

This work was supported in part by a research grant number 5 RO1 DC 00319-11 from the National Institute on Deafness and Other Communication Disorders, National Institutes of Health.

REFERENCES

Assad, J.A., & Maunsell, J.H.R. (1995). Neuronal correlates of inferred motion in primate posterior parietal cortex. *Nature, 373,* 518-521.

Badin, P., Perrier, P., Boe, L.-J., & Abry, C. (1990). Vocalic nomograms: acoustic and articulatory considerations pon formant convergences. *Journal of the Acoustical Society of America, 87,* 1290-1300.

Boliek, C., Hixon, T., Watson, P., & Morgan, W. (forthcoming). Vocalization and breathing during the first year of life. *Journal of Voice, 10.*

Bosma, J. (1976). Discussion of the paper, "Postnatal development of the basicranium and vocal tract region in man" by J.T. Laitman and E.S. Crelin. In J. Bosma, (Ed.), Symposiumon the Development of the Basicranium (pp. 219-220). DHEW Publication No. 76-989, PHS-NIH, Bethesda, MD.

Brookhuijsen, M.L., & van Willigen, J.D. (1983). Factors influencing jaw position sense in man. *Archives or Oral Biology, 28,* 387-391.

Browman, C.P., & Goldstein, L.M. (1986). Towards an articulatory phonology. *Phonology Yearbook, 3,* 219-252.

Browman, C.P., & Goldstein, L. (1988). Some notes on syllabic structure in articulatory phonology. *Phonetica, 45,* 140-155.

Browman, C.P., & Goldstein, L. (1990). Tiers in articulatory phonology, with some implications for casual speech. In J. Kingston & M. Beckman (Eds.), Papers in Laboratory Phonology. *I. Between the Grammar and the Physics of Speech* (pp. 341-376). Cambridge, UK: Cambridge University Press.

Browman, C.P., & Goldstein, L. (1992). Articulatory phonology: An overview. *Phonetica, 49,* 155-180.

Byrd, D. (1995). C-centers revisited. *Phonetica, 52,* 285-306.

Carre, R., & Mrayati, M. (1995). Vowel transitions, vowel systems, and the Distinctive Region Model. In C. Sorin, J. Mariani, H. Meloni, & J. Schoentgen, (Eds.), *Levels in Speech Communication: Relations and Interactions* (pp. 73-89). Amsterdam: Elsevier.

Cherniak, C. (1995). Neural component placement. *Trends in Neuroscience, 18,* 522-527.

Croft, C.B., Shprintzen, R.J., & Rakoff, S.J. (1981). Patterns of velopharyngeal valving in normal and cleft palate subjects: A multi-view videofluoroscopic and nasendoscopic study. *Laryngoscope, 91,* 265-271.

De Nil, L., & Abbs, J.H. (1991). Oral and finger kinesthetic thresholds in stutterers. In H. Peters, W. Hulstijn, & C.W. Starkweather (Eds.), *Speech Motor Control and Stuttering* (pp. 123-130). Amsterdam: Elsevier.

Devlieger, H., Daniels, H., Marchal, G, Moerman, Ph., Casear , P., & Eggermont, E. (1991). The diaphragm of the newborn infant: Anatomic and ultrasonagraphic studies. *Journal of Developmental Physiology, 16,* 321-329.

Duffy, J.R. (1995). *Motor Speech Disorders: Substrates, Differential Diagnosis and Management.* St. Louis, MO: Mosby.

Edelman, G. (1993). Neural Darwinism: Selection and Reentrant signaling in higher brain function. *Neuron, 10,* 115-125.

Fowler, C.A. (1984). Segmentation of coarticulated speech in perception. *Perception & Psychophysics, 36*, 359-368.

Fowler, C. A. (1986). An event approach to the study of speech perception from a direct-realist perspective. *Journal of Phonetics, 14*, 3-28.

Fowler, C.A. (1996). Listeners do hear sounds, not tongues. *Journal of the Acoustical Society of America, 99*, 1730-1741.

Friston, K.J., Tononi, G., Reeke, G.N., Jr., Sporns, O., & Edelman, G.M. (1994). Value-dependent selection in the brain: Simulation in a synthetic neural model. *Neuroscience, 59*, 229-243.

Georgopoulos, A.P. (1995). Current issues in directional motor control. *Trends in Neuroscience, 18*, 506-510.

Gracco, V.L. (1994). Some organizational characteristics of speech movement control. *Journal of Speech and Hearing Research, 37*, 4-27.

Hassler, R. (1966). Thalamic regulation of muscle tone and speed of movements. In D. Purpura & M. Yahr (Eds.), *The Thalamus*. New York: Columbia University Press.

Hirano, M., Kurita, S., & Nakashima, T. (1981). Growth, development and aging of human vocal folds. In D.M. Bless, & J.H. Abbs, (Eds.), *Vocal Fold Physiology: Contemporary Research and Clinical Issues* (pp. 22-43). San Diego: College-Hill Press.

Hirano, M., & Sato, K. (1993). *Histological Color Atlas of the Human Larynx*. San Diego: Singular.

Hoit, J.D., Hixon, T.J., Watson, P.J., & Morgan, W.J. (1990). Speech breathing in children and adolescents. *Journal of Speech and Hearing Research, 33*, 51-69.

Honda, K. (1996). Organization of tongue articulation for vowels. *Journal of Phonetics, 24*, 39-52.

Howell, P., Sackin, S., & Rustin, L. (1995). Comparison of speech motor development in stutterers and fluent speakers between 7 and 12 years old. *Journal of Fluency Disorders, 20*, 243-255.

Huffman, R.F., & Hanson, O.W., Jr. (1990). The descending auditory pathway and acousticomotor systems: connections with the inferior colliculus. *Brain Research Reviews, 15*, 295-323.

Kawato, M., & Gomi, H. (1992). The cerebellum and VOR/OKR learning models. *Trends in Neurosciences, 15*, 445-453.

Kent, R.D. (1986). The iceberg hypothesis: the temporal assembly of speech movements. In J.S. Perkell, & D.H. Klatt, (Eds.), *Invariance and Variability in Speech Processes* (pp. 234-242). Hillsdale, NJ: Lawrence Erlbaum Associates.

Kent, R.D. (in press). Developments in the theoretical understanding of speech and its disorders. To appear in M.J. Ball, (Ed.), *Advances in Clinical Linguistics and Phonetics*.

Kent, R.D., Adams, S.G., & Turner, G. (1996). Models of speech production. In N.J. Lass (Ed.), *Principles of Experimental Phonetics* (pp. 3-45). St. Louis: Mosby.

Kent, R.D., Martin, R.E., & Sufit, R.L. (1990). Oral sensation: A review and clinical prospective. In H. Winitz (Ed.), *Human Communication and its Disorders: A Review - 1990* (pp. 135-191). Norwood, NJ: Ablex Press.

Kent, R.D, and Tjaden, K. (in press). Brain functions underlying speech. To appear in W. Hardcastle & J. Laver, (Eds.), *Handbook of the Phonetic Sciences*. London: Blackwell.

Kent, R.D., & Vorperian, H.K. (1995). Anatomic development of the craniofacial-oral-laryngeal systems: A review. *Journal of Medical Speech-Language Pathology, 3*, 145-190.

Kohler, K.J. (1995). Phonetics -- a language science in its own right? In K. Elenius & P. Branderud (Eds.), *Proceedings of the XIIth International Congress of Phonetics, Vol. 1*, pp. 10-17. Stockholm: Royal Institute of Technology and Stockholm University.

Kroger, B.J. (1993). A gestural production model and its application to reduction in German. *Phonetica, 50*, 213-233.

Kroger, B.J., Shroder, G., & Opgen-Rhein, C. (1995). A gesture-based dynamic model describing articulatory movement data. *Journal of the Acoustical Society of America, 98,* 1878-1889.

Lauter, J.L., & Hirsh, I.J. (1985). Speech as temporal pattern: A psychoacoustic profile. *Speech Communication, 4,* 41-54.

Liberman, A.M., Cooper, F.S., Shankweiler, D.S., & Studdert-Kennedy, M. (1967). Perception of the speech code. *Psychological Review, 72,* 431-461.

Liberman, A.M., & Mattingly, I.G. (1985). The motor theory of speech perception revised. *Cognition, 21,* 1-36.

Lofqvist, A. (1990). Speech as audible gestures. In W.J., Hardcastle, & A., Marchal (Eds.), *Speech Production and Speech Modelling* (pp. 289-322). Dordrecht, Netherlands: Kluwer Academic Publishers.

Logan, C.A. (1992). Developmental analysis in behavioral systems: the case of bird song. In G. Turkewitz (Ed.), Developmental Psychobiology. *Annals of the New York Academy of Sciences, 662,* pp. 102-116.

Lalonde, C.E., & Werker, J.F. (1995). Cognitive influences on cross-language speech perception in infancy. *Infant Behavior and Development, 18,* 459-475.

Marr, D. (1982). *Vision.* New York: Freeman.

Masterton, R.B. (1992). Role of the central nervous system in hearing: the new direction. *Trends in Neuroscience, 15,* 280-285.

Merton, P.A. (1961). The accuracy of directing the eyes and the hand in the dark. *Journal of Physiology (London), 156,* 555-577.

Montague, P.R., Gally, J.A., & Edelman, G.R. (1991). Spatial signaling in the development and function of neural connections. *Cerebral Cortex, 1,* 199-220.

Muller-Preuss, P., & Ploog, D. (1981). Inhibition of auditory cortical neurons during phonation. *Brain Research, 215,* 61-76.

Nittrouer, S. (1993). The emergence of mature gestural patterns is not uniform: evidence from an acoustic study. *Journal of Speech and Hearing Research, 36,* 959-972.

Ploog, D. (1981). Neurobiology of primate audio-vocal behavior. *Brain Research Reviews, 3,* 35-61.

Ploog, D.W. (1992). The evolution of vocal communication. In H. Papousek, U. Jurgens, & M. Papousek (Eds.), *Nonverbal Vocal Communication* (pp. 6-30). Cambridge, UK: Cambridge University Press.

Saltzman, E.L., & Munhall, K.G. (1989). A dynamical approach to gestural patterning in speech production. *Ecological Psychology, 1,* 333-382.

Scammon, R.E. (1930). The measurement of the body in childhood. In J.A., Harris, C.M., Jackson, D.G., Patterson, & R.E., Scammon, (Eds.), *The Measurement of Man* (pp. 173-215). Minneapolis: University of Minnesota Press.

Schneider, J.S., Diamond, S.G., & Markham, C.H. (1986). Deficits in orofacial sensorimotor function in Parkinson's disease. *Annals of Neurology, 19,* 275-282.

Schuller, G. (1979). Vocalization influences auditory processing in collicular neurons of the CF-FM bat, Rhinolophus ferrumequinum. *Journal of Comparative Physiology, 132,* 39-46.

Sharkey, S.G., & Folkins, J.W. (1985). Variability of lip and jaw movements in children and adults: implications for the development of speech motor control. *Journal of Speech and Hearing Research, 28,* 8-15.

Siegel-Sadewitz, V.L., & Shprintzen, R.J. (1986). Changes in velopharyngeal valving with age. *International Journal of Pediatric Otorhinolaryngology, 11,* 171-182.

Skolnick, M.L., Shprintzen, R.J., McCall, G., N., & Rakoff, S.J. (1975). Patterns of velopharyngeal closure in subjects with repaired cleft palate and normal speech: A multi-view videofluoroscopic analysis. *Cleft Palate Journal, 12,* 369-376.

Smith, A., Weber, C.M., Newton, J., & Denny, M. (1991). Developmental and age-related changes in reflexes of the human jaw-closing system. *Electroencephalography and Clinical Neurophysiology, 81,* 118-128.

Smith, B.L. (1995). Variability of lip and jaw movements in the speech of children and adults. *Phonetica, 52,* 307-316.

Sporns, O., & Edelman, G.M. (1993). Solving Bernstein's problem: A proposal for the development of coordinated movement by selection. *Child Development, 64,* 960-981.

Square, P.A., and Martin, R.E. (1994). The nature and treatment of neuromotor speech disorders in aphasia. In R. Chapey (Ed.), *Language Intervention Strategies in Adult Aphasia* (3rd ed.; pp. 467-499). Baltimore: Williams and Wilkins.

Stathopoulos, E.T. (1995). Variability revisited: An acoustic, aerodynamic, and respiratory kinematic comparison of children and adults during speech. *Journal of Phonetics, 23,* 67-80.

Stathopoulos, E.T., & Sapienza, C. (1993). Respiratory and laryngeal measures of children during vocal intensity variation. *Journal of the Acoustical Society of America, 94,* 2531-2543.

Stevens, K.N. (1989). On the quantal nature of speech. *Journal of Phonetics, 17,* 3-45.

Suga, N., & Schlegel, P. (1972). Neural attentuation of responses to emitted sounds in echolating bats. *Science, 177,* 82-84.

Tatham, M.A.A. (1995). The supervision of speech production. In C. Sorin, J. Mariani, H. Meloni, & J. Schoentgen (Eds.), *Levels in Speech Production* (pp. 115-125). Amsterdam: Elsevier.

Thelen, E. (1991). Motor aspects of emergent speech: A dynamic approach. In N.A. Krasnegor et al. (Eds.), *Biological and Behavioral Determinants of Language Development* (pp. 339-362). Hillsdale, NJ: Erlbaum.

Traunmuller, H. (1994). Conventional, biological, and environmental factors in speech communication: A modulation theory. *Phonetica, 51,* 170-183.

Vaadia, E., Haalman, I., Abeles, M., Bergman, H., Prut, Y., Slovin, H., & Aertsen, A. (1995). Dynamics of neuronal interactions in monkey cortex in relation to behavioural events. *Nature, 373,* 515-518.

Van der Merwe, A. (forthcoming). A theoretical framework for the characterization of pathological speech sensorimotor control. In M., McNeil (Ed.), *Sensorimotor Speech Disorders.*

Van Lieshout, P.H.H.M., Hulstijn, W., & Peters, H.F.M. (1996). Speech production in people who stutter: testing the motor plan assembly hypothesis. *Journal of Speech and Hearing Research, 39,* 76-92.

Van Lieshout, P.H.H.M., Peters, H.F.M., Starkweather, C.W., & Hulstijn, W. (1993). Physiological differences between stutterers and nonstutterers in perceptually fluent speech: EMG amplitude and duration. *Journal of Speech and Hearing Research, 36,* 55-63.

Voss, R.F., & Clarke, J. (1975). "1/f noise" in music and speech. *Nature, 258,* 317-318.

Werker, J.F., & Tees, R.C. (1984). Cross-language speech perception: evidence for the perceptual reorganization during the first year of life. *Infant Behavior and Development, 7,* 49-63.

Widmer, R.P. (1992). The normal development of teeth. *Australian Family Physician, 21,* 1251-1261.

Wilhelms-Tricarico, R. (1996). A biomechanical and physiologically-based vocal tract model and its control. *Journal of Phonetics, 24,* 23-38.

Williams, H. (1989). Multiple representations and auditory-motor interactions in the avian song system. In M. Davis, B.L. Jacobs, & R.I. Schoenfeld (Eds.), Modulation of Defined Vertebrate Neural Circuits. *Annals of the New York Academy of Sciences, 563,* (pp. 148-164).

Williams, H.G., & Bishop, J.H. (1992). Speed and consistency of manual movements of stutterers, articulation-disordered children, and children with normal speech. *Journal of Fluency Disorders, 17,*

191-203.

Yairi, E., & Ambrose, N.A. (1992a). A longitudinal study of stuttering in children: A preliminary report. *Journal of Speech and Hearing Research, 35,* 755-760.

Yairi, E., & Ambrose, N.A. (1992b). Onset of stuttering in preschool children: Selected factors. *Journal of Speech and Hearing Research, 35,* 782-788.

Zattorre, R.J., Evans, A.C., Meyer, E., & Gjedde, A. (1992). Lateralization of phonetic and pitch discrimination in speech processing. *Science, 256,* 846-849.

Speech Production: Motor Control, Brain Research and Fluency Disorders
W. Hulstijn, H.F.M. Peters and P.H.H.M. Van Lieshout, editors

Chapter 3

A NEUROMOTOR PERSPECTIVE ON SPEECH PRODUCTION

Vincent L. Gracco

Speech is one of man's most distinguishing traits. At the core of this important communicative behavior is the human nervous system which constantly receives, integrates, and exchanges information on the various operations carried out through a variety of sensorimotor channels. In order to understand speech communication it is essential to understand the machine itself, not only at the level of the physical apparatus but at the level of the physiological components and associated processes. An important assumption is that control principles that govern speech and language production and perception are best understood and unambiguously inferred from a perspective that is grounded in nervous system physiology. The focus of this chapter is to outline a theoretical framework for speech production which explicitly takes into account the contribution of the anatomy and physiology of the speech production mechanism as well as information on general nervous system functions and associated regions known to be involved in speech and language production.

INTRODUCTION

The act of speaking and the processes associated with communication are potentially valuable sources of information on the organization and development of human behavior. Empirical observations are critical for developing an understanding of the fundamental components of communicative behavior, how they develop and how they break down. Empirical observations also can be used to infer nervous system functions associated with this complex and intricate process. Attempts to understand, predict and ultimately formulate a systematic body of scientific knowledge about fundamental aspects of speech and language behavior require two additional elements: models and theories. Since these terms are often inconsistently defined in textbooks they will be defined for the sake of clarity. A model is a set of symbols and associated logical rules for manipulating the symbols. The symbols may be numbers, words, physical objects, or abstract forms. The rules may be explicit or implicit. When the symbols of a model are identified with specific empirical events, the model and set of identifications constitute a theory. A theory specifies the relationship between events for the purpose of explanation or prediction. The level of model description determines, to a large extent, the types of explanations one develops. While often overlooked, models and theories are statements of a philosophical perspective on science and the nature of explanation.

In attempting to understand speech and language one of two philosophical perspectives can be taken. These perspectives have historical roots in natural philosophy. The first approach has its roots in early epistemology and is represented by the philosophical position of Plato, described as substance dualism. Plato's theory postulated two different kinds of substances, one from the mind and one from the material world. For the substance dualist, models of behavior would not need to be constrained by considerations of the form or function of the nervous system, since it is impossible to know about them in an empirical or epistemological sense. As described by Churchland (1986), "Plato is the archetypal antinaturalist and contrasts vividly with contemporary naturalists who argue that the mind is the brain and that empirical science is indispensable to discovering the nature of the mind-brain...". Naturalism, on the other hand, suggests that scientific laws are adequate to account for all phenomena. One important implicit difference between substance dualism and naturalism is a lack of distinction between the mind and brain and the consequence that empirical investigation can be used to learn about the psychological events that are not directly observable. It is the latter perspective that provides the philosophical foundation for much of the current work in contemporary neuroscience and leads quite naturally to "... the possibility of a unified theory of the mind-brain, wherein psychological states and processes are explained in terms of neuronal states and processes." (Churchland, 1986).

An approach in which model constructs and theoretical constraints are grounded in neurobiology represents a reductionistic perspective. Reductionism, as pointed out by Churchland (1986), is a widely misunderstood philosophical position. Reductionism is often identified with an attempt to simply some complex behavior to the point where empirical investigation become tractable. However, in the philosophy of science..., "... reduction is first and foremost a relation between theories" in which "...one theory, the *reduced* theory Tr, stands in a certain relation to another more basic theory Tb." Moreover, "Statements that a phenomenon Pr reduces to another phenomenon Pb are derivative upon the more basic claim that the theory that characterizes the first reduces to the theory that characterizes the second." An example provided by Churchland relates to the theory of optics in which, during the mid-nineteenth century, it was supposed that light and electromagnetic effects were two different kinds of phenomena. By the turn of the century the theory of optics had been reduced to the theory of electromagnetic radiation such that light was now identified as electromagnetic radiation. As more and more information is acquired, due to advances in technology and concomitant changes in experimental design, the expression of psychological theories and model constructs within a neurobiological framework will proceed. From this general philosophical perspective it logically follows that a speech production model should ultimately be reducible to a theory describing how neuronal ensembles work and it should reduce in such a way that the components of the model can be identified with neuronal components. The ultimate reducibility of psychological (or other hypothetical) constructs of speech and language to neuronal processes will only be achieved with considerable time and effort. A necessary first step is the generation of speech production theories and models with a focus on physiological descriptions and behavioral explanations in terms of general nervous system principles and processes.

CONCEPTUAL FRAMEWORK

A current view in the psycholinguistic literature is that two broad processes underlie language formulation (Levelt, 1989; 1992; Garrett, 1991). The first process involves grammatical encoding, or the creation of lexical items within a syntactic frame, and phonological encoding, including the specification of prosodic structure. These two broad processes create the phonetic plan. The phonetic plan interfaces with speech motor processes that generate the sequence of sounds specified in the plan. The phonological structure of the language interfaces seamlessly with the speech motor processes. The framework presented here incorporates a sensorimotor model of speech production with units of production and mechanisms for activating, scaling and sequencing the units for fluent speech. Aspects of the process have been detailed in various forms in a number of related publications (cf. Abbs, Gracco, & Cole, 1984; Gracco, 1987; 1988; 1990; 1991; 1994; Gracco & Abbs, 1987; 1989; Gracco & Löfqvist, 1994). What is of interest is the identification of the fundamental processes or components of the behavior and whether and how they are represented by known nervous system functions. As is often the case, observation of any behavior at one level of organization may yield patterns that emerge from the influence of or organization at another level of observation. Without considering the multiple levels of organization that exist for any behavior, one can easily generate an over-specified model and an unnecessarily detailed theory. One such level in speech production is the patterns and variations in kinematic observables. As a starting point, the structural and biomechanical properties of the vocal tract will be examined as possible contributors to the complex kinematic patterns observed during speech production, followed by some specific examples of how a neuromotor perspective can lead to simple explanations for apparently complex speech production phenomena.

STRUCTURAL PROPERTIES

The human vocal tract displays a number of biophysical properties that may influence speech kinematics. Whereas the tongue and lips are soft tissue structures that undergo substantial viscoelastic deformation during speech, the jaw displays a degree of anisotropic tension (Lynn & Yemm, 1971). Even seemingly homogeneous structures like the upper and lower lips display different stiffness properties (Ho et al., 1982) which may contribute to their differential movement patterns (Gracco & Abbs, 1986; Gracco, 1988). The mandible is a rigid body exhibiting rotational and translational motion while the tongue is a deformable, volume-preserving solid with a complex tissue structure and muscular organization. In addition to the structural arrangement of the vocal tract muscles for valving and shaping actions, mechanical properties of individual vocal tract structures provide insight into the functional organization of the speech motor control system. The dynamic nature of the tissue load against which the different vocal tract muscles contract is extremely heterogeneous. For some structures such as the lips and vocal folds, inertial considerations are minimal, while for the jaw and respiratory structures inertia is a significant consideration.

Considering the structural arrangement of the vocal tract, the different muscular orientations and the vast interconnection of muscles, cartilages, and ligaments, it is clear that complex biomechanical interactions are the rule. Passive or reactive changes due to inherent mechanical coupling is a consequence of almost any vocal tract action, with the relative significance varying according to the specific structural components and conformational change and the speed at which adjustments occur. As a result, a single articulatory action may generate primary as well as secondary effects throughout the vocal tract. It is important to determine the contribution of individual articulatory actions to the sound producing process. However, individual articulatory actions never have isolated effects. The combination of the viscoelastic properties of the tissues, the different biomechanical properties of vocal tract structures, and the complex geometry of the vocal tract comprises a complex biomechanical environment. The kinematic and acoustic variability characteristic of speech production reflects in part the differential filtering of neural control signals by the peripheral biomechanics. Recently, a physiological model of human mandible and hyoid motion (Laboissière et al., 1996) was used to show that certain patterns of intra-articulator coarticulation could be explained, not by active movement planning, but by the dynamics of the system at the level of the biomechanics (Ostry et al., 1996). The clearest example, and the one most relevant to separating active versus passive phenomena, was related to movement variations associated with anticipatory coarticulation. An often reported result is that the maximum articulator position of the C in a VCV sequence varies systematically with the height of the the final V. This variation has been explained as reflecting either an explicit planned response of the speech production system or the result of temporal overlap of central commands. However, simulations of the jaw motion using a physiological model clearly demonstrated that the anticipatory variations in the empirical data were the result of muscle mechanics and jaw dynamics, not central control.

In a study in progress, we have found that in certain other contexts systematic changes in observed jaw kinematics cannot be explained by biomechanical considerations (Gracco et al., in preparation). Empirical observations of the initial jaw position (prior to movement) for the initial C in a CVC sequence revealed that jaw position was being varied in anticipation of the upcoming vowel-related movement.

Shown in Figure 1 is the average pitch of the jaw for six subjects obtained during a steady state associated with the consonants /s/, /t/, /f/, and /k/ when followed by the vowel /a/, /i/, or /o/. As can be seen, the pitch of the jaw is lowest for the vowel /a/, slightly higher for the vowel /o/ and highest for the high vowel /i/. This pattern is consistent for all six subjects suggesting that jaw position for a syllable initial consonant is systematically adjusted for the upcoming vowel in apparent support of a planned response. However, when the task is viewed from a physiological perspective a simpler interpretation is possible that does not rely on a complicated anticipatory or look-ahead (explicit planning) mechanism operating at select

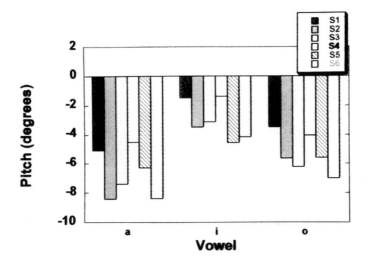

Figure 1. The pitch of the jaw (in degrees relative to the occlusal plane) averaged across the initial consonants /s/, /t/, /f/, and /k/ in a CVC context for six subjects plotted as a function of the medial vowel.

times during production. For almost all consonants and vowels the jaw is activated to position the constriction-producing articulators, in particular the tongue and lips. The muscles involved in positioning the mandible for different syllable-initial consonants and those involved in the production of many of the vowels overlap considerably. One of the characteristics of speech production is the continuous and overlapping nature of the process such that activations for contiguous phonetic gestures are not discrete in time. As such, it is more likely that commands for a syllable-initial consonant and the following vowel overlap in time. Given that the C and following V share some of the same musculature, and hence motoneuron pools, summation would occur and create small but systematic shifts in the consonant-specific spatial positioning of the mandible due to the upcoming vowel. Only by considering potential biomechanical interactions, and explanations of observable phenomena at a physiological level can the control principles and properties of the speech motor control system be realistically interpreted.

SPEECH PRODUCTION UNITS AND THEIR CONTROL

The speech production process, like most functional human behaviors, relies on units of action. From a neurobiological perspective there are a number of potential candidate constructs that may be used in describing the units of action. Two of these, the reflex and fixed action patterns, appear to lack the necessary flexibility to capture the adaptive nature of speech production. In contrast, the concept of functional synergies (Bernstein, 1967), and its elaboration, the coordinative structure (Easton, 1972; Turvey, 1977; Fowler et al., 1980;

Kelso, 1986; Saltzman, 1986), appear to reflect more closely an organizational principle for speech production. While it is clear that coordinative structures, comprised of linguistically-significant gestures, are units of action, it does not necessarily follow that they reflect a distinct level of neural control for speech motor actions. Rather, based on considerations of intergestural resistance to perturbation (Munhall et al., 1994; Löfqvist & Gracco, 1991) and the functional requirements for sound production, it has been suggested that the lowest level of neural control for speech is something on the order of gestural constellations or vocal tract configurations that map onto the phones of the language (see Browman & Goldstein, 1986; 1992; this volume; Gracco, 1990; 1991; Gracco & Löfqvist, 1994). The neuromotor patterns for speech, then, are viewed as characteristic ways of manipulating the vocal tract and are coded according to overall vocal tract goals.

It is also of considerable importance to understand the goal level organization for speech in terms of vocal tract targets and associated control. The concept of spatial targets for speech was suggested by Lashley (1951) in discussing space coordinate systems for controlling serial movements such as those for speech. In spite of the intuitive appeal of speech motion being planned in a spatial reference frame, the notion of spatial targets for speech has received little attention. One reason for the limited attention, again, appears to be related to the presence of variability in the observable signal in which variable vocal tract shapes yield acceptable acoustic signals (cf. Ladefoged et al., 1972). Explanations for the variability range from noise in the system (Perkell, 1990) to systematic adjustments that assure goal acquisition (Gracco & Abbs, 1986; Perkell et al., 1995). These positions rest on a number of assumptions regarding the control of speech movements, the degree of control precision and the goals for speech. The spatial variability that characterizes speech motion can be interpreted as reflecting loosely specified goals in an abstract task space (Abbs et al., 1984; Saltzman, 1986). That is, the details of a task are only specified in a general sense with mechanisms available to assure accurate production. In the present conceptualization, the accuracy is achieved through the integration of somatic sensory afferents and stored central motor commands. An issue of some importance, then, is the amount of variation that can be tolerated in the output. A general perspective can be obtained from consideration of the structure and function of the human nervous system as an information processing device. As pointed out by von Nuemann (1958), the nervous system is an analog device that is ideally suited for reliable operation, not precision. In this context it can be suggested that articulatory performance is good enough without incurring excessive "costs" (Nelson, 1983) with the degree of precision inherently dependent on the listener's ability to extract meaning from the speech code. A recent, conceptually attractive perspective has been offered by Guenther (1994) in which spatial targets for speech are viewed as regions rather than points (convex hulls) in orosensory space. While the available data is limited it is difficult to imagine that speech is not planned to some extent in a spatial coordinate frame since inappropriately placed articulators will produce seriously compromised sounds. Moreover, there is a certain mapping that exists between constriction locations and degrees, and the notion of spatial targets. An example of the apparent looseness in the precision of articulatory control can be found in recent simulation and synthesis results reported by Gay, Böe and Perrier (1992). Parametric manipulation of vocal tract cross sectional area and constriction location was used to determine the acoustic and perceptual boundaries of certain isolated vowels. It was shown that the formants for each of the vowels were more sensitive to changes in cross sectional area than constriction location. Vowel perception, however, was insensitive to both manipulations. From these results it was concluded that the speech production mechanism has "...considerable latitude..." in specifying the articulatory targets.

The data presented in Figure 2 support notions of loosely specified spatial goals and a relatively tolerant control system. Shown are average front and rear tongue paths obtained electromagnetically for productions of the nonsense utterances "aka", "aska", "aksa," and "asa." The asterisks placed over the rear tongue path indicate the maximum tongue height associated with the production of the /k/ in each of the nonsense words. It can be seen that the spatial position of maximum tongue height varies considerably. While the variation is systematic it is clear that the spatial position of the tongue path for /k/ is not precisely specified. Rather, the distribution of tongue positions in the different contexts supports a level of spatial precision or positioning that is best described as stochastic. Other kinematic data reported by Perkell and colleagues (Perkell, 1990; Perkell & Nelson, 1982; Perkell & Cohen, 1989) are also consistent with a relaxed degree of articulatory control.

SENSORY-BASED MOVEMENT ADJUSTMENTS

The conceptualization of stored central commands that represent vocal tract configurations as units of speech motor action requires an adaptive mechanism or process that can adjust the commands to context.

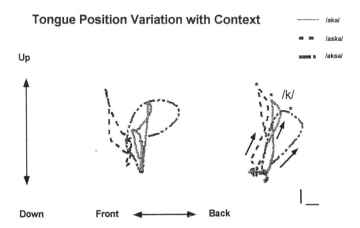

Figure 2. Changes in the point of constriction for the rear of the tongue for /k/ associated with different contexts. Arrows reflect the path of motion for the four contexts. Calibration bars represent 5 mm.

For example, generating a similar set of central commands for a /t/ before a high versus a low vowel will not produce the same desired result, namely, contact with the alveolar ridge. Therefore, some mechanism must be available to adjust the stored commands to changes in the peripheral state of the vocal tract. As argued elsewhere, (Abbs et al., 1984; Gracco, 1987; 1990; 1991; 1995; Saltzman & Munhall, 1989), real-time adaptations to central commands can be easily accomplished through the integration of sensory information. Human and nonhuman studies have shown that sensory receptors located throughout the vocal tract are sufficient to provide a range of dynamic and static information which can be used to signal position, speed, and location of physiological structures on a movement to movement basis (cf. Munger & Halata, 1983; Dubner et al., 1978 for reviews). Studies utilizing perturbation of speech motor output indicate that the rich supply of orofacial somatic sensory afferents interacting with central motor commands have the requisite properties to yield the flexible speech motor patterns involved in oral communication (Abbs & Gracco, 1984; Gracco & Abbs, 1985; Gracco & Abbs, 1988; Kelso et al., 1984).

A schematic of the general manner in which sensorimotor interactions may occur is presented in Figure 3. What is being depicted is a simplified representation of sensory and motor spaces within the nervous system. No attempt has been made to represent the specific anatomical locations of the sensory and motor spaces. Rather, the spaces are a lumped representation of brain stem, subcortical and cortical regions. Structurally, there is strong evidence for the interaction of sensory information from receptors located within the vocal tract with speech motor output at many if not all levels of the neuraxis (cf. Gracco, 1987; Gracco & Abbs, 1987; Barlow & Farley, 1989 for a summary of the vocal tract representation in multiple cortical and subcortical sensory and motor regions).

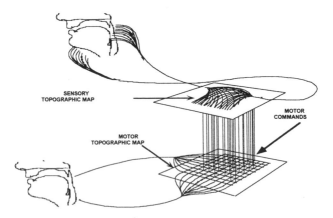

Figure 3. A scheme depicting one possible means of on-line modifications of stored central motor commands resulting from real-time changes in the vocal tract periphery. Topographic somatic sensory information continuously deforms the sensory state space which in turn modifies a topographic representation of the vocal tract in motor state space. The output of the motor space is directed to brain stem motor centers controlling the vocal tract. (Modified from Churchland, 1989).

Further, brain stem organization, evidenced by reflex studies, demonstrates a range of complex interactions in which sensory input from one structure such as the jaw or face is potentially able to modify motor output from other orofacial and lingual regions (Dubner et al., 1978; Smith et al., 1985; Weber & Smith, 1987). A summary of the specific receptor types within the vocal tract can be found in Dubner, Sessle and Storey (1978) and Kent, Martin and Suffit (1990).

It is suggested that as the peripheral conditions change during speaking, the sensorimotor connections continuously change the state of the various motor output regions subserving speech. As such, the same set of central commands for producing a /t/ will have different effects when impinging on a motor region that has been conditioned by a low jaw position compared to a high jaw position associated with the preceding vowel. The speech motor control system apparently adjusts for these movement-to-movement variations by incorporating somatic sensory information from the various muscle and mechanoreceptors located throughout the vocal tract. Sensorimotor connections allow the central commands to be sensitive to a constantly changing peripheral environment in a predictive manner (Gracco & Abbs, 1987; Gracco, 1987). Given the latencies previously reported (50-100 msec; Abbs & Gracco, 1984) and the time necessary for using predictive estimates (based on velocity and/or acceleration) of the dynamic peripheral conditions, it has been suggested that speech motor commands can be updated in real-time from somatic sensory receptor information (Gracco, 1987). That is, during even the most rapid speaking conditions, there is sufficient time available to make simple coordinate transformations between somatic sensory and motor states allowing for continuous modification of descending motor commands. Both empirical and theoretical considerations suggest that somatic sensory interaction is one plausible method to achieve flexibility from relatively stereotypic central motor commands (Gracco, 1987; Gracco, 1990).

A consequence of this conceptualization is that any novel event (the onset of a stuttering episode, for example) or any neurological sequela that change speech motor output parameters will change the sensorimotor environment, such that the same central motor commands will produce different (and possibly maladaptive) vocal tract motion. For example, the onset of a stuttering event, whether movement repetition, prolongation or hesitation, has somatic sensory consequences in which the afferent input onto motor regions will change the overall level of excitability. As a result, the same set of central commands presented to areas associated with speech motor output will result in deviant output until the speech production process is reset in some manner. The fact that it is not easy for an individual who stutters to reset the production process probably reflects the difficulty of on-line modification of sequential central commands for speech and the automatic nature of the speech production process. For neurological disorders such as Parkinson's disease, cerebellar disease, or motor aphasia, there are a myriad of changes that result from the neurological damage that would result from changes in the central commands themselves. Some potential consequences associated with certain movement disorders will be discussed later.

SEQUENCING OF SPEECH MOTOR ACTIONS

Speech is more than the specification of characteristic motor patterns coded to produce vocal tract configurations adjusted for context. An important consideration in speech production is the sequencing of vocal tract actions into communicatively meaningful units of production. An important theoretical issue is determining how the nervous system integrates speech production units into coherent packages for information transfer. As pointed out by Lashley (1951), serial actions such as those for speech, locomotion, typing and the playing of musical instruments cannot be explained in terms of successions of external reflexes. Rather the apparent rhythmicity found in all but the simplest motor activities suggests that some sort of temporal patterning may form the foundation for motor as well as perceptual activities. A number of observations are consistent with the presence of some kind of rhythm generating mechanism as the basis for sequential speech motor adjustments. For example, compensatory adjustments for lower lip perturbations during an oral closing movement demonstrate changes in interarticulator timing consistent with the operation of an underlying oscillatory or rhythm generating mechanism (Gracco & Abbs, 1988; 1989; Saltzman et al., 1991; Saltzman et al., 1995; Saltzman et al., 1992). Other results such as minimal movement durational changes from static (Lindblom et al., 1987) and dynamic perturbation (Gracco & Abbs, 1988) and durational consistencies across experimental sessions (Kozhevnikov & Chistovich, 1965) are consistent with an underlying mechanism in which sequential timing is maintained. However, a strictly isochronous mechanism is not plausible given the different durational requirements for consonants and vowels. Classes of sounds appear to have certain intrinsic temporal properties (or constraints) which must interact with any proposed suprasegmental timing mechanism. Vowels can be categorized as long or short, generally related to their average relative duration, and consequently to different speed and extent of jaw opening actions. High pressure consonants often show faster movements than their voiced low pressure counterparts. It has been suggested that a central rhythm generator provides the timing framework for the sequencing of production units and the general intrinsic requirements of the units in turn modulate the instantaneous frequency of the oscillator such that speech movement timing can be represented as an interaction between extrinsic and intrinsic mechanisms (Gracco, 1990; 1991; 1994).

An important consequence of incorporating a central rhythm generator into a speech production model is the ability to explain rate, stress, and final lengthening changes with manipulation of a single mechanism: global (over the course of an utterance) and local (phone and syllable level) changes in rhythmic frequency. Moreover, the rhythmic nature of the output is potentially available to facilitate speech perception by making signal stream segmentation more predictable (Cutler & Mehler, 1993; Lashley, 1951; Martin, 1972). The rhythmic modulation of speech production would provide the perceptual system with a predictable framework for sampling and parsing the output. The breakdown in the rhythmic structure of speech associated with a number of different speech motor disorders (Kent & Rosenbek, 1982) and the pervasive rhythmicity found throughout the nervous system (Llinas,

1986; Llinas, 1991) strongly suggests that the underlying rhythm is a network property rather than a property of a specific neuroanatomical location.

NEURAL SUBSTRATE

It has been known for over 100 years that multiple regions of the brain are involved in some manner in producing speech and language. The neural substrate for speech has been identified from a variety of sources including human mapping studies using electrical stimulation (Penfield & Roberts, 1959; Ojemann, 1983; Mateer, 1983), positron emission tomography (Petersen et al., 1989; Wise et al., 1991; Petersen & Fiez, 1993), functional magnetic resonance imaging (McCarthy et al., 1993; Shaywitz et al., 1995; Pugh et al., in press) and neuroanatomical studies of nonhuman primates (Muakassa & Strick, 1979; Woolsey et al., 1952). A number of cortical and subcortical regions have been identified in which a representation of the vocal tract can be found (see Barlow & Farley, 1989; Gracco & Abbs, 1987; Kimura, 1993 for reviews). Cortical regions with vocal tract representations include the primary motor and sensory areas (MI and SI, respectively), the so-called nonprimary motor areas including supplementary motor area (SMA) and premotor area (PM; lateral precentral cortex), and a posterior parietal region. The general PM area and posterior parietal regions (including portions of the temporal region in man) comprise the areas associated with Broca's and Wernicke's areas respectively (Penfield & Roberts, 1959; Kimura, 1993). Extensive subcortical representations can also be found in the cerebellar cortex, deep cerebellar nuclei and regions of the basal ganglia.

An interesting aspect of these representations is their extrinsic (and generally reciprocal) interconnections. For example, the different cortical areas are connected to different subcortical structures and contain projections from or project to distinct and (relatively) non-overlapping regions of the thalamus. The PM area receives input from the deep cerebellar nuclei via the thalamus and projects to the primary motor area (MI) as well as contributing direct descending projections to brain stem nuclei. Similar segregated extrinsic connections are found for regions of the basal ganglia and SMA. In addition, SI projects to posterior parietal regions which in turn project to the motor, premotor and temporal regions with descending projections to brain stem nuclei. A summary of neuroanatomical data reported by Schell and Strick (1984) suggests that large regions of the cortex and subcortex are interconnected and maintain relatively segregated modules that ultimately converge at the output. These diverse neural areas, which represent large regions of the nervous system, display an extrinsic organization consistent with the concept of neural modules hypothesized by Mountcastle, suggesting distributed processing functions (Mountcastle, 1978). It should be noted that these large scale networks all have access to peripheral sensory information from somatic receptors as well as the visual and auditory receptors and therefore display "reentrant" characteristics, with changes in one system allowing changes or readjustment in all convergent systems (Edelman, 1987). While this overview leaves out much detail it can be seen that the neuroanatomy underlying speech and language is quite complex and highly specialized to receive, integrate and act on the external and internal environment of the organism.

An additional source of insight into the nervous system organization for speech and language comes from neurological disorders. From a synthesis of various observations some general conclusions can be drawn. A surprising characteristic of almost all lesions involving the central nervous system is the accompaniment of motor impairments with cognitive or linguistic impairments and the converse. It appears, as suggested by Jackson (1875), that the so-called higher centers of the nervous system may be extensions of the lower nervous centers which represent impressions and movements. Consistent with the neuroanatomical substrate outlined above, damage to the cerebellum and/or PM area often results in impairments similar at least in acoustic and perceptual respects (Kent & Rosenbek, 1982). Damage to either of these regions often produces a breakdown in speech that can be characterized as a disruption of the smooth timing of sequential speech movements. Cerebellar patients often show a decomposition of movement, as though the various parts of a complex movement had to be thought out one by one (Holmes, 1922). Dysmetria is also a characteristic of cerebellar damage suggesting that the ability to integrate sensory information to produce appropriately calibrated actions has been affected. These symptoms are generally consistent with those associated with Broca's aphasia (due to anterior premotor lesions). For example, electrical stimulation of the PM area, which receives output from the deep cerebellar nuclei via the thalamus, causes speech arrest (Penfield & Roberts, 1959) and an inability to sequence multiple speech movements (Mateer, 1983). The contribution of the cerebellum to the control of movement is undergoing some modification. While the cerebellum is often considered a motor center, there are multiple sources of relatively new data to suggest that it is also involved in a variety of other behaviors that require more than just motor activities (see Gao et al., 1996 for review). However, it should be remembered that all behaviors are sensorimotor in nature. As such, the cerebellum and the projections to Broca's areas may be appropriately regarded as sensorimotor integration areas in which central commands are modified before the final output. As a module that integrates sensory information on a task-specific basis, the role of the cerebellum and Broca's area appears to be to assist in matching task-specific motor commands to the periphery and the task requirements. The task requirements for communication reflect the phonetic context of the linguistic structure. Because these systems operate together, damage to either produces similar effects that would consist of problems with sequencing successive vocal tract states and adjusting central commands to changes in the peripheral environment.

A similar situation exists for impairments associated with basal ganglia and SMA damage. It is well known that prior to movement SMA activity displays characteristics consistent with movement preparation (Tanji et al., 1980; Deecke & Kornhuber, 1978) while the basal ganglia reflect activity that is consistent with a scaling of motor commands (Horak & Anderson, 1984a, b). Basal ganglia damage, characterized by Parkinson's disease, often results in speech characterized by imprecise consonant production, mono-pitch and loudness, and articulator movements that are reduced in amplitude and speed. SMA damage, on the other hand, results in speech impairments that are similar to and more extreme than those associated with basal ganglia damage, ranging from total speech arrest to imprecise articulation and a reduction in spontaneously generated speech (Laplane et al., 1977; Masdeu et al., 1978; Damasio & Van Hoesen, 1980). In the case of damage to either of these regions, the resulting movement deficits are consistent with a reduced level of activation that accompanies the preparation and modulation of central commands. A reduction in motor preparation and/or a reduction in scaling of motor commands would produce many of the symptoms normally associated with damage to one or the other of these related systems. For example, a lack of modulation of central commands over the course of an utterance would result in a reduction in the ability to produce the movement changes characteristic of emphatic stress (Forrest et al., 1989) and a lack of intonational changes over the course of an utterance. Moreover, a reduction in the scaling of central commands would result in rather consistent articulatory undershoot and consequent bradykinesia. From the present conceptualization, stored central commands that specify characteristic vocal tract configurations are modulated for context by somatic sensory input and scaled based on suprasegmental requirements such as those necessary to produce intonation, loudness, stress and rate manipulations. It is suggested that these neural changes operate through the basal ganglia/SMA system.

A final issue with regard to the neuromotor control of speech is the interpretation of speech movement deficits due to damage to cortical systems traditionally associated with language. The traditional cortical areas often considered to represent linguistic processes and act as the interface between language and speech are Broca's and Wernicke's areas. It has been suggested above that Broca's area, in conjunction with the deep cerebellar nuclei, is involved in the sensorimotor adjustment and timing of segmental phonetic units. Consistent with this position are aphasic data and the theoretical position outlined by Kimura (1993). Kimura (1993) suggests that aphasic patients with anterior lesions have reduced syllable-level fluency (i.e., difficulty with sequencing vocal tract configurations). In contrast, aphasic patients with posterior lesions have difficulty with sequencing syllables into larger multisyllables. Moreover, patients with damage to the posterior speech areas also display output impairments that appear to reflect inappropriate phonological selection compared to the more phonetic errors exhibited by anterior aphasics (Blumstein, 1981). Thus, there are apparently some general functions associated with the hypothetical distributed processing modules known to represent and support motor speech production.

SUMMARY

A conceptual model of speech production has been outlined that provides a framework for investigating the neuromotor characteristics of fluent speech. As noted above, speaking is a communicative act in which the output represents a synthesis of potentially independent but mutually overlapping processes. The processes overlap in time and each stage of the output reflects, to some extent, the influence of any or all contributing levels. Whether one views the communicative process as serial or parallel (or some combination), articulation represents the synthesis of cognitive, linguistic and sensorimotor processes (Levelt, 1989; Bock & Levelt, 1994; Jescheniak & Levelt, 1994). In order to understand and predict this complex process the basic components and the manner in which they interact must be made explicit. In the preceding, an attempt has been made to identify the basic components and properties of a speech production model and the manner in which they might interact to instantiate the communication process.

Summarized in Figure 4 is a schematic representation of the fundamental processes and their interactions hypothesized to underlie the production of fluent speech. A primary component of the speech production process is the preparation of the sensorimotor system for activation. That is, excitability levels associated with sensory and motor regions are increased in a general sense and specific regions involved with communication are tuned for the upcoming motor commands. The overall levels of excitability are dependent on certain pragmatic requirements (emotional content, speaking rate, noisy environment, etc.) that will determine in a general sense the overall level of effort. The stored configurations, which include neural commands that specify the coordination among their gestural components, converge on and interact with the preparatory activations on output areas. The central commands that give rise to specific and neuroanatomically focused motor patterns result in a movement-to-movement tuning of the motor output structures in characteristic ways consistent with the articulatory organization for unique vocal tract configurations. The motor state space is also conditioned by ongoing topographic projections from somatic sensory vocal tract representations which have been made active by the preparatory process.

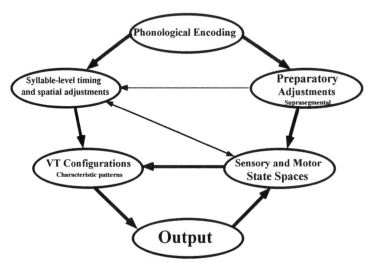

Figure 4. A schematic model of hypothetical speech motor processes. The thickness of the lines reflects the strength of the connections; double headed arrows represent interactive connections. See text for details.

The speech motor system receives input in the form of a phonological code specifying, among other things, the sequence of characteristic neuromotor patterns associated with vocal tract configurations unique for each phone of the language.

At the level of the phonological encoding process the unit of organization is larger than individual phonetic gestures. A level of organization, on the order of a syllable, which may contain one or more phonetic gestures, is hypothesized. This syllable level temporal organization forms the rhythmic basis for all higher level (suprasegmental) temporal phenomena. It is further hypothesized that the rhythmic organization reflects a system property rather than a manifestation of a single rhythmic or oscillatory source. The phonetic composition of each syllable adjusts the instantaneous frequency of the output but does not reset the rhythm. The frequency characteristics of the oscillator can be easily modified by simple tonic inputs as part of the preparatory process that can increase or decrease speaking rate.

In keeping with one of the constraints discussed at the outset, these processes appear to be consistent with known (or inferred) nervous system functions. The motor preparation process involves the SMA/basal ganglia network in which cortical and subcortical sensory and motor areas are activated in preparation for action and tuning the sensorimotor centers in ways that reflect a time scale involving utterance-level and possibly suprasegmental adjustments. It should be noted that while this process may be thought of as motor, it is dependent on the communicative requirements of the situation and involves setting up sensory as well as motor consequences. Hence, all functional speech processes are both sensorimotor and communicative and reflect a synthesis of all available levels of organization. The phonological encoding process involves structures that impart meaning, perhaps lexical items, that are parsed into multisyllabic phonetic codes that are executed on a syllable by syllable basis. In concert with Broca's area, the cerebellar nuclei adjust the spatiotemporal characteristics of the motor commands for sequencing within a syllable and adjust the overall rhythmicity of the system based on phonetic context. The cerebellum has extensive connections onto almost all regions of the nervous system to allow it to play an executive role in sensorimotor integration and motor command adjustment (Arshavsky et al., 1985). Moreover, in contrast to the general setting of sensorimotor excitability levels associated with the SMA/basal ganglia system, the cerebellar/PM system appears to be involved in more specific changes associated with contextual adjustments of motor commands. Hence, it can be suggested that damage to this system will result in a breakdown in the sequencing of successive phonetic gestures, articulatory undershooting as well as overshooting and increased levels of noise or movement variability while damage to the SMA/basal ganglia system will predominantly result in undershooting, decreased speaking rate, a lack of task-specific modulation and a decrease in variability.

The model rests on a number of assumptions about nervous system function and associated organizational principles that, while specific to speech production, may generalize to many other behaviors. First, the level of control for speech is minimally at a level that reflects the smallest functional unit of speech, linguistically-significant vocal tract configurations. These units are ultimately organized into larger units that ultimately represent the communicative function of the task. This conceptualization suggests that speech production is a nested process with function as the organizing principle at each level. Speech movements are contextually variable suggesting that vocal tract configurations for the phonetic segments are only loosely specified reflecting the redundancy of cues available to extract meaning. A fundamental principle that emerges is that the organization for speech and language operates at multiple levels in parallel with communication a synthetic and stochastic process. As a result no one movement component or signal attribute or neural structure is solely responsible for information transfer; the neural control of speech relies on flexible processes and reliable performance rather than invariant principles and rigid tolerances. Finally, a theoretical perspective that focuses on explanations at the level of the anatomy, physiology and fundamental nervous system processes, makes it possible to generate a parsimonious and neurobiologically-plausible model of speech production, in which simple functions interact to produce complex patterns.

ACKNOWLEDGMENTS

Supported by research grant numbers RO1 DC 00595 and P50 DC 00121 from the National Institute on Deafness and Other Communication Disorders, National Institutes of Health.

REFERENCES

Abbs, J.H., & Gracco, V.L. (1984). Control of complex motor gestures: Orofacial muscle responses to load perturbations of the lip during speech. *Journal of Neurophysiology, 51(4)*, 705-723.

Abbs, J.H., Gracco, V.L., & Cole, K.J. (1984). Control of multimovement coordination: Sensorimotor mechanisms in speech motor programming. *Journal of Motor Behavior, 16*, 195-232.

Barlow, S.M., & Farley, G.R. (1989). Neurophysiology of speech. In D.P. Kuehn, M.L. Lemme, & J. Baumgartner (Eds.), *Neural bases of speech, hearing, and language* (pp. 146-200). Boston: College-Hill Press.

Bernstein, N. (1967). The co-ordination and regulation of movements. New York: Pergamon Press.

Blumstein, S.E. (1981). Neurolinguistic disorders: Language-brain relationships. In S.B. Filskov, & T. J. Boll (Eds.), *Handbook of Clinical Neuropsychology*. New York: Wiley.

Browman, C.P., & Goldstein, L. (1986). Towards an articulatory phonology. *Phonology Yearbook, 3*, 219-252.

Browman, C.P., & Goldstein, L. (1992). Articulatory phonology: An overview. *Phonetica, 49(3-4)*, 155-180.

Churchland, P.S. (1986). *Neurophilosophy: Toward a unified science of the mind-brain*. Cambridge: MIT Press.

Churchland, P.M. (1989). *A neurocomputational perspective: The nature of mind and the structure of science*. Cambridge: MIT Press.

Cutler, A., & Mehler, J. (1993). The periodicity bias. *Journal of Phonetics, 21*, 103-108.

Damasio, A.R., & Van Hoesen, G.W. (1980). Structure and function of the supplementary motor area. *Neurology, 30*, 359.

Deecke, L., & Kornhuber, H.H. (1978). An electrical sign of participation of the mesial 'supplementary' motor cortex in human voluntary finger movement. *Brain Research, 159*, 473-476.

Dubner, R., Sessle, B.J., & Storey, A.T. (1978). *The neural basis of oral and facial function.* New York: Plenum Press.

Easton, T.A. (1972). On the normal use of reflexes. *American Scientist, 60*, 591-599.

Edelman, G.M. (1987). *Neural Darwinism.* New York: Basic Books, Inc.

Forrest, K., Weismer, G., & Turner, G.S. (1989). Kinematic, acoustic, and perceptual analyses of connected speech produced by Parkinsonian and normal geriatric adults. *Journal of the Acoustical Society of America, 85*, 2608-2622.

Fowler, C.A., Rubin, P., Remez, R.E. & Turvey, M.T. (1980). Implications for speech production of a general theory of action. In B. Butterworth, (Ed.), *Language production* (pp. 373-420). New York: Academic Press.

Gao, J.-H., Parsons, L., Bower, J., Xiong, J., Li, J., & Fox, P. (1996). Cerebellum implicated in sensory acquisition and discrimination rather than motor control. *Science, 272*, 545-547.

Gay, T., Böe, L.-J., & Perrier, P. (1992). Acoustic and perceptual effects of changes in vocal tract constrictions for vowels. *Journal of the Acoustical Society of America, 92*, 1301-1309.

Garrett, M. (1991). Disorders of lexical selection. In W.J.M. Levelt (Ed.). *Lexical access in speech production* (pp. 143-180). Cambridge, MA: Blackwell.

Gracco, V.L. (1987). A multilevel control model for speech motor activity. In H. Peters, & W. Hulstijn (Eds.), *Speech motor dynamics in stuttering* (pp. 57-76). Berlin: Springer-Verlag.

Gracco, V.L. (1988). Timing factors in the coordination of speech movements. *Journal of Neuroscience, 8*, 4628-4634.

Gracco, V.L. (1990). Characteristics of speech as a motor control system. In G. Hammond (Ed.), *Cerebral control of speech and limb movements* (pp. 3-28). North Holland: Elsevier.

Gracco, V.L. (1991). Sensorimotor mechanisms in speech motor control. In H. Peters, W. Hultsijn, & C.W. Starkweather (Eds.), *Speech motor control and stuttering* (pp. 53-78). North Holland: Elsevier.

Gracco, V.L. (1994). Some organizational characteristics of speech movement control. *Journal of Speech and Hearing Research, 37*, 4-27.

Gracco, V.L. (1995). Central and peripheral components in the control of speech movements. In Bell-Berti, F., & Raphael, L. (Eds.), *Producing speech: Contemporary issues for Katherine Safford Harris* (pp. 417-432). Woodbury: AIP Press.

Gracco, V.L., & Abbs, J.H. (1985). Dynamic control of perioral system during speech: Kinematic analyses of autogenic and nonautogenic sensorimotor processes. *Journal of Neuroscience, 54*, 418-432.

Gracco, V.L., & Abbs, J.H. (1986). Variant and invariant characteristics of speech movements. *Experimental Brain Research, 65*, 156-166.

Gracco, V.L., & Abbs, J.H. (1987). Programming and execution processes of speech movement control: Potential neural correlates. In E. Keller & M. Gopnik (Eds.), *Symposium on motor and sensory language processes* (pp. 163-201). New Jersey: Lawrence Erlbaum Associates, Inc.

Gracco, V.L., & Abbs, J.H. (1988). Central patterning of speech movements. *Experimental Brain Research, 71*, 515-526.

Gracco, V.L., & Abbs, J.H. (1989). Sensorimotor characteristics of speech motor sequences. *Experimental Brain Research, 75*, 586-598.

Gracco, V.L., & Löfqvist, A. (1994). Speech motor coordination and control: Evidence from lip, jaw, and laryngeal movements. *Journal of Neuroscience, 14*, 6585-6597.

Guenther, F.H. (1994). A neural network model of speech acquisition and motor equivalent speech production. *Biological Cybernetics, 73*, 43-53.

Ho, T.P., Azar, K., Weinstein, S., & Bowley, W.W. (1982). Physical properties of human lips: Experimental and theoretical analysis. *Journal of Biomechanics ,15*, 859-866.

Holmes, G. (1922). Clinical symptoms of cerebellar disease and their interpretation. The Croonian lectures I. *Lancet, 1*, 1177-1182.

Horak, F.B., & Anderson, M.E. (1984a). Influence of globus pallidus on arm movements in monkeys. I. Effects of kainic acid-induced lesions. *Journal of Neurophysiology, 52*, 290-304.

Horak, F.B., & Anderson, M.E. (1984b).Influence of globus pallidus on arm movements in monkeys. II. Effects of stimulation. *Journal of Neurophysiology, 52*, 305-322.

Jackson, J.H. (1875). *Clinical and physiological researches on the nervous system.* London: Churchill.

Kelso, J.A.S. (1986). Pattern formation in speech and limb movements involving many degrees of freedom. In H. Heuer, & C. Fromm (Eds.), *Generation and modulation of action patterns* (pp. 105-128). Berlin: Springer-Verlag.

Kelso, J.A.S., Tuller, B., V.-Bateson, E., & Fowler, C.A. (1984). Functionally specific articulatory cooperation following jaw perturbations during speech: Evidence for coordinative structures. *Journal of Experimental Psychology: Human Perception and Performance, 10*, 812-832.

Kent, R.D., & Rosenbek, J.C. (1982). Prosodic disturbance and neurologic lesion. *Brain and Language, 15*, 259-291.

Kent, R.D., Martin, R.E., & Sufit, R.L. (1990). Oral sensation: A review and clinical propsective. In H. Winitz (Ed.), *Human communication and its disorders* (pp. 135-191). Norwood, NJ: Ablex Publishing.

Kimura, D. (1993). *Neuromotor mechanisms in human communication.* New York: Oxford University Press.

Kozhevnikov, V., & Chistovich, L. (1965). *Speech: Articulation and perception.* Joint Publications Research Service, 30,453; U.S. Department of Commerce.

Laboissière, R. Ostry, D., & Feldman, A. (1996). Control of multi-movement systems: Human jaw and hyoid movements. *Biological Cybernetics, 74,* 373-384

Ladefoged, P., DeClerk, J., Lindau, M., & Papcun, G. (1972). An auditory-motor theory of speech production. *UCLA Working Papers in Phonetics, 22*, 48-75.

Laplane, D., Talairach, J., Meininger, V., Bancaud, J., & Orgogozo, J.M., (1977). Clincial consequences of corticectomies involving the supplementary motor area in man. *Journal of the Neurological Sciences, 34*, 301-314.

Lashley, K.S. (1951). The problem of serial order in behavior. In L.A. Jeffress (Ed.), *Cerebral mechanisms in behavior: The Hixon symposium.* New York: Wiley.

Levelt, W.J.M. (1989). *Speaking: from intention to articulation.* Cambridge, MA: MIT Press.

Levelt, W.J.M. (1992). Accessing words in speech production: Stages, processes and representations. *Cognition, 42*, 1-22.

Lindblom, B., Lubker, J., Gay, T., Lyberg, P., Branderal, P., & Holgren, K. (1987). The concept of target and speech timing. In R. Channon, & L. Shockery (Eds.), *In honor of Ilse Lehiste* (pp. 161-181). Dordrecht, The Netherlands: Foris Publications.

Llinas, R.R. (1986). Neuronal oscillators in mammalian brain. In M. J. Cohen & F. Strumwasser (Eds.), *Comparative neurobiology: Modes of communication in the nervous system.* (pp. 279-290). New York: Wiley.

Llinas, R.R. (1991). The noncontinuous nature of movement execution. In D.R. Humphrey, & H.-J.

Freund, (Eds.), *Motor control: Concepts and issues.* (pp. 223-242). New York: Wiley.

Löfqvist, A., & Gracco, V.L. (1991). Discrete and continuous modes in speech motor control. *PERILUS, XIV*, 27-34.

Lynn, A.M.J., & Yemm, R. (1971). External forces required to move the mandible of relaxed human subjects. *Archives of Oral Biology, 16*, 1443-1447.

Martin, J.G. (1972). Rhythmic (hierarchical) versus serial structure in speech and other behavior. *Psychological Review, 79*, 487-509.

Masdeu, J.C., Schoene, W.C., & Funkenstein, H. (1978). Aphasia following infarction of the left supplementary motor area: A clinicopathologic study. *Neurology, 28*, 1220-1223.

Mateer, C.A. (1983). Motor and perceptual functions of the left hemisphere and their interactions. In S. J. Segalowitz (Ed.), *Language functions and brain organization* (pp. 145-170). New York: Academic Press.

McCarthy, G., Blamire, A.M., Rothman, D.L., Gruetter, R., Shulman, R.G. (1993). Echo-planar magnetic resonance imaging studies of frontal cortex activation during word generation in humans. *Proceedings of the National Academy of Sciences, 89*, 5675-5679.

Mountcastle, V.B. (1978). An organizing principle for cerebral function: The unit module and the distributed system. In G.M. Edelman, & V.B. Mountcastle, (Eds.), *The mindful brain: Cortical organization and the group-selective theory of higher brain function* (pp. 7-50). Cambridge: MIT Press.

Muakassa, K.F., & Strick, P.L. (1979). Frontal lobe inputs to primate motor cortex: evidence for four somatotopically organized "premotor" areas. *Brain Research, 177*, 176-182.

Munhall, K., Löfqvist, A., & Kelso, J.A.S. (1994). Lip-larynx coordination in speech: effects of mechanical perturbations to the lower lip. *Journal of the Acoustical Society of America, 96*, 3605-3616.

Nelson, W.L. (1983). Physical principles for economies of skilled movements. *Biological Cybernetics, 46*, 135-147.

Ojemann, G.A. (1983). Brain organization for language from the perspective of electrical stimulation mapping. *The Behavioral and Brain Sciences, 6*, 189-230.

Ostry, D.J., Gribble, P.L., & Gracco, V.L. (1996). Coarticulation of jaw movements in speech production: Is context sensitivity in speech kinematics centrally planned? *Journal of Neuroscience, 16*, 1570-1579.

Penfield, W., & Roberts, L. (1959). *Speech and brain mechanisms.* Princeton, N. J.: Princeton Univ. Press.

Perkell, J.S. (1990). Testing theories of speech production: Implications of some detailed analyses of variable articulatory data. In W. Hardcastle, & A. Marchal, (Eds.) *Speech production and speech modeling,* (pp. 263-288). Dordrecht: Kluwer.

Perkell, J.S. & Nelson, W.L. (1982). Articulatory targets and speech motor control: A study of vowel production. In S. Grillner, A. Persson, B. Lindblom, & J. Lubker, (Eds.), *Speech motor control* (pp. 187-204). Oxford: Pergamon.

Perkell, J.S. & Cohen, M.H. (1989). An indirect test of the quantal nature of speech in the production of the vowels /i/, /a/ and /u/. *Journal of Phonetics, 17*, 123-133.

Perkell, J.S., Matthies, M.L., Svirsky, M.A., & Jordan, M.I. (1995). Goal-based speech motor control: A theoretical framework and some preliminary data. *Journal of Phonetics, 23*, 23-35.

Petersen, S.E., & Fiez, J.A. (1993). The processing of single words studied with positron emission tomography. *Annual Review of Neuroscience, 1*, 509-530.

Petersen, S.E., Fox, P.T., Posner, M.I., Mintun, M., & Raichle, M.E. (1989). Positron emission tomographic studies of the processing of single words. *Journal of Cognitive Nueroscience, 1*, 153-170.

Pugh, K., Shaywitz, B.A., Shaywitz, S.E., Fulbright, R.K., Byrd, D., Skudlarski, P., Shankweiler, D.P., Katz, L., Constable, R.T., Fletcher, J., Lacadie, C., Marchione, K., & Gore, J.C. (in press) Auditory selective attention: An fMRI investigation. *NeuroImage*.

Saltzman, E.L. (1986). Task dynamic coordination of the speech articulators: A preliminary model. In, H. Heuer, & C. Fromm, (Eds.), *Generation and modulation of action patterns* (pp. 129-144). Berlin: Springer-Verlag.

Saltzman, E.L., & Munhall, K.G. (1989). A dynamical approach to gestural patterning in speech production. *Ecological Psychology, 1*, 333-382.

Saltzman, E., Kay, B., Rubin, P., & Kinsella-Shaw, J. (1991). Dynamics of intergestural timing. *Perilus XIV*, 47-56, Institute of Linguistics, University of Stockholm, Stockholm, Sweden.

Saltzman, E., Löfqvist, A., Kinsella-Shaw, J., Kay, B., & Rubin, P. (1995). On the dynamics of temporal patterning in speech. In F. Bell-Berti, & L. Raphael, (Eds.), *Producing speech: Contemporary issues for Katherine Safford Harris.* (pp. 469-488). Woodbury, NY: American Institute of Physics.

Saltzman, E., Löfqvist, A., Kinsella-Shaw, J., Rubin, P.E., & Kay, B. (1992). A perturbation study of lip-larynx coordination. In *Proceedings of the 1992 International Conference on Spoken Language Processing (ICSLP '92): Addendum, Banff, Alberta, Canada* Edmonton, Canada: Priority Printing.

Schell, G.R., & Strick, P.L. (1984). The origin of thalamic inputs to the arcuate premotor and supplementary motor areas. *Journal of Neuroscience, 4*, 539-560.

Shaywitz, B., Pugh, K., Constable, T., Shaywitz, S., Bronen, R., Fullbright, R., Shankweiler, D., Katz, L., Fletcher, J., Skudlarski, P., & Gore, J. (1995). Localization of semantic processing using functional magnetic resonance imaging. *Human Brain Mapping, 2*, 149-158.

Smith, A., Moore, C.A., Weber, C.M., McFarland, D.H., & Moon, J.B. (1985). Reflex responses of the human jaw-closing system depend on the locus of intraoral mechanical stimulation. *Experimental Neurology, 90*, 489-509.

Stevens, K.N. (1972). On the quantal nature of speech: Evidence from articulatory-acoustic data. In E. E. David, & P.B. Denes, (Eds.), *Human communication: A unified view* (pp. 51-66). New York: McGraw-Hill.

Stevens, K.N. (1989). On the quantal nature of speech. *Journal of Phonetics, 17*, 3-45.

Tanji, J., Taniguchi, K., & Saga, T. (1980). Supplementary motor area: Neuronal response to motor instructions. *Journal of Neurophysiology, 43*, 60-68.

Turvey, M.T. (1977). Preliminaries to a theory of action with reference to vision. In R. Shaw, & J. Bransford, (Eds.), *Perceiving, acting and knowing: Towards an ecological psychology*. Hillsdale: Lawrence Erlbaum.

Von Nuemann, J. (1958). *The computer and the brain*. New Haven: Yale University Press.

Weber, C. M., & Smith, A. (1987). Reflex responses of jaw, lip, and tongue muscles to mechanical stimulation. *Journal of Speech and Hearing Research, 30*, 70-79.

Wise, R., Chollet, F., Hadar, U., Friston, K., Hoffner, E., Frackowiak, R. (1991). Distribution of cortical neural networks involved in word comprehension and word retrieval. *Brain, 11*, 1803-1817.

Woolsey, C.N., Settlage, P.H., Meyer, D.R., Spencer, W., Pinto Hamuy, T., & Travis, A.M. (1952). Patterns of localization in precentral and "supplementary" motor areas and their relation to the concept of a premotor area. *Association for Research in Nervous and Mental Disease, 30*, 238-264.

Speech Production: Motor Control, Brain Research and Fluency Disorders
W. Hulstijn, H.F.M. Peters and P.H.H.M. Van Lieshout, editors

Chapter 4

THE GESTURAL PHONOLOGY MODEL

Catherine P. Browman, Louis Goldstein

In the approach to phonology described in this paper, speech is decomposed into units of action and information called gestures. These units provide the basis for a more principled relation between the macroscopic (phonological contrast) and the microscopic (time-varying physical parameters) descriptions of speech than is typically assumed in other approaches. The approach is exemplified, and some results of applying it to the characterization of syllable structure are presented. These results show that hitherto unrelated observations about allophonic variation due to syllable position can follow from general principles when syllable structure is modeled as patterns of gestural configuration.

This paper presents an overview of the model of *gestural* (or *articulatory*) *phonology*, that we have been developing the last several years (e.g, Browman & Goldstein, 1986; 1989; 1992a,b; 1995a). It begins with an introduction that argues for the theoretical desirability of a model that integrates the phonological and physical descriptions of speech, as the gestural model attempts to do. It then presents a tutorial, demonstrating how gestural units can function as phonological primitives, followed by some results that show how characteristic configurations of gestures can instantiate what is usually described as syllable structure. Finally, some conclusions are drawn.

INTRODUCTION

The motivation for developing a gestural phonology comes from a consideration of some problems with the view of speech implicit in traditional linguistic theory and practice. This view (see extended discussion in Browman & Goldstein, 1995a) holds that speech really has two structures: a phonological structure and a physical one. In this view, in its phonological structure, speech is described as a sequence of symbols from a small inventory that can recombine to produce different words. The fact that languages can have large lexicons (with hundreds of thousands of words), and yet require only a very small number of symbols (typically fewer than one hundred), is a testament to the combinatorial possibilities of these units (and is the basis for Hockett's (1955) principle of *duality of patterning*). In its physical structure, speech is described as exhibiting continuous (temporal) variation in a large number of articulatory, aerodynamic, acoustic, and auditory parameters.

Traditionally, the relation between these structures had been held to be complex and uninteresting. The clearest statement of this is probably Hockett's (1955) famous Easter egg analogy. He suggested that the phonological structure of an utterance can be thought of as a row of brightly colored (but unboiled) Easter eggs and that the effect of the activities of speech production can be likened to putting these eggs though a wringer. The result is bits of broken shell, yoke, and albumin, which bears little resemblance to the phonological structure. The listener is then viewed as a kind of forensic specialist who can use the crushed remains to make inferences about the original row of Easter eggs.

There are, in fact, a number of problems with this view. One serious problem is that, if this view were correct, it would be difficult to make measurements of phonological units, as these can be related to observables in only very complex ways. This is particularly problematical for developing concise descriptions of "non-standard" speech (non-fluent, etc.), in terms of units and their coordination: since the units themselves could not (in principle) be observed, we could only make numerous measurements of the physical variables, and hope they are related to the underlying units in a systematic way.

This view also ignores the potentially lawful relation between the phonological and the physical. Specifically, it is possible to view the two structures as low-dimensional (macroscopic) and high-dimensional (microscopic) descriptions of a single complex ("self-organized") system. A hallmark of such systems, which have only recently come under systematic study (e.g., Kugler & Turvey, 1987; Schöner & Kelso, 1988; Kauffman, 1995), is that they exhibit reciprocal constraint between dimensionalities of description. If such reciprocal constraint occurs in the case of speech, this would support the view that speech can be profitably viewed as a single complex system. Browman and Goldstein (1990a) argue that such reciprocal constraint can, in fact, be observed in speech. As is well known, the facts of anatomy, aerodynamics, and acoustics place constraints on the kinds of phonological systems that languages employ (e.g., Lindblom, 1983; Ohala, 1983; Stevens, 1989). These are constraints running from the microscopic to the macroscopic. In addition, there are also constraints running in the opposite direction, from the macroscopic to the microscopic. Examples of this can be found in differences between languages in the detailed physical properties of phonological units, where it is possible to relate those differences to differences in the nature or number of phonological contrasts in the languages' inventories (e.g., Ladefoged, 1982; Manuel & Krakow, 1984; Jongman et al., 1985).

There have been alternatives to the traditional view of strict separation. The framework of *The Sound Pattern of English* (Chomsky & Halle, 1968) ties phonological structure to physical variables in a more principled way. Stevens' Quantal Theory (1972, 1989) provides an account of how physical dimensions can be intrinsically partitioned into regions corresponding to phonological units (features). However, neither of these approaches provides a realistic account of important aspects of the physical structure of speech, particularly with regard to its temporal properties. In addition, most contemporary views reject *The Sound Pattern of English* view, and adhere to the "two-structure" view, positing powerful and unconstrained "implementation rules" to map from phonological structures to physical variables (e.g., Ladefoged, 1980; see discussion in Clements, 1992).

Under the gestural hypothesis that we have proposed, speech has a single structure, not two. Speech can be decomposed into gestures that are simultaneously *units of information* and *units of action*. Gestures are units of information in that they are *distinctive*. That is, different words are signaled by distinct sets of gestures. For example, the word "bad" exhibits a lip closure gesture at the beginning of the word. It is distinct from the word "dad", which exhibits a tongue tip closure gesture at the beginning of the word. Gestures are units of action in that they are *coordinative structures*. (see Turvey, 1977; Fowler, 1980; Kelso et al., 1986). Activities of multiple (potentially independent) articulators and muscles behave in a interdependent fashion to achieve a constriction goal. For example, a lip closure gesture involves coordinated action of three articulators: upper lip, lower lip, and jaw, and as many as fifteen distinct muscles. When a lip closure is active in the vocal tract, all these articulators and muscles are functionally yoked, so their activities cooperate to achieve the goal of lip closure. The goal- (or *task-*) directed coordinated behavior of these articulators has been modeled as a task-dynamical system (Kelso et al., 1986; Saltzman & Munhall, 1989).

Thus, gestures are abstract, combinatorial units of phonological contrast (a macroscopic property), but because they are defined using dynamical systems that guide the coordination of multiple articulators and muscles, they are intrinsically defined with respect to their (microscopic) physical properties. As will be described below, each gesture regulates the formation of a constriction by one of the independently controllable subsets of articulators within the vocal tract. In the formation of utterances, gestures cohere in larger patters, or *constellations*.

GESTURES AS PRIMITIVE PHONOLOGICAL UNITS

Several distinct *effectors* can produce constrictions within the vocal tract. These effectors, divided into *oral* and *non-oral* sets, are shown in (1).

(1)	Oral	LIPS	Lips
		TT	Tongue Tip
		TB	Tongue Body
	Non-Oral	VEL	Velum
		GLO	Glottis

In English, as in virtually all languages, gestures employing different effectors can distinguish words from one another. (2) shows examples of words in English that differ in which of these effectors are involved in constriction gestures at their beginnings. Note that this set of effectors is sufficient to describe most of the gestures employed in languages, although additional effectors are required to handle the contrasts involving the root of the tongue and the height of the larynx (see Ladefoged & Halle, 1988; Browman & Goldstein, 1989; McCarthy, 1994).

(2)	Oral	LIPS	"bought"
		TT	"dot"
		TB	"got"
	Non-Oral	VEL	"not" (vs. "Dot")
		GLO	"tot" (vs. "Dot")

It is important to note that each effector involves a distinct coordinative structure, involving cooperation among a distinct set of articulators (as is shown in Figure 1). Thus, actions using different effectors are intrinsically categorically distinct, and are thus useful in distinguishing utterances. All languages use gestures of distinct effectors to distinguish words.

If employing distinct effectors was the only way of making distinctions, the set of potentially contrastive units would be quite small (five). This is far fewer than the number of distinct gestures employed in languages.

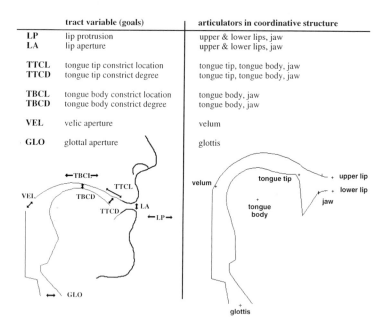

tract variable (goals)		articulators in coordinative structure
LP	lip protrusion	upper & lower lips, jaw
LA	lip aperture	upper & lower lips, jaw
TTCL	tongue tip constrict location	tongue tip, tongue body, jaw
TTCD	tongue tip constrict degree	tongue tip, tongue body, jaw
TBCL	tongue body constrict location	tongue body, jaw
TBCD	tongue body constrict degree	tongue body, jaw
VEL	velic aperture	velum
GLO	glottal aperture	glottis

Figure 1. Tract variables and articulators in the Haskins gestural model. After Browman & Goldstein (1992a).

So there must be additional ways of distinguishing utterances. The added contrastive power comes from the fact that a given effector can produce more than one distinctive type of gesture. Such gestures are typically differentiated along the dimensions of degree (CD) and location (CL) of constriction, produced by the relevant effector. The constriction goals for a given effector can be specified along dimensions referred to as (vocal) *tract variables* (see Browman & Goldstein, 1990b; Saltzman & Munhall, 1989). The inventory of tract variables currently employed in the Haskins computational gestural model, and the articulators associated with each, are shown in Figure 1. In order to see how the gestural units can be used to model the phonological structure of words and larger utterances, it is useful to describe the complete computational model of gestural structure and speech production that has been developed at Haskins Laboratories (see Browman & Goldstein, 1990c; Saltzman & Munhall, 1989; Rubin et al., 1981). The model includes the three submodels shown in the boxes of Figure 2. A transcription of an intended utterance can be input to the *Linguistic Gestural Model*, which contains knowledge of the gestural composition and organization of English words. The output of this model is a gestural score, which specifies what the gestures of the utterance are (in terms of their task-dynamic specifications), and how they are arrayed in time with respect to one another. The task-dynamical specification includes the parameter values for a second order dynamical system that regulates the formation of a constriction by the relevant effector. The specification includes: *equilibrium position* (the tract variable goal), *stiffness* (related to the time constant of constriction formation), and *damping*.

The gestural score is input to the *Task Dynamic Model*, which calculates the response of a set of model vocal tract articulators (those on the right-hand side of Figure 1) to the imposition of that particular dynamical system. In general, gestures (as phonological units)

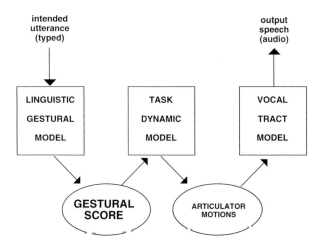

Figure 2. Components of the Haskins computational gestural model. After Browman & Goldstein (1992a).

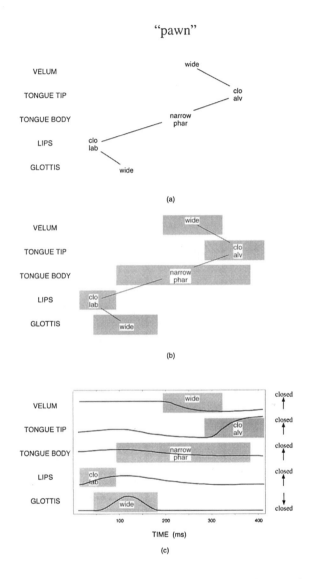

Figure 3. Construction of a gestural score for the utterance "pawn". See text for explanation. After Browman & Goldstein (1995a).

are associated with context-invariant tract variable specifications. However, because of the possibility of temporal overlap of gestures, the movements of the individual articulators will not show context-invariance, because some of the articulators may be part of the coordinative structure of another gesture being produced concurrently. The movements of these model articulators are input to the *Vocal Tract Model*, which calculates the time-varying shape of the vocal tract, the acoustic transfer function, and an output acoustic waveform.

The behavior of the model can be understood by examining gestural scores in more detail, and considering how the (linguistic gestural) model goes about constructing them. For example, if a broad transciption of the utterance "pawn" is input, the linguistic gestural model (LGM) uses its dictionaries to determine that the utterance consists of five gestures. These are shown in Figure 3a. In this, and following displays, the rows represent tiers associated with each of the distinct effectors. The labels associated with each gesture are abbreviations for particular values of the constriction degree and location tract variables that serve as the equilibrium positions for that particular gesture.

In addition to specifying the the gestures themselves, the LGM specifies how the gestures in the utterance are coordinated or *phased* with respect to one another. This information is represented in the lines shown in Figure 3a. Each line specifies that the two connected gestures are critically phased with respect to each other (see Tuller & Kelso, 1984). That is, some point in the ongoing dynamics of one gesture must be synchronous with some point in the other. (The LGM, as discussed in Browman & Goldstein, 1990b, specifies which points in each gesture are synchronized, although that information is not displayed in this figure).

Each gesture is associated with an intrinsic time constant (its stiffness), in addition to the equilibrium positions represented by the labels in Figure 3. Using these stiffnesses, along with the phasing represented by the lines, the LGM calculates an activation interval for each gesture, representing the time during which it has control over the relevant articulators. These activation intervals, shown in Figure 3b, are set by the LGM to be fixed proportions of the underlying (undamped) cycle period of each gesture (for consonant gestures, the proportion is .67, or 230 degrees; for vowel gestures, the proportion is .955, or 340 degrees). When the specifications in Figure 3b are input to the task dynamic model, coordinated motion of the articulators and resulting changes in the tract variables are computed. Figure 3c shows the resulting time functions of the constriction degree tract variables for each of the effectors.

Two points about the gestural score are worth highlighting. One is that the gestures composing the utterance are not strictly sequential; rather they show substantial temporal overlap. This overlap is important, because (as discussed below) it provides the basis for an account of certain patterns of microscopic variation (at the level of the individual articulators), given macroscopic invariance. A second point is that effectors are often left unspecified, and are assumed not to be under active control (these are the intervals in Figure 3 in which no activation box is found on a given row). Note, however, that during such intervals, the relevant tract variables do show (passive) movement; such movement is due to two factors: (a) some of the articulators that are part of the effector's coordinative structure may also be part of another coordinative structure that *is* under active control; (b)

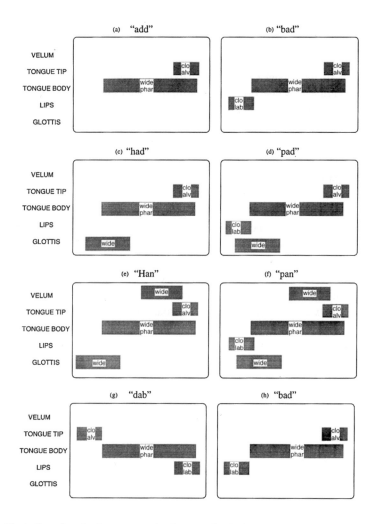

Figure 4. Illustration of contrasts among gestural scores. See text.

when an articulator is not part of any active gesture, it returns to a neutral position.

The macroscopic property of contrast among different words can be defined with reference to properties of gestural scores. A major basis for contrast is the presence vs. absence of particular gestures. For example, in Figure 4, the gestural score for the word "add" is shown in (a). Adding a labial closure gesture (in (b)) yields "bad". Adding a glottal opening-and-closing gesture to the gestural scores in (a) and (b) yields (c) "had" and (d) "pad". Adding a velic opening gesture to these latter words yields, respectively, (e) "Han" and (f) "pan". In addition to the presence and absence of gestures, utterances can differ in the choice of different effectors (e.g. in "ban" vs. "Dan",) or in the particular tract variable parameterization associated with a given effector (e.g., "sad" vs. "shad".). Finally, utterances may contrast with one another in the how the individual gestures are organized (e.g. in Figure 4), (g) "dab" vs. (h) "bad".

The gestural approach can account, in a principled way, for aspects of the relation between the macroscopic and microscopic structure of speech. In particular, certain types of (microscopic) contextual variation in the articulatory and acoustic properties of speech can be seen to follow automatically from the temporal overlap of invariantly specified gestural units. In general, the model predicts different consequences of gestural overlap, depending on the nature of the overlapping gestures. When gestures employing distinct effectors (and tract variables) overlap in time, the model predicts that each of the overlapping gestures will achieve their targets. However, if these overlapping gestures share some articulators in common, the model predicts that the particular pattern of articulator activity used in achieving a gesture's goal (and the resulting acoustics) will vary as a function of the demands of the overlapping gesture. For example, the data of Öhman (1967) show that in the utterances [idi], [ada], and [udu], the position achieved by the tongue tip during the consonant is the same, but the overall shape of the tongue differs substantially at that point in time, essentially mimicking the shape of the tongue during the vowel. In our model, this is accounted for by the overlap of gestures of the consonant and the vowel. Different amounts of tongue tip, tongue body, and jaw activity are automatically recruited to produce the invariant tongue tip constriction in the three contexts (see Saltzman & Munhall, 1989).

When two overlapping gestures share the same tract variables, it is (obviously) not possible for both gestures to achieve their targets, as the gestures are attempting to move the same structures in different ways. In this case, the parameters of the "competing" gestures are blended in the model, and the final position of the tract variables reflects this blending. This is, again, consistent with the data of Öhman (1967) and others. Here, Öhman's data shows that in [igi], [aga], and [ugu], the position of the tongue dorsum during the consonant differs (unlike the case with [d]). This context-dependence of the tract variable positions is also produced by our model (see Saltzman & Munhall, 1989), because the consonants and vowels in this case are defined for the same tract variables (TBCD and TBCL), and therefore blending must occur.

Other kinds of variation, for example the kinds of variation associated with fluent or casual speech, can also be accounted for by gestural overlap (see Browman & Goldstein, 1990c, 1992a). Here, an important point is that as rate and fluency of speaking increase, the amount of overlap of neighboring gestures may increase, and this will result in a variety of consequences of overlap, including cases in which a gesture may be completely hidden by other overlapping gestures, and thus effectively deleted from the acoustic standpoint. Browman and Goldstein (1990c) hypothesize that all the superficially distinct types of variation in casual speech can be described either as changes in gesture magnitude (magnitude reduced as casualness increases) or as changes in temporal overlap (increased overlap as casualness increases).

SYLLABLE STRUCTURE AS GESTURAL CONFIGURATION

In a model in which gestures are the most primitive phonological units, it is possible to analyze other (larger) phonological structures and units in a different (and possibly more satisfactory) way than is done in other approaches to phonology. Browman and Goldstein (1995b) explore this possibility with respect to syllable structure. In the standard view, syllable structure is a hierarchical structure that dominates (groups of) phonological segments (e.g., Anderson, 1974; Kahn, 1976; Selkirk, 1982). In addition, many allophonic rules have been identified that are specific to particular syllable positions. However, as Browman and Goldstein (1995b) argue, in such an approach there is no intrinsic relation between the hypothesized hierarchical structure and the physical (microscopic) properties of speech, nor any obvious connection among these various allophonic rules that occur in a given syllable position.

In contrast, in the gestural view, syllable structure is a characteristic pattern of organization, i.e. a characteristic configuration, of gestural units. Thus, different syllable positions are defined by differences in patterns of gestural overlap. This predicts that there will be lawful microscopic consequences of differences in syllable position, due to the effects of different patterns of gestural overlap (the particular consequences will vary depending on what the gestures are). Thus, processes that seem superficially distinct may have a common basis in the lawful consequences of overlap.

For example, consider the following commonly assumed allophonic rules for English (where $ represents a syllable boundary):

(3) $V \rightarrow [\textit{+nasal}] / \_ [\textit{+nasal}]\ C_0^n\ \$$

(4) $[\textit{+lateral}] \rightarrow [\textit{+back}] / \_ C_0^n\ \$$

(3) states that vowels are nasalized when they precede a nasal that is part of a syllable-final consonant sequence and (4) states that a lateral is velarized (as indicated by the [+back]) when part of a syllable-final consonant sequence. A more extreme version of (4) is sometimes found, in which the lateral ceases to be a lateral altogether and becomes a back vowel:

(5) $[\textit{+lateral}] \rightarrow \begin{vmatrix} \textit{+back} \\ \textit{-lateral} \end{vmatrix} / \_ C_0^n\ \$$

Examining the statement of the rules for nasals and laterals, we find nothing in common in them, apart from the stipulation that they happen in syllable-final position.

Nothing in the rules would suggest that there is any intrinsic connection between these processes. However, as will be elaborated below, these (and other) examples of allophonic variation result automatically from two principles of gestural organization:

(6) principles of gestural organization
   . Syllable positions are defined by different patterns of coordination of consonant gestures.
   . Oral constriction gestures are less extreme in syllable-final position than in syllable-initial position.

Nasals. Krakow (1989, 1993) has shown that the coordination of velum lowering with oral closure for nasal consonants differs qualitatively as a function of syllable position. She tested minimal pairs like "see me" and "seem E", and found that for syllable-initial nasals, the offsets of the relevant gestures (velum lowering and lip closure) are synchronous, while for syllable-final nasals, the offset of velum lowering is synchronous with *onset* of lip closure. Because in final position the velum lowers before the lips start to close, more nasalization during the acoustic vowel interval will be found for syllable-final than for syllable-initial consonants. Thus, the allophonic rule in (3) follows from this coordination principle.

Laterals. Recent articulatory research has found that American English [l] is also a constellation of two gestures, Tongue Tip (TT) raising/fronting and Tongue Body (TB) retraction, with the coordination of the two gestures differing in initial and final positions (Sproat & Fujimura, 1993; Browman & Goldstein, 1995b). In syllable-initial position, the gesture offsets are synchronous while in syllable-final position, the offset of TB retraction is synchronous with the *onset* of TT raising. (The latter statement is due to Browman & Goldstein, 1995b, although it appears consistent with the data presented by Sproat & Fujimura, 1993). The earlier backing of the TB could account for why the [l] sounds more velarized in final position, as is represented in allophonic rule (4).

The behavior of nasals and laterals is apparently parallel. They are both composed of two gestures. One gesture is oral closure (in the data examined, LIPS closure for "m" and TT closure for "l"). The second gesture is less constricted (VEL lowering for nasals, TB retraction for laterals). The two gestures are synchronous initially, and asynchronous finally. Thus, we can posit a generalization about gestural configuration in English that defines syllable positions (as proposed in Browman & Goldstein, 1995b):

(7) Gestural configuration in English
   . Syllable-final linked gestures are phased so that gestures with wider constriction degrees occur earlier.
   . Syllable-initial linked gestures are phased roughly synchronously.

The superficially unrelated allophonic rules in (3) and (4) both follow from this general statement of gestural configuration.

Syllable positions may also be defined with respect to gestural magnitude. In English, at least, syllable-final gestures are generally reduced in magnitude, compared to syllable-initial ones (Browman & Goldstein, 1995b). This general tendency is more extreme for TT (tongue tip) gestures than for Lip or TB gestures. As Browman and Goldstein (1995b) have shown, such TT reduction can result in laterals losing much of their TT constrictions. Such articulations would presumably be perceived as back vowels, as represented in allophonic rule (5).

It is reasonable to question the generality of the apparent parallelism of nasals and laterals. In particular, we can ask if the parallel behavior of nasals and laterals really results from an organizational principle that cuts across very different gesture types, or if it is simply an accidental similarity. If a general principle is at work, then it should be possible to find evidence of the following kinds: (a) across languages, coordination of gestures for nasals and laterals should always pattern together; (b) other types of gestural constellations should exhibit the same kind of bimodal pattern of coordination.

With respect to cross-linguistic evidence, there is not currently enough articulatory data to know whether the syllable structure asymmetry exhibited by both nasals and laterals turns up in a variety of languages. However, Anderson (1995) has argued that if the syllable structure pattern (combined with final reduction) is extreme enough, two historical processes can be expected to occur together: final laterals becoming back glides (8) and vowels becoming nasal vowels with loss of the following (final) nasal consonant (9).

(8)   [l] > [w] (or some back glide)

(9)   [vN] > [ṽ]

Anderson finds that several languages, in fact, exhibit both these processes, occurring at about the same point in their history (e.g., French, Portuguese, and Polish). Such evidence supports the generality of the relation between nasals and laterals.

There is also evidence that at least one other type of gestural constellation exhibits the bimodal pattern of gestural coordination found for nasals and laterals. Articulatory data collected by Gick (1996) suggests that the syllable structure asymmetry in coordination (7) also applies to the glide [w]. The consonant [w] is composed of two gestures: TB retraction and raising and LIPS approximation. These gestures can also be found as the "second" element in various diphthongs (e.g., [aʊ], [oʊ]). Thus, the same pair of gestures is found both syllable-initially and syllable-finally. Gick (1996) found that for syllable-initial [w] (e.g. in "the water"), the two gestures are roughly synchronous, while for the syllable-final glide (e.g., "pow dotter", the TB gesture leads substantially. These patterns are illustrated in Figure 5. Assuming that the LIPS gesture is the more constricted one, then the observed

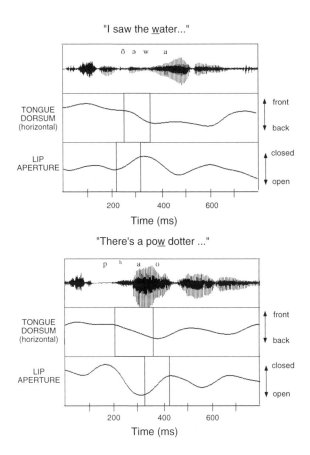

Figure 5. Movements of tongue dorsum and lips in "the water" and in "pow dotter".Shaded areas represent movements for lip closure and tongue body gestures for "w".

pattern fits the general organizational principle in (7). The LIPS gesture also shows reduction in magnitude in final position, compared to initial position, as expected.

CONCLUSIONS

The results that have been obtained to date suggest that important generalizations about the structure of "normal" speech can be uncovered by assuming that phonological units are also units of action, and investigating the organization of those units through measurement of articulatory kinematics. The explicit model of gestural structure that has been developed is a useful tool for helping to analyze such movement data into underlying gestural units, and for investigating the articulatory, acoustic, and perceptual consequences of gestural overlap among different types of gestures. It should be interesting to extend these techniques to the analysis of the speech of individuals with speaking difficulties of various kinds, as van Lieshout(1995), for example, has begun to do.

NOTE

The research summarized in this paper was supported by NSF grant 9112198 and NIH grants HD-01994 and DC-00121 to Haskins Laboratories

REFERENCES

Anderson, S. (1974). *The Organization of Phonology*. Academic Press, New York.

Anderson, S. (1995). *Intra-syllabic gestural relations*. Presented at Haskins Laboratories workshop on Articulatory Phonology.

Browman, C.P., & Goldstein, L. (1986). Towards an articulatory phonology. *Phonology Yearbook, 3*, 219-252.

Browman, C.P., Goldstein, L. (1989). Articulatory gestures as phonological units. *Phonology, 6*, 151-206.

Browman, C.P., & Goldstein, L. (1990a). Representation and reality: Physical systems and phonological structure. *Journal of Phonetics, 18*, 411-424.

Browman, C.P., & Goldstein, L. (1990b). Gestural specification using dynamically-defined articulatory structures. *Journal of Phonetics, 18*, 299-320.

Browman, C.P., & Goldstein, L. (1990c). Tiers in articulatory phonology, with some implications for casual speech. In J. Kingston & M.E. Beckman (Eds), *Papers in laboratory phonology I: Between the grammar and physics of speech*, pages 341-376. Cambridge University Press, Cambridge.

Browman, C.P., & Goldstein, L. (1992a). Articulatory phonology: An overview. *Phonetica, 49*, 155-180.

Browman, C.P., & Goldstein, L. (1992b). Response to commentaries. *Phonetica, 49*, 222-234.

Browman, C.P., & Goldstein, L. (1995a). Dynamics and articulatory phonology. In T. van Gelder & R.F. Port, (Eds.), *Mind as Motion*, pages 175-193. MIT Press, Cambridge, MA.

Browman, C.P. & Goldstein, L. (1995b). Gestural syllable position effects in american english. In F. Bell-Berti F. & L.J. Raphael (Eds.), *Producing speech: Contemporary issues*. For Katherine Safford Harris, pages 19-34. AIP Press, Woodbury, NY.

Chomsky, N., & Halle, M. (1968). The sound pattern of English. Harper and Row, New York.

Clements, G.N. (1992). Phonological primes: features or gestures? *Phonetica, 49*, 181-193.

Fowler, C.A. (1980). Coarticulation and theories of extrinsic timing. *Journal of Phonetics, 8*, 113-133.

Gick, B. (1996). Syllable-based allophony and categorizing english glides. Paper presented at LabPhon 5, Northwestern University.

Hockett, C.F. (1955). A manual of phonology. Waverly Press, Baltimore.

Jongman, A., Blumstein, S., & Lahiri, A. (1985). Acoustic properties for dental and alveolar stop consonants: a cross-language study. *Journal of Phonetics, 13*, 235-251.

Kahn, D. (1976). Syllable-based generalizations in English phonology. PhD thesis, Massachusetts Institute of Technology.

Kauffman, S. (1995). At Home in the Universe: The Search for the Laws of Self-Organization and Complexity. Oxford University Press, Oxford.

Kelso, J.A.S., Saltzman, E.L., & Tuller, B. (1986). The dynamical perspective on speech production: Data and theory. *Journal of Phonetics, 14,* 29-60.

Krakow, R.A. (1989). The articulatory organization of syllables: A kinematic analysis of labial and velar gestures. PhD thesis, Yale University.

Krakow, R.A. (1993). Nonsegmental influences on velum movement patterns: Syllables, sentences, stress, and speaking rate. In M.K. Huffman & R.A. Krakow (Eds.) *Phonetics and phonology,* Volume 5: Nasals, nasalization, and the velum, pages 87-116. Academic Press, New York.

Kugler, P.N., & Turvey, M.T. (1987). *Information, natural law, and the self-assembly of rhythmic movement.* Lawrence Erlbaum Associates, Hillsdale, NJ.

Ladefoged, P. (1980). What are linguistic sounds made of? *Language, 56,* 485-502.

Ladefoged, P. (1982). *A course in phonetics.* Harcourt Brace Jovanovich, New York.

Ladefoged, P., & Halle, M. (1988). Some major features of the international phonetic alphabet. *Language, 64,* 577-582.

Lindblom, B.E. (1983). *Phonetic universals in vowel systems.* In J. Ohala, (Ed.), Experimental phonology. Academic Press, New York.

Manuel, S.Y., & Krakow, R.A. (1984). Universal and language particular aspects of vowel-to-vowel coarticulation. *Haskins Laboratories Status Report on Speech Research,* SR-77/78, 69-78.

McCarthy, J.J. (1994). The phonetics and phonology of semitic pharyngeals. In P. Keating, (Ed.), *Phonological structure and phonetic form: Papers in laboratory phonology III,* pages 191-233. Cambridge University Press, Cambridge.

Ohala, J. (1983). The origin of sound patterns in vocal tract constraints. In P. MacNeilage, (Ed.), *The Production of Speech,* pages 189-216. Springer-Verlag, New York.

Öhman, S.E.G. (1967). Numerical model of coarticulation. *Journal of the Acoustical Society of America, 41,* 310-320.

Rubin, P.E., Baer, T., & Mermelstein, P. (1981). An articulatory synthesizer for perceptual research. *Journal of the Acoustical Society of America, 70,* 321-328.

Saltzman, E.L., & Munhall, K.G. (1989). A dynamical approach to gestural patterning in speech production. *Ecological Psychology, 1,* 333-382.

Schöner, G., & Kelso, J.A.S. (1988). Dynamic pattern generation in behavioral and neural systems. *Science, 239,* 1513-1520.

Selkirk, E.O. (1982). The syllable. In H. van der Hulst & N. Smith, (Eds.), *The Structure of Phonological Representations,* pages 337-383. Foris, Dordrecht.

Sproat, R., & Fujimura, O. (1993). Allophonic variation in english /l/ and its implications for phonetic implementation. *Journal of Phonetics, 21,* 291-311.

Stevens, K.N. (1972). The quantal nature of speech: Evidence from articulatory-acoustic data. In E.E.J. David & P.B. Denes (Eds.), *Human communication: A unified view,* pages 51-66. McGraw-Hill, New York.

Stevens, K.N. (1989). On the quantal nature of speech. *Journal of Phonetics, 17,* 3-45.

Tuller, B., & Kelso, J.A.S. (1984). The timing of articulatory gestures: Evidence for relational invariants. *Journal of the Acoustical Society of America, 76,* 1030-1036.

Turvey, M.T. (1977). Preliminaries to a theory of action with reference to vision. In R. Shaw & J. Bransford (Eds.), *Perceiving, acting and knowing: Toward an ecological psychology,* pages 211-265. Lawrence Erlbaum Associates, Hillsdale, NJ.

Van Lieshout, P. (1995). *Motor planning and articulation in fluent speech of stutterers and nonstutterers.* Nijmegen Institute for Cognition and Information, Nijmegen.

Speech Production: Motor Control, Brain Research and Fluency Disorders
W. Hulstijn, H.F.M. Peters and P.H.H.M. Van Lieshout, editors

Chapter 5

WORD FORM GENERATION IN LANGUAGE PRODUCTION

Antje S. Meyer

Most models of language production assume that word forms are generated in several steps. First, stored lexical representations are decomposed into two independent tiers: a set of phonological segments and a metrical frame. Then the units of these tiers are combined by assigning segments to positions in the metrical frame. Finally, a phonetic representation is created, which governs the articulation of the utterance. This chapter discusses the nature of these representations and the way they are generated and combined. It is argued that the phonological representations speakers create are more abstract than has often been thought (segments may be underspecified for certain features, and the metrical frames capture syllable number and stress pattern, but not the syllable-internal structure) and that the function of the complicated processes of phonological decomposition and reassembly is to make the phonological structure of morphemes visible to the processor and to allow for the generation of contextually appropriate surface forms.

INTRODUCTION

It is a standard assumption in linguistics and psycholinguistics that speakers do not retrieve entire sentences from memory, but create them by retrieving individual words and combining them according to the rules of grammar. It is difficult to explain linguistic productivity -- speakers' ability to produce, and listeners' ability to understand, an indefinite number of different sentences -- in any other way. Curiously, the form of a single word is also generated out of smaller units. It is less obvious than for sentence production why this would be necessary. As there is usually only one word form in the speaker's mental lexicon expressing a given word meaning, it seems much simpler to store and retrieve this form as a unit.

This chapter is organized in the following way. In Section 2, a very general model of word production is outlined. Since its central claims are compatible with almost all existing models of word production (e.g., Dell, 1986; Fromkin, 1971, 1973; Garrett, 1975, 1980; Shattuck-Hufnagel, 1979, 1983), I will call it the Standard Model. In this model, stored form representations are decomposed into phonological constituents before articulatory commands can be selected and carried out. This decomposed phonological representation comprises two independent tiers -- the segmental and the metrical tier. Evidence concerning the nature of these representations will be reviewed in Sections 3 and 4. In Section 5, I will briefly describe the phonetic representation. In Section 6, I will turn to the question of how these representations are generated and combined. Finally, in Section 7, I will discuss why it is necessary to derive the pronunciation of words via intermediate decomposed phonological representations.

AN OVERVIEW OF WORD FORM GENERATION

Speakers frequently commit sound errors, such as "*m*urn my mouth" (instead of "burn my mouth") or "cut my *c*inger" (instead of "cut my finger"), in which the actual utterance differs from the intended one in one or more sounds not corresponding to a complete morpheme. This shows that word forms are not retrieved from the mental lexicon as units but are composed out of smaller building blocks. If word forms were retrieved as units, such sound errors could not arise.

A very important property of sound errors is that listeners usually perceive them as phonetically well-formed (e.g., Boomer & Laver, 1968; Wells, 1951). Very few errors have been reported that violate the phonotactic rules of the language, and misplaced sounds are usually perceived as phonetically accommodated to their new environment (e.g., Fromkin, 1971, 1973; Garrett, 1976, 1980). For example, when an English stop consonant moves from a word-initial to a word-internal position or vice versa, it loses or acquires aspiration, as appropriate for the new environment. The phonetic well-formedness of sound errors suggests that they do not arise during the creation of a phonetic representation or during articulation. Instead they must arise earlier, during the creation of an abstract phonological representation, such that phonetic rules can apply after the error has been committed.

In sound errors the intended and the erroneous utterance typically differ by one or two segments (e.g., Shattuck-Hufnagel, 1983). Errors involving individual phonetic features or entire syllables as error units are very rare. Therefore, it can be concluded that phonological representations are created by retrieving and combining phonological segments and maybe certain segment clusters. Thus, the first main processing component in the generation of word forms is segmental spell-out -- the retrieval of phonological segments.

A particularly important type of sound errors are errors in which two segments trade places (as in "*p*erry *ch*ie" instead of "cherry pie"). These errors suggest that there are positions that exist independently of the segments that take them. This explains how each of the misplaced segments ends up in the position vacated by the other segment rather than elsewhere in the string.

The frames appear to encode the syllabic structure of the utterance because misplaced segments typically move from their target positions to corresponding, rather than different, positions in new syllables (e.g., Boomer & Laver, 1968). For instance, a segment from a syllable onset (the prevocalic part of the syllable) normally moves into a new onset position (as in "*p*ig *b*en" instead of "big pen"), but not into a coda position (the postvocalic part of the syllable). Thus, the second main processing component implicated by analyses of sound errors is the generation of frames representing the syllabic structure of the utterance. As syllables are part of the metrical representation of a word, I will refer to this component as metrical spell-out. The third main component, which must be postulated if segments and metrical frames are retrieved independently of each other, is the association of segments to positions in metrical structures.

The resulting phonological representation must be an abstract characterization of the word form because, as mentioned above, misplaced segments are phonetically accommodated to their new context. Hence, there must be a fourth processing component that computes exactly how the word is to be pronounced.

THE SEGMENTAL REPRESENTATION

In this section two important properties of the segmental representation will be considered, namely, first, that it is constructed out of roughly segment-sized, rather than larger or smaller constituents, and, second, that these constituents are abstract linguistic units.

As mentioned, the most important piece of evidence for the assumption of segment-sized processing units is that the most common error unit has the size of a single segment. In different corpora, 60-90% of the sound errors are single-segment errors (e.g., Berg, 1985, 1988; Boomer & Laver, 1968; Fromkin, 1971; Nooteboom, 1969; Shattuck-Hufnagel, 1983; Shattuck-Hufnagel & Klatt, 1979).

However, errors involving other types of units are regularly observed and require an explanation. First, about 10-30% of the sound errors are sequences of two adjacent segments. The segments constituting such complex error units almost always belong to the same syllable constituent, most frequently to the onset, less often to the nucleus (the vocalic part of the syllable). Coda errors are very rare (e.g., Berg, 1989, 1992, 1994; MacKay, 1972; Picard, 1992; Shattuck-Hufnagel, 1983; Stemberger, 1983). One way to represent the coherence of certain clusters is to assume unitary representations for clusters in addition to, or instead of, representations of the individual segments (see, for instance, Dell, 1986). Interestingly, errors involving entire syllables are extremely rare, indicating that there may be processing units corresponding to syllable constituents but no units corresponding to complete syllables.

Occasionally feature errors are observed, such as Fromkin's (1971) much cited "*g*lear *p*lue sky", but these errors are rare. Probably less than 5% of all sound errors are feature errors. However, there is a much larger class of errors in which the target and the error segment differ by one feature (e.g., "*d*abacco" instead of "*t*abacco"; Berg, 1988; Nooteboom, 1969; Shattuck-Hufnagel, 1986; Shattuck-Hufnagel & Klatt, 1979). MacKay (1970) and Berg (1988) reported that more than 50% of the consonant errors in their German corpora fell into this category. These errors could either be analyzed as feature or as segment errors. However, following Shattuck-Hufnagel (1983; see also Shattuck-Hufnagel & Klatt, 1979) they are usually regarded as segmental errors. Shattuck-Hufnagel examined those sound interaction errors in her English corpus that involved targets differing in two or more features and computed by how many features the error outcomes differed from the target segments. In 67 out of 70 cases the difference was more than one feature. Thus, the large majority of these errors was described more parsimoniously as segmental than as feature errors. Hence, Shattuck-Hufnagel proposed that the ambiguous errors -- those sound errors where target and error segments differ only by one feature -- should also be viewed as segmental errors. However, perhaps feature exchanges are more likely to occur among segments that differ by only one feature than among more dissimilar segments. Thus, it is possible that the frequency of feature errors has been underestimated (see also Browman & Goldstein, 1988).

The second claim to be evaluated concerns the abstractness of the units manipulated during segmental spell-out. As mentioned, the most common argument for abstract planning units is that the error outcomes are usually phonetically well-formed. However, as many investigators have noted, not all sound errors yield phonotactically legal sequences (e.g., Boomer & Laver, 1968; Butterworth & Whittaker, 1980; Stemberger, 1983). It is difficult to estimate the frequency of phonotactic violations since it is unclear how reliably they would be detected and described. Thus, perhaps the phonetic well-formedness of errors arises largely in the listener's ear (or mind) rather than being created by the speaker.

Stemberger (1991a,b; 1992; Stemberger & Stoel-Gammon, 1991; see also Berg, 1991) has argued that the segments retrieved during word form generation are not specified for all of their feature values, which implies that they are fairly abstract. In phonological theory lexical entries specify only those properties of morphemes that are not redundant (e.g., Kenstowicz, 1994). For instance, if in a language all syllable-initial voiceless stops are aspirated, the aspiration of these segments will not be specified in the lexical entries. Some theories assume that also some non-redundant feature values are unspecified in lexical entries (e.g., Archangeli, 1984; Kiparski, 1985; Pulleyblank, 1983). This is possible, if all other values are specified. For instance, if voiced segments are lexically specified, then voiceless ones need not be specified for voicing, since the absence of the feature [+voiced] signals voicelessness. To return to Stemberger's analyses: In general, the segments interacting in errors tend to share more features than expected on the basis of a chance estimate (Fromkin, 1971; García-Albea et al., 1989; Garrett, 1975; Nooteboom, 1969; Shattuck-Hufnagel & Klatt, 1979). In extensive analyses of naturally occurring and experimentally elicited errors Stemberger showed that those features that can be considered underspecified on linguistic grounds are less influential in determining the likelihood of segments to interact in errors than specified features. In addition, asymmetries in segment interactions can be explained by reference to feature (under)specification. Segments specified for a given feature tend to replace segments unspecified for that feature. Stemberger views this as an instantiation of a general addition bias in language production, which is based on the processing principle that activated units tend to "win" in competition against "nothing". Stemberger's analyses support the distinction between an abstract form representation, in which some features are still unspecified, and a more detailed one in which they have been filled in.

Stemberger's arguments for an abstract phonological representation contrast sharply with Mowrey and MacKay's (1990) view who deny the necessity of assuming any abstract sublexical units. They recorded speech motor activity during the production of tongue twisters, such as "Bob flew by Bligh Bay". For each utterance, they determined whether it sounded normal, and whether the pattern of muscle activity was normal. Many utterances were either normal or abnormal in both respects. However, there were also many utterances that sounded perfectly normal, but showed a variety of unusual patterns of muscle activity, which Mowrey and MacKay viewed as blends of the patterns of motor activity typical for different target segments. Thus, the errors were graded events, which did not necessarily affect the entire motor program pertaining to a given segment or feature, but could affect only part of it.

Mowrey and MacKay conclude that their data represent a serious threat to any theory claiming that during speech production discrete linguistic units are selected and combined. They argue that on such a view, the motor patterns should always correspond to those typically found for particular linguistic units, and should not be blends of such patterns.

Mowrey and MacKay's study is important because it reminds us that abnormalities can arise during motor execution that cannot be perceived even by the most attentive listeners (see also Nolan et al. 1996; Stevens, 1972). However, the data probably present less of a challenge for the Standard Model than the authors suggest. First, it is unknown how often motor errors like those found by Mowrey and MacKay occur in more natural speech situations, in which speakers do not produce tongue twisters but sequences of more dissimilar words, and in which there are no EMG needles stuck in their tongue and lips. Second, as Fowler (1995) has pointed out, Mowrey and MacKay only recorded the speech motor activity at a small number of sites. Hence, it is unclear whether the errors affected only small parts of the motor programs, as the authors assume, or larger structures, which would imply that at least some of the alleged motor errors could be regarded as feature or segment errors. Finally, as Mowrey and MacKay note themselves, though the data do not support the Standard Model, they are perfectly compatible with it. Nothing in this model excludes that errors arise during the execution of one normal speech plan or as blends of two competing plans. To exclude the existence of linguistic planning levels, it must be shown that all of the evidence usually explained by reference to these levels can be accounted for purely by reference to motor factors.

THE METRICAL REPRESENTATION

A central claim of the Standard Model is that the segmental and metrical tiers are first retrieved independently of each other, and that only later segments are associated to positions in the metrical representation. Another important claim is that the metrical tier includes a representation of syllable-internal constituents.

A widely used argument to support both claims simultaneously is the syllable-position constraint -- the observation that the interacting segments in sound errors typically stem from corresponding syllable positions. The standard account for this constraint is that there are syllable frames with labelled positions (onset, nucleus, and coda) and that segments are marked with respect to the positions they may take (e.g., Dell, 1986; Shattuck-Hufnagel,

1979, 1983).

Undoubtedly, the syllable-position constraint is observed in the majority of the sound errors (Fromkin, 1971, 1973; García-Albea et al., 1989; MacKay, 1970; Motley, 1973; Nooteboom, 1969; Shattuck-Hufnagel, 1983, 1987; Stemberger, 1982; but see Abd-El-Jawad & Abu-Salim, 1987, on Arabic & Kubozono, 1989, on Japanese errors). However, as Shattuck-Hufnagel (1987, 1992) has pointed out, the lion's share of the evidence for this constraint -- more than 80% of the relevant cases in the English corpora that have been analyzed -- stems from errors involving word onsets (see also Fromkin, 1971; Garrett, 1975, 1980). Thus, word onset consonants are particularly error-prone and prefer to interact with each other rather than with word-internal segments, and this may explain most of the evidence usually taken to support the syllable-position constraint.

Unambiguous evidence for a syllable-position constraint can only come from errors in other word positions. Vowels show a very strong tendency to interact with each other rather than with consonants. This could be due to a syllable-position constraint, but it could also be due to the general tendency of segments to interact with phonemically similar rather than dissimilar segments. In addition, interactions of vowels with consonants may lead to sound sequences that cannot be pronounced and are therefore never observed. Consonantal errors not involving word onsets are too rare to be analyzed for adherence to a positional constraint. In short, the constraints on segment movements do not provide unambiguous evidence for a representation of syllable-internal structure.

Stemberger (1984, 1990) looked for evidence for frames of a slightly different type, namely frames encoding the CV structure of the utterance. Such a structure has been proposed in Autosegmental Phonology (e.g., Clements & Keyser, 1983; Goldsmith, 1990; McCarthy, 1981). This tier captures the number and ordering of vocalic and consonantal elements in a word and their length, as short segments associate to one and long ones to two positions of the CV tier.

Stemberger (1984) examined errors involving segments differing in length. If misordered segments typically acquire the length of the segments they replace, length may be represented independently of segmental content in terms of the number of positions on the CV tier. The analyses of small corpora of German and Swedish errors supported this hypothesis, as misplaced segments usually acquired the length of the segments they replaced. However, in Stemberger's English corpus the misplaced segments showed a strong tendency to maintain their original length, which does not support the view that length is represented independently of segmental content.

In another study, Stemberger (1990) compared the frequencies of segment additions (as in "prich player" instead of "rich player") and substitutions (as in "pich player") and found that additions were more, and substitutions therefore less, likely when the source ("player" in the example) began with a cluster than when it began with a singleton. Thus, there was a tendency towards increased similarity of the CV structures of the interacting words. In the same study he found that the words involved in onset interaction errors ("cook base" instead of "book case") were more likely than expected on the basis of a chance estimate to have the same number of segments in the coda (i.e., either one or two consonants). However, the observed proportion of interacting word pairs with the same number of elements in the nucleus (with long vowels and diphthongs counting as two elements, and short vowels as one element) was not above chance. Thus, Stemberger's evidence is suggestive, but it does not offer very strong support for the assumption of an independent representation of CV structure.

Does this mean that speakers do not create metrical structures at all? Not necessarily. Levelt (1992) has proposed that they do create metrical representations, but that these representations do not capture syllable-internal structure, but only the number of syllables and their stress pattern (and/or weight). Evidence for such metrical frames comes from errors involving vowels stemming from syllables differing in stress value. In these cases, the stress pattern of the utterance is typically maintained (e.g., Shattuck-Hufnagel, 1986), suggesting that the segmental content is separated from the metrical structure. However, such errors are rare, and at least in some cases the perceived constancy of the stress pattern may be created by the listener rather than the speaker.

Firmer support for the assumption of an independent metrical representation comes from recent experiments using the so-called implicit priming paradigm (Roelofs & Meyer, submitted). In this paradigm, participants first learn a small set of word pairs (e.g., "hat-cap", "mouse-cat", "bottle-can"). On each trial of the following test block, the first member of a pair (e.g., "hat") is presented as a prompt, and the participants produce the second member, the target ("cap" in the example), as rapidly as possible. Each pair is tested repeatedly within a block. The targets of a block are either related in form (as in the example) or unrelated. In earlier experiments, response latencies were shorter when the targets shared one or more word-initial segments than when they were unrelated in form. Thus, segmental priming was obtained (see Meyer, 1990; 1991). This priming effect is a preparation effect: In the related blocks, participants create a partial phonological representation of the targets, which includes the shared segments, and maintain it in working memory. Adding to this partial representation after prompt presentation apparently takes less time than creating the phonological representation of a target from scratch.

In the new experiments, this segmental priming effect was replicated. When the targets of a block shared the first two segments, reactions were faster than when they began with different segments. Interestingly, this priming effect was obtained only if the targets also shared the stress pattern and the number of syllables. Apparently the participants had to know the number of syllables and stress pattern of the entire word (and not only the stress value of the first syllable) to be able to use the information about the word-initial segments. This suggests that metrical information is stored and retrieved separately from segmental information. If the stress pattern were coded locally, as diacritics on the vowels, there would be no reason why participants had to know the metrical structure of the entire response word in order to prepare for the first syllable.

In these experiments, constancy of CV structure was not necessary to obtain segmental priming effects. Thus, we assume a metrical representation that encodes only the number of syllables and their stress pattern, but not the syllable-internal structure. Recall that the main reason to postulate frames capturing syllable-internal structure was to account for the syllable position constraint on sound errors. However, as was argued above, other explanations for this constraint are available. In many theories of word production, frames with labelled positions are postulated as an ordering device. Segments are ordered by association to labelled frame positions (e.g., Dell, 1986; Shattuck-Hufnagel, 1979). However, we assume that the segments are ordered before association to syllables (Levelt, 1992; Roelofs, submitted; Roelofs & Meyer, submitted). The association itself is entirely predictable; i.e., it can be achieved by applying universal and language specific syllabification rules. Thus, labelled syllable-internal positions are neither necessary to account for the constraints on segment movements in errors nor for segmental ordering or syllabification.

THE PHONETIC REPRESENTATION

The final step in the creation of word forms is to generate a phonetic representation. The need for this step follows from the abstractness of the phonological representation. In the Standard Model, as in phonological theory, the phonological representation is assumed to be composed of phonological segments, which are discrete (i.e., they do not overlap on an abstract time axis), static (i.e., the features defining them refer to states of the vocal tract or the acoustic signal), and context-free (i.e., the features of a segment are the same in all contexts). By contrast, the actions realizing consonants and vowels may overlap in time, the vocal tract is in continuous movement, and the way features are implemented is context-dependent. Thus, a phonetic representation must be created that defines which movements are to be carried out.

What does this representation look like? Though speakers ultimately carry out movements of the articulators, the phonetic representation most likely does not specify movement trajectories or patterns of muscle activity, but characterizes the speech tasks to be achieved (see, for instance, Fowler, 1995; Levelt, 1989). The main argument for this view is that speakers can realize a given linguistic unit in indefinitely many ways. The sound /b/, for instance, can be produced moving both lips, or only one lip, with or without jaw movement. Most speakers can almost without practice adapt to novel speech situations. For instance, Lindblom et al. (1979) showed that speakers can produce acoustically (almost) normal vowels while holding a bite block between their teeth forcing their jaw in a fixed open position. Abbs and his colleagues (Abbs & Gracco, 1984; Folkins & Abbs, 1975) asked speakers to repeatedly produce an utterance (e.g., "aba" or "sapapple"). On a small number of trials, and unpredictably for the participants, the movement of an articulator (e.g., the lower lip) was mechanically interfered with. Usually, these perturbations were almost immediately (within 30 ms after movement onset) compensated for such that the utterance was acoustically (almost) normal. One way to account for these findings is to assume that the phonetic representation specifies speech tasks to be carried out (e.g., to accomplish lip closure), and that there is a neuro-muscular execution system that computes how the tasks should be carried out in a particular situation (see, for instance, Kelso et al., 1986; Turvey, 1990, for a discussion of the properties of this system). The distinction between a specification of speech tasks and the determination of movements is attractive because it entails that down to a low planning level the speech plan is the same for a given linguistic unit, even though the actual movements may vary.

Very little is known about the creation of the phonetic code. The phonological representation can be viewed as an ordered set of pointers to speech tasks. Levelt (1992) has proposed that speech tasks can generally be derived using segments as critical units. In addition, there may be stored motor templates for entire frequent syllables, which can be retrieved as units from a store, the mental syllabary. The possibility of retrieving precompiled programs for entire syllables would reduce the programming load (relative to segment-by-segment assembly of motor programs), in particular since the syllables of a language differ greatly in frequency. For instance, though Dutch and English have approximately ten thousand different syllable types, the 500 most frequent ones account for more than 80% of the syllable tokens in a large lexical database (see Schiller et al., 1996).

Experimental evidence that is compatible with the notion of a mental syllabary comes from a study by Levelt and Wheeldon (1994), in which a syllable frequency effect was obtained that was independent of word frequency. In one experiment, speech onset latencies were shorter for disyllabic words ending in high-frequency syllables than for otherwise comparable words ending in low-frequency syllables. Thus, high-frequency syllables were accessed faster than low-frequency ones, which implies the existence of syllabic units. However, the syllable frequency effects reported by Levelt and Wheeldon were very small. More importantly, in some experiments, syllable and segment frequencies were correlated. In very recent experiments (Levelt & Meyer, reported in Hendriks & McQueen, 1996), in which a large number of possible confounds were controlled for, neither syllable nor segment frequency effects were obtained. These results do not rule out that speakers retrieve syllables or segments; they only show that the speed of accessing these units does not strongly depend on their frequency, or that frequency-related differences in the speed of access are not reflected in speech onset latencies. The notion of a mental syllabary remains attractive because of the reduction of programming load it offers.

THE TIME COURSE OF WORD FORM GENERATION

The Standard Model would be strengthened by evidence that the different processes it postulates differ in important ways, and that they are ordered as predicted. It should, for instance, be shown that there is a process of segmental retrieval that is distinct from, and precedes, the association of segments to syllables.

Some evidence about the time course of segmental retrieval and the association of segments to syllables comes from implicit priming and picture-word-interference experiments. As mentioned, in implicit priming experiments, participants name sets of target words that are either related or unrelated in form (Meyer, 1990; 1991). Target naming times may be shorter in the related than in the unrelated condition. Importantly, this priming effect is confined to word-initial segments. Thus, participants benefit from overlap in onset and nucleus of monosyllabic targets (as in "cat", "can", "cap"), but not from overlap in their rhymes (as in "cat", "hat", "mat"). Similarly, phonological facilitation is obtained when disyllabic words share the first syllable, but not when they share the second syllable.

In a picture-word interference experiment by Meyer and Schriefers (1991), participants named drawings of objects as quickly as possible while hearing distractor words, which shared word-initial or word-final segments with the targets, or were unrelated to them. The picture of a cat was, for instance, combined with the distractors "cap", "hat", and "tree". Both types of related distractors facilitated target naming relative to unrelated distractors.

Thus, the results from picture-word interference and implicit priming experiments differ in an important way: In the picture-word interference experiment phonological priming effects were obtained from shared word-initial and word-final segments, whereas the facilitatory effect in the implicit priming paradigm was confined to word-initial segments. Roelofs (submitted) has proposed that different processes are tapped in the two paradigms. In the related condition of an implicit priming experiment, participants create partial phonological representations by associating the shared segments to positions in metrical frames. As this process is strictly sequential, preparation effects are found only for word-initial segments. By contrast, the priming effect found in picture-word interference experiments is likely to be due to facilitation of segmental retrieval. The finding that facilitation can be obtained from begin- and end-related distractors suggests that the segments of a word may be activated and selected in any order. Thus, the difference in the results obtained in the two types of experiments can be interpreted by reference to distinct type of processes.

THE NECESSITY OF PHONOLOGICAL DECOMPOSITION

In the preceding sections, it was argued that speakers retrieve a word's segments and metrical structure, then combine them into a phonological representation, and finally generate the corresponding phonetic representation, which specifies the speech motor tasks to be carried out. This may appear to be a cumbersome process. Why can't speakers directly retrieve motor programs for entire morphemes?

The answer has two related parts. First, the stored form representations are likely to be too abstract to determine pronunciation. As mentioned, lexical entries include only non-redundant information, and some theories assume that some non-redundant feature values are also unspecified. Of course, the representations in a speaker's mental lexicon need not be the same as those envisioned by phonologists. Little relevant psycholinguistic evidence is available. Lahiri and Marslen-Wilson (1991) have argued that listeners map spoken input onto fairly abstract underlying representations, but it is not known whether the same representations are used in speech production as in comprehension. The only directly relevant production evidence appears to be Stemberger's research on underspecification discussed above. If the stored lexical representations are not fully specified, processes must be invoked that fill in the missing information. These processes cannot apply to unanalyzed units, but have to "see" individual segments and features. Thus, the purpose of the spell-out processes discussed in the preceding sections is to make the internal structure of morphemes visible to the processor.

A second reason for phonological decomposition is that a given morpheme can be pronounced in many slightly different ways. Importantly, the similarities and differences between the surface forms of a morpheme can best be captured by reference to its internal phonological structure (i.e., its segments, features, and metrical structure). Thus, any model of word form generation in which different pronunciations of a morpheme are generated from a common base form must assume that at some point during word form generation the internal structure of the morpheme becomes visible to the processor and accessible to modification (see Levelt, 1992).

In linguistic theory, alternations of word forms are discussed under the headers of word formation and connected speech rules. I will consider word formation first. The realizations of a morpheme in different morphologically complex words may differ in subtle ways (compare, for instance, the /n/ in "intolerant" and "incapable", or the /n/ in "mantrap" and "mankind", or the phonetic realization of the plural morpheme in "cats", "dogs", and "horses"), or more grossly (compare, for instance, the phonetic realization of the base in "period", "periodic", and "periodicity", or in "divine" and "divinity"; see, for instance, Spencer, 1991, for a systematic introduction to morphology). These differences are systematic, i.e., they can be observed for all lexical items with certain structural properties and can be described as resulting from the application of certain rules to the base forms.

Of course, it can be argued that the mental lexicon perhaps does not (only) include representations of individual morphemes, but (also) complete representations for complex forms. Whether this is the case is an empirical question in need of further study. Reviewing the relevant speech error evidence, Stemberger and MacWhinney (1986) have proposed that the representation of morphologically complex forms may be frequency-dependent. For frequent forms, both unitary and morphologically decomposed forms are available, whereas less frequent forms are composed out of their constituents. Recent experimental evidence (Roelofs, in press) also suggests that at least some morphologically complex forms are assembled out of their constituents.

Let us now consider connected speech rules. Many words can be pronounced in different ways. Some alternations are independent of the context in which the word occurs. English examples are schwa deletion (in "police", "button"), vowel reduction (in "veto the proposal", "potato peeler"), and elision ("and" becoming syllabic /n/, "them" becoming "em"; see Giegerich, 1992). The standard linguistic view is that these forms are generated by applying postlexical rules to the forms retrieved from the mental lexicon. Very frequent surface forms could perhaps be stored in the mental lexicon, side-by-side with the underlying forms. However, though alternations are usually described in categorical terms, many of them are gradual rather than all-or-none, which renders the storage assumption implausible.

There are also changes of word forms that are conditioned by the context in which the words appear. English examples (from Giegerich, 1992) are assimilation (e.g., in "ten pounds", "miss you"), degemination ("call Linda", "weight training") and cliticization ("fish 'n ships", "wonna go", "he'll come"; clitics are the reduced forms of function words that are attached to a preceding or following host). Though frequent clitic-host combination (like "I've") may be stored in the mental lexicon as units, most context-dependent alternations must be computed on-line.

In addition to claiming that morphemes are decomposed into constituents, the Standard Model maintains that the units of the metrical and segmental tier are first retrieved independently and only later combined. There are good linguistic arguments for representing metrical and segmental information on separate tiers, but it does not follow from linguistic theory that the units of the two tiers are at some point not linked (see Frazier, 1995).

Levelt (1992; see also Levelt & Wheeldon, 1994; and Baumann, 1995) has based an argument for unlinked segmental and metrical representations on the fact that the syllabification of words in connected speech often differs from their syllabification in isolation. For instance, when a vowel-initial clitic is appended to a host ending in a consonant, that consonant will become the onset of the next syllable (as, for instance, in "demand it", spoken as "de-man-dit"). In linguistic theory, it is usually assumed that first the individual lexical items are syllabified, and then their syllabification is altered by connected speech rules. Levelt has, however, suggested that speakers directly create the surface forms. Accordingly, they first retrieve the segments and, independently, the metrical structures of lexical items, then combine the metrical structures to larger prosodic units (phonological words), and finally directly associate the segments to positions in these structures following the syllabification rules of the language. For instance, for "demand it", a metrical structure including three syllables is created. Each vowel is associated to a different syllable. Following the Onset Maximization Rule, /d/ is directly associated to the third syllable. This proposal presupposes that in the representation retrieved from the mental lexicon segments are not yet attached to syllable positions.

In summary, the "vertical" decomposition of word forms into segments is necessary in order to give phonological rules a chance to apply. The "horizontal" decomposition into a metrical and segmental tier may be necessary to permit syllabification across lexical boundaries.

SUMMARY AND CONCLUSIONS

I have discussed evidence for the claim that speakers decompose lexical form representations into abstract phonological constituents. The standard argument for the abstractness of the planning units at the segmental level, the phonotactic well-formedness of sound errors, is not convincing, but Stemberger's arguments for underspecified planning units restore confidence. The standard argument for an independent metrical representation, the syllable-position constraint, on sound errors, is not convincing either, but corroborating evidence comes from the results of the implicit priming experiments by Roelofs and Meyer (submitted). These findings suggest that speakers create metrical frames, which encode the number of syllables and the stress pattern, but not the syllable-internal structure. Thus, we assume that the information retrieved from the mental lexicon is more abstract than proposed in most other models of word form generation -- segments may be underspecified and metrical frames do not capture syllable-internal structure. There is preliminary evidence suggesting that segmental retrieval and the association of segments to syllables are distinct processes. Finally, I have presented linguistic arguments for the necessity of phonological decomposition. First, lexical entries are too abstract to guide pronunciation, and, second, the systematic contextual effects on the surface structure of morphemes can best be explained by assuming that certain rules apply to the morphemes' phonological constituents, which therefore must be made accessible to the processor.

Whether the view promoted here is compatible with the gestural framework described by Browman and Goldstein (this volume) remains to be seen. Perhaps a production model couched within the gestural framework can be developed. This would entail, among other things, that the strict distinction between a phonological and a phonetic level of encoding must be given up. Since the psycholinguistic evidence for this distinction is not compelling, this might be a wise move to take. Some findings might then receive a more natural account than in the Standard Model. One of them is that the error units in sound errors are variable: they are usually segments, but they can also be groups of segments or smaller units, corresponding to features or perhaps individual gestures. A related observation that is poorly accounted for in the Standard Model is that features are rarely error units themselves but influence which segments may interact with each other. In a gesture-based model one could view segmental and featural effects as related to different types of units within the same hierarchy. Other findings may be more problematic. For instance, how do sound anticipations and exchanges spanning several intervening sounds arise? And how can we explain Roelofs and Meyer's finding that participants had to know the entire metrical structure of the target words in order to prepare for their initial segments? The available evidence suggests that some of the form representations speakers create in preparing for an utterance are fairly abstract, and an adequate theory of speech planning must capture that.

REFERENCES

Abbs, J.H., & Gracco, V.L. (1984). Control of complex motor gestures: Orofacial muscle responses to load perturbations of lip during speech. *Journal of Neurophysiology, 51,* 705-723.

Abd-El-Jawad, H., & Abu-Salim, I. (1987). Slips of the tongue in Arabic and their theoretical implications. *Language Sciences, 9,* 145-171.

Archangeli, D. (1984). *Underspecification in Yawelmani phonology and morphology.* Doctoral dissertation. MIT: Cambridge, M.A. [Published 1986, New York: Garland]

Baumann, M. (1995). *The production of syllables in connected speech.* Doctoral dissertation. Nijmegen University.

Berg, T. (1985). Is voice a suprasegmental? *Linguistics, 23,* 883-915.

Berg, T. (1988). *Die Abbildung des Sprachproduktionsprozesses in einem Aktivationsfluss-modell:*

Untersuchungen an deutschen und englischen Versprechern. [The representation of the process of language production in a spreading activation model: Studies of German and English speech errors.] Tübingen: Niemeyer.

Berg, T. (1989). Intersegmental cohesiveness. *Folia Linguistica, 23,* 245-280.

Berg, T. (1991). Redundant-feature coding in the mental lexicon. *Linguistics, 29,* 903-925.

Berg, T. (1994). More on intersegmental cohesiveness. *Folia Linguistica, 28,* 257-278.

Boomer, D.S., & Laver, J.D.M. (1968). Slips of the tongue. *British Journal of Disorders of Communication, 3,* 2-12.

Browman, C.P., & Goldstein, L. (1988). Some notes on syllable structure in articulatory phonology. *Phonetica, 45,* 140-155.

Browman, C.P., & Goldstein, L. (this volume). The gestural phonology model. In W. Hulstijn, H.F.M. Peters, & P.H.H.M. Van Lieshout (Eds.), *Speech production: motor control, brain research and fluency disorders.* Amsterdam: Elsevier Science.

Butterworth, B., & Whittaker, S. (1980). Peggy Babcock's relatives. In G.E. Stelmach & J. Requin (Eds.) *Tutorials in motor behavior* (pp. 647-656). Amsterdam: North-Holland.

Clements, G.N., & Keyser, S.J. (1983). *CV-Phonology. A generative theory of the syllable.* Cambridge, MA: MIT Press.

Dell, G. (1986). A spreading-activation theory of retrieval in speech production. *Psychological Review, 93,* 283-321.

Folkins, J.W., & Abbs, J.H. (1975). Lip and jaw motor control during speech: responses to resistive loading of the jaw. *Journal of Speech and Hearing Research, 18,* 207-220.

Fowler, C.A. (1995). Speech production. In J.L. Miller & P.D. Eimas (Eds.), *Speech, language, and communication* (pp. 29-61). San Diego: Academic Press.

Frazier, L. (1995). Issues of representation in psycholinguistics. In J.L. Miller & P.D. Eimas (Eds.), *Speech, language, and communication* (pp. 1-27). San Diego: Academic Press.

Fromkin, V.A. (1971). The non-anomalous nature of anomalous utterances. *Language, 47,* 27-52.

Fromkin, V.A. (1973). Introduction. In V.A. Fromkin (Ed.), *Speech errors as linguistic evidence* (pp. 11-45). The Hague: Mouton.

García-Albea, J.E., del Viso, S., & Igoa, J.M. (1989). Movement errors and levels of processing in sentence production. *Journal of Psycholinguistic Research, 18,* 145-161.

Garrett, M.F. (1975). The analysis of sentence production. In G.H. Bower (Ed.), *The psychology of language and motivation* (Vol. 9, pp. 133-175). New York: Academic Press.

Garrett, M.F. (1976). Syntactic processes in sentence production. In R.J. Wales & E. Walker (Eds.), *New approaches to language mechanisms* (pp. 231-256). Amsterdam: North-Holland.

Garrett, M.F. (1980). Levels of processing in sentence production. In B. Butterworth (Ed.), *Language production: Vol 1. Speech and talk* (pp. 177-210). New York: Academic Press.

Giegerich, H.J. (1992). *English phonology. An introduction.* Cambridge, M.A.: University Press.

Goldsmith, J.A. (1990). *Autosegmental and metrical phonology.* Cambridge, MA: Blackwell.

Hendriks, H., & McQueen, J. (1996). *Annual Report 1995.* Nijmegen: Max Planck Institute for Psycholinguistics.

Kelso, J.A.S., Saltzman, E.L., & Tuller, B. (1986). The dynamical perspective on speech production: data and theory. *Journal of Phonetics, 14,* 29-59.

Kenstowicz, M. (1994). *Phonology in generative grammar.* Cambridge, MA: Blackwell.

Kiparski, P. (1985). Some consequences of lexical phonology. *Phonology Yearbook, 2,* 83-138.

Kubozono, H. (1989). The mora and syllable structure in Japanese: Evidence from speech errors. *Language and Speech, 32,* 249-278.

Lahiri, A., & Marslen-Wilson, W. (1991). The mental representation of lexical form: A phonological approach to the recognition lexicon. *Cognition, 38*, 245-294.

Levelt, W.J.M. (1989). *Speaking: From intention to articulation.* Cambridge, MA.: MIT Press.

Levelt, W.J.M. (1992). Accessing words in speech production: Stages, processes and representations. *Cognition, 42*, 1-22.

Levelt, W.J.M, & Wheeldon, L. (1994). Do speakers have access to a mental syllabary? *Cognition, 50*, 239-269.

Lindblom, B., Lubker, J., & Gay, T. (1979). Formant frequencies of some fixed-mandible vowels and a model of speech motor programming by predictive simulation. *Journal of Phonetics, 7*, 147-161.

MacKay, D.G. (1970). Spoonerisms: The structure of errors in the serial order of speech. *Neuropsychologia, 8*, 323-350.

MacKay, D.G. (1972). The structure of words and syllables: Evidence from errors in speech. *Cognitive Psychology, 3*, 210-227.

McCarthy, J. (1981). A prosodic theory of nonconcatenative morphology. *Linguistic Inquiry, 12*, 373-418.

Meyer, A.S. (1990). The time course of phonological encoding in language production: The encoding of successive syllables of a word. *Journal of Memory and Language, 29*, 524-545.

Meyer, A.S. (1991). The time course of phonological encoding in language production: Phonological encoding inside a syllable. *Journal of Memory and Language, 30*, 69-89.

Meyer, A.S., & Schriefers, H. (1991). Phonological facilitation in picture-word interference experiments: Effects of stimulus onset asynchrony and types of interfering stimuli. *Journal of Experimental Psychology: Learning, Memory, and Cognition, 17*, 1146-1160.

Mowrey, R.A., & MacKay, I.R.A. (1990). Phonological primitives: Electromyographic speech error evidence. *Journal of the Acoustical Society of America, 88*, 1299-1312.

Motley, M.T. (1973). An analysis of spoonerisms as psycholinguistic phenomena. *Speech Monographs, 40*, 66-71.

Nolan, F., Holst, T., & Kuehnert, B. (1996). Modelling [s] to [ʃ] accomodation in English. *Journal of Phonetics, 24*, 113-137.

Nooteboom, S.G. (1969). The tongue slips into patterns. In A.G. Sciarone, A.J. van Essen, & A.A. van Raad (Eds.), *Nomen: Leyden Studies in Linguistics and Phonetics* (pp. 114-132). The Hague: Mouton.

Picard, M. (1992). Syllable structure, sonority and speech errors: a critical assessment. *Folia Linguistica, 26*, 453-465.

Roelofs, A. (in press). Serial order in planning the production of successive morphemes of a word. *Journal of Memory and Language.*

Roelofs, A. (submitted). The WEAVER model of word-form encoding in speech production.

Roelofs, A. & Meyer, A.S. (submitted). Metrical structure in planning the production of spoken words.

Saltzman, E., & Kelso. J.A.S. (1987). Skilled actions: A task-dynamic approach. *Psychological Review, 94*, 84-106.

Schiller, N.O., Meyer, A.S., Baayen, R.H., & Levelt, W.J.M. (1996). A comparison of lexeme and speech syllables in Dutch. *Journal of Quantitative Linguistics, 3*.

Shattuck-Hufnagel, S. (1979). Speech errors as evidence for a serial-ordering mechanism in sentence production. In W.E. Cooper & E.C.T. Walker (Eds.), *Sentence processing: Psycholinguistic studies presented to Merrill Garrett* (pp. 295-342). Hillsdale, N.J.: Erlbaum.

Shattuck-Hufnagel, S. (1983). Sublexical units and suprasegmental structure in speech production planning. In P.F. MacNeilage (Ed.), *The production of speech* (pp. 109-136). New York: Springer.

Shattuck-Hufnagel, S. (1986). The representation of phonological information during speech production planning: evidence from vowel errors in spontaneous speech. *Phonology Yearbook, 3*, 117-149.

Shattuck-Hufnagel, S. (1987). The role of word-onset consonants in speech production planning. New evidence from speech error patterns. In E. Keller & M. Gopnik (Eds.), *Motor and sensory processes of language* (pp. 17-51). Hillsdale, NJ.: Erlbaum.

Shattuck-Hufnagel, S. (1992). The role of word structure in segmental serial ordering. *Cognition, 42*, 213-259.

Shattuck-Hufnagel, S., & Klatt, D.H. (1979). The limited use of distinctive features and markedness in speech production: Evidence from speech error data. *Journal of Verbal Learning and Verbal Behavior, 18*, 41-55.

Spencer, A. (1991). *Morphological theory. An introduction to word structure in generative grammar.* Cambridge, MA.: Blackwell.

Stemberger, J.P. (1982). The nature of segments in the lexicon: Evidence from speech errors. *Lingua, 56*, 43-65.

Stemberger, J.P. (1983). The nature of /r/ and /l/ in English: Evidence from speech errors. *Journal of Phonetics, 11*, 139-147.

Stemberger, J.P. (1984). Length as a suprasegmental: Evidence from speech errors. *Language, 60*, 895-913.

Stemberger, J.P. (1985). *The lexicon in a model of language production.* New York: Garland.

Stemberger, J.P. (1990). Wordshape errors in language production. *Cognition, 35*, 123-157.

Stemberger, (1991). Radical underspecification in language production. *Phonology, 8*, 73-112 (a).

Stemberger, (1991). Apparent anti-frequency effects in language production: The addition bias and phonological underspecification. *Journal of Memory and Language, 30*, 161-185 (b).

Stemberger, J.P. (1992). Vocalic underspecification in English language production. *Language, 68*, 492-524.

Stemberger, J.P, & Stoel-Gammon, C. (1991). The underspecification of coronals: Evidence from language acquisition and performance errors. *Phonetics and Phonology, 2*, 181-199.

Stevens, K.N. (1972). The quantal nature of speech: evidence from articulatory-acoustic data. In E.E. David & P.B. Denes (Eds.), *Human communication: a unified view* (pp. 51-66). New York: McGraw-Hill.

Turvey, M.T. (1990). Coordination. *American Psychologist, 45*, 938-953.

Wells, R. (1951). Predicting slips of the tongue. *Yale Scientific Magazine, 26*, 9-30. (Reprinted in V.A. Fromkin (Ed., 1973). *Speech errors as linguistic evidence* (pp. 82-87). The Hague: Mouton.)

Speech Production: Motor Control, Brain Research and Fluency Disorders
W. Hulstijn, H.F.M. Peters and P.H.H.M. Van Lieshout, editors

Chapter 6

STUTTERING AND MISGUIDED LEARNING OF ARTICULATION AND PHONATION, OR WHY IT IS EXTREMELY DIFFICULT TO MEASURE THE PHYSICAL PROPERTIES OF LIMBS

Karl Th. Kalveram, Ulrich Natke

The speech tract transforms muscle forces exerted on the articulatory system, larynx included, into actual speech sounds. Speaking then means to invert this transformation neurally. The related inverse model can be acquired by auto-imitation. In order to identify the control type of speaking, we tried to measure inertia, stiffness and damping of the jaw during speech. For these purposes, we applied an external force impuls to the jaw and recorded the related acceleration, velocity and position. This is an auto-imitation-like procedure and should provide the parameters looked for. However it turned out that mathematically the problem is ill-posed, whereby small errors in the recorded data will lead to big errors in the parameters to be estimated. Typical regularization methods failed. To get deeper insight into the problem we simulated a threejointed arm and the acquisition of its control. An exact solution of the inverse dynamics could only be obtained under conditions of noiseless feedback lines. However, already under moderate noise, in 5-10 percent of the simulation runs movement control was disrupted, which follows from the ill-posedness also present in this instance. We called this phenomenon 'misguided learning', and concluded that the organism is exposed to the same learning problem when trying to get control of the articulators, larynx included. This holds especially for children of about four years, when they learn to unstress initially stressed, but unimportant syllables. This demands a (second) auto-imitative process which is assumed to be misguided in a manner, that phonation occasionally is prevented. Taking into account models of prosody control and speech planning, it is argued that this could explain iterations of syllables.

INTRODUCTION

What is to be learned in speech production?

Performing a motor task can be considered as "using the own limbs as a tool". In speaking, for instance, this tool can be described by the 'speech tract transformation' (vocal tract transformation), which relates muscle forces exerted on the articulatory system, larynx included, to actual speech sounds defined auditorily. An example is given in Figure 1, which shows the simplified sound spectogram (sonogram) of the first three syllables of the word "supercalifragilisticexpialidocious".

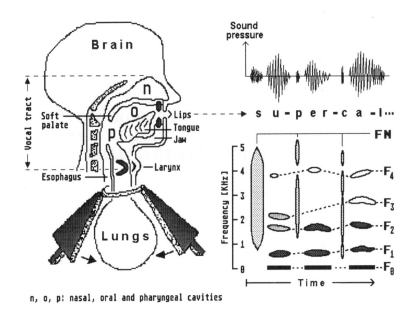

n, o, p: nasal, oral and pharyngeal cavities

Figure 1. Vocal tract, generating "supercalifragilisticexpialidocious", the sound pressure curve of which and the sonogramme of the first three syllables are sketched on the right-hand side. F0: Fundamental frequenency. F1 to F4: Formants. FN: Turbulence noise.

The acoustic outcome is produced by the speech tract consisting of the larynx, and the pharyngeal, oral and nasal cavities. Form and function of the speech tract is 'shaped' by the articulators, which are the vocal folds, soft palate, jaw, tongue and lips. These articulators in turn are driven by different muscles or groups of muscles.

In general, two kinds of tool transformations can be discriminated, namely the inner and the outer tool transformation. The inner tool transformation deals with neurally defined variables. It is that functional unit having the efferences into the muscles as input and exteroceptive afferences due to these efferences as output. The outer tool transformation then deals with physically defined variables and has the forces exerted by the muscles as input and the effect of the tool described in exteroceptive co-ordinates as output. For simplicity, in the present paper both transformations are considered to co-incide.

Speaking however starts with desired speech sounds, whereby the appropriate forces generating these sounds are to be specified subsequently. That is, the auditory targets are given first, and the neural controller has to find forces which influence the articulators so that the targets will be realized. In order to realize acoustic target figures, the speech tract transformation, therefore, must be inverted. Expressed in terms of control theorie: The speaker needs to acquire an internal representation of the inverse model of her or his speech tract.

The purpose of the present paper is to point to a specific difficulty associated with the acquisition of such an inverse model. Because of this difficulty the learning process necessary to acquire the inverse model can be 'misguided', resulting in an inappropriate representation of this model, what then can be related to stuttering.

How the inverse speech tract transformation can be learned

Figure 2b shows the principle of control of a plant by applying an inverse model of it. Expressed in terms of control theory, the tool transformation R describes the system to be controlled by the organism in a forward manner. Referring to figure 2b, this is expressed by $x(t) = R[Q(t)]$, where x represents the produced sound at the point of time t, R the tool transformation and Q(t) the momentary force input vector. x is a vector which has, according to figure 1, the components (F_0, F_1-F_4, F_N). Each component of the vector Q is thought to represent the force by which a distinct muscle is acting upon the articulatory system.

The inverse model of the tool transformation is called R^{-1} and is "stored" in the neural controller.

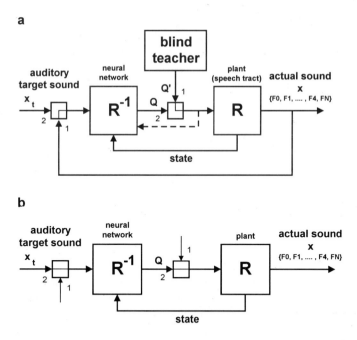

Figure 2: Block diagramme of controlling a plant. (a) learning to control a plant by auto-imitation. The blind teacher puts forces Q' into the plant descripted by the tool transformation R. The neural network observes these forces (dashed arrow) and relates them to the actual outcome x. The network "learns" the law by which the plant's output variable is connected to its input variable. (b) With switches brought into position 2, auditory target sounds xt can be realized.

Its input is the auditory target vector called x_t, and its output is the force vector Q. The inverse model of the speech tract transformation has to be acquired by learning. Figure 2a outlines a learning algorithm called "auto-imitation" (Kalveram, 1990), principally capable of implementing an inverse model of R into the neural controller. The training procedure takes place with all switches in position 1 and requires a "blind teacher" emitting arbitrary force values called Q' into the plant. These forces simultaneously serve also as teaching signals put into the network, as indicated by the dashed line. The network then observes the effect of the forces Q' fed through the plant R and returned by exteroception, and can thus learn the law by which the momentary effect is tied to the value of Q' originating this effect. However, to get an appropriate inverse model of R, the network generally needs to know the momentary physical state of the plant as well. In the present case, this state can be thought to be represented by mechanically defined variables like position and velocity of the articulators, measured by proprioception. Given all these conditions, R^{-1} can principally be acquired, but because of noisy signals the model acquired in this manner may deviate more or less from the true inverse R^{-1}. However, if the inverse model fits well, the unique physical properties of the vocal folds and the other articulators (for instance their mechanical impedance), and all the physical interdependencies between the articulators, vocal folds included, are automatically taken into account.

After learning, the switches are brought into position 2 and the acquired representation of the inverse model is ready to be applied, that is, if an exteroceptively defined target x_t is put in, forces Q appropriate to realize this target are put out. As indicated in figure 2b, also in the application phase the physical state of the plant is needed for proper operation.

Experimental procedure to test inverse modelling really applied in speaking

To analyze the type of control of speaking, we selected the jaw. In order to assess, how the limb under consideration is driven by muscular forces, it is inevitable to know the mechanical properties of the limb. Usually, mass M, (viscous) damping R, stiffness D and equilibrium point x_0 are considered to represent these properties. In a first approximation, the differential equation of the limb can be written as

(1) $M \cdot \ddot{x} + R \cdot \dot{x} + D \cdot (x - x_0) = K + Q$

where $\ddot{x}$, $\dot{x}$, x mean the momentary acceleration, velocity and position of the limb described in appropriate co-ordinates, K an external force (for instance an artificial perturbation) applied to the limb, and Q the resulting muscular force of agonist and antagonist, induced by efferences into these muscles. Thereby, it may happen that also R, D and x_0 are influenced by neural signals into the muscles, that is to say, the mechanical properties R, D and x_0 can also be subject to changes following neural innervation. Therefore, even if K=0 and Q=0 a movement can be initiated and maintained solely by shifting the equilibrium point x_0 from the actual to the desired position and using a stiffness $D > 0$. On the other hand, a movement can be stopped generating a high damping R.

The assessment of such mechanical effects on an ongoing movement demands to the measurement of M, R, D and x_0 while moving the limb. Attempts have been made to assess at least D on the basis of the quotient of maximum velocity/maximum displacement (Cooke, 1980). It should be noted, however, that this is an extremely poor measure, because neither D nor any other of the coefficients in (1) can really be measured unless a known external force K is applied to the limb causing an additional movement component overlaying the undisturbed movement caused by Q.

The method we used was to exert an external impuls K of force with known shape to the jaw and to record the related acceleration, velocity and position. The experimental equipment has already been described in previous papers (Bauer et al., 1995). Analyzing the additional movement due to K should make it possible to get values for the mechanical properties valid at the moment about the onset of the disturbing force: Modifying (1) one yields

$$(2) \quad M \cdot \ddot{x} + R \cdot \dot{x} + D \cdot x - D \cdot x_0 - Q = K$$

Assuming K starts at t_0 and ends at t_4, and t_1, t_2, t_3 being temporal points appropriately inserted between t_0 and t_4, then $\ddot{x}$, $\dot{x}$, x and K must be measured at t_i, $i = 1, 2, 3, 4$. This yields a linear inhomogeneous equation system consisting of four equations with these measured values as coefficients and the unknowns M, R, D and $D.X_0$-Q. Preposing the unknowns are constant during the impuls, it should be possible to compute them. Obviously, the situation is quite similar to auto-imitation, whereby the experimenter plays the role of the "blind teacher" of figure 2a, when he applies the additional known force to the jaw and records the related movement data .

In order to suppress noise, (2) can be integrated by part, for instance:

$$(3) \quad M \int_{t_0}^{t_i} \ddot{x} \cdot dt + R \int_{t_0}^{t_i} \dot{x} \cdot dt + D \int_{t_0}^{t_i} x \cdot dt - D \cdot x_0 \, \Delta t - Q \cdot \Delta t = \int_{t_0}^{t_i} K \cdot dt$$

where t_i ($i = 0, 1, \ldots, 4$) are defined as above, and $\Delta t = t_4 - t_0$ .Again, one gets a system of four inhomogeneous linear equations which should be solvable by standard methods (for other algorithms cf. Natke & Kalveram, 1996).

However, it turned out that the solution of this equation system is a highly 'ill-posed problem' (Hadamard, 1923), which means in the present instance, that the determinant of the 4 by 4 matrix of coefficients describing the system of linear equations derived from (3) is close to zero. This in turn causes that small errors in the coefficients will lead to big errors in the unknowns to be estimated. Typical regularization methods usually diminishing those errors (Baumeister, 1987; Louis, 1989) failed, and we were completely unable to get any plausible values for the mechanical parameters of the jaw using this method.

Simulation experiment using a three-jointed arm

As mentioned above, attributing the external force K to a 'blind teacher' (force Q' in figure 2a), and zeroing additional muscle forces (force Q), reveals that the method we used to destine the physical parameters of the jaw obviously equals auto-imitation learning (see figure 2a). Therefore, the same ill-posed problem should occur in both cases. This was the reason why we switched over to simulations of a three-jointed arm confined in a plane and its control by an artificial neural network (power net, see Kalveram, 1993b) to get deeper insight into the problem.

From a theoretical point of view, the inverse model can be represented using different mathematical methods, and different algorithms can be used to compute an appropriate set of parameters adapting the model to the modelled original. Neilson et al. (1992) proposed, for instance, a method derived from adaptive filter theory. The method used in the present paper is a least squares approximation, applied to a system of linear equations resembling (2), however with much more unknowns, the number of which equalling the number of hidden nodes applied in the power net.

The three-jointed arm was taken because of its redundant degrees of freedom, a matter of fact which also applies to the speech tract, and because we had some experiences concerning a similar plant, the two-jointed arm (Kalveram, 1991b). The architecture of the network was also similar to that in Kalveram (1993a) and consisted of nine inputs (three for the target values of angular acceleration, and six for feedback of angular position and velocity), 48 hidden neurons representing the terms in the related system of three differential equations governing the dynamics of the physical system, and three output neurons providing the forces respectively torques about the three joints. Gravitation has not been taken into consideration. Applying the algorithm called auto-imitative learning (see for instance Kalveram, 1993a), three systems of linear equations, each with 48 unknowns representing the synaptic weights of the respective output neuron, were to be solved. For that, the blind teacher emitted a test movement, during which 100 data vectors were sampled, leading to an overdetermined system of linear equations for each joint. An exact and unique solution of the inverse dynamics, however, could only be obtained without any noise in the feedback lines. The 3x48 synaptic weights yielded without noise were ordered with respect to their absolute values, and the first 44 of the weights ordered in this manner are shown in figure 3 (black boxes). When adding noise, even of low intensity, it turned out, that each run resulted in a different set of weights only partly related to the original ones, but nevertheless enabling movement control in 90-95% of the simulated cases using the same scenario. Noise was normally distributed, with a standard deviation $SD_N = 0.01; SD_0$, where SD_0 means the standard deviation of the angular position respectively velocity values of signals obtained without noise. Figure 3a shows an instance of such a simulation run, where noise was added to the angular position and velocity feedback signals during learning, that is, during data sampling.

In the remaining 5-10% of cases using the same scenario, however, movement control was seriously deteriorated or even disrupted.

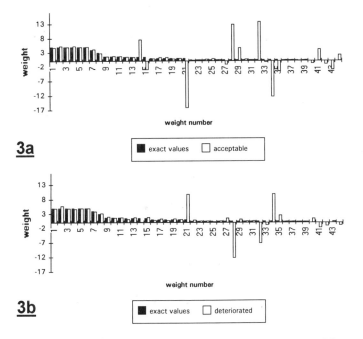

3a

3b

Figure 3. Estimated parameters ("synaptic weights" 1 to 44 of the output layer of the controlling power network) representing the physical (dynamic) properties of the three-jointed arm. Black rectangles: Exact values, obtained without noise and ordered with respect to absolute size. White rectangles: Related values obtained under noisy feedback of the state variables 3a: Control performance acceptable. 3b: Control performance deteriorated. (For more information see text).

Figure 3b outlines an example of a simulation run with such an outcome, though the irregular weights were lower on average than in figure 3a representing acceptable performance. In figure 3a as well as in figure 3b, noisy feedback in the learning stage obviously causes extraordinarily high synaptic weights at locations, where only low values should occur. These locations seemingly were selected at random and varied from one simulation run to another. This phenomenon is likely to be associated with ill-posed learning problems. However, not the absolute magnitude of the irregular weights, but rather their positions determine whether acceptable control performance is given or not. Therefore, at first sight it cannot be decided whether the result of a learning process would lead to an acceptable or a deteriorated performance. If the latter happens, we speak about "misguided learning". We took the notation 'misguided', because it seems to us that noise can occasionally mislead the learning process, such that a local but relative small maximum of performance is reached, which however cannot be left even if the absolute maximum is located in the neighborhood. Thereby, increasing the noise ratio SD_N/SD_0 from 0.001 to 0.05 in different simulation runs didn't essentially enlarge the number of runs with seriously disturbed performance. At present, we are searching for training algorithms capable to overcome these learning difficulties from a theoretical point of view. We suppose that low learning rates, high motor variability, and a large number of repetitions are pre-requisits to prevent faulty estimations of movement related parameters.

DISCUSSION, CONCLUSIONS

Obviously, the organism is exposed to the same kind of ill posed learning problems when trying to get control of limbs (speech tract and larynx), as we were when trying to estimate the parameters of the jaw. We suppose that concerning the problem of generating an invert model of the vocal tract, especially the activity of the vocal folds is very difficult to embedd into the activity of the remaining articulators, subjecting the learning process to particular misguidance. A sometimes occuring incomplete closure of the vocal folds or an adduction too strong to allow airflow may be the result of such a misguided learning. In both instances however the production of phonation is prevented, causing dysfluent speech in a low, but significant number of cases. Thereby, due to the variability of the learning process, each case can have its own "signature". Misguided learning therefore may account for all the various differences between stutterers and nonstutterers on a low level of sensory motor control, reported in great a number of articles (for overview see Van Lieshout, 1995).

In Kalveram (1991b) a model of speech production has been presented making plausible that, when the auditory feedback of the phonation related to the vowel of a syllable is missed, iterations of that syllable can occur - if the syllable is stressed. This relates a typical symptom of stuttering to misguided learning as well as to prosodic features of speaking (cf. Jaencke et al. 1996) and even to higher order speech motor programming and planning processes (Bosshardt, 1993; Peters et al., 1989, Van Lieshout et al., 1991).

Further, there are hints, that regarding the acquisiton of speech, two auto-imitation-like processes are to be expected (Kalveram, 1996). The first is assumed to take place in young children below the age of 3-4 years, enabling the "first speech". First speech when established can be characterized by a very precise articulation, a similar pronunciation of almost all syllables in a word, and - we suppose - auditory feedback of the vowel related phonation always being necessary for proper phonation. Speech rate however is low. Most of the children seem to acquire the first speech, mastering the fluency problems due to misguided learning without considerable remnants. About an age of four years, the "second speech" is acquired, the characteristic feature of which being a rised speech rate obtained by partly automatizing speech, that is, mainly by unstressing less important syllables of words (Allan & Hawkins, 1980; Kalveram, 1996). Unstressing of syllables however means, that a new style of control of the vocal folds respectively the laryngeal muscles must be learnt, by which the effect of auditory feedback on the duration of phonation must be suppressed. In terms of low level learning (Kalveram, 1993), this demands a second auto-imitation process the outcome of which again is subject to misguidance. At this stage of speech development a considerable portion of the children (about 4 per cent) do not succeed completely and will get long lasting fluency problems.

At last, audio-phonatory (audio-phonatoric) coupling is considered. As outlined previously (cf. Kalveram & Jaencke, 1989), in normal speakers shortly delayed auditory feedback (20 to 60 ms) causes a lengthening of the duration of (vowel related) phonation (on-time, vowel duration, OT) of the stressed syllable in a word, compared with the OT under simultaneous auditory feedback. However, the OT of the unstressed syllables is nearly unaffected by delayed auditory feedack. On the other hand, premature auditory feedback shortens the OT for the stressed syllables, but not for the unstressed ones. This can be explained by the assumption that the neural controller responsible for the OT usually must be shifted between two modes of operation during speech. The first mode is applied in stressed syllables. In this mode, auditory feedback from the beginning of the (vowel related) phonation shortens the on-time of the neural timer controlling the duration of the ongoing phonation, and the sooner (with respect to the real beginning of phonation) auditory feedback reaches this timer, the greater is the shortening. In the second mode, which is in operation when the unstressed syllable is being spoken, no auditory feedback is required for the well-timed termination of the OT. In the latter mode, therefore, vowel duration takes place in a preprogrammed (automatical) way, and auditory feedback has no immediate effect on vowel duration. Thus, auditory signals affect the ongoing process of phonation in a reflex-like manner, a phenomenon we called 'audio-phonatory coupling' (APC), the coupling strength being high in stressed and low in unstressed syllables. Stutterers, however, show remarkable delay effects not only on stressed but also on unstressed syllables, which leads to the conclusion that regarding stutterers the coupling strength is very high in stressed and high in unstressed syllables.

These findings can be taken as a clue that stutterers failed to acquire the complete automatization of the utterance of linguistically unstressed syllables (that is, cannot make the utterance of unstressed syllables independent from auditory feedback), and that in stutterers learning of the "second speech" indeed could have been misguided.

REFERENCES

Allen, G.D., & Hawkins, S. (1980). Phonological Rythm: Definition and development. In G.H. Yeni-Komshian, J.F. Kavanagh, & C.A. Ferguson (Eds.), *Child Phonology, Vol. 1: Production* (pp.227-256). New York: Academic Press

Bauer, A., Jäncke, L., & Kalveram, K.Th. (1995). Mechanical perturbation of the jaw movement during speech: Effect on articulation and phonation. *Perceptual and Motor Skills, 80,* 1108-1112

Baumeister, J., Stable (1987). Solutions of Inverse Problems. Braunschweig: Vieweg

Bosshardt, H.G. (1993). Differences between stutterers' and nonstutterers' short term recall and recognition performance. *Journal of Speech and Hearing Research, 36,* 286-293

Cooke, J.D. (1980). The organization of simple skilled movements. In G.E. Stelmach, & J. Requin (Eds.), *Tutorials in motor behavior.* Amsterdam: Elsevier (pp. 199-212)

Jaencke L., Bauer A., & Kalveram K.Th. (this volume). Prosodic disturbances in stuttering adults. In

W. Hulstijn, H.F.M. Peters, & P.H.H.M. Van Lieshout (Eds.), *Speech production motor control, brain research and fluency disorders*. Amsterdam: Elsevier Science.

Hadamard, J. (1923). Lectures on the Cauchy problem in linear partial differential equations. New Haven: Yale University Press

Kalveram, K.Th. (1991a). How pathological audio-phonatoric coupling induces stuttering: A model of speech flow control. In H.F.M. Peters, W.H. Hulstijn, & C.W. Starkweather (Eds.), *Speech motor control and stuttering*. Amsterdam: Elsevier Science Publishers, pp. 163-170

Kalveram, K.Th. (1991b). Controlling the dynamics of a two-jointed arm by central patterning and reflex-like processing. A two-stage hybrid model. *Biological Cybernetics, 65*, 65-71

Kalveram, K.Th. (1993a). A neural-network model enabling sensorimotor learning: Application to the control of arm movements and some implications for speech motor control and stuttering. *Psychological Research, 55*, 299-314

Kalveram, K.Th. (1993b). Power series and neural-net computing. *Neurocomputing, 5*, 165-174

Kalveram, K.Th. (1996). Zur Theorie und Therapie des Stotterns (Engl. titel: Theory and therapy of stuttering). Sprache-Stimme-Gehör (in press).

Kalveram, K.Th., & Jäncke, L. (1989). Vowel duration and voice onset time for stressed and nonstressed syllables in stutterers under delayed auditory feedback condition. *Folia Phoniatrica, 15*, 30-42

Louis, A.K. (1989). Inverse und schlecht gestellte Probleme. Stuttgart: Teubner

Natke, U., & Kalveram, K.Th. (1996). Misguided motor learning as a consequence of illposedness. (in preparation)

Neilson, P.D., Neilson M.D., & O'Dwyer N.J. (1992). Adaptive model theory: Application to disorders of motor control. In J.J. Summers (Ed.), *Approaches to the study of motor control and learning*. Elsevier, Amsterdam: Elsevier Science Publishers

Peters, H.F.M., Hulstijn, W., & Starkweather, C.W. (1989). Acoustic and physiological reaction time of stutterers and nonstutterers. *Journal of Speech and Hearing Research, 32*, 668-680

Van Lieshout, P.H.H.M. Hulstijn W., & Peters, H.F.M. (1991). Word size and word complexity: Differences in speech reaction time between stutterers and nonstutterers in a picture and word naming task. In H.F.M Peters, W. Hulstijn, & C.W. Starkweather (Eds.), *Speech motor control and stuttering* (pp. 311-325). Amsterdam: Elsevier Science Publishers

Van Lieshout, P.H.H.M. (1995) Motor planning and articulation in fluent speech of stutterers and nonstutterers (Thesis University of Nijmegen). Nijmegen: University Press

Speech Production: Motor Control, Brain Research and Fluency Disorders
W. Hulstijn, H.F.M. Peters and P.H.H.M. Van Lieshout, editors

Chapter 7

FUNCTIONAL COMPONENTS OF THE MOTOR SYSTEM: AN APPROACH TO UNDERSTANDING THE MECHANISMS OF SPEECH DISFLUENCY

Michael D. McClean

A functional model of the motor system is described that is intended as a framework for computational modeling and simulation of the neural mechanisms underlying speech disfluency. The central component of the model is pattern generating circuitry (PGC) that regulates motoneuron activity for speech. The PGC is distributed within the motor systems of the brain, and it receives input from a variety of neural systems whose functions include pattern selection, sensory processing, regulation of speech rate, regulation of muscle stiffness, and mediation of emotional-motivational responses. Theory and data relevant to understanding PGC function in speech are reviewed, and various sources of PGC input are considered in order to clarify their relevance to speech disfluency. Normal speech production is assumed to involve the interaction of different inputs within the PGC in order to produce intended speech acoustic patterns. It is suggested that speech disfluency is related to the interaction of various inputs within the PGC primarily during speech movement preparation and initiation. Given the number and complexity of neural systems involved, it is not surprising that high levels of variability are seen in physiologic measures of the fluent and disfluent speech of persons who stutter. The general framework proposed is intended to provide a basis for development of biologically-constrained models that will clarify the sources of this variability.

INTRODUCTION

A central issue for research on stuttering concerns the nature of processes within the CNS that underlie speech disfluency. The goals of this paper are to better define this problem and to present a general hypothesis on the neural mechanisms of speech disfluency. This hypothesis is developed in the context of a simplified model of the speech neuromotor system as schematized in Figure 1. The central component of the model is pattern-generating neuronal circuitry (PGC) whose primary function is coding of the temporal-spatial characteristics of neural spike train patterns affecting motoneuron discharge for speech; that is, production of speech motor commands. The PGC receives input from converging neural systems which involve pattern selection, sensory processing, speech-rate regulation, muscle-stiffness regulation, and mediation of emotional-motivational state. During normal speech production, input from these systems interacts within the PGC in order to produce the intended acoustic patterns in the most efficient manner given the prevailing performance constraints (e.g., body posture and time demands). It should be noted that all possible lines of communication have not been identified in Figure 1. This focus on PGC function reflects the view that current research efforts need to emphasize the nature of PGC involvement in speech production and how different sources of input interact within the PGC to contribute to speech disfluency.

The general hypothesis developed here is that speech disfluency is the result of interactions of the different sources of input within the PGC which lead to conditions that distort or disable the intended speech motor output. This perspective highlights the difficulty in developing simple explanations of how speech disfluency is affected by any single aspect of PGC system input (e.g., speech rate or level of emotional arousal), since it is the interaction of different sources of input and the state of the PGC as a whole that are critical. Given the number and complexity of neural systems involved, it should not be surprising that there is considerable inter- and intra-subject variability in the frequency and form of speech disfluency among individuals who stutter. In order to understand this variability, comprehensive computational models of the speech neuromotor system are required that incorporate the range of systems outlined in Figure 1. Computational neuroscience has reached a stage of development where modeling of this type should be both feasible and productive. This claim is supported by recent progress made in computational modeling of neural processes underlying speech and voice production (Farley, 1994; Guenther, 1994; Perrier et al., 1996) and motor cortical and cerebellar activity regulating limb movement (e.g., Bertheir et al., 1993; Fetz, 1993; Kettner et al., 1993).

PATTERN GENERATING CIRCUITRY FOR SPEECH

There is a long rich history associated with the study of neural pattern generators in motor control. While research in this area has focused on relatively simple forms of

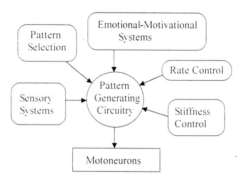

Figure 1. Functional model of the motor system. All possible lines of connection are not indicated, since the emphasis here is on pattern generating circuitry.

invertebrate behavior, there are general principles of pattern-generator organization and function which clearly apply to both vertebrate and invertebrate nervous systems (Pearson, 1993) and are relevant to speech motor control. For example, mechanisms involving neural inhibition are widely observed in pattern generating circuits, and it is likely that they are critical for shaping the patterns of neural activity underlying speech production.

The fact that we can readily repeat any given phonetic sequence in a highly automatic manner suggests that some form of pattern-generating circuitry operates in the neural control of speech production. Interest in pattern generating circuitry with respect to speech motor control is derived in part from parallels drawn with rhythmic animal movements such as locomotion and mastication (Gracco & Abbs, 1988; Grillner, 1981; Lund et al., 1981). It seems unlikely that any of these behaviors involve dedicated neural circuitry; instead, relevant circuits most likely are distributed over large groups of neurons that are altered or reorganized for different behaviors (cf. Morton & Chiel, 1994). Relative to speech, locomotion and mastication have a limited range of behavioral goals, but each must be highly adaptable to sensory input which signals changes in environmental condition (e.g., alterations in terrain or oral contents). In contrast, the critical aspect of adaptability for speech relates to specification of a wide range of phonetic patterns required for language expression, although adaptability to environmental conditions clearly is also required.

It is likely that pattern generating circuity regulating speech production is widely distributed in the motor cortex (Abbs & Welt, 1985); this includes primary motor cortex, Broca's area, and the supplementary motor area (SMA). In addition to the motor cortex, there is good reason to expect a major contribution from the cerebellum. Over the course of human evolution, the lateral cerebellar hemispheres have grown dramatically in size along with the neocortex (Eccles, 1989; Llinas & Walton, 1990). There is anatomical evidence for extensive communication between motor cortex and cerebellum (Allen & Tsukahara, 1974), and this is consistent with the view that the control of volitional movements is achieved by means of parallel cooperative processing in cortical and cerebellar circuits (Cheney et al., 1988; Fetz et al., 1989; Martin & Ghez, 1988). The regulatory effects of these circuits are mediated over cortical and rubral pathways which represent the two major descending tracts of the motor system. PET-scan data show elevated levels of activity in both motor cortex and cerebellum during speech production (Fox et al., 1996; Petersen et al., 1990; Tamas et al., 1993), and as noted in several reports given at this conference, abnormal levels and patterns of cortical and cerebellar activity have been observed during disfluent and fluent speech of persons who stutter.

The view taken here is that Broca's area is especially important in motor pattern selection for speech (see later discussion of pattern selection), while the temporal-spatial fine structure of speech motor programs could be achieved by a variety of other cortical, cerebellar, and midbrain structures. A critical role for cerebellar circuitry in regulation of speech timing is suggested by data on speech motor performance in individuals with cerebellar lesions (e.g., Ackermann et al., 1995; Kent et al., 1979). Also, there is recent evidence that the midbrain periaqueductal gray plays an important role in coordination of

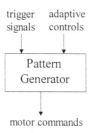

Figure 2. Basic elements of the adjustable pattern generator or APG (adapted from Houk, 1986).

laryngeal, respiratory, and orofacial muscles for vocalization and possibly speech (Zhang et al., 1994).

As suggested above, phonetic encoding for speech production requires a high degree of adaptability of the motor system. In light of this, a general concept which appears well suited for understanding the neural basis of PGC function for speech is the adjustable pattern generator (APG) developed by Houk and his colleagues (Houk, 1987; Houk et al., 1993). As summarized in Figure 2, the APG is seen as an autonomous set of circuits which receive input from triggering and adaptive controls, and which generate outputs in the form of motor commands that regulate motoneuron discharge.

Trigger signals can involve either sensory cues or internal commands. In the case of well-learned movements, adaptive control input involves motor program selection, which presets or tunes the excitability levels of sensorimotor pathways required to execute the intended movement. The PGC for speech production presumably consists of large arrays of APGs which are somatotopically organized in relation to the relevant muscle groups and mechanoreceptor systems.

Houk and his colleagues have utilized the APG concept as a framework for modeling how the motor cortex and cerebellum function to translate motor programs to motor commands. A working hypothesis on how the motor cortex and cerebellum function in parallel to translate motor programs to motor commands has recently been proposed in the form of a computational model that uses the APG concept as the framework for its design (Berthier et al., 1993; Houk et al., 1993). The basic elements of this model are summarized in Figure 3. In this scheme, learned motor programs, acquired under strong control from the climbing fiber system are stored in the cerebellar cortex (Ito, 1993; Llinas & Walton, 1990). The translation of these programs to motor commands requires program selection (adaptive controls in Figure 2) which is mediated over the parallel fiber system. Movement initiation involves the generation of sensory or internal cues (trigger signal in Figure 2) which activate positive feedback in recurrent loops. These recurrent loops are formed between motor cortex, cerebellar nuclei, and red nucleus, and they are assumed to provide the elevated levels of neural activity associated with motor commands. The temporal-spatial patterning of motor commands is determined by inhibitory input from cerebellar Purkinje cells.

The model of Houk et al. (1993) incorporates distinct neurophysiologic mechanisms for

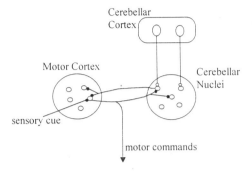

Figure 3. Adjustable pattern generator APG as realized in the interconnection between motor cortex and cerebellum (adapted from Houk et al., 1993). Small filled circles indicate excitatory connections, and small unfilled circles indicate inhibitory connections. The excitatory loop formed between the motor cortex and cerebellar nuclei represents a positive feedback loop whose output is shaped by inhibitory input from cerebellar Purkinje cells.

movement programming and initiation, and this distinction is used to account for certain results from reaction time experiments. Their approach has implications for studies of reaction time in stuttering, because it suggests a way of understanding, in biologic terms, individual differences in reaction time as well as the longer reaction times widely observed in stutterers as a group (e.g., Van Lieshout et al., 1996). With respect to the mechanisms of speech disfluency, if a critical aspect of motor system disfunction relates to problems with movement initiation, then the above model would implicate the triggering function associated with the recurrent loops identified in Figure 3. Another possibility is that disfluent utterances reflect aberrant learned motor programs, which implies anomalies in the adaptive-control function mediated over cerebellar cortex.

Accepting the assumption that the cerebellum is important for normal PGC function in speech production, the question arises as to the specific neuronal mechanisms involved. Recently several computational models of cerebellar-mediated control have been proposed that address this problem in different ways (Berthier, et al., 1993; Buonomano & Mauk, 1994; Chauvet, 1986; Chapeau-Blondeau & Chauvet, 1991). As background for discussion of these models, a brief review is given here of some critical features of cerebellar anatomy. Figure 4 shows the structure of what is often considered the basic unit of the cerebellar cortex, that is, a single Purkinje cell and the set of neurons that are directly and indirectly connected to it. Afferent input to Purkinje units is provided by mossy fibers and climbing fibers, and the sole efferent pathway is established by the Purkinje cell axons. Mossy fibers send excitatory projections to both granule and Golgi cells. Granule cells have excitatory connections to Golgi cells which have reciprocal inhibitory projections back to the granule cells. The granule-Golgi cell loop can be thought of as a distributed negative feedback circuit, with its gain level being controlled by mossy fiber input (Chauvet & Chapeau-Blondeau, 1991). Climbing fiber input to Purkinje cells originates from the inferior olive which receives indirect input from motor cortex, brainstem, spinal cord, and cerebellar nuclei.

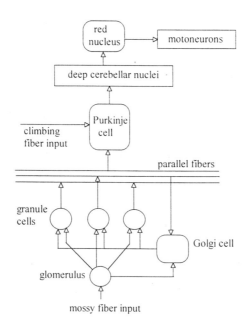

Figure 4. Schematic of cerebellar circuitry associated with a Purkinje unit (adapted from Chapeau-Blondeau & Chauvet, 1991).

Purkinje cells have exclusively inhibitory effects on deep cerebellar nuclei which in turn provide excitatory input to the rednucleus. The basic Purkinje cell unit repeats itself up to 15 million times in humans (Llinas & Walton, 1990) and displays a strong somatotopic organization throughout the cerebellar cortex. Specific regions of cerebellar cortex are given over to orofacial sensorimotor processing and these include cells that are responsive to both somatosensory and auditory input (Bower & Woolston, 1987; Huang et al., 1991). The observations of Huang et al. are particularly relevant to speech control. They observed that auditory-responsive cells are distributed in distinct patches within cerebellar cortex, and these patches tend to be surrounded by cells responsive to mechanical stimulation of the orofacial region.

This supports a role for the cerebellum in integration of auditory and somatosensory input in the motor control of speech and vocalization.

The model of Chauvet and Chapeau-Blondeau is reviewed here to provide an example of how we may come to understand the neural mechanisms of timing control for speech. The model makes explicit use of neural propagation delays and negative-feedback loops within the Golgi-granule cell system to represent temporal patterns. The basic idea underlying their model is that the production of temporal patterns is regulated by the spatial distribution of mossy fiber input to the granule-Golgi cell layer.

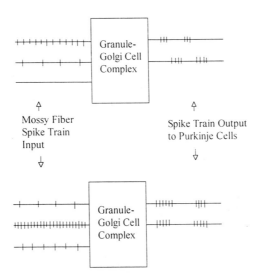

Figure 5. Schematic of how the temporal pattern of granule-cell output to Purkinje cells varies with the pattern of static discharge across different mossy fiber inputs according to model of Chapeau-Blondeau & Chauvet, 1991.

Mossy-fiber input takes the form of static or tonic discharge patterns with a spatial distribution that determines the specifics of temporal-spatial coding at the level of granule cell input to the Purkinje cell layer. This variation in the temporal pattern of granule-cell output emerges from inherent delay properties in the granule-Golgi cell feedback loop. The input-output characteristics of this control system are schematized in Figure 5, which shows how different spatial patterns of tonic input from themossy fiber system produce different temporal patterns of output from granule cells. Within the complete cerebellar system model of Chauvet and Chapeau-Blondeau, learning of actual motor commands occurs at the Purkinje cell level under the control of sensory input mediated over the climbing fiber system. The likely mechanism for such learning, as suggested by Ito (1993) and others, is long-term depression in Purkinje cells due to simultaneous climbing fiber and mossy fiber input. In the case of speech acquisition where the system is still learning what represents the appropriate or intended motor output, patterns of sensory input associated with speech disfluency might have an important conditioning effect on development or "hard wiring" of motor programs.

   Clearly, it is too early to draw definitive conclusions from the above types of model about specific mechanisms of speech disfluency. However, as future work on computational modeling of the motor system progresses, it should provide a framework for modeling PGC function in speech. This could permit simulation of how various inputs to the PGC contribute to the type of output patterns underlying disfluent speech. In the remainder of the paper, the different sources of PGC input outlined in Figure 1 will be discussed briefly in order to clarify their potential relevance for affecting PGC function and the mechanisms of speech disfluency.

MOTOR PATTERN SELECTION

In terms of speech production, motor pattern selection refers to neural encoding that specifies the intended phonetic-prosodic characteristics of speech utterances. This is analogous to the adaptive control process identified in Figure 2, as well as the concept of motor program assembly used by Van Lieshout et al. (1995). As to the neural correlates of pattern selection for speech, it is very likely that the process engages selected regions of the motor cortex and particularly Broca's area (Abbs, 1986; Abbs & Welt, 1985). Accepting the view developed above that the cerebellar cortex is especially important to PGC function for speech, intended phonologic-phonetic strings would be encoded in part in indirect transmission from the motor cortex to the cerebellar cortex. Ultimately, comprehensive computational models of speech motor processing and new empirical data will be required to work out the nature of cerebral-cerebellar communication in terms of what aspects of phonetic encoding and movement-parameter specification are performed in parallel or independently in each brain region.

It is known that phonetic structure is a major variable affecting the probability of speech disfluency (e.g., Peters & Hulstijn, 1987). Here the critical question concerns how pattern selection relative to phonetic structure contributes to the neural mechanisms of disfluency. At least three possibilities present themselves. First, the neural correlates of intended phonetic sequences may be incomplete, resulting in ineffective motor programs. This seems especially likely during language acquisition, and this hypothesis is addressed in part by research on phonologic processing and speech acquisition in young children who stutter (see related papers in this volume). Pattern selection could also contribute to speech disfluency through interaction with sensory input within the PGC. Because of their kinematic and aerodynamic characteristics, particular speech sounds such as voiceless obstruents are likely to contribute to elevated levels of somatosensory input. For individuals with deficits in the regulation of sensorimotor gain, this may result in excessive driving of the PGC and relevant motoneurons. An additional way that pattern selection might contribute to speech disfluency is through interaction with emotional-motivational systems; for example, a history of disfluency with particular speech sounds could contribute to heightened levels of emotional arousal that in turn lead to instability in PGC function. It is plausible that any of these mechanisms might function within a given individual at different times during their stuttering history.

SPEECH RATE CONTROL

Slowing speech rate continues to be a primary means for reducing the frequency of speech disfluency. However, because we have limited understanding of the neuromotor mechanisms of speech rate control, the theoretical basis for speech rate manipulation in stuttering therapy remains limited.

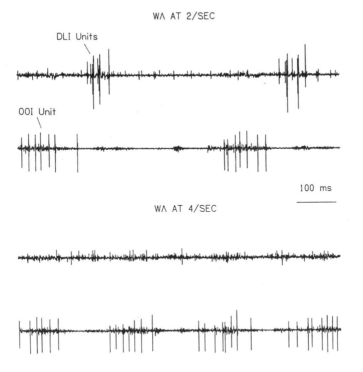

Figure 6. Recordings of lip-muscle EMG showing shutdown in a group of depressor labii inferior (DLI) motor units and continued bursting of an orbicularis oris inferior (OOI) motor unit with increased syllable rate from 2 to 4 syl/s (from McClean & Clay, 1995).

A critical question in efforts to understand rate control function in speech concerns how variations in rate are encoded in the nervous system to affect the overall cycle rate of PGC output. In computer simulations of neural oscillators, this is typically achieved by varying the level of tonic input to some form of PGC. In these cases, the intrinsic structure of the PGC is such that the overall cycle rate of the output pattern varies with the level of tonic input. Several examples now exist in the modeling literature where neural networks have been set up or undergone learning routines to produce control systems of this type (Bullock & Grossberg, 1988; Fetz, 1993; Williams & Zipser, 1989).

Accepting the assumption that rate control signals are encoded as changes in tonic input levels to the PGC, we can gain insight into the neural mechanisms of speech rate control by examining associated muscle activation patterns. Descriptive studies of this type in relation to locomotion indicate that with changes in overall movement rate there are changes in the patterns of muscle activation. This suggests that the peripheral mechanisms of movement control vary markedly across rates (e.g., Smith et al., 1993). Recently we observed similar variation in orofacial muscle activity with changes in the speech rate (McClean & Clay, 1995). EMG recordings of lip muscle single motor units revealed nonlinearities and

discontinuities in system output as subjects repeated simple syllables at rates of 1-4 syl/s. An example of this is given in Figure 6, which shows how a group of phasically active lip opening motor units (DLI) shutdown at high speech rates, while a motor unit activated for lip rounding (OOI) shows distinct bursts associated with each syllable at both rates. It is uncertain whether the control mechanism underlying this type of muscle activation
pattern is due to central (e.g., cerebellar) versus brain stem circuitry, but it does indicate a shift in the mechanism of movement control with variations in speech rate. This interpretation is consistent with the results of recent studies of orofacial movement that show marked differences in kinematic patterns at different speech rates (Adams et al., 1993; McClean, 1996a; Smith et al., 1995). These studies indicate that orofacial kinematics associated with slowed speech are especially distinctive.

Because of its fluency-inducing effects, slowed speech has obvious relevance here. In extreme cases, the temporal structure of slowed speech sounds like the scanning speech associated with cerebellar ataxia. As normal prosody is lost in cases of cerebellar ataxia, multi word utterances tend to be produced as strings of isolated words with retention of normal spatial characteristics for individual speech sounds (Kent et al., 1979). This raises the possibility that fluency-inducing effects of slowed speech are related to an alteration in the mode of interaction between motor cortex and cerebellum in controlling speech motor commands. It may also be that the fluency-inducing effects of slowed speech are related to system interactions with the sensory system. For example, reduced velocities typically are associated with slowed speech, and this presumably would condition reduced levels of somatosensory input with its possibility for perturbing input (cf. Zimmermann, 1980).

SENSORY SYSTEMS

There is now considerable evidence that prior to the onset of voluntary limb movements there is a reduction in the excitability of somatosensory pathways that normally provide feedback to different levels of the motor system (e.g., Cohen & Starr, 1987; Jiang et al., 1991; Kristeva-Feige et al., 1996). It has been suggested that a similar type of sensory modulation in cranial systems prior to speech or voice initiation may reduce the potential disruptive effects of somatosensory input on subsequent movements (Abbs & Cole, 1982; Davis et al., 1993). We recently employed measures of lip-muscle reflexes to assess sensory modulation prior to speech and found a significant tendency for normal speakers to show reduced reflex levels during preparation for speech movement (McClean & Clay, 1995). In a follow-up study (McClean, 1996b), it was observed that, as a group, subjects who stutter show less reflex suppression prior to fluent speech compared with nonstutterers. Also, reflex levels showed significant elevation prior to speech disfluency in some stutterer subjects. While these results may reflect abnormal sensory processing that contributes to speech disfluency in some stutterers (cf. Zimmermann, 1980), their full interpretation will require comprehensive system models that incorporate plausible roles for sensory input in speech motor control.

The computational model of cerebellar control considered earlier (Chauvet & Chapeau-Blondeau, 1993) represents a working example of how temporal programs for speech might be realized. When fully developed, such models are likely to incorporate a variety of functional roles for sensory input. Sensory function in motor control, as outlined by Schmidt (1988), includes parameter selection prior to motor program execution, modification of ongoing motor output, and mediation of motor learning. Consideration is given here to how these different types of sensory processing may affect PGC function and contribute to speech disfluency.

Speech motor output is known to remain relatively invariant under a variety of physical conditions (e.g., Lindblom et al., 1979). Thus, somatosensory input that encodes static variations in peripheral biomechanics (e.g., body position or contents of the mouth) is likely to contribute to selection of movement parameters during speech movement preparation. It has been suggested that mossy fiber input to the granule cell layer performs this type of function by informing the cerebellar cortex of the general status of the body at the time that intended movements are to be executed (Llinas & Walton, 1990). Also, recent PET scan data suggest that the cerebellum is particularly important for movement preparation under some conditions (Horwitz et al., 1995).

Deficits in sensory function for speech-movement preparation in some stutterers are suggested by results of a study involving assessment of the kinesthetic acuity (DeNil & Abbs, 1991). Subjects were asked to make minimal static displacements of the lip, jaw, tongue and finger. As a group, the stutterers showed larger minimal displacements for oral movements but not finger movements, suggesting a selective deficit in orofacial sensorimotor processing among some of the stutterers. For individuals showing such deficits, one would expect sensory contributions to PGC control during movement preparation to be less than optimal. In the future, this might be explored with experiments that assess level of speech disfluency or articulatory imprecision under different peripheral conditions such as changes in body posture. It would also be of interest to evaluate the relative contribution of tonic versus phasic mechanoreceptor input to kinesthetic acuity in orofacial structures.

With respect to modification of ongoing output by sensory input, it is well documented that rapid effective adjustments in orofacial movements are made in response to unpredictable mechanical perturbations (e.g., Abbs & Gracco, 1984). Such data generally indicate that somatosensory input contributes to the integration of neural control signals affecting coordinated movements of multiple speech structures. The type of error detection and multi structure compensation implied by these results is especially well suited for cerebellar processing. Comparable data on spinal muscle systems involving reversible cooling techniques strongly implicate such a role for the cerebellum (Hore & Vilis, 1984). A preliminary study of orofacial load perturbation in persons who stutter indicated reduced levels of load compensation, although considerable intersubject variability was noted (Caruso et al., 1987).

There is little doubt that sensory systems play an essential role in the acquisition of speech motor processes. While it ignores a large amount of biologic detail, Guenther's highly successful model of speech motor acquisition depends inherently on extensive use of both somatosensory and auditory feedback (Guenther, 1994). Questions that might be addressed with models of speech motor acquisition concern the effects of plasticity of sensorimotor pathways during the period when the earliest evidence of speech disfluency emerges. In other words, what is the accumulated effect of disfluent speech events on the developing PGC. If pathways are especially likely to develop strong synaptic connections during early childhood, then they may also be inclined to develop independent, but aberrant, motor programs in response to episodic disfluent speech utterances.

The present discussion of sensory processing has focused on the somatosensory system, but it is known that artificial alteration in auditory feedback, via sidetone delay or frequency shifting, can markedly reduce the frequency of disfluency in persons who stutter (e.g., Howell et al., 1987; Kalinowski et al., 1993; Webster, 1991). Here again, comprehensive system modeling of the speech motor system may prove critical for understanding actual neural mechanisms underlying such effects. Such modeling presumably would incorporate relevant findings from functional brain imaging studies, such as the observation that stutterers show reduced levels of activation in auditory cortex during disfluent speech (Fox et al., 1996).

REGULATION OF MUSCLE STIFFNESS

Muscle stiffness refers to the restoring force generated when a muscle is stretched. It increases systematically with muscle length and extent of muscle contraction as described by the length-tension curve (Lewis, 1981). The concept of stiffness regulation refers here to the setting of tonic or background levels of muscle activity related to postural adjustment. This differs from more phasic forms of muscle activity that underlie voluntary movement. The distinction between tonic and phasic muscle activation is in keeping with a long-held view that the human motor system consists of two functional components that involve tonic and phasic control processes (Humphrey & Reed, 1983). At a more abstract level, muscle stiffness has special status as a regulated parameter with respect to the widely-discussed equilibrium point hypothesis and how it accounts for movement dynamics (Feldman et al., 1990). This perspective may be especially important for understanding how tonic and phasic control systems interact in speech motor control (see Perrier et al., 1996). What is important to keep in mind is that elevated levels of background EMG reflect an increase in excitability of motoneuron pools; this in turn means that the associated muscle system generally is more responsive to different sources of input.

Starkweather (1995) has recently suggested that stutterers display increased levels of both tonic and phasic muscle activity in association with speech production and that this is a primary contributor to speech disfluency. While some stutterers may show elevated EMG levels during their fluent speech, individual differences are likely to be substantial (cf. Van Lieshout et al., 1993; Smith, et al., 1996). As indicated by Smith et al. (1996), available data do not support the conclusion that stutterers show greater EMG levels during disfluent speech. Given our limited understanding of the neural mechanisms of speech disfluency and the paucity of relevant data, it is just as reasonable to predict that increases in background EMG level would reduce, rather than increase, the likelihood of speech disfluency in some stutterers. Clearly, new studies are needed which carefully examine prespeech and inter-utterance background EMG levels. Such work could provide a basis for additional studies of EMG biofeedback like that of Guitar (1975). Future work of this type would benefit from a clearer picture of how stiffness regulatory mechanisms interact with different sources of PGC input in the speech regulatory system.

EMOTIONAL-MOTIVATIONAL SYSTEMS

It has long been recognized that the motor system is subject to influences from regions of the brain that mediate emotional and motivational aspects of thought and behavior. Neurophysiologists are beginning to understand the circuitry and related neurochemistry that underlie these interactions. A general circuit that mediates motivational influences on the motor system now appears to be widely agreed upon (Kalivas & Barnes, 1993). Motivational stimuli influence this circuit via input to the amygdala, and the circuit outputs project to the motor cortex, basal ganglia, and reticulospinal pathways. Dopaminergic afferents are especially important in the function of pathways intrinsic to this motive circuit. These observations are notable in light of movement initiation deficits seen in Parkinson's disease, the documented cases of acquired stuttering following basal-ganglia lesion (Ludlow et al., 1987), and reduced levels of basal ganglia activity during both the fluent and disfluent speech of stutterers (Riley & Wu, this volume).

Brain regions mediating motivation are also associated with those involved in emotional response. For example, there is evidence that the amygdala is especially important in the recognition of fearful expression independent of face recognition (Adolphs et al., 1995). Animal studies have identified specific regions of the CNS that are likely to mediate the patterns of muscle activity required for emotional expression in the voice (Depaulis & Bandler, 1991). Notably, Zhang et al. (1994) provide strong evidence that the midbrain periaqueductal gray has two distinct regions that regulate the patterns of laryngeal, respiratory, and orofacial muscle activity associated different forms of vocalization, one involving expression of intense emotion and the other seen in a greater variety of situations.

The extent and nature of emotional response are correlated with various electro-physiologic measures of autonomic nervous system (ANS) activity. ANS levels vary systematically with anticipation of motor activity, but there can be considerable intersubject variability in this activity (Collet et al., 1994). In general, elevated ANS activity is seen in association with speech production, but stutterers do not show abnormal ANS levels during speech (Peters & Hulstijn, 1984; Weber & Smith, 1990). However, Weber and Smith did find that some stutterers show their highest levels of ANS activity in association with speech disfluency. The relevance of this last finding to speech disfluency may be related to possible interactions of the ANS with sensory pathways and tremororganic mechanisms (Weber & Smith, 1990; Zimmermann, 1980).

TEMPORAL STAGES OF MOVEMENT CONTROL

A widely held view among motor physiologists is that voluntary movements typically involve a progression through different temporal stages of neural activity that underlie movement planning, programming, and execution (Wise et al., 1991). Thus, it is likely that the various components of the motor system considered here will ultimately need to be modeled in relation to how their patterns of activity vary through the time course of these different stages of movement. How stages of movement can be reflected in different neural systems is illustrated by an example from the work of Kien and Altman (1992) on the neural correlates of insect locomotion. Figure 7, which is adapted from their work, shows the time course of neuronal firing rates within widely different regions of an insect's nervous system as it stands, prepares to walk, and walks. It can be seen that there are different types of activity (tonic vs. phasic) in the different neural centers, and these vary in their time of onset across the different stages of motor processing. Data of this type emphasize the parallel-distributed, as opposed to serial-hierarchial, nature of motor system processing. Also, they suggest that motor control processes need to be understood in terms of the ensemble of neural activity across different components of the motor system.

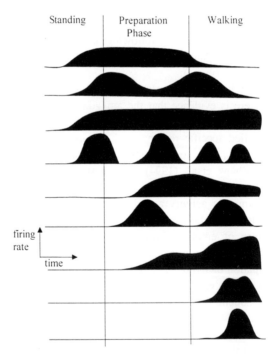

Figure 7. Neuronal firing rate changes associated with a variety of neural centers within an insect nervous system during standing, preparation to walk, and walking (adapted from Kien & Altman, 1993).

For example, when the neuronal activity in Figure 7 is viewed as an ensemble, there is a characteristic activation pattern at the time of movement initiation. The implication of this for speech motor control is that the relative timing of activation across different neural centers may be a critical feature underlying initiation of fluent speech.

There are reasons to suspect that in studying the mechanisms of speech disfluency with respect to PGC function, strong emphasis should be given to processes leading up to the initiation of movement execution. Speech disfluency is known to occur most frequently on the initial sound segments of speech utterances (e.g., Peters & Hulstijn, 1987), and anomalies in orofacial muscle activity in stutterers' fluent speech tend to be associated with the initial words of utterances (Van Lieshout et al., 1993, 1995). In addition, we recently observed that the timing of orofacial movements in adult stutterers was approximately equivalent during fluent and disfluent utterances, where disfluencies occurred on the initial speech sound or during prespeech posturing (McClean et al., 1995). This finding suggests that control processes underlying the execution of speech movements tend to be similar for fluent and disfluent utterances and that the temporal disruptions associated with disfluency are related primarily to the period of movement initiation. Of course, what represents movement initiation within the context of natural speech is not clear, but presumably its temporal boundaries are determined in part by the prevailing unit of speech production.

FINAL COMMENT

Considerable intersubject variability is a characteristic finding in studies involving physiologic, acoustic, and behavioral analyses of the speech of persons who stutter. This represents a central problem in efforts to understand the mechanisms of speech disfluency. The general hypothesis developed here would predict high levels of intersubject variability in terms of almost any single measure of speech motor output. Specifically, because many neural systems contribute to PGC output and affect the control of speech production, the likelihood of intersubject variability becomes substantial. For example, some individuals may have motor systems that are especially sensitive to variations in emotional state; others may employ unusual control strategies for manipulating speech rate; and yet others may have reduced sensory acuity. The implication of such variability for both the laboratory and clinic is that the weighting of factors and how their interactions affect the frequency and specific mechanisms of speech disfluency are likely to differ across individuals who stutter. This emphasizes the importance of continued efforts to develop a valid taxonomy of persons who stutter (cf. Lauter, this volume). But such a taxonomy needs to be based on an understanding of what may be diverse mechanisms underlying speech disfluency (cf. Smith, 1989). A critical tool in such efforts will be biologically-oriented computational models of the speech motor system.

ACKNOWLEDGMENTS

The opinions or assertions contained herein are my private views and are not to be construed as official or as reflecting the views of the Department of the Army or the Department of Defense. Thanks to Charles Larson, Marjorie Leek, Anne Smith, and Brian Walden for their helpful comments on an earlier version of this paper.

REFERENCES

Abbs, J.H. (1986). Invariance and variability in speech production: A distinction between linguistic intent and its neuromotor implementation. In J. Perkell and D. Klatt (Eds.), *Invariance and variability in speech processes* (pp. 202-219). Hillsdale, N.J.: Lawrence Erlbaum.

Abbs, J.H. & Cole, K. (1982). Consideration of bulbar and suprabulbar afferent influences upon speech motor coordination and programming. In S. Grillner, B. Lindblom, J. Lubker, and A. Persson (Eds.), *Speech motor control* (pp. 159-186). Oxford: Pergamon Press.

Abbs, J.H. & Gracco, V. (1984). Control of complex motor gestures: Orofacial muscle responses to load perturbations of the lip during speech. *Journal of Neurophysiology, 52*, 705-723.

Abbs, J.H. & Welt, C. (1985). Structure and function of the lateral precentral cortex: Significance for speech motor control. In R. Daniloff (Ed.), *Speech science: Recent advances*. San Diego: College-Hill Press.

Ackermann, H., Hertrich, I., & Scharf, G. (1995). Kinematic analysis of lower lip movements in ataxic dysarthria. *Journal of Speech and Hearing Research, 38*, 1252-1259.

Adams, S.G., Weismer, G., & Kent, R.D. (1993). Speaking rate and speech movement velocity profiles. *Journal of Speech and Hearing Research, 36*, 41-54.

Adolphs, R., Tranel, D., Damasio, H., & Damasio, A.R. (1995). Fear and the human amygdala. *Journal of Neuroscience, 15*, 5879-5891.

Allen, G., & Tsukahara, N. (1974). Cerebrocerebellar communication systems, *Physiological Reviews, 54*, 957-1006.

Berthier, N.E., Singh, S.P., Barto, A.G., & Houk, J.C. (1993). Distributed representation of limb motor programs in arrays of adjustable pattern generators. *Journal of Cognitive Neuroscience, 5*, 56-78.

Bower, J.M. & Woolston, D.C. (1983). Congruence of spatial organization of tactile projections to granule cell and Purkinje cell layers of cerebellar hemispheres of the albino rate: Vertical organization of cerebellar cortex. *Journal of Neurophysiology, 49*, 745-766.

Bullock, D. & Grossberg, S. (1988). Neural dynamics of planned arm movements: Emergent invariants and speech-accuracy properties during trajectory formation. *Psychological Review, 95*, 49-90.

Buonomano, D.V. & Mauk, M.D. (1994). Neural network model of the cerebellum: Temporal discrimination and the timing of motor responses. *Neural Computation, 6*, 38-55.

Caruso, A.J., Gracco, V.L., & Abbs, J.H. (1987). A speech motor control perspective on stuttering: Preliminary observations. In H. Peters & W. Hulstijn (eds.) *Speech motor dynamics in stuttering* (pp. 244-258). Springer-Verlag: New York.

Chauvet, G. (1986). Habituation rules for a theory of the cerebellar cortex. *Biological Cybernetics, 55*, 201-209.

Chapeau-Blondeau, F., & Chauvet, G. (1991). A neural network model of the cerebellar cortex performing dynamic associations. *Biological Cybernetics, 65*, 267-279.

Cheney, P.D., Mewes, K. & Fetz, E.E. (1988). Encoding of motor parameters by corticomotoneuronal

(CM) and rubromotoneuronal (RM) cells producing postspike facilitation of forelimb muscles in the behaving monkey. *Behavioral Brain Research, 28*, 181-191.

Cohen, L. & Starr, A. (1987). Localization, timing specificity of gating of somatosensory evoked potentials during active movement in man. *Brain, 110*, 654-669.

Collet, C., Deschaumes-Molinaro, C., Delhomme, G., Dittmar, A. & Vernet-Maury, E. (1994). Autonomic responses correlate to motor anticipation. *Behavioural Brain Research, 63*, 71-79.

Davis, P., Bartlett, D. & Luschei, E. (1993). Coordination of the respiratory laryngeal systems in breathing and vocalization. In I. Titze (Ed.), *Vocal fold physiology: Frontiers in basic science* (pp. 189-226). San Diego: Singular Publishing Group.

De Nil, L.F. & Abbs, J.H. (1991). Kinesthetic acuity of stutterers and non-stutterers for oral and non-oral movement. *Brain, 114*, 2145-2158.

Depaulis, A., & Bandler, R. (1991). *The midbrain periaqueductal gray matter: Functional, anatomical and immunohistochemical organization*, Plenum Press, New York.

Eccles, J.C. (1989). *Evolution of the brain*, Routlidge: London.

Farley, G. (1994). Control of voice F_0 by an artificial neural network. *Journal of the Acoustical Society of America, 96*, 1374-1379.

Feldman, A.G., Adamovich, S.V., Ostry, D.J. & Flanagan, J.R. (1990). The origin of electromyograms - explanations based on the equilibrium point hypothesis. In J.M. Winters & S.L-Y. Woo (Eds.), *Muscle systems: Biomechanics and movement organization* (pp. 195-213). New York: Springer-Verlag.

Fetz, E.E. (1993). Dynamic neural network models of sensorimotor behavior. In D. Gardner (Ed.), *The neurobiology of neural networks* (pp. 165-190). MIT Press: Cambridge, Mass.

Fetz, E.E., Cheney, P.D., Mewes, K., & Palmer, S. (1989). Control of forelimb muscle activity by populations of corticomotoneuronal and rubromotoneuronal cells. *Progress in Brain Research, 80*, 437-449.

Fox, P.T., Ingham, R.J., Ingham, J.C., Hirsch, T.B., Downs, J., Martin, C., Jerabek, P., Glass, T., & Lancaster, J. (1996). A PET study of the neural systems of stuttering. *Nature, 382*, 158-162.

Gracco, V.L. & Abbs, J.H. (1988). Central patterning of speech movements. *Experimental Brain Research, 71*, 515-526.

Grillner, S. (1981). Possible analogies in the control of innate motor acts and the production of sound in speech. In S. Grillner, B. Lindblom, J. Lubker, & A. Persson (Eds.), *Speech motor control* (pp. 217-230). New York: Pergamon Press.

Guenther, F.H. (1994). A neural network model of speech acquisition and motor equivalent speech production. *Biological Cybernetics, 72*, 43-53.

Guitar, B. (1975). Reduction of stuttering frequency using analog electromyographic feedback. *Journal of Speech and Hearing Research, 18*, 672-685.

Hore, J. & Vilis, T. (1984). Loss of set in muscle responses to limb perturbations during cerebellar dysfunction. *Journal of Neurophysiology, 51*, 1137-1148.

Horwitz, B., Deiber, M., Ibanez, Sadato, N., & Hallet, M. (1995). Cerebellar involvement in motor preparation: A PET-Reaction Time (RT) study. *Society for Neuroscience Abstracts, 21*, 364.7.

Houk, J.C. (1987). Model of the cerebellum as an array of adjustable pattern generators. In M. Glickstein, C. Yeo, & J. Stein (Eds.), *Cerebellum and neuronal plasticity* (pp. 249-260). New York: Plenum Press.

Houk, J.C., Keifer, J. & Barto, A.G. (1993). Distributed motor commands in the limb premotor network. *Trends in Neuroscience, 16*, 27-3

Howell, P., El-Yaniv, N., & Powell, D.J. (1987). Factors affecting fluency in stutterers when speaking under altered auditory feedback. In H.F. Peters & W. Hulstijn (Eds.), *Speech motor dynamics in stuttering* (pp. 361-369). New York: Springer-Verlag.

Huang, C.M., Liu, G.L., Yang, B.Y., Mu, H., & Hsiao, C.F. (1991). Auditory receptive area in the cerebellar hemisphere is surrounded by somatosensory areas. *Brain Research, 15*, 252-256.

Humphrey, D.R., & Reed, D.J. (1983). Separate cortical systems for control of joint movement and joint stiffness: Reciprocal activation and coactivation of antagonist muscles. In J.E. Desmedt (Ed.), *Advances in neurology: Motor control mechanisms in health and disease* (pp. 347-372). New York: Raven Press.

Ito, M. (1993). Synaptic plasticity in the cerebellar cortex and its role in motor learning. *The Canadian Journal of Neurological Sciences*, Suppl. 3, S70-S74.

Jiang, W., Chapman, C.E. & Lamarre, Y., (1991). Modulation of the cutaneous responsiveness of neurones in the primary somatosensory cortex during conditioned arm movements in the monkey. *Experimental Brain Research, 84*, 342-354.

Kalinowski, J., Armson, J., Roland-Mieszkowski, M, Stuart, A. & Gracco, V.L. (1993). Effects of alterations in auditory feedback and speech rate on stuttering frequency. *Language and Speech, 36*, 1-16.

Kalivas, P.W. & Barnes, C.D. (1993). *Limbic motor circuits and neuropsychiatry*, CRC Press: Boca Raton.

Kent, R.D., Netsell, R, & Abbs, J.H. (1979). Acoustic characteristics of dysarthria associated with cerebellar disease. *Journal of Speech and Hearing Research, 22*, 627-648.

Kettner, R., Marcario, J., & Port, N. (1993). A neural network model of cortical activity during reaching. *Journal of Cognitive Neuroscience, 5*, 14-33.

Kien, J. & Altman, J.S. (1992). Preparation and execution of movement: Parallels between insect and mammalian motor systems. *Comparative Biochemistry and Physiology, 103A*, 15-24.

Kristeva-Feige, R., Rossi, S., Pizzella, V., Lopez, L., Erne, S.N., Edrich, J., & Rossini, P. (1996). A neuromagnetic study of movement-related somatosensory gating in the human brain. *Experimental Brain Research, 107*, 504-514.

Lauter, J. (this volume). Brain imaging in speech production: choices and challenges. In W. Hulstijn, H.F.M. Peters, & P.H.H.M. Van Lieshout (Eds.), *Speech production: motor control, brain research and fluency disorders*. Amsterdam: Elsevier Science.

Lewis, D.M. (1981). The physiology of motor units in mammalian skeletal muscle. In A.L. Towe & E.S. Luschei (Eds.), *Handbook of behavioral neurobiology: Volume 5 motor coordination* (pp. 1-67). New York: Plenum Press.

Lindblom, B., Lubker, J., & Gay, T. (1979). Formant frequencies of some fixed-mandible vowels and a model of speech motor programming by predictive simulation. *Journal of Phonetics, 7*, 147-161.

Llinas, R.R. & Walton, K.D. (1990). Cerebellum. In G. Shepherd (Ed.), *The synaptic organization of the brain* (pp. 214-245). New York: Oxford Univ. Press.

Ludlow, C., Rosenberg, J., Salazar, A., Grafman, J., & Smutok, M. (1987). Site of penetrating brain lesions causing chronic acquired stuttering. *Annals of Neurology, 22*, 60-66.

Lund, J., Appenteng, K., & Sequin, J.J. (1981). Analogies and common features in the speech and masticatory control systems. In S. Grillner, B. Lindblom, J. Lubker, & A. Persson (Eds.), *Speech motor control* (pp. 231-245), New York: Pergamon Press.

Martin, J.H. & Ghez, C. (1988). Red nucleus and motor cortex: parallel motor systems for the initiation and control of skilled movement. *Behavioural Brain Research, 28*, 217-223.

McClean, M.D. (1996a). Individual differences in orofacial movement coordination with variations in speech rate. *Society for Neuroscience Abstracts, 22*, 643.16.

McClean, M.D. (1996b). Lip muscle reflexes during speech movement preparation in stutterers. *Journal of Fluency Disorders, 21*, 49-60.

McClean, M.D. & Clay, J.L. (1994). Evidence for suppression of lip-muscle reflexes prior to speech. *Experimental Brain Research, 97*, 541-544.

McClean, M.D., Cord, M.T., & Levandowski, D.R. (1995). Timing of lip, jaw, and laryngeal movements following speech disfluencies. In F. Bell-Berti and L.J. Raphael (Eds.), *Producing speech: Contemporary issues (for Katherine Safford Harris)* (pp. 65-76). New York: American Institute of Physics.

McClean, M.D. & Clay, J.L. (1995). Activation of lip motor units with variations in speech rate and phonetic structure. *Journal of Speech and Hearing Research, 38*, 772-782.

Morton, D.W., & Chiel, J. (1994). Neural architectures for adaptive behavior. *Trends in Neuroscience, 17*, 413-420.

Pearson, A. (1993). Common principles of motor control in vertebrates and invertebrates. *Annual Reviews of Neuroscience, 16*, 265-297.

Perrier, P., Ostry, D.J., & Laboissiere, R. (1996). The equilibrium point hypothesis and its application to speech motor control. *Journal of Speech and Hearing Research, 39*, 365-378.

Peters, H.F. & Hulstijn, W. (1984). Stuttering and anxiety: The difference between stutterers and nonstutterers in verbal apprehension and physiologic arousal during the anticipation of speech and non-speech tasks. *Journal of Fluency Disorders, 9*, 67-84.

Peters, H. F. & Hulstijn, W. (1987). Programming and initiation of speech utterances in stuttering. In H. Peters & W. Hulstijn (Eds.), *Speech motor dynamics in stuttering* (pp. 185-195). New York: Springer-Verlag.

Petersen, S.E., Fox, P.T., Posner, M.I., Mintun, M. (1990). Positron emission tomographic studies of the processing of single words. *Journal of Cognitive Neuroscience, 1*, 153-170.

Riley, G. & Wu, J.C. (this volume). Pet scan evidence of parallel cerebral systems related to treatments effects. In W. Hulstijn, H.F.M. Peters, & P.H.H.M. Van Lieshout (Eds.), *Speech production: motor control, brain research and fluency disorders*. Amsterdam: Elsevier Science.

Schmidt, R.A. (1988). *Motor control and motor learning*, Champaign, Il.:Human Kinetics.

Smith, A. (1989). Neural drive to muscle in stuttering. *Journal of Speech and Hearing Research, 32*, 252-264.

Smith, A., Luschei, E., Denny, M., Wood, J., Hirano, M. & Badylak, S. (1993). Spectral analyses of activity of laryngeal and orofacial muscles in stutterers. *Journal of Neurology, Neurosurgery, and Psychiatry, 56*, 1303-1311.

Smith, A., Goffman, L., Zelaznik, H.N., Goangshiuan, Y., McGillem, C. (1995). Spatiotemporal stability and patterning of speech movement sequences. *Experimental Brain Research, 104*, 493-501.

Smith, A., Denny, M., Shaffer, L.A., Kelly, E.M., & Hirano, M. (1996). Activity of intrinsic laryngeal muscles in fluent and disfluent speech. *Journal of Speech and Hearing Research, 39*, 329-348.

Smith, A.M., Dugas, C., Fortier, P., Kalaska, J. & Picard, N. (1993). Comparing cerebellar and motor cortical activity in reaching and grasping. *Canadian Journal of Neurologic Sciences, 20* (Suppl. 3) 53-61.

Smith, J.L., Chung, S.H., & Zernicke, R.F. (1993). Gait-related motor patterns and hindlimb kinetics for the cat trot and gallop. *Experimental Brain Research, 94*, 308-322.

Starkweather, C.W. (1995). A simple theory of stuttering. *Journal of Fluency Disorders, 20*, 91-116.

Tamas, L.B., Shibasaki, T., Horikoshi, S., & Ohye, C. (1993). General activation of cerebral metabolism with speech: a PET study. *International Journal of Psychophysiology, 14*, 199-208.

Van Lieshout, P.H., Peters, H.F., Starkweather, C.W., & Hulstijn, W. (1993). Physiological differences between stutterers and nonstutterers in perceptually fluent speech: EMG amplitude and duration. *Journal of Speech and Hearing Research, 36*, 55-63.

Van Lieshout, P.H., Starkweather, C.W., Hulstijn, W., & Peters, H.F. (1995). Effects of linguistic correlates of stuttering on EMG activity in nonstuttering speakers. *Journal of Speech and Hearing Research, 38*, 360-372.

Van Lieshout, P.H., Hulstijn, W., & Peters, H.F.M. (1996). Speech production in people who stutter: Testing the motor plan assembly hypothesis. *Journal of Speech and Hearing Research, 39*, 76-92.

Weber, C.M. & Smith, A. (1990). Autonomic correlates of stuttering and speech assessed in a range of experimental tasks. *Journal of Speech and Hearing Research, 33*, 690-706.

Webster, R.L. (1991). Manipulation of vocal tone: Implications for stuttering. In H. Peters, W. Hulstijn, C.W. Starkweather (Eds.), *Speech motor control and stuttering* (pp. 535-545). Amsterdam: Elsevier.

Williams, R.J. & Zipser, D. (1989). A learning algorithm for continually running fully recurrent neural networks. *Neural Computation, 1*, 270-280.

Wise, S.P. and others (1991). Group report: What are the specific functions of the different motor areas? In D.R. Humphrey & H.J. Freund (Eds.), *Motor control: concepts and issues* (pp. 463-485). New York: John Wiley & Sons.

Zhang, S.P., Davis, P.J., Bandler, R., & Carrive, P. (1994). Brain stem integration of vocalization: Role of the midbrain periaqueductal gray. *Journal of Neurophysiology, 72*, 1337-1356.

Zimmermann, G. (1980). Stuttering: a disorder of movement. *Journal of Speech and Hearing Research, 23*, 122-136.

Speech Production: Motor Control, Brain Research and Fluency Disorders
W. Hulstijn, H.F.M. Peters and P.H.H.M. Van Lieshout, editors

Chapter 8

PRINCIPLES OF HUMAN BRAIN ORGANIZATION RELATED TO LATERALIZATION OF LANGUAGE AND SPEECH MOTOR FUNCTIONS IN NORMAL SPEAKERS AND STUTTERERS

William G. Webster

The search for an understanding of brain mechanisms associated with stuttering has long been influenced by models and theories attributing the disorder to an anomaly of lateralization of speech and language function in people who stutter or, more generally, to an anomaly in some aspect of interhemispheric relations. This paper reviews the evidence pointing to such anomalies and considers principles of human brain organization that bear on the interpretation of that evidence. Drawing upon contemporary research initiatives, a neuropsychological model of stuttering is reviewed that has three major tenets: i) The usual and normal pattern of left hemisphere lateralization of speech motor mechanisms in people who stutter; ii) left hemisphere speech motor mechanisms (specifically involving the supplementary motor area) in people who stutter that are fragile and susceptible to interference from other on-going brain activities, especially those of the right hemisphere; and iii) an unusually labile pattern of hemispheric activation in people who stutter.

INTRODUCTION

During the past twenty years a growing body of literature in speech pathology and neuropsychology has pointed to a significant role for biological factors underlying stuttering. Noteworthy in this regard are studies of the inheritance of stuttering, particularly those that allow for inferences to be made about genetic factors (Howie, 1981; Kidd, 1984) and those that have focussed on brain mechanisms. It is this latter body of literature on which I have been asked to comment today. Because of the breadth of the topic and the constraints of time and space, I decided to limit myself in at least three ways. First, I am going to emphasize speech production more than language. Second, I am going to anticipate some of the papers that will be presented in the later sessions on brain imaging but *not* attempt to include reference to them (or directly related research) in my remarks on stuttering. And third, I am going to focus on just certain aspects of lateralization that have influenced my own research and my thinking about brain mechanisms and stuttering. In approaching this, I thought I would take the opportunity to share with you some ideas about the nature of interhemispheric relations that I believe underlie stuttering. I hope this may provide some framework for interpreting the brain imaging papers that follow in the conference.

In order to put my remarks into context, let me begin by saying that my research program has been shaped by the experiences I have had as a person who stutters. Like most people who stutter, I have stuttered since childhood; others in my family stutter; I have experienced all the interpersonal, social, and emotional difficulties of growing up and living with a stutter; and I have found the severity of my stuttering to have varied enormously over the years, and indeed it still does vary from one time to another and from one situation to another. Although variability is what makes stuttering such a frustrating disorder for those of us who stutter, it is also what makes it such an interesting phenomenon from a scientific perspective. The variability implies to me that the underlying mechanisms are dynamic in nature rather than being ones which reflect a relatively static structural defect or structural anomaly. In other words, I suspect that the problem will *not* prove to be that people who stutter have a hole in the brain, or the equivalent. Instead, I suspect there will prove to be some peculiarity in how information is integrated and processed in different regions of the brain. Furthermore, I suspect that part of that peculiarity will involve how the two hemispheres interact with one another.

My research began some years ago out of my interest in what might underlie the variability in stuttering severity. Two very general and related questions then drove my research agenda: First, what is it that is different about the brain of the person who stutters compared with the brain of the person who does not stutter? Second, what is it that changes in the brain of the person who stutters as he or she goes from periods of fluency to periods of dysfluency?

TOWARD A MODEL OF BRAIN MECHANISMS AND STUTTERING

Bilateral vs. Unilateral Speech Motor Control

One of the earliest theories of brain mechanisms and stuttering was proposed in the late 1920's by Samuel Orton, a neurologist, and Lee Travis, a psychologist and speech pathologist. It held that stuttering is due to an anomaly or peculiarity in interhemispheric relations. More specifically, Orton (1928) and Travis (1931) argued that, in contrast to the fluent speaker whose speech and language processes are controlled by the left hemisphere, the person who stutters has bilateral speech control, in other words, has speech centers in both hemispheres rather than just one. According to their model, which is illustrated conceptually in Figure 1, this results in two sets of commands being sent to the speech musculature resulting in discoordination when those commands are slightly out of synchrony.

Before elaborating on this, let me comment briefly on the pattern of *lateralization* found in the normal human brain.

Two interchangeable terms are used to describe the nature of interhemispheric relations in human brain organization: *lateralization* and *hemispheric specialization*. These

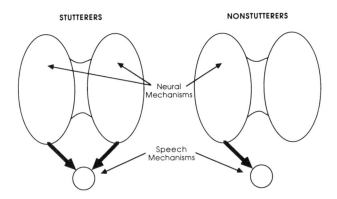

Figure 1. Schematic diagram of the Orton/Travis model of stuttering. In contrast to the normal fluent speaker with brain mechanisms for speech, language, and fine motor control lateralized in the left hemisphere, the brain of the person who stutters has, under this model, such mechanisms in both hemispheres (from Webster, 1993).

terms refer to the fact that although the two hemispheres look more or less the same,certain cognitive and behavioral functions are mediated primarily by one or the other hemisphere. In this sense the functions are lateralized. The best documented of these functions is speech and language, mediated mainly by the left hemisphere in most individuals. As has been known for well over a century (Young, 1970), damage to the left hemisphere results in changes in speech and language function not found following comparable damage to the right hemisphere.

In my own view, the complementary nature of hemispheric specialization has been most dramatically demonstrated in those individual patients with intractable epilepsy who have had the corpus callosum sectioned in the midline (Sperry, 1974). Because of how the sensory systems are connected to the two hemispheres of the brain, it is possible to restrict sensory information to one hemisphere or the other and hence, since cutting the callosum has the effect of disconnecting the hemispheres, to test the capabilities of each hemisphere in relative isolation. When this is done, the complementarity of hemispheric specialization becomes readily apparent within individuals. In general terms, tasks involving speech and language are far better performed when the person is using the left hemisphere rather than the right. In contrast, tasks that involve visuoconstructional skills, such as arranging blocks in certain spatial configu-rations, are far better performed when the person is using the right hemisphere rather than the left.

Of particular relevance for today is the fact that the patients can talk only about information directed to the left hemisphere (Sperry, 1974). Although there may be some debate about the linguistic capability of the right hemisphere in these split-brain cases (Gazzaniga, 1983; Zaidel, 1983) and in neurologically normal people (Perecman, 1983; Searleman, 1977), there is little debate about speech. The mechanisms have access only to information processed in the left hemisphere.

This then leads to a first principle of human brain organization:

The two cerebral hemispheres are specialized for certain forms of cognitive proces sing. In most people, the left hemisphere is usually the one specialized for speech and language functions and the right hemisphere for visuospatial functions, among other things.

Contrary to some out-dated but persisting popular notions of cerebral dominace, this principle applies to both right- and left-handers. As is evident in the results of assessment of hemispheric specialization for speech and language through injections of sodium amytal into one carotid artery or the other, virtually all right-handers demonstrate evidence of left-hemisphere dominance for speech and language. Although less predictable, the majority of left-handers do so as well (Milner et al., 1966).

Although the two cerebral hemispheres are of similar size and shape, a number of consistent anatomical asymmetries between the hemispheres probably underlie these functional asymmetries. One of these can be seen easily if one first cuts through the brain in the plane of the Sylvian fissure that separates the temporal lobe from the rest of the brain, and then views the cut brain from above. Along the upper surface of the temporal lobe is a pair of transverse sulci which define Heschl's gyrus, the primarily auditory cortex. Lying immediately posterior to this gyrus is an area called the *planum temporale* which continues along the upper surface of the temporal lobe until tissue merges into parietal cortex.

In their classic paper, Geschwind and Levitsky (1968) reported that in about two-thirds of the 100 brains they examined, the planum temporale was larger in the left hemisphere than the right. It was larger in the right hemisphere than the left in about 10% of the brains, and it was of similar size in the two hemispheres in the remaining 25%. The general finding has been well replicated using both post-mortem material (Wada et al., 1975) and imaging of intact brains (Foundas et al., 1995; Karbe et al., 1995; Steinmetz et al., 1990). It has also been reported in neonatal brain tissue (Wada et al., 1975; Witelson & Pallie, 1973). What makes the asymmetry of the planum temporale so provocative is that it is part of the classical posterior language area referred to as Wernicke's area (Galaburda et al., 1978). Damage to that area results in receptive aphasias or difficulties in language comprehension.

Anatomical asymmetries of the anterior classical speech and language area, Broca's area, have been somewhat more difficult to demonstrate than those in the posterior region (Wada et al., 1975). However, once certain methodological difficulties in defining Broca's area were resolved, asymmetries of gross morphology (Albanese et al., 1989; Foundas et al., 1995) and cytoarchitectonics (Hayes & Lewis, 1995) became evident.

It is important to understand that what was reported originally amounts in effect to a weak form of correlation between various anatomical differences between the hemispheres and various functional differences. However, an extensive body of literature (Foundas et al., 1995; Galaburda et al., 1978; Steinmetz et al., 1990) now suggests that the covariation is sufficiently close that we can have considerable confidence that the anatomical asymmetries in fact underlie the functional asymmetries in individuals.

Accordingly, a second principle of brain organization is that,

> *although the two hemispheres are of the same general size and shape, there are a number of consistent anatomical asymmetries which are generally thought to be related to functional asymmetries in speech and language processing in individual normal fluent speakers.*

The Orton (1928) and Travis (1931) model of stuttering postulated that people who stutter have a rather different brain organization than that described in the first two principles. My own research began with an attempt to test this model. Our approach was indirect and involved the study in people who stutter of hand and finger movements rather than speech. The rationale for this approach has been described elsewhere (Webster, 1990a, 1993) and so let me simply state without elaboration that because of the overlap of neural mechanisms involved in the control of speech with those involved in the control of other fine motor movements (Kimura, 1993), we hope to discern something about the neural mechanisms associated with stuttering by studying the control of other fine motor movements.

Our first experiment (Webster, 1985) built upon the observation that most people, right- and left-handers, tap the fingers of the right hand faster and more accurately than the fingers of the left hand (Denckla, 1973; Peters, 1980; Todor & Kyprie, 1980). This effect is apparent with both single finger tapping as well as sequential finger tapping in which subjects are required to tap telegraph keys repeatedly in a particular order. The usual interpretation of the right hand advantage (Kinsbourne & McMurray, 1975; Peters, 1980; Wolff et al., 1977) is that the right hand has direct access to the left hemisphere mechanisms of movement sequencing and fine motor control. In contrast, the motor cortex controlling the left hand has access to these commands only after they have crossed the callosum. The prediction under the Orton and Travis model was that, if stutterers in fact have bilateral speech motor control mechanisms, they may also have bilateral control of other fine motor movements. Accordingly, they should not show a right hand advantage but show similar finger tapping performance by the two hands.

When adult stutterers and normal speakers were tested on this sequential finger tapping task, the performance was almost identical for the two groups: both groups showed a right hand advantage, and there was similar overall performance indicating that stutterers are not generally uncoordinated and slow. There was, however, a very small but nonetheless reliable difference between the groups in errors, a finding I'll come back to momentarily.

Our interpretation of the data was that they provided no evidence that the neural mechanisms for sequencing (and by implication those of speech) are bilaterally represented as in the Orton/Travis model. We saw the data instead as constituting evidence of normal left hemisphere lateralization in stutterers. This is a conclusion similar to that reached from studies assessing cerebral dominance for speech and language in people who stutter by using injections of sodium amytal into one carotid artery or the other. This procedure, used routinely in neurosurgical contexts, results in a short-term anesthetization of the ipsilateral hemisphere and allows one to identify readily which hemisphere is specialized for speech and language. As described by Andrews, Quinn, and Sorby (1972) and Luessenhop (1973), people who stutter respond to these right- and left-sided injections in the same way as do fluent speakers, suggesting again a normal pattern of hemispheric specialization for speech.

Hence I would suggest that a principle of cerebral lateralization related to stuttering is that

people who stutter have normal left hemisphere lateralization of the neural mechanisms for the control of speech and other forms of sequential movement.

Two general points need to be made about this principle. First, it is unknown whether people who stutter have the normal pattern of anterior and posterior cortical anatomical asymmetries found in fluent speakers (Geschwind & Levitsky, 1968), but to the extent that the principle in neurobiology holds that "structure and function covary", we would expect that they should. As will be discussed later, the peculiarity in brain organization probably relates more to the supplementary motor area.

Second, let me make very clear that I am not suggesting that there is no right hemisphere involvement in speech or other fine motor movements. The evidence is clear that there is. A number of studies of the neural correlates of movement have been reported using methodologies including regional cerebral blood flow (Roland, 1984a, 1984b, 1985), positron emission tomography (Herholz et al., 1994; Petersen et al., 1988), and the analysis of DC cortical potentials recorded from the right and left hemispheres prior to and during movement (Wohlert, 1993). They have all demonstrated clearly that areas of primary motor cortex associated with movements of the face, tongue and jaw in both the right and left hemisphere are active during speech. They have also demonstrated, however, that the same primary sensorimotor areas show increased activity during non-speech oral movements, suggesting it is a motor movement effect, not a speech effect per se, that is bilaterally represented.

A second type of involvement of the right hemisphere in speech may relate to prosody. A number of studies of patients with unilateral anterior damage to the right hemisphere (e.g., Behrens, 1988; Ross, 1981; Shapiro & Danly, 1985) suggest that while such damage may leave speech more or less intact it can affect the use of prosody and intonation in both speech production and speech comprehension. What is not so clear is whether this effect is primary or secondary to alterations in emotionality commonly observed following right hemisphere damage (Gainotti, 1972, 1984). I mention these observations because, in the context of what I shall be saying shortly about right hemisphere activation in people who stutter, they may prove to have special significance for conceptualizations of stuttering as a prosodic disorder (Wingate, 1984).

What we are really concerned with in the principle, however, are the neural mechanisms associated with the organization and control of coordinated motor movements of a sequential nature, including speech. It is those that we believe are lateralized in the left hemisphere in stutterers just as they are in normal fluent speakers.

Despite normal lateralization, we have found evidence that the left hemisphere mechanisms underlying speech in stutterers may not be as efficient as they are in fluent speakers. This was first suggested in the slightly elevated error rate on sequential finger tapping noted above. It was more dramatically suggested in a study (Webster, 1986b) in which we asked subjects to tap, not the same sequences over and over again but a new sequence on each trial. On this sequence reproduction task, we found stutterers to be slower in initiating their responses and to make more errors in carrying out the first sequence, but once they got started, their performance was just as fast and accurate as the nonstutterers. The implication of these data is that people who stutter have difficulty not only with the initiation of speech utterances but also with the initiation of non-speech sequential movements. This appears to be related to response planning and organization. We found in a separate study (Webster, 1989a) that even when subjects were not under time pressure, stutterers still made significantly more errors than fluent controls in reproducing the sequences.

This finding, together with others that I shall describe below, led us to hypothesize (Webster, 1988) that a key area of the brain that is implicated in stuttering is the Supplementary Motor Area (SMA). A similar conclusion was reached by Caruso, Abbs and Gracco (1988) based on their analysis of the sequential organization of lip and jaw movements in stutterers and nonstutterers. Before I elaborate on this hypothesis in more detail, let me remind you of what I suggested at the outset: The variability in stuttering severity that is so characteristic of the disorder implies an underlying mechanism that is dynamic rather than one that reflects a static structural defect. In a number of experiments we have explored the possibility that these dynamic processes are ones that involve interference of the left hemisphere by on-going neural activity in the right.

Interhemispheric Interference

We began to explore the issue of interference by developing and testing the Interhemispheric Interference Model (Webster, 1986a) shown conceptually in Figure 2. The model implied normal left hemisphere lateralization of speech and language processes, normal right hemisphere organization and function, but an overflow of activity from the right to the left hemisphere, producing interference in some area of the left hemisphere (an area that we now suspect is the SMA). Within this model, variation in stuttering severity would reflect variations in the amount of overflow from the right to the left hemisphere.

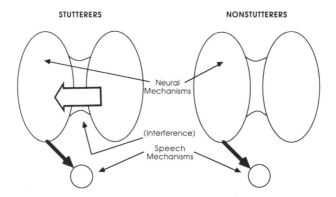

Figure 2. Schematic diagram of the Interhemispheric Interference model. Under this model, people who stutter differ from fluent speakers with respect to overflow of activity from the right to the left hemisphere which in turn interferes with speech processes (from Webster, 1993).

To test the model, we exploited the fact that each hemisphere controls the opposite hand and developed experimental analogues of the old parlor game of rubbing your stomach and patting your head at the same time. If under the model there is an excess of overflow from the right to the left hemisphere, we should expect people who stutter will have more difficulty in performing different activities with the two hands at the same time. This is precisely what we found in a number of experiments. Subjects were required to perform either the repetitive sequential finger tapping task (Webster, 1986a) or the sequence reproduction task (Webster, 1989b) using the right hand and to perform concurrently a second task that required them to turn a knob back and forth with the left hand whenever a tone sounded.

Not surprisingly, all subjects, stutterers and fluent controls, showed an interference effect whereby the knob turning interfered with finger tapping.

The critical finding, however, was that the stutterers showed significantly more interference than did the fluent controls. We found a similar differential interference effect in a bimanual handwriting task (Webster, 1988) that required the subject on each trial to write with both hands simultaneously the first letter of four words that had been read aloud. The stutterers not only took longer than the controls to write the four letters, but they made more errors, particularly mirror reversal errors, than the controls.

The results were consistent with the model, and we took this as evidence of either an excess overflow or a susceptibility of the left hemisphere to interference from activity in the right hemisphere. And so perhaps we could add to the earlier principle of normal lateralization of neural mechanisms for speech and language in stutterers the principle (or really the hypothesis) that

these left hemisphere mechanisms are "fragile" and susceptible to interference from other on-going neural activities, particularly those of the right hemisphere.

An Anomaly of Hemispheric Activation

We have completed two experiments (Webster, 1990b; Forster & Webster, 1991) the results of which have indicated that superimposed on this fragile left hemisphere system that is susceptible to interference is an anomaly in stutterers with respect to attentional mechanisms. Aspects of these studies have suggested that these attentional mechanisms may relate in particular to peculiarities in hemispheric activation.

A large literature in neuropsychology (Bradshaw & Nettleton, 1983; Bryden, 1982) leads to a distinction between *hemispheric specialization* and *hemispheric activation*. On the one hand, the concept of *hemispheric specialization* refers to the underlying structural specializations of the hemispheres that I discussed earlier. We believe it is these underlying structural specializations that are similar in people who stutter to those of fluent speakers. On the other hand, the concept of *hemispheric activation* refers to hemispheric arousal, either an enduring bias or temporary and task-specific, and the differential arousal or activation is manifest in the distribution of attentional resources favoring one side of the body or the other or one side of space or another (Bryden, 1982). This distinction and the evidence for it underlines another principle of lateralization in normal brain function:

the two cerebral hemispheres can be differentially engaged or activated to reflect the attentional demands of the situation (and this differential activation can be independent of structural specializations)

Related to the concept of hemispheric activation is the concept of an *inherent bias towards left hemisphere activation*. A number of lines of evidence, mainly from experimental neuropsychology (Annett, 1978; Bryden, 1978; Cohen, 1982), and in particular from the study of perceptual asymmetries (Bryden, 1991, 1993; Mondor & Bryden, 1992) suggest that *right-handers* have a predisposition for the left hemisphere to be in a state of greater readiness to process information and to respond. I stress *right-handers* because of the evidence that left-handers, or at least some left-handers, do not have this bias but appear to be able to direct their attention equally readily to right and left perceptual space. One clear demonstration of this phenomenon was provided by Peters (1987) who developed a task that required subjects to tap a key twice for every single tap of a key by the other hand. Peters reported that right-handers (nonstutterers) performed this task better when it was the right hand that tapped twice (R2/L1 condition) rather than the left hand (L2/R1 condition). Among left-handers, however, performance was similar under the two lead hand tapping conditions. Drawing upon Annett's (1978) single gene model of handedness which suggests that right-handers but not left-handers have an inherent directional bias, Peters has argued that the differences he observed between right- and left-handers reflect the role of attention in the expression of handedness. More specifically, he argued that right-handers have an attentional bias to the right hand that facilitated performance in the R2/L1 condition, but left-handers are more flexible in focusing lateralized attention and can attend with equal facility to the right or left hand when leading. Underlying this right side attentional bias in right-handers is thought to be a tonic left hemisphere activation not found in left-handers who show a greater lability of hemispheric activation.

This kind of evidence on hemispheric activation bias and handedness in normal fluent speakers leads to a further principle of lateralization that I believe is particularly germane to the issue of stuttering:

> *an inherent bias towards left hemisphere is found in in right-handed fluent speakers; a more equal distribution of activation is found in left-handed fluent speakers..*

When we repeated the Peters (1987) study with stutterers (Webster, 1990b), we found that both left- and right-handed stutterers performed like the left-handed nonstutterers, in other words, there was similar performance under the two lead hand conditions. Following from Peter's interpretation of the performance asymmetry, the results suggested that stutterers lack a left hemisphere activation bias and have a greater lability or flexibility of hemispheric activation or biasing than do nonstutterers.

We reached a similar conclusion in another experiment (Forster & Webster, 1991) that had a very different purpose and methodology. The study was designed to determine whether the dual task interference results obtained previously were specific to tasks that involved the opposite hemispheres, as implied by the Interhemispheric Interference Model, or whether the results would also be obtained when any two tasks are performed concurrently, including those mediated by a single hemisphere. The paradigm used was similar to that described by Webster (1986a) involving one hand performing finger tapping and the other a concurrent stimulus-contingent knob turning task. Specifically, in this case, the participants were tested on a sequential finger tapping task with one hand while either the contralateral or ipsilateral foot pressed a pedal in response to a periodic tone onset. The results indicated similar interference for the intra- and inter-hemispheric conditions. More germane for the present discussion, however, was the fact that among non-stutterers, responding with the left foot interfered more with finger tapping (with either hand) than did responding with the right foot, a finding we interpreted in attentional terms whereby a response with the left foot required a rapid switch in attention from the left hemisphere to the right. The fact that stutterers demonstrated similar interference with responding with either foot led us again to the conclusion that stutterers lack a left hemisphere attentional bias and can switch hemispheric attention or engagement more readily than nonstutterers.

The convergence of conclusions from the two studies with very different purposes and methodologies provides some basis for confidence that the hypothesized mechanisms reflect a principle of brain organization in stutterers, namely that

> *people who stutter (right- and left-handed) do not demonstrate a left hemisphere*

activation bias but are similar to fluent left-handers by showing a distribution of hemispheric activation that is more equal and more labile.

This principle of a lack of activation bias in stutterers is consistent with the results of many experiments reported in the literature of perceptual asymmetries in people who stutter. The performance of stutterers on dichotic listening tasks (e.g., Blood, 1985; Brady & Berson, 1975; Curry & Gregory, 1969; Rosenfield & Goodglass, 1980) and tachisto-scopic half field recognition tasks (e.g., Johannsen & Victor, 1986; Moore, 1976) indicate ear or visual field asymmetries, respectively, that are attenuated and more variable than those found in normal fluent speakers. Our interpretation of the differences is that they do not reflect differences in hemispheric specialization between stutterers and fluent speakers but differences in hemispheric activation biases.

A TWO-FACTOR WORKING MODEL OF NEURAL MECHANISMS UNDERLYING STUTTERING

We have now incorporated this idea of a labile pattern of hemispheric activation into the working model. The first two elements of the model are the same as earlier: a) normal left hemisphere lateralization of neural mechanisms for speech and motor sequencing; and b) a left hemisphere system for speech and motor sequencing that is inefficient or fragile and susceptible to interference from other on-going neural activities. To this we have added a third element, a lack of left hemispheric activation bias. The idea is illustrated conceptually in Figure 3. The left hemisphere speech motor control area is represented by the circle, and the vulnerability of the area to interference from other brain activity is represented by the "pores" in the circles as well as in the varying number of interference arrows, of both intra-hemispheric and inter-hemispheric origin. Hemispheric activation is represented by the arrows from the midbrain activating systems, and the bias in normal fluent right-handers is represented by the differing widths of the arrows.

STUTTERERS   NONSTUTTERERS

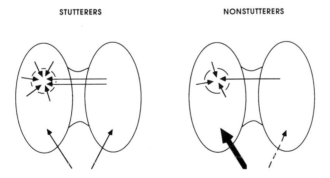

Figure 3. Schematic diagram of the Two-factor Model of Stuttering.

The Supplementary Motor Area

We believe at this time that the critical area of the left hemisphere with respect to stuttering is the supplementary motor area (SMA). Part of Brodmann area 6, the premotor cortex, the SMA is located on the medial bank of the hemispheres just above the cingulate cortex and anterior to the hind limb region of primary motor cortex (Tanji, 1994).

Called the supplementary motor area first by Penfield and Welch (1949) based on their clinical research involving electrical stimulation of exposed cerebral cortex of human patients, the area has been the subject of a great deal of research attention during the past decade. A number of methodologies have been used, including the analysis of regional cerebral blood flow, positron emission tomography, DC electrical potentials (the motor readiness potential or *Bereitschaftspotential*), single cell recordings, electrical stimulation, neuropsychological analysis of lesions in both humans and animals, together with basic research on neuroanatomy. Goldberg (1985), Tanji (1994), and Wise (1984) have reviewed the research literature in the area, and a number of consistent sets of findings have emerged that point to its function in the normal organization of behavior. I would mention only four that seem especially germane for our present purposes.

First, as evidenced in single unit studies of nonhuman primates (Mushiake et al., 1990; Tanji & Shima, 1994) as well as in brain imaging studies of human subjects (Roland, 1984a,b), activity in the SMA is associated with the planning of complex sequential movements of either the limbs or the speech musculature (Ikeda et al., 1995). The critical words here are *planning* and *complex* or *sequential.* The area does not seem critically involved in the execution of well practiced or simple movements but shows evidence of increased activity both when the person is simply thinking about carrying out an action or when the movement involves a number of components (Simonetta et al., 1991; Wohlert, 1993). These findings are consistent with reports from human patients that electrical stimulation of the area results in a feeling of intention to move (Penfield & Welch, 1949), but does not result in movement as such. Electrical stimulation also interferes with speech, specifically resulting in slowing, hesitation, and an inability to initiate speech sounds (Ojemann, 1994).

The second point is that there are very rich inter- and intra-hemispheric connections associated with the SMA. In fact, most interhemispheric connections between the motor areas go through the SMA (Rouiller et al., 1994).

The third set of findings, and this is not surprising in light of the rich interhemispheric connections, implicates the area as being crucial in bimanual coordination (Lang et al., 1990). Damage to the SMA interferes with the ability to coordinate hand movements and to do two different things with the hands at the same time (Brinkman, 1984). The fact that damage in humans also results in temporary mutism (Jonas, 1981) is consistent with a possible role in the bilateral coordination of the speech musculature.

And finally, there is some evidence that the area is crucial for the planning of self-initiated and internally guided movements rather than ones that are externally signaled and externally guided (Halsband et al., 1994; Passingham, 1989).

We were attracted to the SMA as a critical locus for stuttering for three principal reasons. First, the basic research on SMA that I have just summarized has linked the area to speech and non-speech motor functions, both of which are anomalous in people who stutter. Second, our sequence reproduction findings (Webster, 1986b) suggested a particular problem in the planning and initiation of new sequences of movements, a function that seems to be well associated with the SMA, but not in the execution of practiced movements, a function more associated with other premotor areas. And finally, the anomalies in bimanual coordination we have found in people who stutter (Webster, 1986a; 1988) also point to the SMA as a potential locus of difficulty.

The Lack of Left Hemisphere Activation Bias in People Who Stutter
   The second factor in the model is the lack of hemispheric activation bias discussed earlier. This lack of bias may lead to a relative periodic overactivation of the right hemisphere, an idea that is not new but which has attracted considerable interest over the years (Boberg et al., 1983; Moore, 1993; Moore & Haynes, 1980; Rastatter & Dell, 1987). What is perhaps original is the idea that the overactivation contributes to stuttering by being a source of interference with left hemisphere processes. Although the basis for this interference may include anomalous processing of linguistic information by the right hemisphere (Moore, 1993; Rastatter & Dell, 1987), let me comment briefly on another possible basis related to emotions.
   Patterns of electrical activity recorded from the frontal cortical areas of the left and right hemispheres suggest that when we experience positive emotions that motivate us to approach a situation, the left hemisphere becomes increasingly active (Ahern & Schwartz, 1985; Davidson, 1984; Davidson & Fox, 1982; Fox & Davidson, 1988). In contrast, when we experience negative emotions like fear and anxiety and apprehension, emotions that motivate us to withdraw from a situation, the right hemisphere becomes increasingly active. What all this then leads to is the suggestion (Webster, 1993) that the apprehension associated with stuttering affects the speech of people who stutter by being associated with right hemisphere activation, and this activation in turn interferes with the left hemisphere SMA. There is therefore an interplay between neurology and psychology. The anomalous brain mechanisms of the left hemisphere lead to speech disfluency, and this disfluency in turn leads to and reinforces negative emotional reactions to speech. These reactions in turn evoke greater right hemisphere activity which, in turn, interferes more with the fragile left hemisphere mechanisms resulting in disfluency, and so on.

Independence of the Factors
   I should comment in light of the extensive interhemispheric connections through the SMA that we have some evidence that the two factors are independent. Forster (1996) has recently examined the model in some detail and, in doing so, explored possible mechanisms for recovery from stuttering. Very briefly, he compared the performance of i) adults who stutter, ii) adults who reported having once stuttered but no longer do so ("ex-

stutterers"), and iii) adults who reported never having stuttered on two sets of behavioral tasks. One set was motor control tasks intended to assess the integrity of the SMA; the other was visual half-field tasks intended to detect hemispheric activation biases. Without elaborating here on the rationale, let me simply say that Forster (1996) hypothesized that non-stutterers and ex-stutterers would perform in a similar manner on the motor control tasks and do better than the stutterers. On the visual half-field tasks he expected to find that stutterers and ex-stutterers would be similar in showing markedly reduced or even reversed perceptual asymmetries compared to those of normal fluent speakers, a finding that was consistent with the idea of an anomaly in hemispheric activation. In other words, Forster was testing the idea that recovery from stuttering entails a maturation of the SMA despite a persistence in anomalous hemispheric activation. Put simply, the hypotheses were confirmed. While these data are interesting from the perspective of recovery from stuttering, the only point I wish to make with them here is that they indicate independence of the factors: Compared to the normal fluent speakers, the stutterers showed impairments on both the SMA motor tasks and on the hemispheric activation tasks while the ex-stutterers showed impairments only on the hemispheric activation tasks.

CONCLUDING COMMENTS

Emerging out of these ideas about brain mechanisms associated with stuttering are two comments that relate to the treatment and management of the disorder. First, the model suggests that successful therapy (or management) must have two components, one corresponding to each of the factors. The first is to remove sources of interference with speech motor control mechanisms. Implicit in what I have been saying is that a major source of interference is right hemisphere activity. Because one source of heightened activity can relate to negative emotions, it becomes critical that therapy include strategies for dealing with apprehension, avoidance, and withdrawal. As we overcome these tendencies, the right hemisphere activation associated with them decreases and then the interference with the left hemisphere SMA decreases. The second component must be to counteract the fragility of the left hemisphere system. I think we do this when we use fluency skills like gentle onsets and rate control which simplify speech and bring it within the capability of the fragile speech motor system.

Most treatment programs today include both factors (Boberg & Webster, 1990), and I think both are critical. If you deal only with speech motor control, the fears and apprehensions associated with right hemisphere activation will continue to provide a source of interference with the fragile system. If you deal only with fears, you still have a fragile speech motor control system that cannot handle the demands placed upon it.

The second concluding point I would like to leave you with is that although it is now clear that there is a biological basis to stuttering, *biological does not mean inevitable,* even when biological is the brain.

Let's look briefly at the brain, and let me tell you first how it does not work.

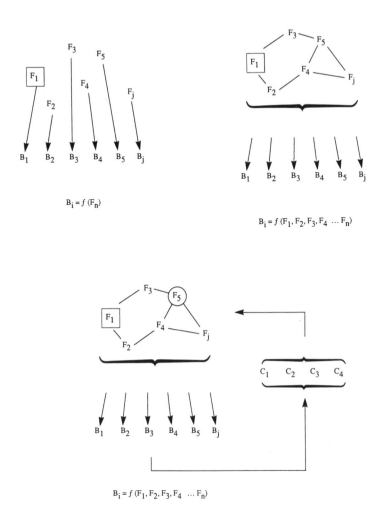

Figure 4. Three conceptual models of brain function and behavior. (Upper left) A model derived from phrenology which holds that each separate part of the brain (F1, F2, etc.) is responsible for some specific behavior or trait. (Upper right) A model which holds that brain parts are interconnected, and behavior emerges from the combined activity of many brain parts none of which is responsible entirely for any one behavior. (Lower) A model which holds that not only do behavior, thought, and feelings emerge from the combined activity of many parts of the brain, but that these consequences of brain activity can in turn can influence and alter brain activity.

One of the oldest general models of brain function (phrenology) held that each specific part of the brain (shown as F1, F2, etc. in Figure 4, upper left) has a specific behavioral or cognitive function. If there is something wrong with a part of the brain, it will show up in the associated behavior or cognitive function. Within that framework, stuttering would be inevitable if a part, like the SMA, were dysfunctional.

A more contemporary conceptualization of brain-behavior relations is that the parts ofthe brain interact and behavior emerges from the functioning of many parts of the brain (upper right portion of Figure 4). Indeed, the anomaly in the SMA of people who stutter shows up not just in speech but in various manual sequencing tasks as well. Even this framework implies inevitability, but instead of there being just one inevitable behavioral anomaly, there may be many.

Most important, it is now clear that, as illustrated schematically in the lower portion of Figure 4, not only is the brain the origin of behavior and cognition, but behavior and cognition are the origin of brain function. In other words, there are consequences of brain activity which can in turn affect brain activity. Not only does consciousness emerge from brain function, but consciousness affects brain function. Not only does thinking result from brain activity, but thinking itself affects brain activity. Not only do our emotions emerge from the activity of the brain, but our emotions drive the activity of the brain.

I would suggest that when we voluntarily control our speech through monitoring, regulating speed, controlling breathing and voice onsets, and being deliberate in our speech (R.F. Webster, 1980), we are in effect controlling left hemisphere activity. I would similarly suggest that when we voluntarily control our fears and apprehensions by using techniques like progressive relaxation and positive self-talk (Webster & Poulos, 1989), and when we systematically go into feared situations so we become less fearful, we are doing things that will affect our right hemisphere. And when we control the right hemisphere, we minimize interference with the left and we minimize stuttering. In other words, I am suggesting that when we use techniques to control our speech and to control our emotions, we are using techniques to control our brains. And when we control our brains, we are bringing an appropriate balance to the interhemispheric relations within them, a balance that enhances fluency and faciliates communication.

REFERENCES

Ahern, G.L., & Schwartz, G.E. (1985). Differential lateralization for positive and negative emotion in the human brain: EEG spectral analysis. *Neuropsychologia, 23,* 745-755.

Albanese, E., Merlo, A., Albanese, A., & Gomez, E. (1989). Anterior speech region: Asymmetry and weight-surface correlation. *Archives of Neurology, 46,* 307-310.

Andrews, G., Quinn, P.T., & Sorby, W.A. (1972). Stuttering: an investigation into cerebral dominance for speech. *Journal of Neurology, Neurosurgery and Psychiatry, 35,* 414-418.

Annett, M. (1978). *A single gene explanation of right and left handedness and brainedness.* Coventry: Lanchester Polytechnic.

Behrens, S.J. (1988). The role of the right hemisphere in the production of linguistic stress. *Brain and Language, 33,* 104-127.

Blood, G.W. (1985). Laterality differences in child stutterers: Heterogeneity, severity levels, and statistical treatments. *Journal of Speech and Hearing Disorders, 50,* 66-72.

Boberg, E., & Webster, W.G. (1990) Stuttering: Current status of theory and therapy. *Canadian Family Physician, 36,* 1156-1160.

Boberg, E., Yeudall, L.T., Schopflocher, D., & Bo-Lassen, P. (1983). The effect of an intensive behavioral program on the distribution of EEG alpha power in stutterers during the processing of verbal and visuospatial information. *Journal of Fluency Disorders, 8,* 245-263.

Bradshaw, J.L., & Nettleton, N.C. (1983). *Human cerebral asymmetry.* Englewood Cliffs: Prentice-Hall.

Brady, J.P., & Berson, J. (1975). Stuttering, dichotic listening, and cerebral dominance. *Archives of General Psychiatry, 32,* 1449-1452.

Brinkman, C. (1984). Supplementary motor area of the monkey's cerebral cortex: Short- and long-term deficits after unilateral ablation and the effects of subsequent callosal section. *Journal of Neuroscience, 4,* 918-929.

Bryden, M.P. (1978). Strategy effects in the assessment of hemispheric asymmetries. In G. Underwood (Ed.), *Strategies of information processing.* New York: Academic Press.

Bryden, M.P. (1982). *Laterality: Functional asymmetry in the intact brain.* New York: Academic Press.

Bryden, M.P., & Mondor, T.A. (1991). Attentional factors in visual field asymmetries. *Canadian Journal of Psychology, 45,* 427-447.

Caruso, A.J., Abbs, J.H., & Gracco, V.L. (1988). Kinematic analysis of multiple movement coordination during speech in stutterers. *Brain, 111,* 439-455.

Cohen, G. (1982). Theoretical interpretations. In J.G. Beaumont (Ed.), *Divided visual field studies of cerebral organization.* New York: Academic Press.

Curry, F.K.W., & Gregory, H.H. (1969). The performance of stutterers on dichotic listening tasks thought to reflect cerebral dominance. *Journal of Speech and Hearing Research, 12,* 73-82.

Davidson, R.J. (1984). Hemispheric asymmetry and emotion. In K.R. Scherer & P. Ekman (Eds.), *Approaches to emotion.* Hillsdale, NJ: Erlbaum.

Davidson, R.J., & Fox, N.A. (1982). Asymmetrical brain activity discriminates between positive versus negative affective stimuli in ten month old infants. *Science, 218,* 1235-1237.

Denckla, M.B. (1973). Development of speed in repetitive and successive finger-movements in normal children. *Developmental Medicine and Child Neurology, 15,* 635-645.

Forster, D.C. (1996). *Speech-motor control and interhemispheric relations in recovered and persistent stuttering.* Ph.D. dissertation, Carleton University, Ottawa, Canada.

Forster, D.C., & Webster, W.G. (1991). Concurrent task interference in stutterers: Dissociating hemispheric specialization and activation. *The Canadian Journal of Psychology, 45,* 321-335.

Foundas, A.L., Leonard, C.M., & Heilman, K.M. (1995). Morphologic cerebral asymmetries and handedness. *Archives of Neurology, 52,* 501-508.

Fox, N.A., & Davidson, R.J. (1988). Patterns of brain electrical activity during facial signs of emotion in 10-month-old infants. *Developmental Psychology, 24,* 130-136.

Gainotti, G. (1972). Emotional behavior and hemispheric side of the lesion. *Cortex, 8,* 41-55.

Gainotti, G. (1984). Some methodological problems in the study of the relationships between emotions and cerebral dominance. *Journal of Clinical Neuropsychology, 6,* 1-10.

Galaburda, A.M., LeMay, M., Kemper, T.L., & Geschwind, N. (1978). Right-left asymmetries in the brain. *Science, 199,* 852-856.

Gazzaniga, M.S. (1983). Right hemisphere language following brain bisection. *American Psychologist, 38,* 525-537.

Geschwind, N., & Levitsky, W. (1968). Human brain: Left-right asymmetries in temporal speech region. *Science, 161,* 186-187.

Goldberg, G. (1985). Supplementary motor area structure and function: Review and hypotheses. *The Behavioral and Brain Sciences, 8,* 567-616.

Halsband, U., Matsuzaka, Y., & Tanji, J. (1994). Neuronal activity in the primate supplementary, pre-supplementary and premotor cortex during externally and internally instructed sequential movements. *Neuroscience Research, 20,* 149-155.

Hayes, T.L., & Lewis, D.A. (1995). Anatomical specialization of the anterior motor speech area: Hemispheric differences in magnopyramidal neurons. *Brain and Language 49,* 289-308.

Herholz, K., Pietrzyk, U., Karbe, H., Würker, M., Wienhard, K., & Heiss, W.-D. (1994). Individual metabolic anatomy of repeating words demonstrated by MRI-guided positron emission tomography. *Neuroscience Letters, 182,* 47-50.

Howie, P.M. (1981). Concordance for stuttering in monozygotic and dizygotic twin pairs. *Journal of Speech and Hearing Research, 24,* 317-321.

Ikeda, A., Lüders, H.O., Shibasaki, H., Collura, T.F., Burgess, R.C., Morris, H.H., & Hamano, T. (1995). Movement-related potentials associated with bilateral simultaneous and unilateral movements recorded from human supplementary motor area. *Electroencephalography and clinical Neurophysiology, 95,* 323-334.

Johannsen, H.S., & Victor, C. (1986). Visual information processing in the left and left hemispheres during unilateral tachistoscopic stimulation of stutterers. *Journal of Fluency Disorders, 11,* 285-291.

Jonas, S. (1981). The supplementary motor region and speech emission. *Journal of Communication Disorders, 14,* 349-373.

Karbe, H., Würker, M., Herholz, K., Ghaemi, M., Pietrzyk, U., Kessler, J., & Heiss, W.-D. (1995). Planum temporale and Brodmann's Area 22. *Archives of Neurology, 52,* 869-874.

Kidd, K.K. (1984). Stuttering as a genetic disorder. In R.F. Curlee & W.H. Perkins (Eds.), *The nature and treatment of stuttering: New directions* (pp. 149-169). San Diego, CA: College-Hill Press.

Kimura, D. (1993). *Neuromotor mechanisms in human communication.* Oxford: Oxford University Press.

Kinsbourne, M., & McMurray, J. (1975). The effect of cerebral dominance on time sharing between speaking and tapping by preschool children. *Child Development, 46,* 240-242.

Lang, W., Obrig, H., Lindinger, G., Cheyne, D., & Deecke, L. (1990). Supplementary motor area activation while tapping bimanually different rhythms in musicians. *Experimental Brain Research, 79,* 504-514.

Luessenhop, A.J., Boggs, J.S., Lororwit, L.J., & Walle, E.L. (1973). Cerebral dominance in stutterers determined by Wada testing. *Neurology, 23,* 1190-1192.

Milner, B., Branch, D., & Rasmussen, T. (1966). Evidence for bilateral speech representation in some non-right-handers. *Transactions of the American Neurological Association, 91,* 306-308.

Mondor, T.A., & Bryden, M.P. (1992a). On the relation between visual spatial attention and visual field asymmetries. *The Quarterly Journal of Experimental Psychology, 44,* 529-555.

Moore, W.H. (1976). Bilateral tachistoscopic word perception of stutterers and normal subjects. *Brain and Language, 3,* 434-442.

Moore, W.H. (1993). Hemispheric processsing research. In E. Boberg (Ed.), *The neuropsychology of stuttering* (pp. 39-72). Edmonton: University of Alberta Press.

Moore, W.H., & Haynes, W.O. (1980). Alpha hemispheric asymmetry and stuttering: Some support for a segmentation dysfunction hypothesis. *Journal of Speech and Hearing Research, 23,* 229-247.

Mushiake, H., Inase, M., & Tanji, J. (1990). Selective coding of motor sequence in the supplementary motor area of the monkey cerebral cortex. *Experimental Brain Research, 82,* 208-210.

Ojemann, G.A. (1994). Cortical stimulation and recording in language. In A. Kertesz (Ed.), *Localization and neuroimaging in neuropsychology* (pp. 35-55). New York: Academic Press, 1994.

Orton, S.T. (1928). A physiological theory of reading disability and stuttering in children. *New England Journal of Medicine, 199,* 1046-1052.

Passingham, R.E., Chen, Y.C., & Thaler, D. (1989). Supplementary motor cortex and self-initiated movement. In M. Ito (Ed.), *Neural Progamming (Taniguchi Symposia on Brain Sciences No. 12)* (pp. 13-24). Basal: S. Karger.

Penfield, W., & Welch, K. (1949). The supplementary motor area in the cerebral cortex of man. *Transactions of the American Neurological Association, 74,* 79-84.

Perecman, E. (1983). (Ed.) *Cognitive Processing in the right hemisphere.* New York: Academic Press.

Peters, M. (1980). Why the preferred hand taps more quickly than the non-preferred hand: Three experiments on handedness. *Canadian Journal of Psychology, 34,* 62-71.

Peters, M. (1987). A nontrivial motor performance difference between right-handers and left-handers: Attention as intervening variable in the expression of handedness. *Canadian Journal of Psychology, 41,* 91-99.

Petersen, S.E., Fox, P.T., Posner, M.I., Mintun, M., & Raichle, M.E. (1988). Positron emission tomographic studies of the cortical anatomy of single-word processing. *Nature, 331,* 585-589.

Rastatter, M.P., & Dell, C.W. (1987). Reaction times of moderate and severe stutterers to monaural verbal stimuli: Some implications for neurolinguistic organization. *Journal of Speech and Hearing Research, 30,* 21-27.

Roland, P.E. (1984a). Organization of motor control by the normal human brain. *Human Neurobiology, 2,* 205-216.

Roland, P.E. (1984b). Metabolic measurements of the working frontal cortex in man. *Trends in Neuroscience, 7,* 430-435,

Roland, P.E. (1985). Cortical organization of voluntary behavior in man. *Human Neurobiology, 4,* 155-167.

Rosenfield, D.B., & Goodglass, H. (1980). Dichotic testing of cerebral dominance of stutterers. *Brain and Language, 11,* 170-180.

Ross, E.D. (1981). The aprosodias: Functional/anatomical organization of the affective components of language in the right hemisphere. *Archives of Neurology, 38,* 561-569.

Rouiller, E.M., Babalian, A., Kazennikov, O., Moret, V., Yu, X.-H., & Wiesendanger, M. (1994). Transcalloal connections of the distal forelimb representations of the primary and supplementary motor cortical areas in macaque monkeys. *Experimental Brain Research, 102,* 227-243.

Searleman, A. (1977). A review of right hemisphere linguistic capabilities. *Psychological Bulletin, 84,* 503-528.

Shapiro, B.E., & Danly, M. (1985). The role of the right hemisphere in the control of speech prosody in propositional and affective contexts. *Brain and Language, 25,* 19-36.

Simonetta, M., Clanet, M., & Rascol, O. (1991). Bereitschaftspotential in a simple movement or in a motor sequence starting with the same simple movement. *Electroencephalography and clinical Neurophysiology, 81,* 129-134.

Sperry, R.W. (1974). Lateral specialization in the surgically separated hemispheres. In F.O. Schmitt & F.G. Worden (Eds.), *The Neurosciences: Third Study Program* (pp. 5-20). Cambridge, Mass.: MIT Press.

Steinmetz, H., Volkmann, J., Jancke, L., & Freund, H.-J. (1990). Anatomical left-right asymmetry of language-related temporal cortex is different in left- and right-handers. *Annals of Neurology, 29,* 315-319.

Tanji, J. (1994). The supplementary motor area in the cerebral cortex. *Neuroscience Research, 19,* 251-268.

Tanji, J., & Shima, K. (1994). Role for supplementary motor area cells in planning several movements ahead. *Nature, 371,* 413-416.

Todor, J.I., & Kyprie, P.M. (1980). Hand differences in the rate and variability of rapid tapping. *Journal of Motor Behavior, 12,* 57-62.

Travis, L.E. (1931). *Speech pathology.* New York: Appleton.

Wada, J.A., Clarke, R., & Hamm, A. (1975). Cerebral hemispheric asymmetry in humans. *Archives of Neurology, 32,* 239-246.

Webster, R.L. (1980). Evolution of a target-based behavioral therapy for stuttering. *Journal of Fluency Disorders, 5,* 303-320.

Webster, W.G. (1985). Neuropsychological models of stuttering -- I. Representation of sequential response mechanisms. *Neuropsychologia, 23,* 263-267.

Webster, W.G. (1986a). Neuropsychological models of stuttering -- II. Interhemispheric interference. *Neuropsychologia, 24,* 737-741.

Webster, W.G. (1986b). Response sequence organization and reproduction by stutterers. *Neuropsychologia, 24,* 813-821.

Webster, W.G. (1988). Neural mechanisms underlying stuttering: Evidence from bimanual handwriting. *Brain and Language, 33,* 226-244.

Webster, W.G. (1989a). Sequence reproduction deficits in stutterers tested under nonspeeded response conditions. *Journal of Fluency Disorders, 14,* 79-86.

Webster, W.G. (1989b). Sequence initiation by stutterers under conditions of response competition. *Brain and Language, 36,* 286-300.

Webster, W.G. (1990a). Motor performance of stutterers: A search for mechanisms. *Journal of Motor Behavior, 22,* 553-571.

Webster, W.G. (1990b). Evidence in bimanual finger tapping of an attentional component to stuttering. *Behavioural Brain Research, 37,* 93-100.

Webster, W.G. (1993). Hurried hands and tangled tongues: Implications of current research for the management of stuttering. In E. Boberg (Ed.), *The neuropsychology of stuttering* (pp. 73-127). Edmonton: University of Alberta Press.

Webster, W.G., & Poulos, M. (1989). *Facilitating Fluency: Transfer strategies for adult stuttering treatment programs.* Tucson, Arizona: Communication Skill Builders.

Wiesendanger, M. (1986). Initiation of voluntary movements and the supplementary motor area. In H. Heuer & C. Fromm (Eds.), *Generation and modulation of action patterns* (pp. 3-13). (*Experimental Brain Research Series,* Vol. 15). Berlin: Springer-Verlag.

Wingate, M. (1984). Stuttering as a prosodic disorder. In R.F. Curlee and W. H. Perkins (Eds.), *Nature and treatment of stuttering: New directions* (pp. 215-235). San Diego: College-Hill Press.

Wise, S.P. (1984). The nonprimary motor cortex and its role in the cerebral control of movement. In G.M. Edelman, W.E. Gall, & W.M. Cowan (Eds.), *Dynamic aspects of neocortical function* (pp. 525-555). New York: John Wiley & Sons.

Witelson, S.F., & Pallie, W. (1973). Left hemisphere specialization for language in the newborn: Neuroanatomical evidence of asymmetry. *Brain, 96,* 641-646.

Wohlert, A.B. (1993). Event-related brain potentials preceding speech and nonspeech oral movements of varying complexity. *Journal of speech and hearing research, 36,* 897-905.

Wolff, P.H., Hurwitz, I., & Moss, H. (1977). Serial organization of motor skills in left- and right-handed adults. *Neuropsychologia, 15,* 539-546.

Young, R.M. (1970). *Mind, brain and adaptation in the nineteenth century.* Oxford University Press.

Zaidel, E. (1983). A response to Gazzaniga: Language in the right hemisphere, an empirical perspective. *American Psychologist, 38,* 542-546.

Motor control in speech production and fluency disorders

Speech Production: Motor Control, Brain Research and Fluency Disorders
W. Hulstijn, H.F.M. Peters and P.H.H.M. Van Lieshout, editors

Chapter 9

DYNAMIC INTERACTIONS OF FACTORS THAT IMPACT SPEECH MOTOR STABILITY IN CHILDREN AND ADULTS

Anne Smith

We view stuttering as a multifactorial, dynamic disorder that emerges from the nonlinear interactions of many heterogeneous systems. In individuals who stutter, speech motor performance is unusually vulnerable to influences from factors traditionally viewed as remote from the speech motor system. Thus a challenge to experimentalists is to find methods by which links between variables operating at many different levels may be uncovered. For example, speaking rate is a variable that is often used therapeutically, but there is little understanding of how rate changes actually affect speech motor output. In addition, there has been increasing interest in experiments that integrate linguistic and motor factors in stuttering. To explore links between such variables, our laboratory has developed a new index of speech motor stability, the spatiotemporal index or STI. In series of experiments we show how global variables such as rate affect the STI in subjects who do and do not stutter. In addition, data from experiments on children and adults suggest that the stability of execution of speech movement sequences is affected by the syntactic complexity and/or length of the utterance to be spoken.

INTRODUCTION

This chapter is comprised of two sections: (1) a brief statement of the theoretical framework underpinning our experimental work, and (2) a discussion of a set of experiments on speech motor stability that address some of the questions raised within this framework.
I. A Dynamic, Multifactorial Approach to Stuttering

We have suggested that a major shift in paradigm is necessary for progress in understanding stuttering (Smith, 1996; Smith & Kelly, 1996). We encourage a move from a focus on static units of disfluency that are counted and used to define stuttering, to a dynamic, multifactorial model accounting for the full continuum of fluency experienced by individuals who stutter. A comprehensive theory of stuttering should account for fluency and fluency failures in a multidimensional space that includes family history, social context, linguistic processes, emotional/autonomic factors, speech motor organization, and other factors. In other words, a theory of stuttering should not be focused on how to explain a repetition of a perceptually defined unit, such as a sound or syllable repetition, rather it must account for all of the complex phenomena associated with the disorder. These phenomena may be observed and analyzed at many different levels, from cognitive and linguistic to physiological levels. Ultimately data from each level of analysis must be interpreted in relation to a global theory of stuttering.

Considering these multiple factors in terms of the neurophysiological processes involved, it is clear that there are multiple, heterogeneous neural systems interacting during speech production. These systems are characterized by plasticity, interactiveness, and highly parallel operations. Within dynamic models of neural systems, patterned output is an emergent property of these interactive components. We (Smith & Kelly, 1996) have proposed that stuttering be viewed as an emergent, dynamical disorder (Mackey & Milton, 1987). This implies that stuttering refers to processes that change in time, rather than to compartmentalized, static events.

Many features of stuttering fit well with dynamic systems theory. First, the concept of emergent property helps us to understand the behavior of complex systems. Specifically, the output behavior of a system is viewed as an "emergent property" of the nonlinear interactions of components; as such, properties of the output are not necessarily isomorphic with features of the input (Thelen & Smith, 1994). The factors that interact to produce stuttering may bear little resemblance to descriptions of disfluency (e.g., part-word repetition, silent block). Thus classification of disfluency types may tell us little about the dynamic interplay of factors that contribute to stuttering. Also significant for the area of stuttering is that dynamic theories help us to reject the seductive simplicity of linear explanations that attribute stuttering to a single, core, causal factor. In other words, it is a misconception that the "cause of stuttering" will be found by identifying the one experimental variable present in all individuals who stutter and absent in all who do not stutter. Stuttering emerges in individuals when complex, multileveled, and dynamic processes interact to produce failures in fluency that the individuals and their culture judge to be aberrant. There is no core factor - - a brain lesion, a DNA sequence, a type of disfluency, a feedback loop-- that generates all the phenomena associated with stuttering.

Dynamic theories incorporate the feature of nonlinearity (very small changes in one component of a dynamic system may produce very large changes in the output of the system); stuttering is an extremely nonlinear disorder. That is, the "output" of the system, e.g., fluency, may change dramatically with small changes in underlying factors. Finally, the dynamical systems literature suggests new methods to examine the dynamic behavior of systems (Bassingthwaighte et al., 1994). While the experiments described below are not derived from the dynamic literature directly, the novel approach to kinematic analysis that we developed was prompted by dynamic principles, which suggest that, instead of measuring a signal at single points in time, the entire signal be entered into the analysis.

II. Experiments in Spatiotemporal Stability.

One of the overall goals of our work has been to develop novel ways to assess fluency. A new metric might reveal subtle performance characteristics of the system and could provide a more sensitive means of assessing the stability of patterning of speech movement production. Our theoretical framework suggests that factors seemingly removed from speech motor systems have an impact on speech motor stability. Therefore, a critical experimental challenge is to relate traditionally disparate variables, such as linguistic complexity and emotional arousal to speech motor output. If a speaker has a speech motor system that is either inherently unstable, or relatively stable but vulnerable to breakdown when conditions are altered, a sensitive index of stability could reveal the effects of increased demands operating on the system. We would not expect to see the effects of factors such as linguistic complexity on the traditional measures employed in motor control experiments, e.g., on measures of peak velocity or displacement. Finally one constraint we placed upon ourselves in developing this new metric was that the measurement must be applicable to very young children, as stuttering is a developmental disorder.

In a recent paper, we introduced the method of computing the Spatiotemporal Index, or STI (Smith et al., 1995). We computed this index in normally speaking adults and determined the effects of changes in speaking rate. The basic idea underlying the STI is as follows. In normal, adult speakers, speech is a highly practiced, extremely stable motor behavior. Given this, we suggested that, when adult speakers generate an utterance repeatedly, their movement output will be highly reliable. Further, if amplitude- and time-normalization procedures were applied to the movement records, waveforms from a repeated utterance would fall upon a single core template. The STI is a measure of how well the movement waveforms from a repeated utterance converge onto a single template: the higher the STI the greater the deviation from a single template.

A complete description of the methods has been published (Smith et al., 1995). Briefly, the movement of the lower lip is recorded while subjects repeat a phrase (we have used "buy bobby a puppy" as the target phrase in our work to date). Fifteen displacement waveforms for each subject are amplitude- and time-normalized. Standard procedures of amplitude normalization (z-score transformation) are used. For time-normalization the fast Fourier transform of each amplitude-normalized displacement record is computed after the linear trend is removed. The displacement waveforms are then resynthesized on a time base of 1000 points by adding the first 10 harmonics with the fundamental of each Fourier series fixed as 1 Hz. Finally, the linear trend is added to the resynthesized displacement records. Figure 1 shows examples of the original and normalized displacement waveforms.

For the sets of 15 time- and amplitude-normalized displacement waveforms for each subject in each condition, a standard deviation is computed across the 15 samples at one point in relative time. The standard deviations are computed successively at 2% intervals. The standard deviation function is shown in Figure 1 in the bottom plot of each panel. These 50 standard deviations are summed, and the result, which reflects the overall spatiotemporal stability across 15 repetitions of the utterance, is the spatiotemporal index. As shown in Table 1, for normal adult speakers producing "buy bobby a puppy" at their habitual rate, the STI seems to be a very reliable measure.

Consider now the questions we have addressed using the STI as an index of the stability of patterning of speech motor performance. First, what happens to the stability of movement output when speakers change their rates?

146   *A. Smith*

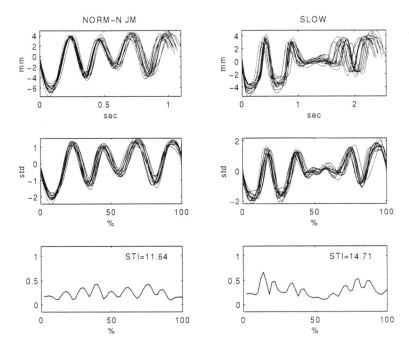

Figure 1. Lower lip displacement for a normal adult speaker producing "buy Bobby a puppy" at normal (left panel) and slow (right panel) speech rates. The three plots from top to bottom are: the original displacement waveforms, the amplitude- and time-normalized displacement waveforms, and the standard deviation computed at 2% intervals in relative time. The STI is the cumulative sum of these 50 standard deviations.

In our first study of normal adult speakers (Smith et al., 1995), the results were consistent across subjects. Normal and fast rates of speech produced STIs that were not significantly different, while slow speech rate was characterized by significantly higher STI values. Typical results for the normal and slow rates are shown for one subject in Figure 1. Our findings suggest that for normal adult speakers, slowing rate of speech produces less stable speech motor performance.

Table 1. STI for normal adult speakers producing "buy Bobby a puppy" at their habitual rate and loudness.

Study	n	STI (mean)	s.d.
Smith et al. (1995)	7	12.5	2.3
Smith & Goffman (submitted)	8	13.5	2.5
Maner & Smith (In progress)	8	13.0	2.7

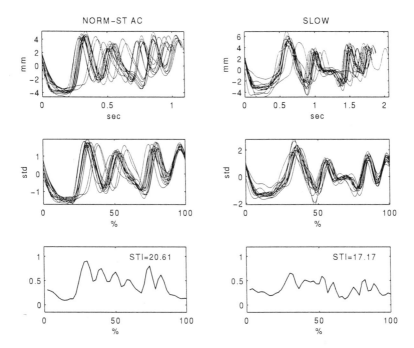

Figure 2. Lower lip displacement for a adult who stutters producing "buy Bobby a puppy" at normal (left panel) and slow (right panel) speech rates. All productions were judged to be fluent. In each vertical panel, the three plots (top to bottom) are: the original displacement waveforms, the amplitude- and time-normalized displacement waveforms, and the standard deviation computed at 2% intervals in relative time. The STI is the cumulative sum of these 50 standard deviations.

In a second study of rate change (Smith et al., In progress), we asked fifteen adults who stutter to produce habitual, fast, and slow speech rates. Sample data from one adult who stutters are shown in Figure 2. In this case, the normal rate STI is relatively high, and the slower rate of speech does not produce the expected increase in the STI, rather there is a slight decrease. We are in the process of testing a matched, normally speaking, control group. However, our preliminary analyses suggest that, as a control parameter, rate change operates differently in some adult stutterers. Further, there is evidence that some, but not all adults who stutter, are inherently less stable, even at their preferred, normal rates.

In another set of experiments, we employ the STI as an index of changes in speech motor performance as a function of age of speaker and of syntactic complexity of the utterance. First the simpler question, does the STI decrease as children mature? Assuming that stability of oral movement is a goal of the mature system, we predicted that 4- and 7-year-old children would have higher STIs compared to those of young adults. This prediction was confirmed (Smith & Goffman, submitted); the 4-year-old group had a mean STI that was twice that of the young adult group.

Finally, turning to the last topic of this chapter, we note that there is a great divide between those engaged in language research and those engaged in research on speech production, especially on speech motor control. Is this gap appropriate, reflecting the true independence of the neurophysiological processes underpinning language formulation and speech production? Or is it more a reflection of our narrow training, which confines our studies to certain realms, a division of experimental inquiry that belies the true interdependence of language and speech motor processes in the brain? We conducted a preliminary experiment that attempts to bridge the language/motor gap (Maner & Smith, In progress). If linguistic processes, specifically syntactic complexity, impact speech motor processes, we reasoned that increased syntactic complexity might be reflected in higher values on the STI. Our approach was to embed "buy Bobby a puppy " in four sentences of varying syntactic complexity (e.g., "you buy Bobby a puppy now if he wants one") and to compare subjects' STI values on the baseline condition ("buy Bobby a puppy" alone) with those calculated form the phrase embedded in the four sentences. Two groups of subjects were

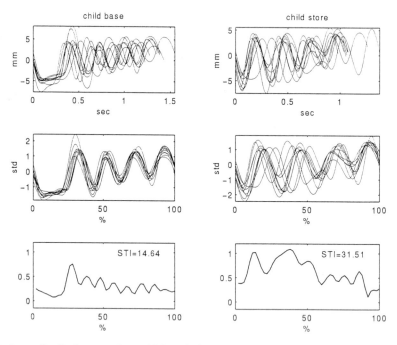

Figure 3. Lower lip displacement for a child producing "buy Bobby a puppy" (left panel) and "he wants to buy Bobby a puppy at my store" (right panel). The three plots from top to bottom are: the original displacement waveforms (in the right panel, the displacment associated with "buy bobby a puppy" has been extracted from the longer sentence), the amplitude- and time-normalized displacement waveforms, and the standard deviation computed at 2% intervals in relative time. The STI is the cumulative sum of these 50 standard deviations. The increase in the value of the STI when the phrase was embedded in the longer sentence was typical of both child and adult subjects.

tested: typically developing children aged 5 years and young adults. As shown in Figure 3, the results of this study supported our hypothesis: embedding the phrase in complex sentences significantly increased the STI both for children and adults. The design of this study was intended to allow us to disambiguate the effects of syntactic complexity and length of utterance. This aspect of the experiment was not successful, as the STI was higher on all embedded conditions. The details cannot be discussed in the present context, however, we must recognize that the increased STI could reflect the impact of syntactic complexity and/or utterance length. In any case, we find these results very promising, as they provide evidence that processes traditionally envisioned as well removed from speech motor performance, such as syntactic complexity and utterance planning, may in fact have observable effects on the execution of speech movement sequences.

REFERENCES

Bassingthwaighte, J.B., Liebovitch, L.S., & West, B.J. (1994). *Fractal physiology*. New York: Oxford University Press.

Glass, L., & Mackey, M.C. (1988). *From clocks to chaos*. Princeton, NJ: Princeton University Press.

Mackey, M.C., & Milton, J.G. (1987). Dynamical diseases. In S.H. Koslow, A.J. Mandell, & M.F. Shlesinger (Eds.), *Perspectives in biological dynamics and theoretical medicine* (pp. 16-32). New York: The New York Academy of Sciences.

Smith, A. (1996). Stuttering and volcanoes: Beyond classification to a global theory. A paper presented at the Third Annual Leadership Conference, *"Research and Treatment: Bridging the Gap,"* ASHA Division of Fluency and Fluency Disorders, Monterey, CA, May, 1996.

Smith, A., & Goffman, L. (1996). Stability and patterning of speech movement sequences in children and adults: A preliminary study. Manuscript submitted for publication.

Smith, A., Goffman, L., Zelaznik, H., Ying, G., & McGillem, C. (1995). Spatiotemporal stability and patterning of speech movement sequences. *Experimental Brain Research, 104*, 493-501.

Smith, A., & Kelly, E. (1996). Stuttering: A dynamic, multifactorial model. In *Nature and Treatment of Stuttering: New Directions*. R. Curlee, & G. Siegel (Eds.), Boston: Allyn & Bacon.

Thelen, E., & Smith, L.B. (1994) *A Dynamic Systems Approach to the Development of Cognition and Action*. Cambridge, MA: MIT Press/Bradford.

Speech Production: Motor Control, Brain Research and Fluency Disorders
W. Hulstijn, H.F.M. Peters and P.H.H.M. Van Lieshout, editors

Chapter 10

SPATIAL AND TEMPORAL VARIABILITY IN OBSTRUENT GESTURAL SPECIFICATION BY STUTTERERS AND CONTROLS: COMPARISONS ACROSS SESSIONS.

Peter J. Alfonso, Pascal H.H.M. van Lieshout

Assumptions made about invariant control schemes are gleaned from data collected from a single point in time, that is, data collected from a single session. Thus, we know relatively little about the magnitude of the day-to-day articulatory variability that underlies an invariant percept. The aims of this study are to: 1) explore further the short- and long-term flexibility in normal speech kinematics, and 2) identify relatively stable spatial and temporal characteristics that could function as appropriate experimental and control group comparative parameters. Movements of the tongue, lips, and jaw were transduced by electromagnetic midsagittal articulography. Seven stutterers and matched controls completed three sessions at two week intervals. Results indicate that neither traditional spatial nor temporal organizational characteristics are stable across sessions for all control subjects and thus are not appropriate group comparative parameters because of natural long-term flexibility. Only motor equivalence covariability is consistently correlated with the invariant percept even in the case of unstable spatial and temporal characteristics. Natural flexibility is compatible with the notion of coordinative structures within a task-dynamic point of view.

INTRODUCTION

An implicit notion in many dynamical models of movement is that there is an underlying invariance in the motor control scheme despite the observed surface variations in performance (e.g., Saltzman, 1991; Saltzman & Munhall, 1989). However, and in spite of the decades-long search for the so-called invariant characteristics that underlie normal speech production (e.g., Gracco & Abbs, 1986), the majority of the often cited motor characteristics of speech (e.g., Gracco, 1994) are much more variable in repeated-trial tasks than they are invariant. Further, the assumptions that we make about invariant control schemes are gleaned from data collected from a single point in time, that is, data collected from a single session and usually within a single speech rate. Thus, we know less about the magnitude of the day-to-day articulatory variability that underlies an invariant percept. The focal point that we make in this paper is that the field's poor understanding of the short- and long-term variability associated with normal speech output posses a special problem in regard to the ultimate understanding of stutterers' speech production, in general, and of treatment effects on stutterers' fluency, in particular. Thus, the overall purpose of the experiment described here is to explore further the saliency of certain presumed invariant motor characteristics of speech, and by extension, the notion of coordinative structures, by comparing certain spatiotemporal characteristics of tongue-jaw and lip-jaw movements for stops and fricatives across multiple sessions and across speech rate. Another aim of the project is to identify relatively stable spatial and temporal characteristics that could function as appropriate group comparative parameters.

METHODS

The movements of the tongue blade, lips, and jaw were transduced by electromagnetic midsaggital articulography. A single session included at least twenty perceptually fluent repetitions of /pap/, /tat/, and /sas/ imbedded in a carrier phrase at normal, slow, and fast speech rates. The 60 phrases were blocked by rate and produced first at a normal speech rate, than again at a fast rate, and finally at a slow rate resulting in a minimum of 180 phrases per session. Seven stutterers and seven matched controls completed three sessions, and the interval between sessions was about two weeks. Only perceptually fluent utterances, which were classified as such by the subject, the experimenters, and two experienced speech-language pathologists who later rated the audio tapes, were included in the analysis shown here. Analysis of the complete data set is ongoing and only data associated with syllable initial /p/ closure during the normal rate condition are discussed here.

RESULTS

General trends in the spatial stability for /p/ closure were estimated by comparison of the normalized vertical displacement across sessions. The comparisons show that organizational patterns differ across control subjects. For example, subject 6 achieves closure primarily by jaw and upper lip displacement, 45 and 32 percent respectively, the lower lip contributing the least with 23 percent of the total displacement. On the other hand, Subject 5 achieves closure predominately by jaw displacement (62 percent) with relatively less contribution of the lips (18 and 20 percent). Next, the relative displacement patterns are generally stable across sessions for 4 of the 7 subjects. As a first approximation of across session stability, inconsistencies across sessions in the primary articulator, that is, the articulator that contributed the most toward closure, were noted. Three of the seven control subjects showed inconsistencies across sessions. In the case of Subject 3, /p/ closure is achieved primarily by the jaw in session 1 but by the lower lip in sessions 2 and 3. Subjects 1 and 7 show a shift in the predominate articulator from the jaw in session 1 to equal contribution of the jaw and upper lip in session 2. In absolute terms, these differences can be large. For Subject 2, for example, average vertical displacements of the non-dominate upper and lower lips vary 200 percent across sessions, from about 2 to 4 mm, while total displacement of the jaw and lips synergy vary from 10 to 14 mm across sessions.

The same comparisons of the normalized vertical displacement across sessions were made for the stutterers. First, stutterers, like the control subjects, demonstrate idiosyncratic control strategies, that is, different subjects elect to achieve closure with varying contributions of jaw and lip displacement. Second, and again like the controls, four of the subjects demonstrate stable control strategies whereas three of the stutterers use varying contributions of jaw and lip displacements across sessions, most notably Subject 6, who achieves closure primarily by lower lip displacement in session 1, the jaw in session 2, and equal contribution of the jaw and upper lip in session 3. Subjects 3 and 4 enlist a different primary articulator for one of the sessions compared to the other two. With two important caveats in mind, that is, intersubject variability is greater for the stutterers as a group, and more sophisticated measures of across session stability need to be carried out, the main point that arises from the comparisons of the normalized vertical displacement across sessions is this: spatial organizational patterns are not invariant across time for all members of the control population, and until the magnitude of the normal variability can be quantified and understood, relative displacement patterns should not be considered an appropriate group comparison parameter. In fact, the analysis we have completed thus far do not appear to indicate a group difference in regard to long-term stability but rather show that the same number of subjects from both groups are either consistent or variable across session.

Turning next to temporal stability, Figure 1 shows the relative distribution of the upper lip, lower lip, and jaw sequence patterns across sessions for /p/ closure in control subjects. The black portions of the bars represent the upper lip, lower lip, and jaw sequence, the white portions represent the lower lip, upper lip, and jaw sequence, and the striated portions represent all others.

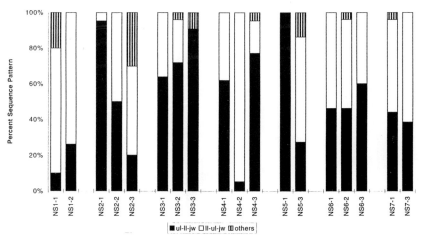

Figure 1. Control subjects, /p/ Closure across sessions and subjects. Relative distribution of each sequence re peak velocity.

By far, the predominant sequences are those in which lip movement occurs first and jaw movement occurs last. First, the figure shows that either lip lead sequence is equally likely to occur. For example, Subject 1 prefers the lower lip lead sequence while Subject 3 prefers the upper lip lead sequence. Second, the figure shows that some subjects, for example Subjects 6 and 7, show no clear preference for either lip lead sequence. Third, two of the subjects, 2 and 4, show a clear reversal in the lip lead sequence across sessions.

One of the reasons that the sequence pattern is not stable across time is that it does not reflect interarticulator relative time. Subjects who demonstrate tight coupling of lip movements, for example, would have a higher probability of producing both lip-lead sequences compared to subjects who demonstrate longer relative timing of the lip movements. This is demonstrated for control subjects in Figure 2, which shows the lip relative time in black and the lagging lip to jaw relative time in striation for the session average sequences. A session average sequence represents the ensemble averaged trajectories associated with the movements of the lips and jaw. Note that the relative time for lip movements in the case of Subjects 6 and 7 is less than five ms. Recall that Figure 1 showed that these subjects demonstrate nearly equal probability of producing either lip-lead sequences. Thus, a temporal invariancy criterion based on consistent sequence patterns would exclude Subjects 6 and 7 whereas a criterion based on tight interarticulator timing would include the same subjects.

Figures 3 and 4 show the same temporal parameters for the stutterers. Trends indicated in Figure 1 for controls are observed also in Figure 3 for stutterers, namely that lip lead sequences are predominate and that either lip lead sequence can occur, although the lower lip lead sequence, shown by the white bars, is prevalent in the stutterers' data whereas the upper lip lead sequence, shown by the black bars, is prevalent in the control data. Perhaps a more meaningful distinction is that there is a greater prevalence of sequences in the stutterers' data compared to the controls where the jaw did not move last, shown by the striated bars.

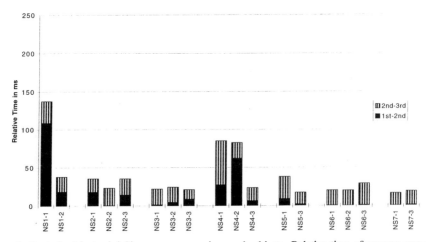

Figure 2. Control subjects. /p/ Closure across sessions and subjects. Relative time of average sequence re peak velocity.

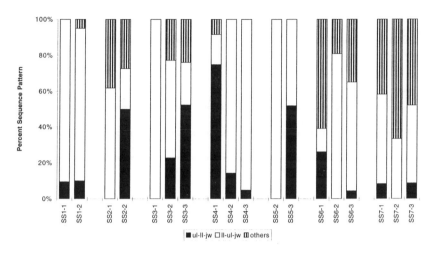

Figure 3. PWS subjects. /p/ Closure across sessions and subjects. Relative distribution of each sequence re peak velocity.

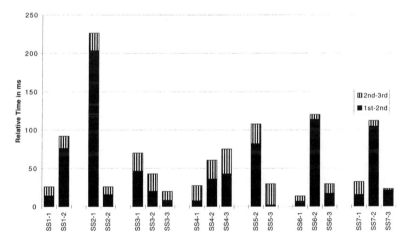

Figure 4. PWS subjects. /p/ Closure across sessions and subjects. Relative time of aevrage sequence re peak velocity.

However, it is still difficult to interpret the significance of the sequence patterns with respect to the integrity of the speech motor system without considering relative time. For example, note that Subject 5 shows a clear preference for the lower-lip lead sequence in Session 1 but that in Session 2 either lip lead sequence occurs equally often. The relative time measures shown in Figure 4 for this subject, Subject 5, show a relatively long average lower lip lead for Session 1 but short lip interarticulator time for Session 2.

Table 1. Control subjects. /p/ Closure across sessions and subjects. Relative time of average sequence re peak velocity.

	NS1-1	NS1-2	NS2-1	NS2-2	NS2-3	NS3-1	NS3-2	NS3-3	NS4-1	NS4-2	NS4-3	NS5-1	NS5-3	NS6-1	NS6-2	NS6-3	NS7-1	NS7-3
1st ul-ll			17.9			1.5	4.6	8.8						0.5	0.0	0.8		
2nd ll-jw			17.8			20.6	20.0	12.5						19.4	19.6	28.0		
1st ll-ul	108.9	18.3		0.4	14.3				27.5	62.1	6.5	9.3	2.1				0.3	1.0
2nd ul-jw	28.6	19.8		22.8	21.4				57.4	20.4	17.1	28.8	15.1				15.9	17.6

Table 2. PWS subjects. /p/ Closure across sessions and subjects. Relative time of average sequence re peak velocity.

	SS1-1	SS1-2	SS2-1	SS2-2	SS3-1	SS3-2	SS3-3	SS4-1	SS4-2	SS4-3	SS5-2	2S5-3	SS6-1	SS6-2	SS6-3	SS7-1	SS7-2	SS7-3
1st ul-ll				16				7.75										
2nd ll-jw				10				19.63										
1st ll-ul	14.49	76.52		46.88	20.21	8.42			36.25	42.79	82.24	2.25		114	17.14			21.25
2nd ul-jw	11.63	15.63		23.5	22.63	11.32			24.63	32.63	25.63	27.38		6.13	12.25			1.88
1ST ll-jw			203.8													15.69	104.8	
2ND jw-ul			22.7													16.48	7.25	
1st jw-ll													7.06					
2nd ll-ul													6.61					

Thus, sequence patterns alone are not appropriate group comparison parameters because of: 1) the high intrasubject variability in the control population, and 2) the relationship between the sequence pattern and interarticulator relative time (Van Lieshout et al., 1994).

Tables 1 and 2 show both the average sequence pattern and relative time. Table 1 shows that three of the control subjects are inconsistent in at least one of the two temporal parameters across sessions. Control Subject 2 shows a sequence reversal and Control Subjects 1 and 4 show relatively large differences, that is, greater than 50 ms across sessions, in interarticulator relative time.

Table 2 shows that the combined relative time for average sequence analysis for stutterers is different from that of the controls, at least more so than that observed for the group comparisons based on relative displacements patterns. Like the controls, the average sequence that occurs most often is the lower lip, upper lip, and jaw sequence. The upper lip, lower lip, and jaw average sequence occurs only twice. Second, note that a total of four sequence patterns occur; in addition to the two lip lead sequences, the lower lip, jaw, and upper lip sequence occurs in Subjects 2 and 7, and the jaw, lower lip, and upper lip sequence occurs in Subjects 6. Third, note that sequence reversals occur in four subjects; Subjects 2, 4, 6, and 7. And fourth, note that differences in interarticulator time greater than 50 ms across sessions occur in five subjects; Subjects 1, 2, 5, 6, and 7. Only one subject, Subject 3, compared to four in the control group, is stable for both temporal parameters.

While the combination of two temporal measures appears to differentiate the groups better than the single spatial measure, the validity of the former measure as a group comparison estimate remains unclear because of the inherent variability in the control population. Next, we turn to an analysis that reflects both space and time, that is, motor equivalence

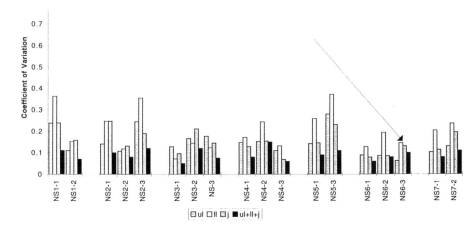

Figure 5. Control subjects. /p/ Closure. Coefficient of variation. Synergies that do not meet motor equivalence covariability are indicated by arrows.

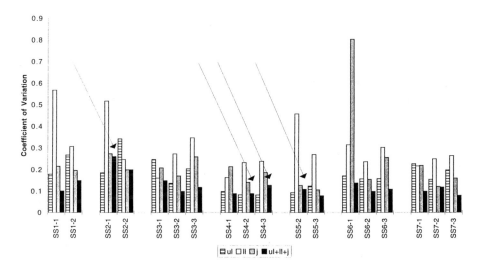

Figure 6. PWS subjects. /p/ Closure. Coefficient of variation. Synergies that do not meet motor equivalence covariability are indicated by arrows.

covariability. Relative time is preserved in the way that motor equivalence covariability is calculated here in that the peak displacement for each of the articulators is used rather than the relative displacement of the lips at the time of the peak displacement of the jaw. Figure 5 shows the coefficient of variation, appearing left to right, for the upper lip in striation, the lower lip in white, the jaw in gray, and the total displacement in black across sessions for the control subjects. The figure shows that while spatial and temporal control strategies can and do vary across sessions for some control subjects, the movements of the lips and jaw are well coordinated in each of the sessions save one and for all subjects. Motor equivalence covariability is stable even in the case of Subjects 1, 3, and 7 who demonstrated instability across sessions. Only in the case of the third session for Control Subject 6 is motor equivalence covariability not observed. On the other hand, well-coordinated movements of the lips and jaw in the case of stutterers is less consistent.

Figure 6 shows that three of the stutterers do not show consistent motor equivalence covariability across sessions, namely Subjects 2, 4, and 6 with Subject 4 failing to show motor equivalence covariability in two of the three sessions. The data in Figures 5 and 6 demonstrate that motor equivalence covariability is relatively stable within the control population, that this measure of gestural coordination would therefore represent the most valid group comparison parameter of the candidates examined here, and that the movements of the lips and jaw for /p/ closure for three of the seven stutterers are consistently less well coordinated compared to the control group.

DISCUSSION

The results thus far indicate that traditional spatial organizational characteristics, such as displacement and velocity profiles, and that traditional temporal organizational characteristics, such as temporal order and interarticulator relative time, are not stable across sessions for all control subjects. Only motor equivalence covariability is consistently correlated with the invariant percept even in the instances of unstable spatial and temporal characteristics. Thus, motor equivalence covariability represents the only appropriate group comparative parameter of the possibilities that we have examined.

One of the interesting questions to arise from these data is the nature of the precursors to the differing control strategies demonstrated by some of the subjects. Speech articulation is inherently variable due to a large number of time varying demands upon the speech motor control system such as speech rate and articulatory precision. With regard to the relationship between speech rate and spatiotemporal stability: in sessions 2 and 3, subjects were asked to model the rate that they self selected in session 1. In most cases, differences in phrase durations were relatively small at about 15 percent. The relationship between rate variation and spatiotemporal stability is not straightforward and does not appear to account for all of the across session instability. For example, Control Subject 2, who consistently demonstrates varying control strategies in /t/ and /s/ closure in addition to that shown here, was very successful in maintaining a similar rate across sessions. With regard to articulatory precision, we are assessing other kinematic measures to estimate better the precision in which articulatory gestures are achieved, and how target accuracy bears on the spatiotemporal instability shown here.

In conclusion, the results support the notion that there is an inherent long-term variability in speech motor output that reflects the natural flexibility of the motor system in meeting the time varying demands of rapid conversational speech. Further, the observed stability in the coordination index, namely motor equivalence covariability, even in the case of instability of the displacement and velocity profiles, temporal order, and interarticulator relative timing is in agreement with the idea that spatial and temporal organization of functionally linked articulators is secondary to gestural specification. This is precisely what the coordinative structure notion within a task-dynamic framework would predict; that the spatial and temporal organization of the articulators that comprise an articulatory complex represent the natural consequence of gestural specification and therefore would not demonstrate stability across sessions. Thus, some of the variability observed in speech motor output is indeed "normal" and is reflective of natural flexibility.

In my view, the inherent and natural flexibility associated with normal speech motor output represents the core of the problem that remains unresolved in the study of speech articulation in stutterers, which is to devise appropriate protocols and to select appropriate measures that best identify the stutterers ability to cope with the varying demands of conversational speech. The solution to the problem rests with our ability to disassociate the components of the output variability that reflect natural flexibility with the components of the output variability that are most often associated with abnormal speech motor output. We have shown here that many of the traditional measures of spatiotemporal organization are not appropriate for this purpose. We will present and discuss a novel approach that we hope will prove fruitful (Van Lieshout et al., this volume).

ACKNOWLEDGEMENT

Research Supported in part by a Fulbright Research Award and by a University of Illinois Research Board Grant to the first author, and by NIH Grant DC-00121 to Haskins Laboratories.

REFERENCES

Gracco, V.L. (1994). Some organizational characteristics of speech movement control. *Journal of Speech and Hearing Research, 37*, 4-27.

Gracco, V.L., & Abbs, J.H. (1986). Variant and invariant characteristics of speech movements. *Experimental Brain Research, 65*, 156-166.

Saltzman, E. (1991). The task dynamic model in speech production. In H.F.M. Peters, W. Hulstijn, and C.W. Starkweather (Eds). *Speech motor control and stuttering* (pp. 37-52). Amsterdam: Excerpta Medica.

Saltzman, E., & Munhall, K. (1989). A dynamical approach to gestural patterning in speech production. *Ecological Psychology, 1*, 333-382.

Van Lieshout, P.H.H.M., Hulstijn, W., Alfonso, P.J., & Peters H.F.M. (this volume). Higher and lower order influences on the stability of the dynamic coupling between articulations. In W. Hulstijn, H.F.M. Peters, & P.H.H.M. Van Lieshout (Eds.), *Speech production: motor control, brain research and fluency disorders*. Amsterdam: Elsevier Science.

Van Lieshout, P.H.H.M., Alfonso, P.J., Hulstijn W., & Peters H.F.M. Electromagnisctic midsagital articulography (EMMA). In F.J. Maassen, A.E. Akkerman, A.N. Brand, L.J.M. Mulder, & M.J. Van der Stilt, (Eds.), *Computers in psychology 5: Applications, methods and instrumentation*. Lisse, the Netherlands. Swetz & Zeitlinger (pp. 62-76).

Speech Production: Motor Control, Brain Research and Fluency Disorders
W. Hulstijn, H.F.M. Peters and P.H.H.M. Van Lieshout, editors

Chapter 11

HIGHER AND LOWER ORDER INFLUENCES ON THE STABILITY OF THE DYNAMIC COUPLING BETWEEN ARTICULATORS

Pascal H.H.M. van Lieshout, Wouter Hulstijn, Peter J. Alfonso, Herman F.M. Peters

In this paper, data will be presented on the stability of relative phasing between articulators in speech. In testing the model of Articulatory Phonology it was hypothesized that closing the lips in the context of a speech-related task would require the formation of a coordinative structure evidenced by a functional relatively stable coupling between upper lip and lower lip that would not or to a lesser extent occur in non-speech lip closing tasks. In varying the execution rate during a trial of repetitive sequences, the stability of such an interlip coupling was tested. Furthermore, the influence of higher order factors on the stability of interlip coupling was tested by varying the complexity of the syllabic structure of the verbal sequences that had to be repeated. The results clearly showed that, in line with the predictions, lip closing gestures in speech-related tasks generally showed evidence for a more stable coupling than in non-speech tasks as expressed in the variability of relative phase. Particularly, VCV syllables, as opposed to more reduced syllabic structures (C, VC, or CV), showed the most stable coupling behavior, without clear influences of execution rate. Thus, it seems that the phasing of upper lip and lower lip is most tightly constrained when the consonantal gesture of lip closure is embedded in vowel articulations. These data are interpreted in terms of recent ideas on different modes of coordination in dynamic patterns.

INTRODUCTION

Articulation in speech is characterized by fast sequences of movements of articulators as the lips, jaw and tongue. Both speed and accuracy in speech motor production require a high level of verbal motor skill to control the potentially many available degrees of freedom in the speech effector system. As indicated by Van Lieshout (1995), for people who stutter this may be a problem given the assumption that they are at the low end of the verbal motor continuum. This reduced skill might force them to look for alternative motor control strategies which in particular would show up in the way they coordinate individual moment patterns in speech production. However, simply making group comparisons between people who stutter and control speakers in their ability to coordinate speech movements can be a rather fruitless enterprise as shown by Alfonso (1991) who indicated that "We need to make group comparisons based on relatively stable spatial and temporal characteristics of normal speech motor dynamics, for example, those that best reflect organizational principles of speech motor control." (p. 80).

An interesting approach towards describing these organizational principles in speech motor control can be found in the Articulatory Phonology model (Browman & Goldstein, 1993; see also this volume). At the articulatory level of this model the degrees of freedom are controlled by neuro-muscular organizations or coordinative structures that functionally constrain the combined movement patterns of the individual articulators that are activated for a specific speech task (cf. Saltzman & Munhall, 1989). Control parameters are assumed to determine the kinematic behavior of a coordinative structure. For example, by scaling kinematic stiffness (indexed by the ratio between peak velocity and peak amplitude of a movement signal) the speed by which the articulators move can be influenced. The constraints on individual movements that emerge from the control parameter settings within the boundaries of a coordinative structure can be examined by an analysis of the behavior of so-called order parameters like relative phase (cf. Kelso et al., 1986). This was most recently restated by Kelso (1995) in saying that "To understand coordinated behavior as self-organized, new quantities have to be introduced beyond the ones typical of the individual components. Also, we need a variable that captures not only the observed patterns but transitions between them. Only the phase relation appears to fulfill these requirements" (p. 42).

Thus, one might say that the strength or stability of an articulatory coupling is reflected by the amount of variability in relative phase, either calculated at discrete selected points in time (cf. Ward, this volume), or on a sample to sample basis as a continuous estimate (cf. Scholz & Kelso, 1989, for an example in non-speech movement tasks). A test for the stability of a coupling can be found in scaling the kinematic stiffness control parameter by instructing subjects to increase their rate of task execution up to and beyond the point where amplitude fluctuations in relative phase indicate a decrease in or loss of stability (Tuller & Kelso, 1990). Other studies have shown that besides execution rate other variables, such as linguistic structure, may influence the stability of articulatory phasing, at least at the gestural level (Nittrouer et al., 1988; Shaiman & Porter, 1991). In the present experiment, a continuous estimate of relative phase was used to quantify the upper lip and lower lip coupling behavior in lip closing gestures. To this end, non-speech and speech tasks were compared and furthermore, for the speech tasks, the linguistic structure was varied to assess its effect on the interlip coupling.

METHOD

Subjects

Four normal speaking subjects (age range 21-28 years), two males (RO, MA) and two females (MH, SH), all native speakers of Dutch, participated in the experiment.

Tasks and procedure

Each subject had to perform eight different tasks, that is, two non-speech tasks and six speech tasks. For the non-speech tasks, the subjects were instructed to: 1) move their jaw up and down from open to closed mouth position (JAW task), and 2) with their front teeth clenched together to immobilize the jaw, to close and open their lips (LIPS task). For these two tasks functional constraints on the combined action of the upper and lower lip were not apparent a-priori because the lips were unspecified as regards their contribution to close and open the mouth (JAW), or because they were used in a relatively unfamiliar task (LIPS).

For the speech tasks, the selected verbal sequences differed in the complexity of their syllabic structure as follows:

- single [p] consonant lip closing gesture, without phonation (/p/ task)
- monosyllabic CV string ['pi] (/pi/ task)
- monosyllabic VC string ['i p] (/ip/ task)
- bisyllabic VCV string ['i .pi] (/ipi/ task)
- bisyllabic VCV string ['i .pa] (/ipa/ task)
- bisyllabic VCV string ['a .pi] (/api/ task)

The VCV sequences used different phonetic contexts to assess their effect on relative phase within a particular linguistic structure. The subjects were instructed to repeat each sequence for twelve seconds, while increasing the rate in two different ways: a) continuously, and, b) in 4 steps of 3 second intervals.

Data recording

Movement and acoustic data were recorded simultaneously using the AG100 (Carstens Medizinelektronik GmbH), an Electromagnetic Midsagittal Articulography (EMMA) device. Movement data were sampled at 400 Hz (after adequate low-pass filtering) and smoothed with a 11 point triangular filter (effective low pass frequency 27.5 Hz) before data processing. After cutting off the first 1500 ms and the last 1000 ms of a trial, down sampling the data from 400 to 100 Hz, and high-pass filtering (188 point Hamming window FIR filter, cut-off frequency of 0.5 Hz) to remove slow varying drifts, position and derived velocity signals (normalized between -1 and +1) were used to calculate a continuous estimate of relative phase, using an algorithm described by Heuer (1993), shown below Figure 1. Using this algorithm relative phase angles can vary between 0 (in-phase) and 180 (out-phase) degrees, i.e. it always takes the smaller angle, thus ignoring differences in the sequence of upper and lower lip. Figure 1 shows an example of a typical '/api/ task' trial with position and velocity signals for upper lip and lower lip for lip closure, and the continuous estimate of relative phase, together with the acoustic signal and its wide-band spectrogram.

The relative phase signal was used to calculate the average variation around the mean,

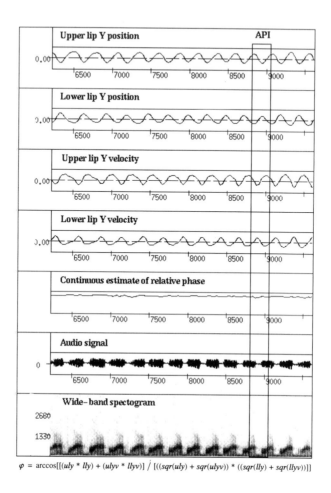

$$\varphi = \arccos[[(uly * lly) + (ulyv * llyv)] \, / \, [((sqr(uly) + sqr(ulyv)) * ((sqr(lly) + sqr(llyv))]]$$

Figure 1. Typical trial illustrating upper lip position (ULY) and velocity (ULYv) signals, lower lip position (LLY) and velocity (LLYv) signals, the derived continuous estimate of relative phase, the acoustic signal, as well as its wide-band spectrogram. A single /api/ sequence is indicated within the borders of the rectangle. Below the figure is the equation (Heuer, 1993) used for calculating a continuous estimate of relative phase.

expressed in the amplitude variability index (AVI, cf. Deal & Emanual, 1978), a $\log_{10}$ transformed coefficient of variation. The relative phase signal was divided into three equally long intervals minus the first 500 msec of the signal. As shown in Figure 2, these intervals represent estimates of relative phase in three different rate conditions. For this trial interval 1 includes cycle frequencies from approximately 2 to 3 Hz, interval 2 includes frequencies from 3 to 4 Hz, and finally, interval 3 includes frequencies from 4 to

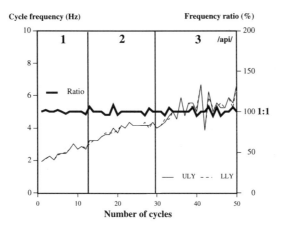

Figure 2. Typical trial showing cycle frequency (Hz) for upper lip (UL) and lower lip (LL) and the corresponding ratio (in %) as well as the demarcation lines of the rate intervals that were used to calculate the amplitude variability index (AVI).

6 Hz. In general, these intervals represent rate conditions varying from relatively slow (interval 1) to relatively fast (interval 3) rates. For each rate interval an AVI value was calculated. Each task was performed three times in the continuous speed-up mode and three times in the step-wise speed-up mode. Since there were no clear differences in relative phase between these modes, and subjects for both modes actually used a consistent quasi-continuous speed-up strategy, the distinction was not maintained in the data analysis. Thus, we have one "speed-up" mode with 6 repetitions for all eight tasks.

RESULTS

Figure 3 shows the AVI values for the two non speech and the six speech tasks for the three rate intervals and their average separated for each subject. For the non-speech tasks all four subjects clearly show the highest variability in relative phase for the JAW task. For the LIPS task, it is interesting to notice that for the male subjects (RO, MA) relative phase was only slightly less variable than in the JAW task, whereas for the female subjects (MH, SH), the variability in relative phase was more similar to that of the single consonant (/p/) and monosyllabic (/pi/ and /ip/) speech tasks. For the speech tasks, the single consonant and monosyllabic tasks showed a similar amount of variability in relative phase, except for subject RO. Most interestingly however, the least variability in relative phase was found for the bisyllabic sequences, in particular for the /api/ task. Also the effect of rate was smaller for the bisyllabic tasks, in particular for /api/, as compared to the single consonant and monosyllabic tasks. For the latter tasks higher rates seem to destabilize the interlip coupling, as shown in Figure 3 by higher AVI values for interval 2 and in particular interval 3.

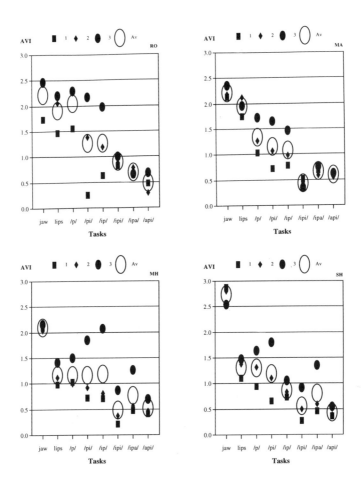

Figure 3. Mean amplitude variability index (AVI) values per task for individual subjects for the three rate intervals and their average.

For the JAW condition even at slow rates there was no apparent stable coupling behavior, indicating a lack of functional constraints on lip
movements.   Figure 4 shows AVI values for each subject, averaged across the three rate intervals. Although there are some individual variations, it is apparent that in particular for the speech tasks, there is very little inter-subject variability. As already suggested by the data in Figure 3, there appear to be three clusters regarding AVI values; higher values for the non-speech tasks (but notice the already mentioned sex difference for the LIPS task), lower values for the single consonant and monosyllabic tasks, and the lowest values for the bisyllabic tasks.

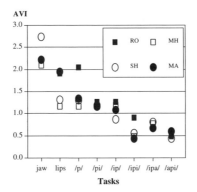

Figure 4.   AVI values averaged across rate intervals per subject for non-speech and speech tasks.

The results of an analysis of variance on AVI show for all four subjects significant main effects for task and rate interval, as well as a significant interaction effect. A post-hoc test (Tukey HSD-procedure) confirms the observations made from Figures 3 and 4, that for all subjects the bisyllabic sequences form a more or less coherent group in terms of relative phase variability. For the other tasks, there was more individual variation, in particular regarding the differences between monosyllabic and single consonant or LIPS data. Finally, relative phase data for the JAW task always show significantly higher AVI values than any other task.

A closer look at the maximum cycle frequency that a subject obtained for each task while the lips were in a frequency locked state (ratio of 1:1, see Figure 2), revealed that for most subjects there is no consistent relationship between this measure and type of task. That is, subjects in general were not slower or faster for a particular type of task. Pearson product moment correlations between AVI values and maximum cycle frequencies ranged from -.15 to .19, which were all non-significant. In general, for most tasks subjects reached a maximum frequency between 4.5 and 5.5 Hz, centering around 5 Hz.

DISCUSSION

In this study evidence was found that if the lips were not intended to be functionally coupled, as in the JAW task, the relative phase signal was unstable regardless the movement rate, suggesting a low or non-existing constraint on lip movements in terms of a synergy. Also, for the LIPS task in which the lips were functionally but in an unfamiliar way coupled, the variability in relative phase was relatively high. However, in the slow rate condition, subjects seemed more able to constrain lip movements in this task, illustrating the fact that unfamiliar (non-automated) movements are better to control if movement rate is not too high.

For the speech tasks, differences in linguistic structure had a clear influence on the variability in relative phase. AVI values for relative phase in single consonant and monosyllabic sequences were not only clearly higher compared to bisyllabic VCV sequences, but in particular with higher rates the interlip coupling showed transitions to instability, which were not seen for any of the VCV tasks. This finding might suggest that constraints on degrees of freedom for articulators are more effective in a vowel-to-vowel articulation (cf. Tuller & Kelso, 1984). This adheres to the claim that regarding motor control, stress- or syllable timed languages, like English and Dutch, are characterized by a vowel-to-vowel model of organization (cf. Tuller et al., 1982; Smith, 1993).

An interesting aspect of this type of study and its methodology lies in its potential to reveal mechanisms of coordination in both normal and speech disordered populations. Based on the work of the German physiologist Erik von Holst (1908-1962) Kelso (1995) makes a distinction between different modes of coordination, as expressed in the behavior of order parameters like relative phase.

The perhaps intuitively most appealing but also by far the less common mode is *absolute coordination*. Under absolute coordination, articulators are both frequency and phase locked, showing a single stable solution to the degrees of freedom problem. This stable solution is often referred to as an attractor. By an active process (e.g., by changing control parameter settings) the system can be switched from one stable solution to another (bifurcation).

On the other hand, there is *relative coordination*, which seems a more usual mode, in particular with reference to non-symmetric coupling. Because of a broken symmetry, the system "is poised near critical points where it can spontaneously switch in and out" (p. 99, Kelso, 1995), a process referred to as intermittency. In contrast to absolute coordination, the system is near (attracted by) but not in a phase locked state, offering both metastability and flexibility at the same time.

Another mode of coordination is *desynchronization*. Actually, this mode refers to the process of loss of entrainment between individual components. At critical frequencies, one of the components is suddenly decoupled as a consequence of broken symmetry, as in the case of relative coordination. However, as already mentioned, in the latter mode the coupling relationship may change but it is maintained!

Finally, there is a mode of coordination that represents *uncoordinated behavior*, which of course is a kind of contradiction in terms. It means that the components (articulators) behave in a strictly independent, i.e. uncoupled way, similar to what is seen in the relative phase data of the JAW task presented in this study.

Using the paradigm as described in this study to study both normal and disordered speech motor production, we hope to find evidence that people exploit these different modes of coordination in order to maximize the efficiency of motor control with a minimum of effort. Or, as it was recently stated by Bongaardt (1996), addressing the work of Nikolai Aleksandrovitsj Bernstein (1896-1966):

In Bernstein's later works it becomes more and more clear that the freezing and releasing of degrees of freedom can be understood as an active process of exploring new and better ways to move. Varying the couplings between degrees of freedom allows for exploration, just as freezing out or stabilizing the couplings between degrees of freedom renders movement control possible. Thus, in Bernstein's views, variability is controlled. It is constrained with respect to the goals of the movement, whereas the system lets go with respect to the remaining variability. (p. 95)

NOTES

[1] This research was supported in part by the Netherlands Organization of Scientific Research (NWO-SGW), Grant 575-59-048.

REFERENCES

Alfonso, P.J. (1991). Implications of the concepts underlying task-dynamic modelling on kinematic studies of stuttering (pp. 79-100). In H.F.M. Peters, W. Hulstijn, & C.W. Starkweather (Eds.), *Speech motor control and stuttering*, Amsterdam, The Netherlands: Elsevier Science Publishers.

Bongaardt, R. (1996). *Shifting focus: The Bernstein tradition in movement science*. Unpublished doctoral dissertation, Free University Amsterdam.

Browman, C.P., & Goldstein, L. (1993). Dynamics and articulatory phonology. *Haskins Laboratories Status Report on Speech Research, SR-113* , 51-62 (also in T. van Gelder, & B. Port (Eds.), *Mind as motion*. Cambridge, MA: MIT Press).

Deal, R.E., & Emanuel, F.W. (1978). Some waveform and spectral features of vowel roughness. *Journal of Speech and Hearing Research, 21*, 250-264.

Heuer, H. (1993). Structural constraints on bimanual movements. *Psychological Research, 55*, 83-98.

Kelso, J.A.S. (1995). *Dynamic patterns: The self-organization of brain and behavior*. Cambridge, MA: MIT press.

Kelso, J.A.S., Saltzman, E.L., & Tuller, B. (1986). The dynamical perspective on speech production: data and theory. *Journal of Phonetics, 14*, 29-59.

Nittrouer, S., Munhall, K., Kelso, J.A.S., Tuller, B., & Harris, K.S. (1988). Patterns of interarticulator phasing and their relation to linguistic structure. *Journal of the Acoustical Society of America, 84*, 1653-1661.

Saltzman, E.L., & Munhall, K.G. (1989). A dynamical approach to gestural patterning in speech production. *Ecological Psychology, 1*, 333-382.

Shaiman, S., & Porter, R.J. (1991). Different phase-stable relationships of the upper lip and jaw for production of vowels and diphthongs. *Journal of the Acoustical Society of America, 90*, 3000-3007.

Scholz, J.P., & Kelso, J.A.S. (1989). A quantitative approach to understanding the formation and change of coordinated movement patterns. *Journal of Motor Behavior, 21*, 122-144.

Smith, C.L. (1993). Prosodic patterns in the coordination of vowel and consonant gestures. *Haskins Laboratories Status Report on Speech Research, SR-115/116*, 45-55.

Tuller, B., & Kelso, J.A.S. (1984). The timing of articulatory gestures: Evidence for relational invariants. *Journal of the Acoustical Society of America, 76(4)*, 1030-1036.

Tuller, B., Kelso, J.A.S., & Harris, K.S. (1982). Interarticulator phasing as an index of temporal regularity in speech. *Journal of Experimental Psychology: Human Perception and Performance, 8*, 460-472.

Tuller, B., & Kelso, J.A.S. (1990). Phase transitions in speech production and their perceptual consequences. In H. Jeannerod (Ed.), *Motor representation and control* (pp. 429-452). Hilldale, NJ: Lawrence Erlbaum Associates.

Van Lieshout, P.H.H.M. (1995). *Motor planning and articulation in fluent speech of stutterers and nonstutterers*. Unpublished doctoral dissertation, University of Nijmegen.

Ward, D. (this volume). Stuttering and articulator sequencing: Intrinsic and extrinsic timing perspectives. In W. Hulstijn, H.F.M. Peters, & P.H.H.M. Van Lieshout (Eds.), *Speech production: motor control, brain research and fluency disorders*. Amsterdam: Elsevier Science.

Speech Production: Motor Control, Brain Research and Fluency Disorders
W. Hulstijn, H.F.M. Peters and P.H.H.M. Van Lieshout, editors

Chapter 12

STUTTERING AND ARTICULATOR SEQUENCING: INTRINSIC AND EXTRINSIC TIMING PERSPECTIVES

David Ward

This paper reports a recent attempt to define articulator timing relationships amongst stuttering speakers in terms of two competing models of motor speech control; intrinsic timing, measured by phase angles and extrinsic timing, measured by peak velocity articulator sequencing (Ward submitted). Principle findings which focused on the timing relationships between upper lip, lower lip and jaw for a bilabial closure task, found persons who stutter to be more variable than nonstuttering speakers when parameterised by the phase angle analysis, across rate and stress conditions. However, when extrinsic timing data were analysed independent of articulator sequence type (sequence period), variability was found to be similar to that of the phase angle analysis. The present paper also considers to what extent increased articulatory stability amongst the nonstuttering speakers is represented differentially by the sequence period and phase angle measurements, and difficulties in categorically defining data as extrinsic or intrinsic are discussed.

INTRODUCTION

A significant problem in attempting explanations of the motor disruptions in the speech of persons who stutter (PWS) lies in the fact that there are opposing views on how normal speech production may be characterized. Fowler (1980; 1986) has questioned some beliefs surrounding the extent of cognitive dominance of the vocal tract musculature. In an "action theory" perspective, rather than a timing element being metered out by a neural timing device (usually modeled as a central pattern generator) the relational timing of articulatory movement for a given articulatory gesture occurs as a consequence of the relevant muscle groups' dynamics. Using a task dynamic modeling (TDM) approach (Kelso et al., 1986; Saltzman, 1991) in which phase plane portraits are constructed, it is possible to test the extent to which the control of gestural timing is undertaken at the level of the vocal tract: albeit with simple articulatory sequences such as bilabial closure tasks. Articulatory timing, in the phase portrait conceptualization is modeled without reference to extrinsic (or clock) time. Instead, the moment that the upper lip commences movement toward closure is represented as an angle on a 360° jaw cycle.

Kelso et al. (1986) found upper lip phase angles (PAs) remained constant across both segmental and suprasegmental contingencies for /V bilabial/ sequences, however subsequent studies have failed to replicate these findings. Nittrouer et al. (1988) found that phase angle of upper lip onset with the jaw was affected systematically by syllable identity (closed vs open syllable), medial consonant identity (/p/ vs /m/) as well as rate differences (fast vs normal) and differences in stress patterning (target syllable stressed vs unstressed). Nittrouer (1991) found similar data with tongue/jaw phase angle relations, with consonant effects again producing systematic phase angle differences. Shaiman and Porter (1991) noted a strong increase in both phase angle onset and jaw cycle duration when comparing diphthong productions to either of the tested vowels (/i/ or /a/), and in comparing the diphthongs /ei/ to /ai/.

Extrinsic timing theory and the measurement of articulatory movement in real time forms the implicit underpinning of the majority of interpretations of motor speech activity seen in stuttering behavior (eg. Caruso et al., 1988; De Nil, 1992; De Nil, 1995; De Nil & Abbs, 1991; Gracco, 1991, 1994; Zimmermann, 1980,a,b), although work by Alfonso (1991), Alfonso and Van Lieshout (this volume) and Van Lieshout et al. (this volume) provide notable exceptions. Caruso et al. (1988) found that across hundreds of tokens, normal speakers produced specific peak velocity sequencing profiles of upper lip, lower lip, jaw, (UL-LL-J) during oral closure tasks. PWS, on the other hand were found to be inconsistent in this regard and demonstrated many reversals of this sequence. Although subsequent investigations have failed to uncover the reported near invariance of nonstuttering persons sequence profiles, the UL-LL-J sequence has generally be found to be more prevalent amongst nonstuttering persons than PWS (De Nil, 1995; Van Lieshout et al., 1993). This finding has led researchers to reconsider the role of articulator sequencing and the potential neurological correlates of PWSŝ speech.

PHASE ANGLE AND SEQUENCE PERIOD DATA

Ward (submitted) analyzed upper lip (UL) lower lip (LL) and jaw (J) peak velocity sequence profiles and phase angle relations of a group of five PWS and five control speakers for an intervocalic bilabial closure task ['pæpæp], embedded in a carrier phrase. Mean PA relationships were found to be similar for both groups across three rate conditions (fast, normal and slow) and when a reversed stress pattern ([pæ'pæp]) was required however the PWS group phase angles were produced with greater variability for all conditions. These differences were significant amongst conditions of altered stress (p < .005) and increased rate (p < .05) which are known to be difficult for PWS. No strong UL-LL-J sequencing effect was uncovered, but when the elapsed time between the moment the first articulator reached peak velocity and the moment that the last articulator reached peak velocity (irrespective of sequence "type") was also analyzed, between group variability for this measure, which Ward (1995) called sequence period (SP), was found to closely resemble that of the phase angle data. Increased variability was associated with fast rate and destressed syllables, and variability associated with normal and slow rate data was more similar to that seen in the control group. As was the case with the phase angle analyses, between group mean differences were found to be similar. Findings indicate that both intrinsic and extrinsic analyses may reflect differential performance in articulatory control, when a sequencing component is removed. One possibility is that a (UL-LL-J) sequencing hypothesis, though holding true for some speakers, may be insufficient to explain the variety of aberrant motor activity in stuttering speakers' speech. Thus, both PA and SP data would reflect a generalized instability in articulator sequencing in PWS speech, but that variability is not necessarily confined to within-sequence errors for either stuttering or nonstuttering speakers.

Whilst it is clear that between group variability is similar for both PA and SP analyses, there is considerable variability at subject level between the two data sets (figure 1). 1 way Anovas showed significant intragroup SD variability for both groups for all SP analyses (p < .01) with the exception of the control group, normal rate ([4,140] F=2.297, p=.062) and the stuttering group, stress condition ([4,115] F=3.365, p=.0121). Similar analyses for the PA data revealed homogeneity of variance for the control speakers (p > .05) for all conditions but significant variability for all conditions amongst the stuttering speaker group (p < .01). SP and PA methods do not reflect articulatory variability from similar perspectives, but the finding of homogeneity amongst nonstuttering speakers might suggest that PA analyses may potentially tell us more about articulatory timing relationships than those from SP data: The PA standard deviation data indicate that nonstuttering speakers are able to control articulatory variability within acceptable limits (by definition, those which result in fluent speech) on an individual basis when such action is necessary, whereas stuttering speakers experience a reduced ability to do so. It could be tentatively suggested that an individual may have some canonical mean phase angle figure for a certain articulatory gesture (here, the bilabial closure task) which can only tolerate certain variability (indicated in the stress condition as around 10°) before coordination breaks down.

A further feature of the stuttering groups' data (consistent for both PA and SP analyses) is the heterogeneous within-subject data across all conditions. That is, no subject demonstrates any consistency in articulatory performance across the conditions tested (also see Alfonso & Van Lieshout; this volume, on this issue). One possibility is that this might reflect a greater range of articulatory strategies utilized by the stuttering subjects in an attempt to maintain and maximize fluency. Fluent speakers, on the other hand, may only require a limited repertoire (Harrington; personal communication). Further studies with larger data samples are needed to provide some more concrete answers.

SEQUENTIAL COMPONENTS IN PHASE ANGLE AND SEQUENCE PERIOD DATA

To this point, timing relationships among nonstuttering speakers and PWS have been considered from three different perspectives; sequential peak velocity; nonsequential peak velocity (SP); (nonsequential) phase angle (PA). One problem in explaining PWS' speech in terms of PA findings, as suggested above, concerns the difficulty in defining to what extent the SP and PA analyses genuinely reflect different articulatory activity with regard to the sequential vs nonsequential differences. Firstly, the PA procedure does not consider

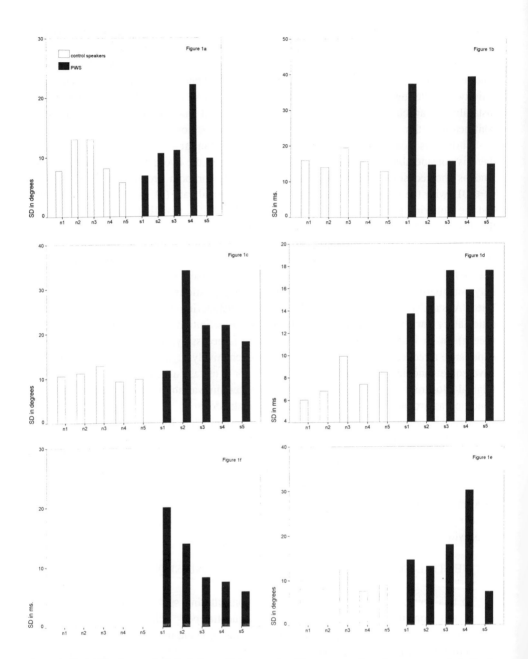

Figure 1. Variability in standard deviations of phase angles (figures a, c, e), and sequence periods (b, d, f) for three conditions; normal rate (a, b), altered stress (c, d) and fast rate (e, f).

movement of the lower lip. With relationships being confined to the activity of two more remote articulators it could be that the data are still reflecting an analytical procedure that is still less constrained than the sequence period data, rather than a procedure which models time as an intrinsic property. The problem is, that although the SP analysis does away with a sequencing component, the PA analysis (in which, conceptually, extrinsic timing phenomena such as sequencing are not considered) in fact, does not. Taking a hypothetical example, we might see two upper lip phase angles calculated at 160° and 200°. As functions of a sinusoidal jaw motion, these different phase angles could appear as identical SP (clock time) time-frames. Thus a relational element is preserved in the phase angle description, dependent on jaw turnaround time, which does not appear explicitly in the phase angle calculation (as defined by Kelso et al., 1986). Similarly, the case for SP data being considered exclusively as extrinsic timing phenomena can be questioned. Measuring variability of upper lip, lower lip and jaw PV time frames irrespective of sequence pattern does not account for any variability in the relative timing of different SP periods, and points at which the SP time-frames occur during oral closure are not specified with relation to one-another. A second hypothetical example might see one subject's SP data (or set of peak velocities) occur consistently closer to the moment of oral closure than for another subject, whilst maintaining similar mean scores and SD variability.

Although PA descriptions have been associated with action theory (Kelso et al., 1986) we are not convinced that even if a phase angle description of stuttering were to be developed, that this would necessarily exclusively reflect an AT approach (see above; Ward, submitted). There are difficulties, in practical terms, of differentiating intrinsic and extrinsic data, and also there seems much of some extrinsic theory which overlap with AT. Similarly, a TDM/PA approach does not appear inconsistent with some current extrinsic theories. For the present, however, findings do suggest that at the very least, phase angle descriptions can play an important role in capturing differences in articulatory performance between normal and disordered speech. Data from larger samples, attempting to associate physiological (PA and SP) events with acoustic correlates, are needed to indicate the potential these procedures might hold for increasing our understanding of motor speech performance among both normal speaking and speech disordered populations.

REFERENCES

Alfonso, P.J. (1991). Implications of the concepts underlying task-dynamic modelling on kinematic studies of stuttering. In H.F.M. Peters, W.J. Hustijn, & C.W. Starkweather (Eds) *Speech Motor Control and Stuttering* North Holland: Elsevier Science Publishers.

Alfonso, P.J., & Van Lieshout, P.H.M.M. (this volume). Spatial and temporal in obstruent gestural specification by stutterers and controls: comparisons across sessions. In W. Hulstijn, H.F.M. Peters, & P.H.H.M. Van Lieshout (Eds.), *Speech production: motor control, brain research and fluency disorders*. Amsterdam: Flsevier Science.

Caruso, A.J., Abbs, J.H., & Gracco, V.L. (1988). Kinematic analysis of multiple movement coordination during speech in stutterers. *Brain, 111*, 439-455.

De Nil, L.F. (1992). *Articulatory sequencing revisited: do stutterers and nonstutterers differ?* Paper presentation at the 1992 Annual Convention of the ASHA, San Antonio, Texas.

De Nil, L.F. (1995). The influence of phonetic context on temporal sequencing of upper-lip, lower-lip and jaw peak velocity and movement onset during bilabial consonants in stuttering and nonstuttering adults. *Journal of Fluency Disorders, 20.*

De Nil, L.F., & Abbs, J.H. (1991). The influence of speaking rate on the upper lip, lower lip and jaw peak velocity sequencing during bilabial closing movements. *Journal of the Acoustical Society of America, 89,* 845-849.

Fowler, C.A. (1980). Coarticulation and theories of extrinsic timing control. *Journal of Phonetics, 8,* 113-133.

Fowler, C.A. (1986). An event perception approach to the study of speech perception from a direct-realist perspective. *Journal of Phonetics, 14,* 3-28.

Gracco, V.L. (1988). Timing factors in the coordination of speech movements. *Journal of Neuroscience 8* , 4628-4639.

Gracco, V.L. (1991). Sensorimotor mechanisms in speech motor control. In H. Peters, W.J. Hustijn & C.W. Starkweather (Eds) *Speech Motor Control and Stuttering* North Holland: Elsevier Science Publishers.

Gracco, V.L. (1994). Some organizational characteristics of speech movement control. *Journal of Speech and Hearing Research, 37,* 4-27.

Kelso, J.A.S., Saltzman, E.L, & Tuller, B. (1986). The dynamical perspective on speech production: Data and theory. *Journal of Phonetics, 14,* 29-59.

Nittrouer, S. (1991). Phase relations of jaw and tongue tip movements in the production of VCV utterences. *Journal of the Acoustical Society of America, 90,* (4), 1806-1815.

Nittrouer, S., Munhall, K., Kelso, J.A.S., Tuller, B., & Harris, K. (1988). Patterns of interarticulator phasing and their relation to linguistic structure. *Journal of the Acoustical Society of America, 84,* (5) 1653-1661.

Saltzman, E. (1991). The task dynamic model in speech production. In H.F.M. Peters, W. Hustijn & C.W. Starkweather (Eds). *Speech Motor Control and Stuttering* Amsterdam: Elsevier Science Publishers.

Shaiman, S., & Porter, R.J. (1991). Different phase-stable relationships of the upper-lip and jaw for the production of vowels and diphthongs. *Journal of the Acoustical Society of America, 90,* 3000-3007.

Van Lieshout, P.H.H.M., Peters, H.F.M., Starkweather, C.W., & Hulstijn, W. (1993). Physiological differences between stutterers and nonstutterers in perceptually fluent speech: EMG amplitude and duration. *Journal of Speech and Hearing Research, 36,* 55-63.

Van Lieshout, P.H.H.M., Hulstijn, W., Alfonso, P.J., & Peters, H.F.M. (this volume). Higher and lower order influences on the stability of the dynamic coupling between articulators. In W. Hulstijn, H.F.M. Peters, & P.H.H.M. Van Lieshout (Eds.), *Speech production: motor control, brain research and fluency disorders.* Amsterdam: Elsevier Science.

Ward, D. (1995). *Intrinsic timing, extrinsic timing and stuttered speech.* PhD thesis. The University of Reading, UK.

Ward, D. (submitted). *Intrinsic and extrinsic timing in stuttering persons' speech: Data and implications.*

Zimmermann, G. (1990a). Articulatory behaviors associated with stuttering. *Journal of Speech and Hearing Research, 23,* 108-121.

Zimmermann, G. (1990b). Stuttering: A disorder of movement. *Journal of Speech and Hearing Research, 23,* 122-136.

1997 Elsevier Science B.V.
Speech Production: Motor Control, Brain Research and Fluency Disorders
W. Hulstijn, H.F.M. Peters and P.H.H.M. Van Lieshout, editors

Chapter 13

ANALYSIS OF LIPS AND JAW MULTI-PEAKED VELOCITY CURVE PROFILES IN FLUENT SPEECH BY STUTTERERS AND NONSTUTTERERS

Claudio Zmarich, Emanuela Magno Caldognetto

It is well known that changes in the rate of movement of the speech articulators can modify the bell-shaped profile of a typical velocity curve. In this experiment, four stutterers and four nonstutterers produced 10 sequences of /papapapa.../ and 10 of /bababa.../ at comfortable rate, and then at maximal rate. The kinematics of the opening and closing phonetic gestures was investigated using ELITE, a fully automatic, real-time system for 3D kinematic data acquisition. Analyses was performed only on the "dynamic" portion of the curves of the gestures perceived to be fluent, thereby excluding the steady state portions of the movement pattern. For both subjects groups, the comfortable rate condition is associated with a greater number of multi-peaked velocity curves than is the fast condition (most for the upper lip). However, stutterers realize a significantly greater percentage of multi-peaked curves than do nonstutterers.

INTRODUCTION

It has recently been suggested that "single-peaked velocity profiles may serve as an index for coordinated multi-articulator systems" (Alfonso 1991, 83), and the "combined movement" profile (referred to in this paper as interlabial vertical distance) represents the most important factor, as it describes the synergistic nature of goal-directed speech movements. Ideally, the degree of departure in terms of the number of velocity peaks for any unique speech gesture could thus be attributed to a possible articulatory disorder. However, this index may also be affected by changes in speech rate, as a recent finding has revealed a relationship between speech rate and the peak velocity number (Adams et al., 1993). On the other hand, the kinematics of fluent speech by stutterers and nonstutterers may be affected by changes in speech rate in a different manner. This would suggest that it may be appropriate to establish first of all which rate is more critical for stutterers and why.

METHOD

Four stutterers (mean age : 25.25) and four nonstutterers (mean age 28.50) took part in this experiment. All the subjects under examination featured negative case histories relating to neurological, speech, language and hearing problems, except for stuttering. Stuttering severity, which was assessed by means of the Stuttering Severity Instrument (Riley, 1972), was classified as mild in one subject and severe for the other three stutterers.

All the subjects were asked to pronounce 40 sequences lasting 2 seconds each, with evenly stressed syllables and in random order, including: 10 /pa/ sequences at a comfortable rate, 10 /ba/ sequences at comfortable rate, 10 /pa/ sequences at maximal rate and 10 /ba/ sequences at maximal rate (Zmarich et al., 1995). The max. rate factor was the fastest rate at which the subject was able to perform the task without altering the perceptual characteristics of the phones. Thus each subject produced 40 sequences, except for one stutterer, who produced only 20 sequences (i.e. 5 of each kind).

The kinematics of the opening and closing phonetic gestures was measured by using ELITE, a fully-automatic, real-time, 3D kinematic data acquisition system (Magno Caldognetto et al., this volume). The positions of small, non-obtrusive passive markers, situated at the central points of the upper lip (UL), lower lip (LL) and jaw (J), and the interlabial vertical distance between UL and LL (C, i.e. combined movement), were sampled at 100 Hz together with the acoustic signal (16 kHz A/D).

After the movements of each of the above mentioned articulatory parameters had been detected by the ELITE system, two low-pass filters were alternatively applied to the original movement sequences, depending on the speech rate. After visual inspection of the acoustic waveforms to determine the higher articulatory frequencies, gestures performed at a comfortable rate were fed through a low-pass filter with a 6 Hz cut-off frequency, while gestures performed at a maximal rate were filtered through a 12 Hz low-pass filter. Movement velocities were calculated automatically by evaluating the first derivative of the movement curve. Appropriate movement points (i.e. peak opening and closing positions) and velocity points (i.e. the peak velocities of opening and closing gestures) were automatically tabulated as a sequence of min. and max. values by assessing the zero-axis crosspoints of the velocity and acceleration curves, respectively. In addition, a movable cursor on the PC screen could be positioned over critical points of the movement and velocity profiles. With reference to C, each sequence was considered starting from the first min. value (i.e. closed mouth position) and ending at the final min. value. All gestures preceding or following these points were excluded. The criterion chosen for comparison consisted in the presence of more than one peak in the velocity curve of each gesture for each single articulator (Figure 1).

As our purpose was to analyze only perceptively fluent gestures, we focused our attention on signs of non-fluency and defective articulations, thereby enabling us to eliminate 9 gestures that were seen as slurred speech in several different sequences produced by one of the stutterers. Furthermore, as we felt that a number of velocity peaks may have been caused (besides random noise) by the narrow range oscillation of the velocity curve around the zero-axis associated to a state of relative articulatory immobility, and

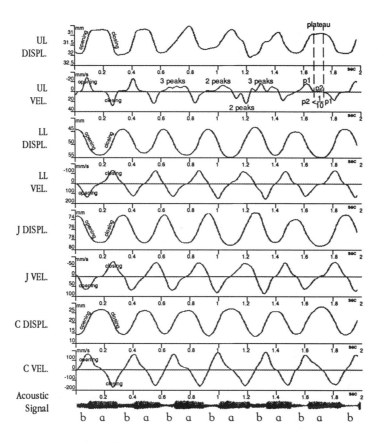

Figure 1. Displacement and velocity profiles *vs*. time for each articulator, here represented together with the acoustic signal. Critical analysis points are also highlighted in UL profiles.

since these peaks could not always be related to either the preceding or subsequent gestures, we chose to examine only the dynamic portions of the curves, thus excluding the steady state sections, or *plateaux*. An articulatory plateau was said to *"occur"* when the velocity curve crossed the zero-axis more than once within a single gesture and the part of the curve lying between the first and final cross-points did not depart notably (i.e. one-tenth of the maximal velocity along the same direction of movement) from the zero-axis (Figure 1). An additional criterion for exclusion consisted in the case where the movement rate of a particular speech articulator differed considerably from the rate of C. Five sequences performed by 2 stutterers were eliminated due to high rates (approx. 15 Hz) of UL oscillatory movements.

A number of other UL sequences were eliminated when the displacement range was limited to within 0.5 mm, thus producing a practically immobile articulator. Finally, whenever a UL velocity peak occurred simultaneously with a LL peak closing position and the C displacement value for this same instant turned out to be lower than the value associated to the mean rest position (measured twice during the recording session), then the occlusion formed by UL and LL was identified as a compression, and the UL peak velocity was considered to be a possible mechanical alteration due to the action of LL (Figure 2). Nevertheless, these gestures were included in the general count of multi-peaked velocity curves.

The presence of extrapeaks on the velocity curves of the speech gestures sufficed to qualify the gesture affected as irregular, no matter whether featuring one, two or three extrapeaks.

All counts were therefore divided by the total number of gestures relating to each kind of sequence and expressed as a proportion of multi-peaked velocity gestures out of the total. Sequence kinds were determined by the following variables: subjects (8), number of repetitions (10), status (2), rates (2), consonants (2) and gestures (2).

In order to normalize the variance of the dependent variable, i.e. the proportion of multi-peaked gestures out of the total number of gestures of the same kind, the means of ten repetitions were transformed according to the *formula* : $x1 = 2$ arcsin (square root of x); cfr. Winer, 1971:400).

The statistical analysis was done separately for each articulator using an ANOVA mixed model, where status (2) was the between factor and rate (2), consonant (2) and gesture (2) were the within factors (repeated measurements factors).

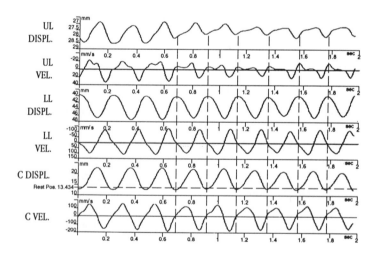

Figure 2. UL, LL and C displacement and velocity curves *vs*. time. UL profiles are clearly altered by the compression caused by LL.

Table 1. Articulation frequency (gestures/sec.) at each speech rate for subjects belonging to the two groups

Stutt.	Pref.rate	Max. rate	Mean	Nons.	Pref.rate	Max.rate	Mean
1 CZ	2.00	2.67	2.33	1 MC	1.60	3.55	2.57
2 LF	3.00	4.65	3.82	2 GA	1.70	5.52	3.61
3 DS	2.50	6.00	4.25	3 PP	3.00	4.50	3.75
4 MC	2.80	6.15	4.47	4 GB	3.00	6.71	4.85
Mean	2.57	4.86	3.71	Mean	2.32	5.07	3.69

RESULTS

The total number of gestures analyzed for each articulator was 1,972 in the case of nonstutterers and 1,628 for stutterers. The average number of gestures per second performed by each subject at the two rates is listed in Table 1.

In the following, data have been re-transformed to percentages of multi-peaked gestures out of the total number of gestures of the same kind.

For each articulator, the grouping factor (status) yelded no significant result at any reasonable p level.

Upper lip: the kind of gesture (a repeated measurements factor), that distinguished opening (mean value: 48.9%) from closing movements (25.0%), was the only one that exhibited statistical significance [$F(1,6)=12.503$, $p=0.012$]. As to status factor, stutterers scored 33.9% and nonstutterers 40.1%.

Lower lip: rate [$F(1,6)=11.138$, $p=0.016$; preferred: 12.4% vs. max.: 1.3%] and consonant-gesture interactions [$F(1,6=9.119$, $p=0.023$; /b/ consonant * closing gesture scored the highest (12.0%)] were significant factors. As to status factor, stutterers scored 10.7% and nonstutterers 3.0%.

Jaw : rate [$F(1,6)=8.551$, $p=0.026$; preferred: 8.7% vs. max.: 0.6%] was the only significant factor. The comparison in the status factor between stutterers and nonstutterers was 7.6% vs. 1.6%, respectively.

Combined movements : rate [$F(1,6)=12.041$, $p=0.013$; preferred: 9.5% vs. max.: 1.1%] and consonant-gesture interactions [$F(1,6)=17.681$, $p=0.006$; /b/ consonant * closing gesture scored the highest (10.4%)] were significant factors. As to status factor, stutterers scored 8.9% and nonstutterers 1.6%.

DISCUSSION

Although statistical analysis failed to reveal a significant effect for the grouping factor "status" (stutterers vs nonstutterers), these absence could be ascribed to the low effect-size and power for the tested model (group size is only 4 subjects). When looking at the mean values of percentages of multi-peaked gestures, a clear trend appears: at preferred rate, in fluent utterances, stutterers perform LL, J and C opening and closing movements with a greater number of multi-peaked velocity curves than nonstutterers.

Jaw movements were considered the most reliable speech articulator for analysis, due to the fact that unlike UL, this articulator was not affected by mechanical alterations caused by other articulators. Furthermore, jaw movements were more accurately defined than LL movements, as LL data were processed by the ELITE system as the joined product of lower lip and jaw movements. Combined movements (C) may also be rather important, mainly for theoretical reasons, but they could be affected by UL movement alterations.

The most important result that emerges from our analysis is that, for both subject groups, the comfortable rate condition is associated to a significantly greater number of multi-peaked velocity curves than the fast speech condition (mostly for UL). However, except for the case of UL data, stutterers performed a greater percentage of multi-peaked curves than nonstutterers. These results are temporarily open to two broad hypotheses, though not mutually exclusive, namely : (1) stutterers "must talk with a speech mechanism that is muscularly more tense than that of nonstutterers [...], so the system would have a lower threshold for free vibration" (Starkweather, 1995), and (2) stutterers make a greater resort to articulatory feedback mechanisms (assuming that "multiple peaks reflect a sequence of overlapping sub-movements that are used to make spatial and temporal adjustments during movements", Adams et al., 1993).

ACKNOWLEDGEMENTS

Many thanks to Edda Farnetani and Eraldo Nicotra for their insight and invaluable suggestions.

REFERENCES

Alfonso, P.J. (1991). Implications of the concepts underlying task-dynamic modelling on kinematic studies of stuttering. In H.F.M. Peters, W. Hulstijn, & C.W. Starkweather (Eds.), *Speech motor control and stuttering, 79-100*, Amsterdam, Excerpta Medica.

Adams, S.G., Weismer, G., & Kent, R.D. (1993). Speaking rate and speech movement velocity profiles. *Journal of Speech and Hearing Research, 36*, 41-54.

Magno Caldognetto, E., Zmarich, C., Bettini, F., & Ferrigno G. (this volume). Simultaneous analysis of lip, jaw and tongue movements with an integrated optical tracking and EPG system.

Riley, G.D. (1972). A stuttering instrument for children and adults. *Journal of Speech and Hearing Disorders, 37*, 314-322.

Starkweather, C.W. (1995). A simple theory of stuttering. *Journal of Fluency Disorders, 20*, 91-116.

Winer, B.J. (1971). *Statistical Principles in experimental design*. New York, McGraw-Hill.

Zmarich, C., Magno Caldognetto, E., & Vagges, K. (1995). Variability in the articulatory kinematics of lips and jaw in repeated /pa/ and /ba/ sequences in Italian stutterers. *Proceedings XIIIl International Congress of Phonetic Sciences*, 536-539, Stockholm, Vol.4.

Speech Production: Motor Control, Brain Research and Fluency Disorders
W. Hulstijn, H.F.M. Peters and P.H.H.M. Van Lieshout, editors

Chapter 14

GESTURE MIRRORS SPEECH MOTOR CONTROL IN STUTTERERS

Rachel I. Mayberry, Rosalee C. Shenker

The relationship of stuttered disfluency to manual gesture during spontaneous speech was investigated in three studies. In the first study, adult stutterers produced fewer narrative details with simpler sentence structures compared to fluent controls matched for age and sex. Similarly, their speech was accompanied by fewer gestures and these gestures were simpler in form and meaning than those of the controls. Stuttered disfluencies were negatively correlated with the frequency and complexity of gesture; no such relationship was observed for normal disfluencies. The second study demonstrated that these effects are not caused by a motor-shutdown of hand and arm movement during stuttering. The third study investigated these effects in children. Like adults, children who stuttered accompanied significantly less of their spontaneous speech with gesture than controls matched for age and sex. We interpret these results to mean that the gesture-to-speech ratio during spontaneous expression reflects linguistic processing capacity.

INTRODUCTION

Are gesture and speech linked together in spontaneous expression? In order to shed light on this complex question, we have been investigating the gesture-speech relationship in adults and children who stutter. Before describing our work, it is important that we contextualize it by briefly summarizing current work in this area.

There are two competing theories as to how gesture and speech are related during the act of spontaneous, linguistic expression. The traditional and most commonly held hypothesis is that gesture and speech are autonomous and separate communication systems (Butterworth & Beattie, 1978; Butterworth & Hadar, 1989). In the *compensatory* framework, gesture functions as an backup or auxiliary system for the temporary absence or failure of speech, such as in coughing, having a mouth full of food, or being unable to put words to thoughts. Note that this hypothesis requires speech to fail in order for gesture to appear in the speech stream. The compensatory explanation of how gesture and speech are related predicts that stuttered speech will be accompanied by more gestures than will fluent speech.

An alternative hypothesis is that gesture and speech work together to form an integrated system for the single purpose of linguistic expression (Kendon, 1980; McNeill, 1985, 1992). In the *integrated system* framework, gesture is linked to the structure, meaning, and timing of spoken language. Thus, speech and gesture will always be co-expressed. The integrated system hypothesis predicts that stuttered speech will be accompanied by fewer gestures than fluent speech.

It is important to know that gesture occurs primarily during the act of speaking spontaneously and much less frequently, or rarely, in rehearsed, memorized, or read language (Krauss, 1996). This may be because, as McNeill (1992) has postulated, gesture is the product of putting thoughts to sentences and not simply uttering speech without meaning.

It is also important to note that by the term gesture we are referring specifically to the non-purposive movements of the hands and arms that accompany spontaneous speech. We are not referring to the more global concept used in stuttering research of what is commonly called *nonspeech behavior* where bodily actions, such as head and eye movement and lip, have been observed and documented to co-occur with and become incorporated into the stuttered disfluencies of children (Conture & Kelly, 1991; Schwartz et al., 1990).

Recent research has shown that gesture is linked to the structure of language in many ways. For example, American speakers typically produce 80 to 90% of their gestures simultaneously with speech at a rate of approximately 1.5 gestures per minute. Kendon (1980) and McNeill (1992) have observed that three different kinds of gesture are used to mark discourse structure across languages. These kind of gestures are *deitics*, or points at either real or abstract locations, *beats*, or up and down movements of the hand that are void of meaning, and *representational gestures*, which are gestures that depict, either concretely and abstractly, actions, people and objects, and spatial relationships. The meaning of the gesture that co-occurs with speech is either redundant with or supplementary to the meaning expressed in spoken language.

Data on the timing of gesture and speech production are limited, but Nobe (1996) has recently found that English speakers produce the stroke, or central and salient, movement of representational gestures such that it coincides with the peak stress of the phrase being spoken. Although the peak of the gesture movement and the peak phrasal stress are co-produced, the hand can be observed to prepare to gesture well before the particular phrase begins, sometimes in the silent pauses between clauses.

Thus, stuttering provides us with an opportunity to investigate the nature of the gesture-speech relationship when speech production is disrupted by stuttered disfluency. The question is whether gesture will show comparable disruptions, as the integrated-systems hypothesis predicts, or whether gesture will increase in frequency to compensate for disruptions in speech production caused by stuttered disfluency, as the compensation hypothesis predicts.

STUDY I

The goal of our first study was to analyze and describe the gesture-speech relationship in disfluent as compared to fluent speech in order to test these two hypotheses about the nature of the gesture-speech relationship (Mayberry et al., 1996; Scoble, 1993; Shenker et al., 1995). We used a 'cartoon narration task' to elicit spontaneous speech from subjects who identified themselves as stutters along with matched control subjects.

Study I Methods

Each subject was tested individually and watched a 7 minute animated cartoon. After watching the cartoon, the subject narrated the story line to an unfamiliar listener. The listener made few comments other than, "anything else," and never gestured. We videotaped the subject's narration and then began the time-consuming task of transcribing and coding it.

The transcription and coding consisted of three steps. First, the gestures were transcribed without the sound track. We noted the location and kind of gestures and along with their probable meanings. Next the speech was transcribed verbatim without the video picture and all speech disfluencies were noted and described. Third, the two transcripts were assembled by noting which gestures co-occurred with which words, clauses, and speech disfluencies. Although the transcriptions were done by hand, the actual counting and tabulating was computerized (Miller & Chapman, 1984).

Study I Subjects

The subjects were 12 English speaking adults. Six subjects identified themselves as stutterers, five males and one female ranging in age 21 to 51 years. Their stuttering severity according to the Iowa Scale was mild for two subjects, moderate for two, and severe for two (Johnson & Darley, 1963). We matched the subjects by age, sex, and level of education to 6 control subjects with no history of stuttering[1].

Study I Results and Discussion

The subjects who stuttered tended to say less using simpler sentence structure in more time than the controls. This was true for number of words, clauses, embedings and narrative details. Although the greatest difference between the groups was in the number of stuttered disfluencies produced, there were no differences in the number of normal disfluencies produced.

The subjects who stuttered produced significantly fewer total gestures than the controls. However, gesture production was not a simple function of how much the subjects talked. The ratio of gesture to speech was significantly different for the two groups. The controls accompanied 84% of their words with gesture and gestured 68% of the total time they spoke. By contrast, the subjects who stuttered accompanied only 34% of their words with gesture and gestured for only 23% of the total time they spoke.

These findings clearly support the *integrated system* hypothesis. Gesture production is highly associated with the fluent expression of spoken language and not with speech breakdown as the *compensatory* hypothesis predicts. This is further demonstrated by the high and positive correlations between the structure and content of the subjects' speech and the structure and content of their gesture. The number of words and clauses spoken were highly and positively correlated to the number of gestures produced [$r = +0.53$ (df=11, $p < .05$) and $r = +0.94$ (df=11, $p < .01$)]. Moreover, the number of narrative details given in the spoken discourse was highly correlated with the meaning complexity of the gestures [$r=+0.62$ (df=11, $p<.05$)]. Finally, the number of gestures produced while speaking was positively correlated with normal speech disfluencies [$r=.57$, $p<.05$] but negatively correlated with stuttered disfluencies [$r=-.31$, n.s.].

The dependency of gesture production upon fluent speech production is clearly shown by an analysis of normal as compared to stuttered disfluencies. By stuttered disfluencies we mean disfluencies that fragment word production, such as sound and syllable repetitions and prolongations. By normal disfluencies we mean word and phrase repetitions that do not fragment word production. Both groups produced gesture simultaneously with normal speech disfluencies with equal frequency. Importantly, however, gesture was rarely co-produced with stuttered disfluencies, as Figure 1 shows. In those rare instances when a gesture was co-produced with a stuttered disfluency, the gesturing hand could be readily observed to fall to rest during the moment of stuttering and then to rise again and resume the gesture within milliseconds of the resumption of fluency. Less frequently, the gesturing hand would stop moving during the moment of stuttering and resume moving within milliseconds of speech fluency resumption.

These results provide striking evidence of how gesture and speech are fundamentally and deeply linked for the single purpose of linguistic expression. The structure and content of gesture mirrors the structural and semantic properties of the co-expressed spoken language. This mirroring is also evident in the tight temporal relationship between the two. Smith and her colleagues (Franz et al., 1992; Smith et al., 1986) have shown that cyclic movements of the mouth and arm and fingers harmonize with one other in motor repetition tasks and that speech amplitude correlates with finger movement. Our findings show that the synchronization of dynamic gesture and speech motor patterns during spontaneous language production are all ultimately coordinated with the single linguistic meaning being expressed simultaneously by both modes (Tuite, 1993).

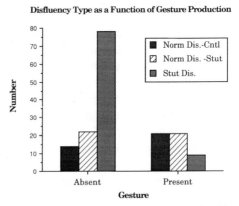

Figure 1. Gesture production accompanies the normal disfluencies of subjects who stutter and fluent controls with equal frequency. By contrast, gesture production seldom accompanies stuttered disfluencies.

Stuttered disfluency never disrupts this co-expression principle.

STUDY II

In order to rule out out a purely motor-shutdown explanation for this phenomenon, we asked three subjects who participated in the first study to participate in a second one where they narrated a second cartoon under three dual-task conditions. In the first dual task, the subject narrated a cartoon and simultaneously pressed a button continually. In the second dual task, the subject pressed a button to signal that he or she was stuttering. And in the third task, the subject took a pencil and wrote the word being stuttered. The subjects were able to carry out the simultaneous hand and speaking tasks without any disruption to their manual motor patterns during moments of stuttering. These findings demonstrate that stuttered disfluency, per se, does not impede hand and arm movement. Thus, the effects of stuttered disfluency on manual gesture cannot be explained by a simple manual-motor-shutdown explanation.

This means that gesture production is attenuated and/or interrupted by stuttered disfluency, not because the hand is unable to move, but because gesture expression is always concordant with speech expression. Gesture-speech concordance is evident in the coordination of structure, meaning, and motor execution timing. If gesture expression were to continue while speech was disfluent, the result would be a temporal asynchrony and semantic anomaly between gesture and speech. Such asynchronous anomalies never occurred in any of our three data sets.

STUDY III

In the third study, we replicated the results of the first study with two pairs of preadolescent boys who were 11 years old (DeDe, 1996). Two subjects were rated as showing a severe level of stuttering and two control subjects were matched by age, sex, and handedness.

The gesture-speech expression of the child subjects paralleled that of the adult subjects except that both pairs of children did not gesture as frequently as did the adults. However, the control children produced many more total gestures than did the children who stuttered at a ratio of nearly 3:1. The control children accompanied 26% of their words with gesture while the children who stuttered accompanied only 8% of their words with gesture. Again, the attenuated gesture production of the children who stuttered was accompanied by attenuated expression of spoken language. This was evident in terms of fewer words and clauses and simpler sentence structures. Like the adults who stuttered, the children who stuttered never used gesture to compensate for stuttered disfluencies. Also like the adults, the children primarily co-expressed gesture with fluent speech and normal disfluencies and almost never with stuttered disfluencies.

Comparing the gesture-speech ratios of the adults with those of the children reveals a very clear trend in the developmental relationship of gesture to speech, as Figure 2 shows.

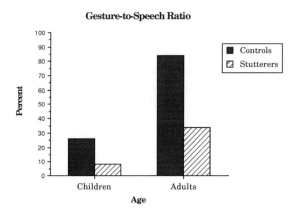

Figure 2. The amount of speech (measured in total number of words) that is accompanied by manual gesture (measured in total gestures) increases dramatically between the ages of 11 and adulthood and, moreover, is highly attenuated by stuttering in both children and adults.

The gesture-to-speech ratio increases four-fold between preadolescence and adulthood. This is true for both the controls and the subjects who stutter.

This developmental trend suggests to us that gesture production is constrained by the overall capacity to process language. Although 11-year olds have acquired nearly all of their grammar and have a very large lexicon, their capacity to process language is nevertheless limited in comparison to that of adults. At the same time, their gesture-to-speech ratio is four times less than that of adults. We interpret these substantial differences in the gesture-to-speech ratio to reflect the greater capacity of adults to process language than preadolescents. In other words, we propose that increases in linguistic processing capacity are marked by concomitant increases in the gesture-to-speech ratio during the act of spontaneous language expression.

GENERAL DISCUSSION

The results of these studies lead directly to the question of why stuttered disfluency so dramatically attenuates the gesture-to-speech ratio in the spontaneous language production of adults as well as children. Our working hypothesis is that the gesture-to-speech ratio is a reliable and valid indicator of language processing capacity. This explanation means that that gesture decreases with increases in stuttered disfluency because stuttering drains linguistic processing resources.

In our proposed framework, the frequency and duration with which gesture appears in the speech stream may indicate how much mental processing space and processing resources are being used to produce the spoken portion of the linguistic message. When the spoken portion of the message absorbs most of the available processing capacity, few resources remain for the gestural portion of the linguistic message to be expressed. This would mean that the spoken portion of the message has priority on linguistic processing resources while the gestured portion of the message gets any processing resources that remain.

In conclusion, our findings demonstrate clearly that the relationship of gesture to speech is a highly principled one of integrated co-expression of a single linguistic message. Because gesture production is characteristic of fluent (and we hypothesize 'easy') speech and not of disfluent (or 'difficult') speech, we believe that it provides a potentially powerful and meaningful new tool with which the disorder of stuttering can be observed, evaluated, and potentially, treated.

ACKNOWLEDGEMENTS

This research was supported by a grant from the Natural Sciences and Engineering Research Council of Canada (Grant #171239) to R. Mayberry. Additional funds were provided by the Fonds de la recherche en santé du québec through the McGill University Faculty of Medicine (Program étudiants d'été, #921182-103). We thank J. Jaques for help collecting and analyzing the adult data, K. White for help collecting the child data, and G. DeDe for help analyzing the child data.

NOTE

[1]   Subjects were unpaid volunteers. The experimental protocol of this study was approved by the Ethics Committee of the School of Communication Sciences & Disorders of McGill University.

REFERENCES

Butterworth, B., & Beattie, G. (1978). Gesture and silence as indicators of planning in speech. In R. N. Campbell & P. T. Smith (Eds.), *Recent advances in the psychology of language: Formal and experimental approaches* (pp. 347-360). New York: Plenum Press.

Butterworth, B., & Hadar, U. (1989). Gesture, speech, and computational stages: A reply to McNeill. *Psychological Review, 96,* 168-174.

Conture, E., & Kelly, E.M. (1991). Young stutterers' nonspeech behaviors during stuttering. *Journal of Speech and Hearing Research, 34,* 144-1056.

DeDe, G. (1996). The gesture-speech relationship in children: A preliminary study. *Unpublished undergraduate honors thesis,* McGill University.

Franz, E., Zelaznik, H., & Smith, A. (1992). Evidence of common timing processes in the control of manual, orofacial, and speech movements. *Journal of Motor Behavior, 24,* 281-287.

Johnson, W., Darley, F., & Spriesterbach, D. (1963). Iowa Scale of Stuttering Severity, in *Diagnostic methods in speech pathology.* New York· Harper & Row.

Kendon, A. (1980). Gesticulation and speech: Two aspects of the processes of utterance. In M. R. Key (Ed.), *The relation between verbal and nonverbal communication* (pp. 207-227). The Hague: Mouton.

Krauss, R. (1996). Gesture, speech and lexical access. To appear in A. Kendon, D. McNeill & S. Wilcox

Mayberry, R., Jaques, J., & Shenker, R. (1996). The disruption of gesture by stuttering: Insights into the nature of gesture-speech integration. To appear in A. Kendon, D. McNeill & S. Wilcox (Eds.), *Gestures: An emerging field of study.*

Mayberry, R., Jaques, J., & Shenker, R. (n.d.). The co-expression principle in gesture-speech production: Evidence from stuttering. Manuscript under review.

McNeill, D. (1985). So you think gestures are nonverbal? *Psychological Review, 92,* 350-371.

McNeill, D. (1992). *Hand and mind: What gestures reveal about thought.* Chicago: Univ. of Chicago Press, 1992.

Miller, J.F., & Chapman, R.S. (1984). *SALT: Systematic analysis of language transcripts.* Madison: Univ. of Wisconsin.

Nobe, S. (1996). Cognitive rhythms, gestures, and acoustic aspects of speech: Are most spontaneous representational gestures caused by problems in linguistic processes? To appear in A. Kendon, D., McNeill & S. Wilcox (Eds.), *Gestures: An emerging field of study.*

Schwartz, H.B., Zebrowski, P.M., & Conture, E.G. (1990). Behaviors at the onset of stuttering. *Journal of Fluency Disorders, 15,* 77-86.

Scoble, J. (1993). Stuttering blocks the flow of speech and gesture: The speech and gesture relationship in chronic stutterers. *Unpublished masters thesis,* McGill University.

Shenker, R., Mayberry, R., Scoble, J., Grothe, M., & White, K. (1995). The gesture-speech relationship in stuttering: Preliminary findings and applications to treatment. *First world congress on fluency disorders, 1,* 116-118.

Smith, A., McFarland, D., & Weber, C.M. (1986). Interactions between speech and finger movements: An exploration of the dynamic pattern perspective. *Journal of Speech and Hearing Research, 29,* 471-480.

Tuite, K. (1993). The production of gesture. *Semiotica, 93,* 83-105.

© 1997 Elsevier Science B.V. All rights reserved.
Speech Production: Motor Control, Brain Research and Fluency Disorders
W. Hulstijn, H.F.M. Peters and P.H.H.M. Van Lieshout, editors

Chapter 15

MECHANICAL PERTURBATION OF THE JAW DURING SPEECH IN STUTTERERS AND NONSTUTTERERS

Anne Bauer, Lutz Jäncke, Karl-Theodor Kalveram

10 stuttering and 10 nonstuttering adults uttered the testword [sasasar] repeatedly with normal or with slow speech rate and with stress either on the first or on the second syllable. In 17% of the trials of each condition (randomly chosen), an unexpected and unpredictable mechanical perturbation was applied to the jaw during the utterance of the first syllable of the testword. In these trials, the jaw was suddenly loaded with 80 g by means of a spatula lying on the lower front teeth. This load was applied during the jaw opening movement at the moment when the jaw reached 70% of maximal opening as determined for the first syllable of the preceding utterance.
Assuming that stuttering is a temporal discoordination of speech movements, we hypothesized that the mechanical perturbation of the jaw would lead to a greater discoordination between jaw movement and phonation in the stutterers than in the nonstutterers. A semiautomatic analysis of the jaw movement and phonation signals showed that the reaction to the perturbation varied for both stutterers and nonstutterers from trial to trial and that in most cases, the perturbation was integrated into the ongoing opening movement of the jaw. In some trials, the application of the load evoked overshooting compensatory movements of the jaw in stutterers as well as in nonstutterers. Only two severe stutterers showed cases of complete destruction of the jaw movement but preserved phonation. In some severe stutterers, there were cases of disturbed jaw movements in unperturbed trials following trials with perturbation. These results show that the sensorimotor speech control of both stutterers and nonstutterers is subject to temporary fluctuations and that most of the time, the reactions to the mechanical perturbation of the jaw are not different for both groups. On the other hand, occasionally the sensorimotor speech control of some severe stutterers is especially prone to disturbances.

INTRODUCTION

The investigation of the sensorimotor speech control system in normal speakers with the method of unexpectedly and unpredictably loading the jaw or the lower lip during speech demonstrated that such perturbations are compensated for by all articulators involved in the ongoing speech task (e.g. Gracco & Abbs, 1985; Shaiman, 1989; Kollia et al., 1992). Studies of our research group showed that this compensatory behavior is stress-dependent because a mechanical perturbation of the jaw during speech prolonged the duration of the jaw movement and the phonation only in unstressed but not in stressed syllables. Furthermore, our results indicated a functional coupling between articulation and phonation (Bauer et al., 1995a,b). Investigating the speech motor control of stutterers with this method, we found no prolongation of the jaw movement but signs of a discoordination between articulation and phonation (Bauer et al., 1995b). Because of the great inter- and intraindividual variability of our results, we suggested that the perturbation effects might be quite different from trial to trial. Therefore, in the present study, the reactions of stutterers and nonstutterers to a mechanical perturbation of the jaw during speech are investigated not only by automatic analysis of jaw movement and phonation parameters but also by visual inspection of the respective signals for each trial. Furthermore, we developed a method that enabled us to apply the perturbation at relatively fixed phase points of the jaw movement. In the above mentioned studies of our research group, the load was applied at the time of phonation onset which might vary with stress. In the present experiment, we applied the perturbation at a fixed phase point of the jaw opening movement some time around phonation onset to test whether the stress-dependent reactions could be replicated with this method.

METHOD

Subjects

10 stuttering adults (3 female, 7 male), aged 23 to 42 years (mean: 31.1 years) participated in this study. Stuttering severity was assessed by two speech pathologists. According to the Stuttering Severity Instrument of Riley (1972), the stuttering behavior was judged as mild in 3 Ss, as moderate in 4 Ss and as severe in 3 Ss. All stutterers had previously participated in various speech therapies. The control group consisted of 10 normally speaking Ss (3 female, 7 male), aged 23 to 38 years (mean: 28.4 years). All Ss were native German speakers and none of them had a neurological or a speech disorder. For participating in this investigation lasting about one hour all Ss were paid.

Speech task

Ss had to utter the testword [sasasar] in 2 different speech rates [slow / normal] with stress either on the first or on the second syllable. Under each of the resulting 4 conditions, they uttered the testword 30 times. At the beginning of each trial, a sequence of 3 tones (400 Hz, sine, 70 dB) indicating stress pattern and speech rate was presented by loudspeaker (duration of tones representing unstressed syllables = 150 ms [normal], and 200 ms [slow]; duration of tones representing stressed syllables = 300 ms [normal], and 400 ms [slow]). Ss were instructed to adjust their utterance to this pattern and to keep the speech intensity shown on a monitor constant. The order of experimental conditions for each subject was randomized by Latin Square.

Mechanical perturbation

In 5 randomly selected trials under each condition, the jaw was suddenly loaded during the utterance of the first syllable of the testword. The load of 80 g was applied during the jaw opening movement at the moment when the jaw reached 70% of maximal opening as determined for the first syllable of the preceding utterance. Between two experimental trials with load application, there were at least two trials without perturbation. The load that persisted for the rest of the trial (10 ms rise time) was automatically realized by means of a spatula connected to a torque motor and lying on the lower front teeth. This perturbation resulted in an additional force acting in movement direction. During the whole time of the experiment, the spatula followed the jaw movement with a load of 5 g in order to keep contact with the lower front teeth.

Data acquisition

Ss were seated in a sound insulated chamber on a chair which was equipped for the purposes of this study. In order to prevent head movements, the Ss' head was fixed to a device mounted at the back of the seat. A selspot-like optical tracking system (TS-3423, Optoelectronic) was used to record jaw position data during utterance production. During production by each speaker, the camera tracked the movement of an infrared light emitting diode (LED, diameter=4.15mm, wavelength=950nm, emitting angle=60 degrees) placed at the point of the chin in a location that yielded negligible artefact from skin movement. This LED was attached to the skin using high-quality adhesive plaster minimizing vibrations of the probes during movement. The vertical position of the LED was transformed into voltage data by the system. Each speaker was seated 30 cm aside of the camera with his face parallel to the camera's focal plane. A microphone (Ramsa WMS 10) was positioned in front of the speaker's face (mouth to microphone distance 15 cm) so that it did not occlude the LED. The auditory speech signal was lowpass filtered (400 Hz, 24 dB/octave), rectified and again lowpass filtered (40 Hz, 24dB/octave). The filtered and rectified speech waves and the position data from the LED were digitized at a rate of 1000 Hz (12-Bit resolution) and stored in computer memory. Experimental control, the delivering of the tones and the storage of data was managed by a laboratory computer (VME-bus computer Eltec Eurocom 7).

Data analysis

The original movement signals were digitally lowpass filtered (upper corner frequency 50 Hz / 6 dB octave). The velocity of the jaw movement signal was obtained by digitally differentiating the position signal. A computer algorithm identified several measures of the first syllable that were stored and from which the following dependent variables were computed with the SPSSPC program: displacement of the jaw for opening and closure movement, duration of jaw movement, and duration of phonation. [As a measure of movement onset we used the point where 10% of maximum displacement was reached. In this way, irrelevant small jaw movements were excluded from analysis. Jaw opening displacement was measured as the distance from the so defined movement onset to maximum opening. Jaw closing displacement was defined as the distance from maximum opening to 90% of maximum closing for the second [s], and jaw movement duration as the time from movement onset to 90% of maximum jaw closing.] Only fluent utterances were included in the analysis. The data for trials with perturbation, the trials before and after perturbation and the remaining trials were averaged for each subject and each experimental condition. These values were subjected to a four-way analysis of variance (ANOVA) with repeated measurements (speech rate: slow, normal; stress pattern: stressed, unstressed; load: pre, load, post, other) and one between-subjects factor (group: stutterer, nonstutterer). As suggested by O'Brien and Kaiser (1985), all repeated measurements effects involving more than two levels were tested using the multivariate test statistic (Wilks' lambda) generated in the repeated measurements ANOVA output of SPSSPC. Furthermore, Wilcoxon-tests were performed to test the effect of the perturbation by comparing the perturbed trials with the preceding unperturbed trials. For each trial, the jaw movement and phonation signals were inspected visually and the effect of the perturbation was classified by two raters.

RESULTS AND DISCUSSION

The durations of the jaw movement and of the phonation showed that stutterers as well as nonstutterers realized the required prosodic patterns of the testword quite precisely. The ANOVA yielded highly significant effects for the factors 'stress' and 'speech rate' concerning these variables ($p < 0.001$).

The effects of the perturbation on the duration of the jaw movement and of the phonation were tested by means of the Wilcoxon-test. As Figure 1 shows, only 1 out of the 2 x 8 comparisons reached significance ($p < 0.05$). Furthermore, there was no interaction of the factors 'speech rate', 'stress', or 'group' with the factor 'load' (all $p > 0.05$). These results are in contrast to previous findings of our research group (Bauer et al., 1995b), but they can

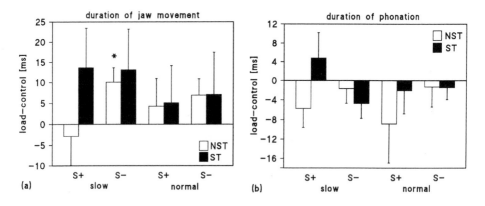

Figure 1. Effects of the mechanical perturbation on the duration of jaw movement and phonation for the different prosodic conditions; shown are the differences of the values for perturbed trials and the preceding unperturbed trials; NST: nonstutterers, ST: stutterers; *: $p < 0.05$; vertical lines: SEM

be explained by different characteristics of the mechanical perturbation in both studies. The most important difference may be that in the present study, the load was applied at relatively fixed phase points of the jaw movement cycle, whereas in the previous study, the load was applied at the time of phonation onset. Calculating the phase angles of phonation onset and offset showed that the phonation started earlier in stressed syllables than in unstressed syllables related to the phase of the jaw movement (p=0.001, interaction between 'stress' and 'speech rate': p=0.002). Furthermore, in stressed syllables stutterers tended to start phonation earlier than nonstutterers (an interesting finding that will be investigated in more detail). Therefore, the stress-dependent and group-dependent reactions to the perturbation in the previous study might be explained by the phase-dependency of compensatory reactions (e.g. Forssberg et al., 1975).

As indicated by the great variability of the perturbation effects, the visual inspection of the jaw movement and phonation signals showed that the reaction to the loading of the jaw varied for both stutterers and nonstutterers from trial to trial and that in most cases, the perturbation was integrated in the ongoing opening movement of the jaw. In some trials, the perturbation evoked overshooting compensatory movements in both groups. Only two severe stutterers showed cases of complete destruction of the jaw movement but preserved phonation (Figure 2). In some severe stutterers, there were cases of disturbed jaw movements in unperturbed trials following trials with perturbation (Table 1).

These results show that the sensorimotor speech control of both stutterers and nonstutterers is subject to temporary fluctuations and that most of the time, the reactions to the mechanical perturbation of the jaw are not different for both groups. On the other hand, occasionally the sensorimotor speech control of some severe stutterers is especially prone to disturbances.

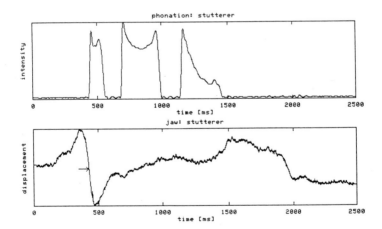

Figure 2. Jaw movement and phonation signal of a severe stutterer in a trial with perturbation; the arrow indicates perturbation onset; the extreme impairment of the jaw movement occured only twice during the whole experiment

Table 1. Number of different reactions to the mechanical perturbation; judged by visual inspection of the jaw movement and phonation signals.

	stutterer	nonstutterer
- visible effect of the load (increase of movement amplitude)	1	0
- visible overcompensation	5	5
- jerk in jaw movement in an unloaded trial after a loaded trail	6	0
- extreme impairment of the jaw movement	2	0

NOTE

This study was supported by grant Ka117/13-2 from the Deutsche Forschungsgemeinschaft.

REFERENCES

Bauer, A., Jäncke, L., & Kalveram, K.Th. (1995a). Mechanical perturbation of jaw movements during speech: Effects on articulation and phonation. *Perceptual and Motor Skills, 80,* 1108-1112.

Bauer, A., Jäncke, L., & Kalveram, K.Th. (1995b). Mechanical perturbation of the jaw during stutterers' and nonstutterers' fluent speech. In C.W. Starkweather, & H.F.M. Peters (Eds.), *Stuttering: Proceedings of the First World Congress on Fluency Disorders* (pp. 31-34). The International Fluency Association.

Forssberg, H., Grillner, S., & Rossignol, S. (1975). Phase dependent reflex reversal during walking in chronic spinal cats. *Brain Research, 85,* 103-107.

Gracco, V.L. & Abbs, J.H. (1985). Dynamic control of the perioral system during speech: Kinematic analyses of autogenic and nonautogenic sensorimotor processes. *Journal of Neurophysiology, 54,* 418-432.

Kollia, H.B., Gracco, V.L., & Harris, K.S. (1992). Functional organization of velar movements following jaw perturbation. *Journal of the Acoustical Society of America, 91,* 2474.

O'Brien, R.G. & Kaiser, M.K. (1985). MANOVA method for analysing repeated measures designs: An extensive primer. *Psychological Bulletin, 97,* 316-333.

Riley, G.D. (1972). A stuttering severity instrument for children and adults. *Journal of Speech and Hearing Disorders, 37,* 314-322.

Shaiman, S. (1989). Kinematic and electromyographic responses to perturbation of the jaw. *Journal of the Acoustical Society of America, 86,* 78-88.

Speech Production: Motor Control, Brain Research and Fluency Disorders
W. Hulstijn, H.F.M. Peters and P.H.H.M. Van Lieshout, editors

Chapter 16

IS STUTTERING CAUSED BY FAILING NEUROMUSCULAR FORCE CONTROL?

Marc Grosjean, Gerard P. van Galen, Peter de Jong, Pascal H.H.M. van Lieshout, Wouter Hulstijn

This study investigated whether force control is less efficient in stutterers than in fluent speakers, and whether this can be detected with nonspeech tasks. To do so, an isometric force production task (with and without visual feedback) was used. Force control was studied with effectors actively used in speech, i.e. the lips, and assessed by measuring bilabial closing pressure. Dependent variables were mean error of force, force signal-to-noise ratio and neuromotor noise present in force production. The latter variable was obtained by applying a power spectral density analysis (PSDA) to the jerk profile derived from the force signal. Results generally showed no group differences when visual feedback was absent. However, when visual feedback was present, the stutterers proved to have significantly greater mean errors of force than the nonstutterers and to have a tendency to show worse signal-to-noise ratios. In terms of PSDA, the stutterers showed more energy in the lower frequency bands (1-4 Hz) which correspond to corrective control, while the nonstutterers had more energy in the higher bands (7-9 Hz) which represent neuromotor tremor. Taken together, these results suggest that stutterers have less efficient and more noisy force control than nonstutterers. The Dynamic Noise Filtering Model of motor control proposed by Van Galen and De Jong (1995) can account for these results in terms of less efficient biomechanical filtering strategies in the force production of stutterers.

INTRODUCTION

Recent studies have shown that inefficient motor control strategies can perhaps be more important than psycho linguistic deficiencies in understanding the causes of stuttering. For example, Van Lieshout (1995) proposes that control strategies in the coordination of the speech musculature discriminate between stutterers and fluent speakers. Much of this evidence is based on the use of speech tasks. In this study, we wanted to test how efficient stutterers and nonstutterers are in controlling their speech musculature when performing a nonspeech task, i.e. isometric force production. Although other researchers have not defended the idea that stutterers differ from matched controls when they produce and maintain force over a fixed period of time (e.g., Zelaznik et al., 1994), it might still be premature to conclude that no differences exist on these type of tasks and this for two main reasons. First, these studies used non-oral effectors. It could be that stutterers' deficit in force production may be restricted to the orofacial region. Second, in the Zelaznik et al. (1994) study, the data analysis was limited to only a few measures of performance (i.e. means, standard deviations and root mean squared errors of force). These measures have the disadvantage of giving a restricted picture of the processes underlying performance.

In light of these problems, it seems reasonable to reinvestigate the proposal that stuttering is related to a force control deficit. This will be done in light of the Dynamic Noise Filtering Model of motor control proposed by Van Galen and De Jong (1995). This model posits that "... the psychomotor system is an inherently noisy mechanical system for which spatial demands should be formulated in terms of a desired signal-to-noise ratio between goal-related propulsion of the limb (signal) and stochastic error (noise). Adequate movements would, from this point of view, result from the optimization between the application of muscle forces to the limb system and the noise reducing effects of biomechanical properties, such as stiffness, viscosity, or friction due to surface contact." (Van Galen & De Jong, 1995; p. 539). In other words, for a movement to be accurate, efficient biomechanical filtering strategies must be employed to reduce the inherent noisiness of the movement signal, and thereby lessen noise-related movement variability. The natural degree of movement variability or "neuromotor noise" has various sources, ranging from higher order (cognitive) planning errors to low level (peripheral) mechanical oscillations of the effector system.

Because neuromotor noise superimposes itself on the intended movement signal, it is important to distinguish these two signals from one another if one is to understand motor performance. Van Galen et al. (1990) were the first to apply a power spectral density analysis (PSDA) to the acceleration profiles of movement signals and were able to extract the energy of the noise components in the signal. The use of this method to understand motor performance has been illustrated in a series of studies by Van Galen and his colleagues (for example, see Van Galen et al., 1993). They showed that disorders in motor behavior can be equated with an excessively noisy motor output system, inefficient biomechanical strategies used to "filter out" the noise, or a combination of the two.

In this study it is proposed that stutterers have a more noisy speech motor output system than fluent speakers and/or less efficient biomechanical filtering strategies used to reduce the inherent noisiness of their system. To test this, two versions of an isometric force production task were used: with and without on-line visual feedback. This latter version was added in order to test a proposal made by De Nil and Abbs (1991) that stutterers may have deficient kinesthetic feedback or deficient processing of that feedback.

METHODS

Subjects

Eleven adult male stutterers (mean age = 24.0, range 17-30) and the same number of adult male nonstutterers (mean age = 24.2, range 18-42) were paid to participate in this experiment. One subject in each group was left-handed. Subjects were approximately matched for age, sex, education and handedness, and apart from a stuttering problem in the experimental group, no subjects had a history of neurological, speech, language, visual, or hearing disorders. Stuttering severity classifications were based on ratings of experienced speech-language pathologists using the Stuttering Severity Instrument (SSI, Riley, 1984). There were 3 moderate, 5 moderate/severe and 3 severe stutterers.

Task and conditions

Before the isometric force production task was run, a maximum voluntary closing force (*MVCF*) measure of bilabial pressure was taken for each subject. This was done by asking the subjects to produce a continuously increasing force until they could "no longer go higher". To help them with this, the height of an on-line cursor was displayed on a computer screen indicating the force being produced. The isometric force production task was a "ramp-and-hold" force control task (for a review of these tasks, see Barlow & Burton, 1990). The target forces were represented on a computer screen by the height of a color bar. By applying lip pressure on a force transducer, subjects had to move a visible cursor onto the bar and maintain it there for 10 seconds. There were two versions of this task. First, a *visual* version in which subjects were given visual feedback for the entire length of the trial, i.e. they saw the cursor under their control continuously. Second, a *kinesthetic* version, which was similar to the first except that visual feedback was withdrawn immediately after the cursor was stabilized on the bar, i.e. the cursor disappeared with the sound of a tone that signaled the beginning of the 10 second recording. Five levels of submaximal force were tested: 10, 20, 30, 40, and 50% of *MVCF*.

Instrumentation

The force-transducer used for measuring bilabial muscle force production was designed explicitly for this experiment, as was the software used for recording and translating the force signal into on-line cursor movement feedback. The transducer was light and small enough to be held easily in the mouth. When lip force was measured, the jaw was immobilized by inserting a bilateral bite-block between the subject's teeth. (For a description of a similar type of apparatus, see Barlow & Abbs, 1983.) The feedback was displayed on a color monitor.

Procedure

Before assessing maximum voluntary closing force (*MVCF*), the positioning of the bite-block was adjusted in the subject's mouth, as was the force-transducer. When a correct and comfortable position was attained, the subject was told to "always position the bite-block and transducer in the same way" and to "only use the lips when producing force". *MVCF* was measured and the isometric force production task was then administered. Both versions were preceded by practice trials in order to familiarize the subjects with the stimuli and material, and to make sure that they understood the task. Every condition of both versions of the task was measured 4 times, and in the same order for all subjects. For both versions, four blocks of either increasing (i.e. 10, 20, 30, 40, 50% of *MVCF*: order A) or decreasing (order B) force levels were administered. The blocks were balanced in an ABBA fashion.

Data analysis

A descriptive analysis was performed on the "raw" force data of 10 subjects in each group. The middle 8 seconds (out of the 10 s recorded) of each trial were selected for analysis. The following parameters were computed for each subject and condition (i.e. level of force). First, the absolute and normalized mean (*Mn*) and standard deviation (*SD*) of force. The normalized values refer to the absolute values divided by the subjects' *MVCF*. On this basis, mean errors of force were calculated by subtracting from normalized mean force the required target force. Thus, mean errors of force were represented in percentages of *MVCF*. Second, a signal-to-noise ratio (*SNR*) was computed by dividing mean normalized force (*MnNF*) by the standard deviation of normalized force (*SDNF*) for each subject and condition (*SNR = [MnNF/SDNF]*). Third, a power spectral density analysis (PSDA) was performed on the jerk profiles (i.e. the time rate change of force, obtained by a derivation of the force signal) for each subject and level of force. In this situation, a more direct estimate of the noise energy is obtained by using jerk. A Fast Fourier Transform was employed to derive absolute power spectral density functions (PSDFs). These functions correspond to the distribution of energy in each of the extracted frequency bands. Finally, normalized spectra were obtained by normalizing the area under each power spectrum to one. The Nyquist frequency of the reduced signal was 31.25 Hz and that was also the highest frequency of the highest band of each spectrum. In all, 32 bands were derived, each of which had a width of approximately 1 Hz. Although the match was not perfect, band numbers correspond rather well to frequencies of jerks of about the same number of Hertz.

RESULTS AND DISCUSSION

Maximum voluntary closing force (MVCF)

This measure was initially obtained so that all target forces would be relative to each subject's *MVCF* and would thus offer a better basis of comparison. Nonstutterers showed a significantly higher mean *MVCF* overall (*Mn*=8.29 Newtons, *SD*=1.1) than stutterers (*Mn*=6.96 Newtons, *SD*=1.1; $t=2.70$, $df=18$, $p<.05$). Because in isometric force production tasks the signal to noise ratio is dependent on the produced level of force (see Van Galen & De Jong, 1995) in the following ANOVA's stutterers and nonstutterers were matched for individual MVCF's.

Mean error of force

Figure 1 depicts the absolute mean error of force as a function of target force for stutterers and nonstutterers. Both groups performed the task rather well (absolute mean errors are never greater than 4% of *MVCF*) and showed an increase in mean error as the target force increases. What is also clear is that stutterers were less accurate in performing the task. This was confirmed by an ANOVA which showed a main effect for group ($F(1,18)=7.31$, $p<.05$). There was also a large effect of target force upon mean error of force ($F(4,72)=41.11$, $p<.001$). This could be expected as the difficulty of the task increases with the amount of force to be produced.

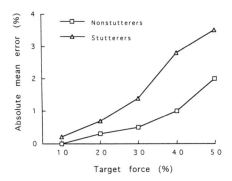

Figure 1. Absolute mean error of force as a function of target force for stutterers and nonstutterers in the *visual* version of the isometric force production task.

Finally, there was a group by target force interaction ($F(4,72) = 4.44$, $p < .05$). These results do not replicate the findings found by Zelaznik et al. (1994) in which there were no differences in the accuracy of force control between stutterers and nonstutterers.

Signal-to-noise ratio (SNR)

Figure 2 presents *SNR* as a function of target force for the two groups. Stutterers' force signal relative to their variability was not as high as the nonstutterers'. In the overall analysis this result was highly significant ($p < 0.001$) but in a step down analysis this result appeared to be mainly caused by the visual condition (see figure 2). When visual feedback was withdrawn the stutterers produced only slightly worse than the nonstutterers. There was a significant decrease of *SNR* as a function of target force for both groups ($F(4,72)=5.26$, $p < .05$). Finally, no interaction between groups and force level was found ($F(4,72)=4.07$, *NS*). Thus, there seems to be a tendency for stutterers' *SNR* to be worse than that of nonstutterers, implying that the former have somewhat more noisy force control than the latter.

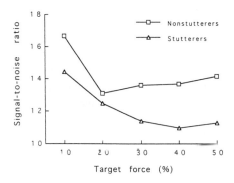

Figure 2. Signal-to-noise ratio as a function of target force for stutterers and nonstutterers in the *visual* version of the isometric force production task.

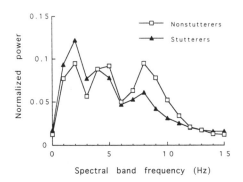

Figure 3. Normalized power spectral density functions of the normalized jerk profiles for stutterers and nonstutterers in the *visual* version of the isometric force production task. Each spectrum represents an average taken across the 5 PSDFs (one for each target force) of each group.

Power spectral density analysis (PSDA)

Figure 3 shows the power spectral density functions (PSDFs) of the normalized jerk profiles for stutterers and nonstutterers. Each spectrum is based on an average taken across the 5 PSDFs (one for each target force) of each group. The spectral band frequencies end at 15 because after this point the spectra for stutterers and nonstutterers did not change in form and contained very little energy. Band numbers correspond rather well to frequencies of jerks of about the same number of Hertz. In reality though, all band numbers correspond to a frequency slightly higher than their number, which explains why the 0 spectral band frequency contains some energy.

Although stutterers and nonstutterers seem to show a similar pattern of noise distribution, they do not have the same energy in all frequency bands. Systematic testing at each band frequency showed that stutterers had significantly more energy in the 3 Hz-band region ($F(1,18)=5.04$, $p<.05$) and less energy in the 8 Hz-band region ($F(1,18)=4.73$, $p<.05$). This implies that stutterers showed more noise in the corrective loops region of the spectrum (i.e. in the 3 Hz region) while nonstutterers had more neuromotor tremor (i.e. in the 8 Hz region). It should be noted that a similar pattern of results was obtained for the *kinesthetic* version of the task.

One could argue than the results obtained in the PSDA are due to the fact that the two groups were performing at different overall levels of force (see MVCF results). In order to test this, a series of ANOVAs were performed on the normalized jerk profiles using the *actual* required level of force. The results in the new analysis did change somewhat, with a few differences becoming significant and others disappearing. However, the general tendency was the same, with stutterers having more noise in the corrective loops region of the spectra and nonstutterers having more neuromotor tremor.

GENERAL DISCUSSION

The main purpose of this study was to test whether stuttering is related to a deficit in speech musculature control and whether this can be detected with a nonspeech task. The results obtained suggest that stutterers do have less efficient, and more noisy, force control than nonstutterers. This finding is all the more noteworthy as in our study stutterers were working at overall lower force levels than the fluent speakers. Stutterers were less accurate in their force production than the matched controls (at least in the *visual* version of the task). This does not replicate the result found by Zelaznik et al. (1994) and suggests that stutterers' deficiency in force control might be restricted to the orofacial region. Stutterers also showed a tendency to have worse signal-to-noise ratios and differed in the amount of neuromotor noise present in specific regions of the spectrum. They had more noise related to kinesthetic corrective control, while nonstutterers had more neuromotor tremor. Based on the Dynamic Noise Filtering Model of motor control (Van Galen & De Jong, 1995), we propose that stutterers may have less efficient biomechanical filtering strategies than nonstutterers. Because of this, each group may have been using a different general motor control strategy when producing force. In particular, stutterers may try to compensate for their more variable motor output system by relying more on kinesthetic control loops. This would explain why they have more noise for the control loop region of the spectra. Although our data do not allow us to prove this hypothesis directly, it is in line with an idea developed by Van Lieshout (1995) which states that people who stutter use different motor control strategies than people who do not stutter. These strategies are developed in order to compensate for their impairment and may allow them to achieve stable patterns of speech articulator coordination.

Taken together, these results tend to suggest that stuttering may be caused by failing neuromuscular force control. The disorder may be due to the stutterers' noisier neuromotor system and/or less efficient biomechanical filtering strategies which are used to reduce the inherent noisiness of their system. In order to cope with this deficiency, stutterers may have developed motor control strategies in which they rely more on kinesthetic information than fluent speakers. This would naturally slow down their speech rate and could perhaps be responsible for some of the typical motor events that are observed in their speech production (Van Lieshout, 1995).

REFERENCES

Barlow, S.M., & Abbs, J.H. (1983). Force transducers for the evaluation of labial, lingual, and mandibular motor impairments. *Journal of Speech and Hearing Research, 26*, 616-621.

Barlow, S.M., & Burton, M.K. (1990). Ramp-and-hold force control in the upper and lower lips: Developing new neuromotor assessment applications in traumatically brain-injured adults. *Journal of Speech and Hearing Research, 33*, 660-675.

De Nil, L.F., & Abbs, J.H. (1991). Kinesthetic acuity of stutterers and non-stutterers for oral and non-oral movements. *Brain, 114*, 2145-2158.

Riley, G.D. (1984). *Stuttering severity instrument for children and adults*. Portland, OR: C.C.

Publications.

Van Galen, G.P., & De Jong, W.P. (1995). Fitts' law as the outcome of a dynamic noise filtering model of motor control. *Human Movement Science, 14,* 539-571.

Van Galen, G.P., Portier, S.J., Smits-Engelsman, B.C.M., & Schomaker, L.R.B. (1993). Neuromotor noise and poor handwriting in children. *Acta Psychologica, 82,* 161-178.

Van Galen, G.P., van Doorn, R.R.A., & Schomaker, L.R.B. (1990). Effects of motor programming on the power spectral density function of finger and wrist movements. *Journal of Experimental Psychology: Human Perception and Performance, 16,* 755-765.

Van Lieshout, P.H.H.M. (1995). *Motor planning and articulation in fluent speech of stutterers and nonstutterers* (Ph.D.-thesis University of Nijmegen). Nijmegen: NICI.

Zelaznik, H.N., Smith, A., & Franz, E.A. (1994). Motor performance of stutterers and nonstutterers on timing and force control tasks. *Journal of Motor Behavior, 26,* 340-347.

Speech Production: Motor Control, Brain Research and Fluency Disorders
W. Hulstijn, H.F.M. Peters and P.H.H.M. Van Lieshout, editors

Chapter 17

A COMPARISON OF NORMALS' AND APHASICS´ ABILITY TO PLAN RESPIRATORY ACTIVITY IN OVERT AND COVERT SPEECH

Philip Hoole, Wolfram Ziegler

Disturbances of aphasic patients in the planning of spoken utterances have hitherto mainly been investigated through patterns of paraphasic errors, the scope of these errors usually not involving more extensive units than the word. In contrast, comparatively little is known about disturbances at the level of larger planning units. In the present study we focus on respiratory activity, asking how normals and one apraxic aphasic link the linguistic-phonetic demands of an utterance in terms of length, loudness, and tempo to appropriate patterns of respiratory motor activity. We further wished to determine the extent to which covert speech may take account of the airflow requirements of the planned utterance and speculated that inclusion of this experimental condition could help to throw more precise light on the levels of the speech production system where planning deficiences can occur in apraxic speakers.

INTRODUCTION

The question of how aphasic patients prepare for the articulatory realisation of a grammatically encoded sentence has so far been studied mainly on the background of lexical retrieval and segmental-phonological encoding processes. Only few authors have looked at suprasegmental aspects of utterance planning (e.g. Danly & Shapiro, 1982). Although speech breathing parameters are considered valuable in the analysis of speech planning processes (cf. Winkworth et al., 1995), they have to our knowledge not been used in the study of aphasic output disorders.

We present here our experience with the development of a speech breathing paradigm, illustrating its application to a group of normal subjects and a first clinical case (apraxia of speech). The paradigm focussed on the influence of loudness level and sentence length in overt and covert speech.

METHODS

Subjects

The experimental subject of this study was a male patient, 49 years, with an infarction of the left middle cerebral artery. Time since onset was 14 months. The patient had a mild non-classifiable aphasia with good comprehension, mild naming impairment, mild agraphia, and mild-to-moderate apraxia of speech. This patient was chosen as a first clinical subject on the following grounds: Assuming that apraxic speakers have no basic motor problems in the control of respiratory activity it is of interest whether such patients´ presumed speech motor programming deficit would show-up in their speech breathing pattern.

A group of five healthy males (28-46 yrs) served as controls.

Procedure

The speech material consisted of 10 short sentences (5 syllables; e.g. "Der Fuchs streicht durch´s Gras") and 10 long sentences (29-31 syllables; e.g. "Die beiden unbekannten Taschendiebe flohen aus der Lebensmittelabteilung eines Hamburger Kaufhauses"). The syntactic structure of long and short sentences was as homogeneous as possible, e.g no long sentences employed subordinate clauses. These 20 sentences were each elicited in all combinations of 3 Delivery Modes: Normal, Fast, Loud and 2 Speech Modes: Overt, Covert.

The resulting 120 utterances were elicited in random order using the following procedure:

1. *Familiarization*: Orthographic presentation of the sentence to the subject on display terminal; subject scans sentence for as long as desired; subject operates push-button to terminate this phase.
2. *Prompt*: On the expiratory phase of the following cycle of quiet breathing investigator prompts subject verbally with required combination of Speech- and Delivery Mode.
3. *Speech Task*: Subject speaks / reads sentence exactly once; operates push-button again on completion.
4. *Return to quiet breathing*: Investigator allows one cycle of quiet tidal breathing to be completed before triggering next item.

For the covert speech condition the subject was asked to imagine the tempo and loudness he would employ if speaking the utterance aloud.

Stimulus presentation and data collection was performed under computer control. The following signals were acquired: speech signal, thoracic and abdominal respiratory activity monitored by means of Respiratory Inductive Plethysmography, push-button activation. The respiratory signals were monitored online by the investigator. In addition to the speech tasks, the subjects also performed calibration tasks with a pneumotach to allow least-squares prediction of total lung-volume changes from a weighted combination of the two Respitrace signals.

Rationale for the design

The paradigm we employed can be regarded as maximizing the opportunity for pre-planning. A first purpose of the investigation was thus to establish to what extent the inspiratory volumes of normal subjects anticipate the volume demands of the spoken utterance under such conditions. Increased loudness has been reliably reported to be accompanied by increased magnitudes of inspiratory volumes (e.g Stathopoulos & Sapienza,

1993). Somewhat surprisingly, the relation between utterance length and inspiratory volume is less clear (Winkworth et al., 1994). The inclusion of the fast delivery mode was related to this concern. It was hypothesized that the fast rate could favour pre-planning activity since to achieve a fast rate speakers might need to minimize the necessity for within-utterance inspirations (cf. Grosjean & Collins, 1979). With regard to covert speech, and following on from observations of Conrad and Schönle (1979), we asked whether normals and aphasics would differ in the extent to which covert speech could shift breathing activity towards a speech-breathing pattern.

RESULTS

For reasons of space we will confine our attention here to the thoracic signal, since this was the respiratory signal showing the most consistent effect of the experimental variables. For the analysis of overt (i.e spoken) speech, the focus will be on inspiratory amplitude prior to the utterance, as an index for anticipation of the ensuing expiratory volume demands. For covert speech, analysis was conducted primarily in terms of the ratio of inspiratory to expiratory duration for the breath cycle following the prompt given by the investigator. Conrad and Schönle (1979) had used this ratio to demonstrate a continuum of respiratory behaviour from quiet tidal breathing via sub-vocal speech tasks to normal spoken utterances.

Overt speech
Table 1 summarizes the results of ANOVAs carried out to examine the effect of Sentence Length and Delivery Mode on inspiratory amplitude.

These results suggest firstly, and much as expected, that sentence length and delivery mode have a consistent influence on inspiratory amplitude (for subject N3 , who was the only one not to show an effect of delivery mode, this was due to several major outliers for the long sentences. For the short sentences, delivery mode was highly significant). They indicate secondly the absence of any drastic differences between patient and normal subjects.

Relating the inspiratory volume to the volume actually expired during speech reveals more precisely the relative potency of "Sentence Length" and "Delivery Mode" in influencing inspiratory activity. Figure 1 shows this relationship for the average values of each of the 6 experimental conditions.

Table 1. Effects of 'Sentence Length' and 'Delivery Mode' on inspiratory amplitude for each subject (ANOVA;**:p<0.01;*:p<0.05; ns: not significant)

Subject	N1	N2	N3	N4	N5	PAT
Sentence length	**	**	**	*	**	*
Delivery Mode:	**	**	ns	**	**	**

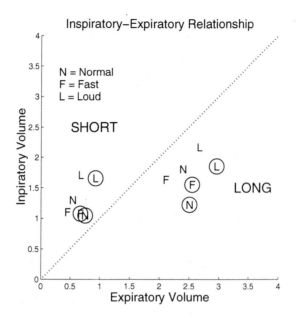

Figure 1. Amplitude (normalized units) of inpiratory and expiratory activity for the two 'Sentence Length' and the three 'Delivery Mode' conditions. Averaged normal-speaker data (without circles); patient data (with circles).

(Each subject's data was first normalized by the standard deviation of expiratory amplitude.)

The figure includes a dashed line with a gradient of +1. Data points would be located on this line under the "simple-minded" hypothesis that subjects inspire by an amount corresponding to the expected volume requirements. Looking first at the values averaged over all 5 normal subjects (data points without circles), it will be observed that short utterances are located above the diagonal: Virtually all utterances are initiated at volume levels greater than the end-inspiratory level of tidal breathing, and short utterances do not occupy the totality of the ensuing expiratory limb. Long utterances are below the diagonal: they typically encroach on the expiratory reserve volume below the end-expiratory level of tidal breathing. The figure shows that the effect of sentence length on inspiratory volume is really quite modest when seen in relation to the substantial change in expiratory volume going from short to long utterances.

The patient (data points with circles) conforms to the basic pattern of short and long utterances on opposite sides of the +1 gradient. The increase in inspiratory volume for long vs. short utterances is less pronounced than that found for the averaged normal subjects, however; the effect of sentence length only just reached statistical significance.

(A note on the fast delivery condition: This does not in fact appear to reinforce preplanning. This would have been visible in a disproportionately large inspiratory volume. On the contrary, but perfectly logically, the normal speakers inspired less, anticipating the lower expiratory volumes of fast utterances.

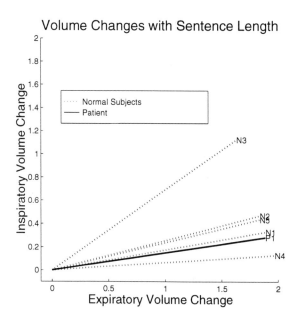

Figure 2. Inspiratory and expiratory volume changes shown separately for each subject for short vs. long sentences (normalized units as in figure 1).

The patient does not show this pattern, but little importance should be attached to this, since due to articulatory difficulties he had only a
limited capacity to accelerate his speech rate in the first place.)

The next two figures leave fast delivery out of consideration and aim firstly to drive home the fact that loudness contrasts on the one hand and length contrast on the other hand differ markedly in the strength of their influence on inspiratory activity. Secondly they allow a closer look at the extent to which the patient falls within the range of the normal subject. Figure 2 places the average of each subject's short utterances at the origin and shows by a vector the changes in inspiratory and expiratory volume associated with a transition to long utterances. Clearly, only a small proportion of the increased volume demands of long utterances are anticipated in the pre-utterance inspiration.

Figure 3 places normal-delivery utterances at the origin and shows by a vector the changes in inspiratory and expiratory volume associated with a transition to loud delivery. Thus, the increase in inspiratory amplitude may well *exceed* the increase in the air actually expired in the utterance. This could be interpreted as exploitation of larger recoil forces to help generate loud speech. Regarding the patient, the most interesting issue is whether his comparatively limited inspiratory anticipation of the volume requirements of long utterances is indeed so weak as to be outside the normal range: The shallower the gradient, the weaker the anticipation.

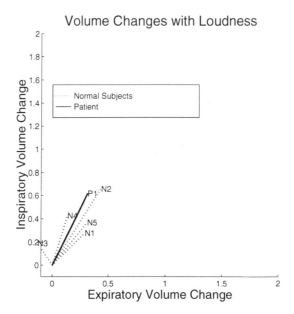

Figure 3. Inspiratory and expiratory volume changes shown separately for each subject for normal delivery vs. loud utterances (normalized units as in figure 1).

Clearly such a conclusion would be premature on the basis of the limited data available at present.

Covert speech

The majority of normal subjects showed for long sentences quite consistent departures from the non-speech tidal breathing pattern. Three normal subjects (N1, N2 and N4) showed highly significant differences between long and short sentences with respect to the ratio of inspiratory to expiratory duration. One normal subject (N3) showed no effect there but did show a highly significant difference in inspiratory *volume* for long vs. short sentences. (In addition, these four subjects all showed a highly significant effect of *delivery* with respect to inspiratory volume.) One normal subject (N5) showed no tendency whatsoever to depart from tidal breathing patterns during the covert speech tasks. He was remarkable for extremely fast completion of the tasks, even long-sentence stimuli often being terminated before the end of the inspiratory phase following the prompt.

The patient showed similar behaviour to this normal subject in showing negligible departure from tidal breathing in the covert speech tasks, but nonetheless differed markedly both from him as well from all other normal subjects in that long-sentence stimuli typically required more than one respiratory cycle for completion (whereas his *spoken* utterances were with very few exceptions produced on a single expiratory limb).

To round off this section the following speculation is offered: Covert speech normally requires activation of the complete speech motor system with subsequent inhibition of the articulatory and laryngeal subsystems to avoid actual sound generation. Due to a lower degree of subsystem integration in the apraxic speaker the respiratory system does not become activated at all.

CONCLUSIONS - OUTLOOK

Taking into account the fact that the current investigation is still at an exploratory stage the following conclusions can be advanced: (i) Combination of length and loudness variation appears to offer a promising framework for examining respiratory activity, with potential application to quite a wide range of speech disorders; (ii) Observation of respiratory activity in overt and covert speech may extend current knowledge on the organisation of mental motor activity and on the status of inner speech within speech production models. In further work, additional kinematic analysis of respiratory behaviour will be supplemented by more linguistically-oriented analysis of within-utterance inspirations and their relation to syntactic boundaries, repairs etc.

REFERENCES

Conrad, B., & Schönle, P. (1979). Speech and respiration. *Archives of Psychiatrische Nervenkrankheit*, *226*, 251-268.

Danly, M., & Shapiro, B. (1982). Speech Prosody in Broca's aphasia. *Brain and Language*, *16*, 171-190.

Grosjean, F., & Collins, M. (1979). Breathing, pausing and reading. *Phonetica*, *36*, 98-114.

Stathopoulos, E., & Sapienza, C. (1993). Respiratory and laryngeal function of women and men during vocal intensity variation. *Journal of Speech and Hearing Research*, *36*, 64-75

Winkworth, A., Davis, P., Ellis, E., & Adams, R. (1994). Variability and consistency in speech breathing during reading: lung volumes, speech intensity and linguistic factors. *Journal of Speech and Hearing Research*, *37*, 535-556.

Winkworth, A., Davis, P., Adams, R., & Ellis, E. (1995). Breathing patterns during spontaneous speech. *Journal of Speech and Hearing Research*, *38*, 124-144.

Speech Production: Motor Control, Brain Research and Fluency Disorders
W. Hulstijn, H.F.M. Peters and P.H.H.M. Van Lieshout, editors

Chapter 18

APPLICATIONS OF MOTOR LEARNING THEORY TO STUTTERING RESEARCH

Anthony J. Caruso, Ludo Max

Most individuals who stutter show a decrease in stuttering frequency during repeated readings of the same material (adaptation effect). There is little agreement, however, as to which theoretical explanation accounts best for the extant descriptive data with regard to this phenomenon. Results from a recent replication of a study by Frank & Bloodstein (1971) indicate that adaptation is primarily the result of repeated reading rather than repeated stuttering. It is hypothesized that the decrease in stuttering frequency during adaptation readings is an effect of *practice* of speech movements and may be considered a result of *motor learning*. Motor learning may prove to be a valuable theoretical framework to interpret changes in stuttering frequency during repeated readings or other conditions involving practice of articulatory/phonatory movements. In order to stimulate development of comprehensive models regarding the importance of this framework for stuttering, some neurobiological correlates of motor learning are briefly discussed.

INTRODUCTION

Numerous studies have shown that the speech of most individuals who stutter becomes remarkably more fluent under conditions such as delayed auditory feedback, masking noise, metronome-timed speech and unison reading. Consequently, investigators have attempted to document observable changes in the speech production of stuttering (e.g., Andrews et al., 1982) as well as nonstuttering individuals (e.g., Stager & Ludlow, 1993) under such fluency-enhancing conditions. An alternative, and for some fluency-enhancing conditions possibly more valuable, approach may be to focus on the question *why* changes occur in subjects' dysfluency levels under the given conditions. For example, most individuals who stutter show a gradual decrease in stuttering frequency during repeated readings of the same material (i.e., adaptation) but there is little agreement as to which theoretical explanation (e.g., Johnson et al., 1963; Wingate, 1986; Wischner, 1950) accounts best for the tremendous amount of empirical data regarding this phenomenon (see Bloodstein, 1995).

The lack of insight into factors underlying the decrease in stuttering frequency during repeated readings is particularly unfortunate in light of previous suggestions that "factors that help to explain the adaptation of stuttering could be important in understanding the nature of the disorder and its treatment" (Prins & Hubbard, 1990, p. 494). The purpose of this paper is to re-evaluate published findings and hypotheses regarding the adaptation effect in stuttering and to offer a new perspective based on a theoretical framework that is widely used to explain phenomena of nonspeech motor control and learning.

EFFECTS OF REPEATED READING ON SPEECH PRODUCTION IN INDIVIDUALS WHO STUTTER

One of the theoretically most important studies regarding the adaptation effect was reported by Frank and Bloodstein (1971). Briefly, those authors investigated whether the reduction in stuttering frequency during repeated readings is due to repeated *stuttering* or to repeated *reading*. A paradigm was used in which stuttering subjects performed six repeated readings (1) in a conventional adaptation series and (2) in a series of five unison readings followed by one independent reading. The results clearly indicated that stuttering frequency after five relatively fluent unison readings was similar to that after five conventional adaptation readings. Frank and Bloodstein (1971) concluded that adaptation does not require overt stuttering and that the effect is a result of "oral rehearsal of the motor plan" (p. 523).

To our knowledge, there have been no published replications of Frank and Bloodstein's (1971) work. Recently, the present authors replicated and extended this study (Max et al., in press). Eight male and two female adults who stutter, all native speakers of Dutch, performed repeated readings under two conditions. In Condition I, subjects performed six consecutive readings of the same text. Condition II consisted of ten consecutive readings of another text: the first five readings were performed in unison with the investigator, readings 6-10 were performed independently. Findings from this study were in agreement with those of Frank and Bloodstein (1971) and showed no statistically significant difference in stuttering frequency after five relatively fluent unison readings versus five more dysfluent independent readings

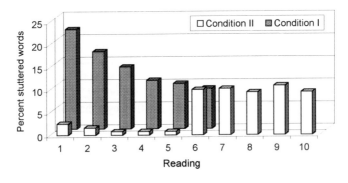

Figure 1. Mean percent stuttered words during repeated readings by 10 individuals who stutter in a conventional adaptation procedure (Condition I) and 5 unison readings followed by 5 independent readings (Condition II).

(Figure 1). Thus, despite the difference between the two conditions in stuttering frequency during the readings 1-5, stuttering frequency was similar in the sixth reading of both conditions. In addition, no significant increase in stuttering frequency was observed after the sixth reading in Condition II. These findings support the hypothesis that oral motor rehearsal is a major component underlying the adaptation effect. In particular, it was speculated that the decreased stuttering frequency observed during repeated readings is induced by repeated *practice* of the speech movements and may be considered a result of *motor learning* (Max et al., in press).

Although in need of further confirmation, the hypothesis that adaptation is primarily the result of practicing a set of articulatory and phonatory motor sequences may explain various previously reported findings regarding the adaptation effect. For example, it has been found that adaptation either does not occur (Peins, 1961; Robbins, 1971) or occurs to a lesser degree (Besozzi & Adams, 1969; Moss, 1976) during silent rehearsal without oral movements. Moreover, with the exception of findings obtained by Robbins (1971), investigations have also shown a reduced amount of adaptation during repeated readings with silently performed speech movements (Moss, 1976) or when whispered speech is used (Bruce & Adams, 1978; Moss, 1976). Also noteworthy, although not obtained in an adaptation paradigm, are results reported by Brenner et al. (1972). Those authors asked individuals who stutter to recite individual sentences from memory after silent rehearsal, silent rehearsal with lip movements, whispered rehearsal or speech motor rehearsal. Their results showed that only speech motor rehearsal resulted in a significant decrease in stuttering frequency. In conclusion, the present authors speculate that the ineffectiveness of silent and whispered speech in eliciting the adaptation effect may be due to the fact that these conditions are associated with a distinct reduction in the complex spatiotemporal organization of the supralaryngeal and laryngeal movements involved in speech. As such, practice of a simplified speech pattern may not result in improved performance when more complex coordination of articulatory and phonatory movements is required.

A classic study by Crossman (1959) on nonspeech motor learning is frequently cited as evidence that increased motor skill for a certain task is often associated with increased speed of performance. This observation has been confirmed for practice of nonspeech movements around single (e.g., Gottlieb et al., 1988) as well as multiple joints (e.g., Shea & Morgan, 1979). Preliminary results from an acoustic study currently in progress in our own laboratory show similar changes in the speech production of stuttering individuals during six repeated readings of the same material. In particular, all seven subjects whose speech has been analyzed so far, increased speed of performance (i.e., decreased word duration) for fluently produced words in reading 6 versus reading 1. It should be emphasized that for these analyses only words were selected that were produced fluently in *both* the first and the sixth reading and that measures of word duration were used to obtain information regarding articulation rate. This procedure eliminates the confounding effects of instances of dysfluency as well as within-sentence pause duration. Thus, these acoustic analyses seem to provide further support for the hypothesis that improved motor performance, due to practice, may explain the beneficial effects of repeated readings on the speech of individuals who stutter.

CHANGES IN MOTOR PERFORMANCE AS INDICATIONS OF MOTOR LEARNING

It is well documented in the nonspeech literature that not all improvements in motor *performance* are indicative of motor *learning*. Changes in motor performance may occur as mere temporary effects of factors such as fatigue or motivation. Motor learning, on the other hand, requires the occurrence of relatively permanent changes in subjects' motor performance as a result of repeated practice (Schmidt, 1988). A widely-used criterion to distinguish between temporary changes in motor performance and relatively permanent changes indicative of motor learning is to observe subjects' behavior during a *retention* test after a sufficiently long rest interval has been provided to allow temporary effects to dissipate (Schmidt, 1988).

At first glance, application of this criterion to the stuttering literature might seem to argue against an interpretation of the adaptation effect as a result of motor learning. Bloodstein (1995), for example, claims that complete "spontaneous recovery" occurs within a few hours after the repeated readings. This conclusion seems to be based on several studies reporting a significant increase in stuttering frequency from the last reading in an adaptation series to the first reading after a subsequent rest interval. However, a closer look at the results from these studies (Max et al., in press) reveals that, although stuttering frequency does indeed increase after a rest interval, this increase rarely results in dysfluency levels similar to those observed during the subjects' *first* reading in the adaptation series (i.e., spontaneous recovery was incomplete). Hence, the decreased stuttering frequency during subjects' repeated readings can be described as at least *relatively* permanent. In fact, this observation argues for a fairly strong *learning* effect considering that speech movements, as compared with the novel nonspeech tasks typically used in motor learning research, may be expected to be more susceptible to *interference* by competing (dysfluent) motor responses that have been learned prior to the practice trials. Indeed, most adult stuttering subjects have been using (i.e., "practicing") dysfluent speech patterns since childhood, and it has been previously suggested that "Whatever pattern of activity is practiced is the pattern that will be developed. [...] volitional excitation causes that pattern to occur in the manner in which it has been practiced" (Kottke et al., 1978, p. 569). Therefore, long-term changes in stuttering frequency are unlikely to result from the minimal amount of practice (see Kottke et al., 1978) provided by five or six adaptation readings.

NEUROBIOLOGICAL CORRELATES OF MOTOR LEARNING

Although various neural centers are important in speech production, the cerebellum is thought to be associated with the timing of highly skilled volitional acts as well as have a major role in motor learning. Through its role in movement timing, the cerebellum may be involved in the speech timing problems underlying stuttering (Wu et al., 1995). Regardless of whether or not this hypothesis is correct, the reviewed data regarding stuttering adaptation suggest that individuals who stutter show at least some degree of motor learning during repeated readings. Thus, understanding the role of the cerebellum in motor learning seems necessary in order to develop comprehensive models regarding the importance of motor learning for the reduction of stuttering.

Based on ideas first formulated by Marr (1969) and Albus (1971), current theories regarding the neurobiological basis of motor learning propose that the cerebellum constitutes the primary neuroanatomical substrate for motor skill acquisition and refinement (e.g., Ghez, 1991). Obviously, the cerebellar circuitry is by no means the *only* neural mechanism involved in motor learning. Mechanisms for motor learning have also been situated in, for example, basal ganglia (e.g., Rolls, 1994) and motor cortex (e.g., Kimura et al., 1994). Nevertheless, recent neurobiological accounts of motor learning have emphasized the role of cerebellar plasticity in this process. According to the most widely accepted theory, the cerebellum acts as a comparator which compensates for movement error by continuously comparing performance with intention (e.g., Ghez, 1991). The cerebellum is able to fulfill this function through a combination of specific connections: (1) the cerebellum receives information about movement *plans* (i.e., internal feedback) from those brain structures concerned with movement programming and execution, (2) it receives peripheral sensory feedback about the actual motor *performance* (i.e., external feedback) during the course of the movements, and (3) its output projects to the direct motor pathways originating in the motor and premotor areas of the cerebral cortex. The cerebellum is thought to use this internal and external feedback for *on-line* adjustments of ongoing movements as well as for modifications in *future* performance of these movements.

Cerebellar involvement in the optimization of future performances of a given movement is possible through the capacity of inputs to the cerebellum to modify cerebellar circuits for long periods of time (i.e., long-term depression or LTD), allowing "storage" of movement-related information. The sites for cerebellar LTD are the synapses from parallel fibers onto Purkinje cell dendrites. The main hypothesis of cerebellar models of motor learning is that the strength of parallel fiber synapses onto Purkinje cells is modified through the firing of climbing fibers, which also synapse onto Purkinje cells, during the period of movement adjustments (Gilbert & Thach, 1977). In essence, the LTD permits increased firing from the cerebellar nuclei to the motor cortex thus facilitating motor learning.

CONCLUSION

If confirmed by future research, *motor learning* may prove to be a valuable theoretical framework to interpret changes in stuttering frequency during repeated readings or other conditions involving practice of speech movements. The present authors wish to encourage investigators in the area of stuttering to develop research designs which include practice conditions followed by retention tests to differentiate between temporary changes in speech performance versus relatively permanent changes indicative of speech motor learning. Several suggestions for future research regarding the role of motor learning in the reduction of stuttering have been made elsewhere (Max et al., in press).

REFERENCES

Albus, J.S. (1971). A theory of cerebellar function. *Mathematical Biosciences, 10,* 25-61.

Andrews, G., Howie, P., Dozsa, M., & Guitar, B. (1982). Stuttering: speech pattern characteristics under fluency-inducing conditions. *Journal of Speech and Hearing Research, 25,* 208-216.

Besozzi, T.E., & Adams, M.R. (1969). The influence of prosody on stuttering adaptation. *Journal of Speech and Hearing Research, 12,* 818-824.

Bloodstein, O. (1995). *A handbook on stuttering* (5th ed.). San Diego, CA: Singular Publishing Group.

Brenner, N.C., Perkins, W.H., & Soderberg, G.A. (1972). The effect of rehearsal on frequency of stuttering. *Journal of Speech and Hearing Research, 15,* 483-486.

Bruce, M.C., & Adams, M.R. (1978). Effects of two types of motor practice on stuttering adaptation. *Journal of Speech and Hearing Research, 21,* 421-428.

Crossman, E.R.F.W. (1959). A theory of the acquisition of speed-skill. *Ergonomics, 2,* 153-166.

Frank, A., & Bloodstein, O. (1971). Frequency of stuttering following repeated unison readings. *Journal of Speech and Hearing Research, 14,* 519-524.

Ghez, C. (1991). The cerebellum. In E.R. Kandel, J.H. Schwartz & T.M. Jessell (Eds.), *Principles of neural science* (pp. 626-646). Norwalk, CT: Appleton & Lange.

Gilbert, P.F.C., & Thach, W.T. (1977). Purkinje cell activity during motor learning. *Brain Research, 128,* 309-328.

Gottlieb, G.L., Corcos, D.M., Jaric, S., & Agarwal, G.C. (1988). Practice improves even the simplest movements. *Experimental Brain Research, 73,* 436-440.

Johnson, W., Darley, F.L., & Spriestersbach, D.C. (1963). *Diagnostic methods in speech pathology.* New York: Harper & Row.

Kimura, A., Caria, M.A., Melis, F., & Asanuma, H. (1994). Long-term potentiation within the cat motor cortex. *NeuroReport, 5,* 2372-2376.

Kottke, F.J., Halpern, D., Easton, J.K.M., Ozel, A.T., & Burrill, C.A. (1978). The training of coordination. *Archives of Physical Medicine and Rehabilitation, 59,* 567-572.

Marr, D. (1969). A theory of cerebellar cortex. *Journal of Physiology (London), 202,* 437-470.

Max, L., Caruso, A.J., & Vandevenne, A. (in press). Decreased stuttering frequency during repeated readings: a motor learning perspective. *Journal of Fluency Disorders.*

Moss, S.E. (1976). The influence of varying degrees of voicing on the adaptation effect in the repeated oral readings of stutterers. *Australian Journal of Human Communication Disorders, 4,* 127-132.

Peins, M. (1961). Adaptation effect and spontaneous recovery in stuttering expectancy. *Journal of Speech and Hearing Research, 4,* 91-99.

Prins, D., & Hubbard, C.P. (1990). Acoustical durations of speech segments during stuttering adaptation. *Journal of Speech and Hearing Research, 33,* 494-504.

Robbins, M.G. (1971). The effect of varying conditions of rehearsal on the frequency of stuttering. *Dissertation Abstracts International, 32B-6,* 3692

Rolls, E.T. (1994). Neurophysiology and cognitive functions of the striatum. *Revue Neurologique, 150,* 648-660.

Schmidt, R.A. (1988). *Motor control and learning.* Champaign,IL: Human Kinetics Publishers.

Shea, J.B., & Morgan, R.L. (1979). Contextual interference effects on the acquisition, retention, and transfer of a motor skill. *Journal of Experimental Psychology: Human Learning and Memory, 5,*

179-187.

Stager, S., & Ludlow, C.L. (1993). Speech production changes under fluency-evoking conditions in nonstuttering speakers. *Journal of Speech and Hearing Research, 36,* 245-253.

Wingate, M.E. (1986). Adaptation, consistency and beyond: II. An integral account. *Journal of Fluency Disorders, 11,* 37-53.

Wu, J.C., Maguire, G., Riley, G., Fallon, J., LaCasse, L., Chin, S., Klein, E., Tang, C., Cadwell, S., & Lottenberg, S. (1995). A positron emission tomography [18F] deoxyglucose study of developmental stuttering. *NeuroReport, 6,* 501-505.

1997 Elsevier Science B.V.
Speech Production: Motor Control, Brain Research and Fluency Disorders
W. Hulstijn, H.F.M. Peters and P.H.H.M. Van Lieshout, editors

Chapter 19

SPEECH PRODUCTION LEARNING IN ADULTS WITH CHRONIC DEVELOPMENTAL STUTTERING

Christy L. Ludlow, Kathleen Siren, Mary Zikria

Speech learning for novel pseudowords was compared in adults who stutter and control subjects. Subjects performed 11 test recall trials which were interspersed with modeling practice trials for two novel pseudowords associated with meaningless idiographs. The number of phonemes correctly achieved on each of the 11 test trials were scored by the same listener. The adults who stuttered were impaired in their rate of learning as well as the overall accuracy of their word productions. The results suggest that the speech production learning is less efficient in those affected by chronic stuttering and may contribute to their less efficient and unstable speech production capabilities throughout adult life.

INTRODUCTION

Several characteristics are novel to stuttering in comparison with other speech and language disorders. Stuttering only occurs when the speaker must encode speech to convey language meaning. Thus dysfluency is difficult to study in the laboratory in contrast with other speech disorders such as phonological disorders and dysarthria. In these latter disorders, single words or nonsense syllables can be used to test a subject's speech errors in a way that is representative of symptom characteristics during spontaneous speech. Such approaches cannot be used in stuttering because symptoms only occur when meaningful language information must be conveyed to listeners. However, this is not to say that those who stutter have language processing disorders (Nippold, 1990). Rather, it is the *interface* between language formulation and speech production that engenders stuttering symptoms, not either task alone.

As reviewed recently by Bernstein Ratner (Bernstein Ratner, 1997), increases in language and speech production processing demands render persons who stutter more prone to symptom production during speech containing: more complex utterances (Bernstein Ratner & Sih, 1987), less familiar words (Hubbard & Prins, 1994), open class content words (Johnson & Brown, 1935; Brown, 1838), or words containing longer more complex phonological sequences (Brown, 1945; Taylor, 1966; Soderberg, 1967; Soderberg, 1966; Silverman, 1972). The neurobiology of the speech/language production system in those who stutter renders it more fragile and susceptible to disruption, particularly when the complexity of language processing increases.

Speech dysfluency often appears during the period of rapid speech and language development, between 30 and 42 months of age (Yairi & Ambrose, 1992a; Yairi & Ambrose, 1992b). In most young children this seems to represent a period of instability in the evolution of an efficient speech and language system. This period of developmental stuttering is transient in most children to varying degrees (Yairi & Ambrose, 1992b). In some, the instability is momentary as the child's developing speech/language system continues to evolve due to developmental neuroplasticity. Limited information is available on the processes which underlie the development of an efficient speech and language production system. Possibly those processes that are essential in the development of speech/language production are no longer operative in adults. In adults who continue to stutter, however, the emergence of an efficient speech/language processing system has not occurred within the critical period of speech/language development. The evolution of an efficient speech/language processing system may have been disrupted due to impairment in processes essential to developing fluent speech production.

We hypothesized that one component in the development of an efficient speech/language processing system may be the ability to learn to produce new phonological patterns as words. This may involve the interface of speech motor control systems and language phonology in establishing new production patterns. To examine whether some of the processes which are involved in the establishment of an efficient speech/language production system may be affected in those with chronic stuttering, we examined the ability of adults who stutter to learn to produce new words. Because we did not want to study their perception of new speech sounds, but rather the development of new speech sound production patterns, we examined subjects' abilities to learn novel combinations of English sounds in words associated with novel idiographic symbols.

METHODS

Subjects

The study involved 7 controls (4 females and 3 males) and 5 males who stuttered. All were adults with normal language skills and gainfully employed. All subjects had a normal medical history and physical examinations by a physician. All subjects who stuttered were videotaped during spontaneous conversation and paragraph reading. The videotapes were scored later by a speech pathologist on the Stuttering Severity Instrument -3 (SSI) (Riley, 1994).

After reading and signing the informed consent, the subjects were told that this was a study of their ability to learn to produce new words. An Articulograph AG100 with 5 transducers was placed on each subject before beginning the study, although these data will not be reported here. Miniature transducers were applied to the tongue blade, tongue tip, lower incisors and the upper and lower lips in the midline.

Tasks

Two novel speech "words" each involving 11 English phonemes in 4 syllables were used, "abisthwoychleet" /abɪsθwɔ͞ɪtʃlit   / and "eepashfwujbok" /ipæʃfwudʒbok   /. Both "words" began with a VCV cluster containing a stop consonant. The third and fourth syllables included consonant clusters; involving lingual and labial stops, fricatives, liquids and glides. Subjects first listened to an audio recording of the first word while being presented with a written transcription and an idiograph for that word. They repeated the word twice during the first two modeling trials. The same procedure was then used for the second word. A distraction task required that the subject listen to the examiner read a paragraph of approximately 200 words and then answer 2 or 3 questions on its content. The distraction task was followed by a test trial for the first word when only the idiograph was presented and the subject was asked to say the "word" for that symbol. This was followed by two modeling trials for the first word. The test trial and modeling trials for the second word were then presented. The sequence of distraction task, test trial for the first word and 2 modeling trials, the test trial for the second word and 2 modeling trials for the second word, was repeated 8 times. Finally, two test trials for each word were alternated when the symbols were presented. This sequence resulted in 11 test trials for each of the two words. The order of the two words presented was alternated across subjects. Subjects were allowed 10 seconds to respond between trials, if more time was required, the tape was stopped unless the subject indicated that they forgot the word entirely and wanted to proceed.

One of the experimenters (KS) transcribed each of the subjects' productions phonetically from audio tape. The proportion of phonemes produced correctly out of the 8 phonemes contained in the third and fourth syllables, was the measure of speech learning. Errors due to stuttering were not deducted in the scoring. That is, if a subject produced syllable repetitions or vowel prolongations or had a severe block, the subject was given credit based on his ability to produce each of the sounds in the correct order. Stuttering occurred usually only on the early training and test trials.

RESULTS

Group Learning Score Comparisons

To determine if the groups differed in their speed and learning accuracy, repeated MANOVAs were conducted for each of the two words to examine the repeated effects of test trials on speech production accuracy along with group effects, and factor interactions (Table 1). Because the same analysis was conducted twice, a .025 probability was used as criterion for statistical significance.

For "abisthwoychleet", group effects were not statistically significant, trial effects were significant across groups ($p \le .0005$) and there was a significant trial by group interaction ($p = .016$). The controls were accurate by the fourth trial averaging .8 of the phonemes correct while the subjects who stuttered averaged .56 of the phonemes correct for the remainder of the study (Figure 1). For the word "epashfwujbok", group effects were statistically significant

Table 1. Results of repeated MANOVAs examining the effects of group, learning trial (repeated), and learning trial by group interactions on the accuracy of speech production for each word.

For "abisthwoychleet"	df	F ratio	p value
Between Subjects			
Group	1	1.550	.245
Within Subjects			
Learning Trial	10	7.304	$\leq$.0005
Trial * Group	10	2.360	.016
For "epashfwujbok"	df	F ratio	p value
Between Subjects			
Group	1	7.337	.024
Within Subjects			
Learning Trial	10	6.753	$\leq$.0005
Trial * Group	10	1.766	.078

(p=.024), trial effects were significant across groups (p≤ .0005) and there was not a significant trial by group interaction (p=.078). (Table 1). When individual results were evaluated, all of the normal subjects reached .80 proportion accuracy. None of the adults who stuttered reached this level of accuracy on the word "epashfwujbok" (Figure 2).

Group Learning Characteristics

The learning characteristics of the two subject groups were also contrasted. No significant word differences were found in either group.

The ability to learn each of the phonemes in the two words was also evaluated to determine

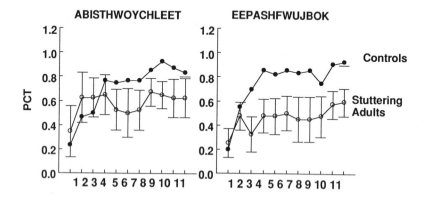

Figure 1. Mean proportion of phonemes produced accurately in the third and fourth syllables for both the adults who stuttered (open circles) and the control subjects (filled circles) on each learning trial. The horizontal bars are the standard errors for each group.

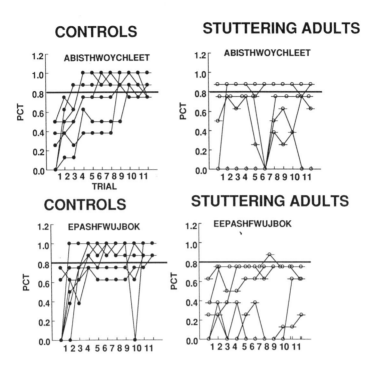

Figure 2. The proportion of phonemes produced accurately in the third and fourth syllables on each test trial for both the adults who stuttered, in the right hand graphs, and the control subjects, in the left hand graphs. The top two graphs are for the pseudoword "abisthwoychleet", the two bottom graphs are for the pseudoword "epashfwujbok".

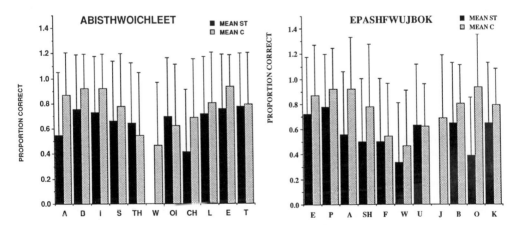

Figure 3. The group means and standard deviations for each phoneme in each word across all 11 test trials.

if subjects in the two groups differed in their speech learning patterns (Figure 3).

Repeated MANOVAs were conducted for each word to examine the repeated effects of phonemes on speech production accuracy along with group effects, and within subject phoneme effects and group by phoneme interactions (Table 2). Because the same analysis was conducted twice, a .025 probability was used as criterion for statistical significance. For "abisthwoychleet", group effects were not statistically significant, phoneme effects were significant across groups (p ≤ .0005) and there was not a significant phoneme by group interaction (p=.260). For the word "epashfwujbok", group effects were statistically significant (p=.02), phoneme effects were significant across groups (p ≤ .0005) but there was no significant phoneme by group interaction (p=.970). (Table 2).

None of the subjects who stuttered had any correct productions of the "w" in "abisthwoychleet" and on the "j" in "epashfwujbok" and the adults who stuttered were reduced in comparison with the controls on "o" in "epashfwujbok" (Figure 3).

Relationship Between Speech Learning and Stuttering Severity

To relate the subjects' abilities on the speech learning task with symptom severity, the SSI scores were used to rank order the subjects. The relationship between stuttering severity and subjects' total accuracy score on the speech learning task on each of the two words was examined (Figure 4). The resulting Pearson Correlation Coefficient was not statistically significant (r= -.447, p=.195).

Two of the subjects who stuttered were entirely unable to learn the two words with any approximation. One subject with an SSI of 38, was unable to produce the words reliably by the end of the study. Therefore, the entire study was repeated to determine how many trials he needed but he was unsuccessful even with an additional 22 training and 11 test trials for

Table 2. Results of repeated MANOVAs examining the effects of group, phoneme type (repeated), and group by phoneme interactions on the accuracy of speech production for each word.

For "abisthwoychleet"			
Between Subjects	df	F ratio	p value
Group	1	0.917	.363
Within Subjects			
Phoneme Type	7	6.620	≤ .0005
Phoneme * Group	7	1.311	.260
For "epashfwujbok"			
Between Subjects	df	F ratio	p value
Group	1	8.341	.020
Within Subjects			
Phoneme Type	7	5.416	≤ .0005
Phoneme * Group	7	0.252	.970

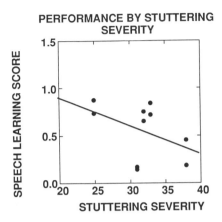

Figure 4. The relationship between the Stuttering Severity Index scores in each of the 5 adults who stuttered and their total speech production accuracy on all test trials for each word.

each word. Another stuttering subject, with an SSI of 31, was unable to learn "epashfwujbok" and continued to produce parts of "abisthwoychleet" in response to the "epashfwujbok" symbol, although the symbols and training trials were presented correctly. Although the least affected adult who stuttered (SSI =25) learned to approximate the words quickly, he never produced them accurately. He consistently omitted at least one sound in each word and seemed unaware of his errors. None of the adults who stuttered achieved the normal level of accuracy ($\geq$.80) on the word, "epashfwujbok".

DISCUSSION

This was only a preliminary study of the question of whether learning to produce phonological combinations for new words might be affected in adults who stutter in comparison with controls who had no history of childhood stuttering based on self report. The perceptual scoring of subjects' learning of new phonological sequences suggested that they were both slower to learn new sequences and less accurate overall. Even the least affected adult who stuttered, made errors although he seemed unaware of them. We did not test the subjects' accuracy in perception by having them transcribe the words. This we plan to do when we replicate the study with a larger cohort.

In addition, we collected movement data on the tongue, lip and jaw in both groups using the Articulograph. Although these data have not yet been formally analyzed, they do suggest that the normal subjects progressively differentiated their movement patterns as they learned the words (Siren et al., 1996). That is, they started out with a gross movement pattern and gradually added more detailed movement for particular sounds within the pattern.

We plan to examine the movement changes in both groups to determine if the adults who stutter follow the same trends.

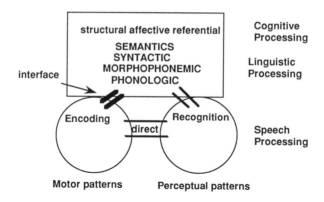

Figure 5. A proposed model illustrating the independence of the direct connections between speech production and speech perceptual processing independent from the linguistic and cognitive processing systems. The interface between linguistic and cognitive processing systems and the speech production system is labeled as the point of disruption in stuttering.

The results suggest that chronically affected adults who stutter have difficulty learning new sequences of speech sounds in comparison with unaffected controls. None of the adults who stuttered had language processing deficits that interfered with their everyday language functioning. Thus, the word learning difficulties may be a residual of impairment in some processes that play a role in the development of a fluent speech production system for expressin g language.

None of the pseudo words used in this experiment were assigned any significant meaning of either referential or emotional significance. They were only tied with a meaningless idiographic symbol. Therefore it is not surprising that very little stuttering behavior was elicited during the testing situation. This was likely because the pseudo words had no meaning to the subjects and therefore would not have communicative or language content. In spite of this, however, the subjects who stuttered had greater difficulty than normal in learning to produce these new phonological patterns.

What then do these results suggest about the interface among speech and language processes and which aspects of this interface may be affected in adults who stutter and during their speech development? A model is proposed in Figure 5. This suggests that speech processing per se and speech perception per se may not be affected in those who stutter rather only their interface with language and cognitive processing. One of the aspects of stuttering that is most salient is the ability to be fluent during choral reading. During choral reading subjects can repeat others' speech without language processing. Thus they need only process the "surface" components of the graphic to phonologic translation process. Only the direct link between speech production and speech perception processing is employed and no interface with language or cognition is required.

Transcortical sensory aphasia also suggests a direct link between speech production and speech perception processes independent from linguistic and cognitive processing. These aphasic patients can repeat because the speech production and speech perception systems and their direct link are spared. Linguistic and cognitive processes are severely affected in this form of aphasia due to diffuse brain injury, while Broca's area, the arcuate fasciculus and the temporal lobe functioning seem unaffected (Goodglass & Kaplan, 1972).

The separability of speech production and perception processing from linguistic and cognitive processing is suggested by both transcortical sensory aphasia and stuttering. In stuttering both the speech production and speech perception and the central linguistic and cognitive processing systems are intact and functioning normally. Rather the interconnections between the input-output speech system and semantic and cognitive processing seem less efficient in those who stutter. Our results suggest that phonological word learning may have proceeded differently in those with persistent stuttering into adulthood rendering their ability to produce fluent speech for language expression inefficient and unstable.

ACKNOWLEDGMENTS

The authors wish to thank Ms. Lucila San José and Dr. Geralyn Schulz for assistance with data collection and processing and Dr. Paul Smith for statistical advice.

REFERENCES

Bernstein Ratner, N. (1997). Stuttering: A psycholinguistic perspective. In: R. Curlee & G. Siegel, (Eds.) *Nature and treatment of stuttering: New directions* 2nd Ed. Boston,MA: Allyn and Bacon.

Bernstein Ratner, N., & Sih, C.C. (1987). Effects of gradual increases in sentence length and complexity in children's disfluency. *Journal of Speech and Hearing Disorders*, *52*, 278-287.

Brown, S.F. (1838). Stuttering with relation to word accent and word position. *Journal of Abnormal and Social Psychology*, *33*, 112-120.

Brown, S.F. (1945). The loci of stutterings in the speech sequence. *The Journal of Speech Disorders*, *10*, 181-192.

Goodglass, H., & Kaplan, E. (1972). *The Assessment of Aphasia and Related Disorders*. Philadelphia: Lea and Febiger.

Hubbard, C.P., & Prins, D. (1994). Word familiarity, syllabic sttress pattern, and stuttering. *Journal of Speech and Hearing Research*, *37*, 564-571.

Johnson, W., & Brown, S. (1935). Stuttering in relation to various speech sounds. *Quarterly Journal of Speech*, *21*, 481-496.

Nippold, M.A. (1990). Concomitant speech and language disorders in stuttering children: A critique of the literature. *Journal of Speech and Hearing Disorders*, *55*, 51-60.

Riley, G.D. (1994). *Stuttering Severity Instrument for Children and Adults*. 3rd Ed. Austin, TX: Pro-Ed.

Silverman, F.H. (1972). Disfluency and word length. *Journal of Speech and Hearing Research*, *15*, 788-791.

Siren, K.A., Zikria, M., & Ludlow, C.L. (1996). *Speech motor learning: Movement and perceptual analyses*. Amelia Island, FLA: Paper presented at the Speech Motor Control Conference. (UnPub)

Soderberg, G.A. (1966). The relations of stuttering to word length and word frequency. *Journal of Speech and Hearing Research, 9,* 584-589.

Soderberg, G.A. (1967). Linguistic factors in stuttering. *Journal of Speech and Hearing Research, 10,* 801-810.

Taylor, I.K. (1966). What words are stuttered? *Psychological Bulletin, 65,* 233-242.

Yairi, E., & Ambrose, N. (1992a). Onset of stuttering in preschool children: selected factors. *Journal of Speech and Hearing Research, 35,* 782-788.

Yairi, E., & Ambrose, N. (1992b). A longitudinal study of stuttering in children: a preliminary report. *Journal of Speech and Hearing Research, 35,* 755-760.

Brain research in speech production and fluency disorders

Speech Production: Motor Control, Brain Research and Fluency Disorders
W. Hulstijn, H.F.M. Peters and P.H.H.M. Van Lieshout, editors

Chapter 20

NONINVASIVE BRAIN IMAGING IN SPEECH MOTOR CONTROL AND STUTTERING: CHOICES AND CHALLENGES

Judith L. Lauter

A thousand questions regarding the neural foundations of human speech production and its disorders present challenges to researchers, therapists, and clients alike. Over the past decade, new techniques have become available which allow us to begin to answer those questions -- simply because their *noninvasive* nature now makes it possible to look *inside* the living, behaving human brain. Techniques such as computerized tomography (CT) and magnetic resonance imaging (MRI) provide new "windows" on brain structure, while evoked potentials (EPs), quantitative electroencephalography (qEEG), magnetoencephalography (MEG), single-photon emission computed tomography (SPECT), positron emission tomography (PET), and functional MRI (fMRI) render brain function in a variety of complementary ways. In addition, the *spatial and temporal resolution* of these new methods provide unique means for quantifying the exquisite, "fingerprint" detail of individual brains, assessed either in a resting state or during activation. As we learn to make use of the complementarity of the new techniques, and interpret the richness of detail in dynamic brain/behavior relations observed at the individual level, we can expect new insights into the *repertoire* of ways in which human brain structure and function are reflected in behaviors such as speech production. This should lead to basic revisions of our concepts of normality and dysfunction, and have revolutionary implications for more sensitive diagnostics, customized therapy, and individualized outcome assessment.

INTRODUCTION

In 1891, in his book *Zur Auffassung der Aphasien,* Sigmund Freud reviewed contemporary views on the neurological aspects of speech production, and concluded that the neural organization underlying human speech was of a "complexity beyond comprehension" (quoted in Finger, 1994). In the one hundred years since this despairing comment was written, very little has changed regarding the degree to which the neural correlates for speech are understood -- largely because during most of that time, the means of access to brain/behavior correlates in humans have remained virtually the same as they were in the 19th century.

During just the last decade, an array of *noninvasive* methods for assessing both structure and function in the human brain, have come to maturity. Together they offer remarkable advances in means for visualizing both anatomy and physiology in living brains. The techniques are so new in fact that researchers are still in the process of discovering how best to make use of their powers of spatial and temporal resolution -- providing unprecedented access to healthy as well as disordered brains, for observing brains under resting and activation conditions, and most of them appropriate for use in subjects of all ages. Thus on the centenary anniversary of Freud's book on aphasia, students of human speech found themselves on the threshold of finally being able to begin to untangle the complexity of its neural organization.

This chapter will provide a brief introduction to the noninvasive methods for "human neuroscience" which are available as of the last decade of the 20th century, with one or more examples for each illustrating the possibilities for its application to the study of human speech motor behavior and fluency disorders. Space constraints will restrict us to research reported only during the first half of the "Decade of the Brain;" additional details regarding each method along with more comprehensive reviews of related research are provided in three companion chapters: 1) a more comprehensive introductory tutorial to the methods (Lauter, in Press); 2) a review of applications of brain imaging to a broader spectrum of issues in speech and language (Lauter, 1995); and 3) an overview of similar applications in human hearing and vestibular function (Lauter, in Press).

BRAIN ANATOMY

Overview of methods

Details of brain structure may be imaged with two techniques, computerized tomography (CT) and magnetic resonance imaging (MRI). CT makes use of X-rays to image the brain, and thus involves the risks associated with radiation; in contrast, MRI depends on manipulated magnetic fields and radio-frequency pulses, neither of which is considered to pose any health hazard. As a result, CT is generally restricted to use in patients, while MRI has enjoyed a wide range of applications in healthy as well as disordered humans, ranging in age from neonates to the elderly. The underlying physics of the two techniques also accounts for the fact that they provide *complementary* anatomical views: the X-ray basis of CT makes it most sensitive to hard tissues, such as bone, while the basis of MRI -- which is actually a version of chemical spectroscopy, in this case analyzing the distribution of protons (hydrogen atoms) -- makes it most sensitive to distinctions in soft tissues, such as contrasts among grey matter, white matter, cerebrospinal fluid, and abnormal states of neural tissue associated with injury or disease.

As both methods are currently used, they can render images in the form of slices ("tomography" from Greek *tomos*, "slice"), in quasi-relief surface renderings, or as three-dimensional arrays which can be computer-manipulated in space as though turning an actual brain. CT and MRI can be used to image any part of the body including the central nervous system (CNS). For brain imaging, all levels are revealed, from brainstem into the cortex. MRI's resolution of 1 mm is fine enough to enable visualization of individual cranial nerves and identification of subcortical structures related to speech motor control, such as the basal ganglia and brainstem nuclei.

Computerized tomography (CT)

The X-radiation involved in CT dictates that it is used primarily in patients, for whom the procedure can be very important. While we will see that MRI has generally superseded CT in terms of flexibility and resolution, CT is still utilized for brain imaging in many centers, even those in which MRI is also available.

With regard to imaging related to speech motor control disorders, CT was employed in some of the pioneering imaging studies of the 1980s, for example the research by the Callier group on spasmodic dysphonia (Finitzo et al., 1987), and in many papers reporting correlations between the appearance of brain insults as shown by CT and behavioral deficits such as aphasia (Lauter, 1995). However, for the purposes of this overview, we will focus on MRI as a tool for studies of the neuroanatomical correlates of speech motor control.

Magnetic resonance imaging (MRI)

The physics of MRI does not require that the subject be exposed to any type of radiation, either from external sources (as in CT), or from internal ones (such as are required for methods such as SPECT and PET). For scanning, the individual is placed within a strong, controlled magnetic field which acts to align atoms in body tissues. Then radiofrequency pulses are employed to tip the atoms off their aligned axes of spin, and as they return to their original orientation, they give off a "resonance" which can be detected as a signal. The nature of the resonance depends on several factors, including the atom, the tissue in which it is located, the nature of the radio pulse, and other testing parameters. The beautiful "anatomical" images which can be produced with MR are actually chemical plots of the distribution of hydrogen atoms captured within different body tissues; scanning parameters can be manipulated to highlight different contrasts between the tissues. Thus for example, a tumor can appear and disappear in the images, depending on how the scanning is done.

Although subjects are not exposed to radiation for MR, there are two aspects of the testing which must be considered to present a certain amount of "invasivity." First, current MR scanners require the patient to be totally enclosed within a whole-body cylinder. This evokes claustrophobia in many individuals, and potential anxiety reactions must be counselled for, along with suggestions for strategies for adjusting to the threatening situation. Second, during testing there is a loud series of sounds, which are the perceptual expression of the radiofrequency pulses. Clients must also be prepared for this component of the exam, which can exacerbate the feelings of anxiety.

MRI has enjoyed most use in imaging the anatomical signs of frank neurological disorders, such as stroke, tumor, and results of traumatic injury, including instances of these related to problems with speech motor control. However, it can also reveal striking abnormalities which may be due to developmental causes. For instance, Boey and colleagues (Boey et al., 1995) reported a case of a 22-month-old child with the only presenting symptoms those of a history of congenital stridor and dyspnea, subsequently managed with

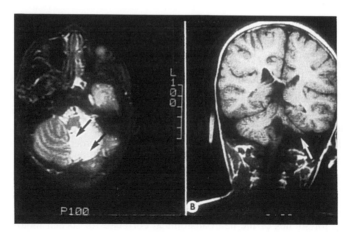

Figure 1. MRI scans of a child originally diagnosed with severe laryngomalacia, who was found on examination to have a marked underdevelopment in the left cerebellum. Areas of deficit are marked with arrows in the axial (left panel) and coronal (right panel) planes. (Reprinted with permission from Boey et al., 1995.)

tracheotomy. Although the child's condition had originally been diagnosed as severe laryngomalacia, fiberoptic laryngeal examination by the reporting authors revealed *bilateral paralysis of the true vocal folds,* resulting in a very narrow glottal aperture. Although developmental milestones for the child were reported to be normal, a magnetic resonance imaging scan revealed "impressively abnormal findings" consisting of marked hypoplasia of the *left cerebellum* (Figure 1). Other portions of the child's CNS as imaged with MRI appeared to be normal. The authors emphasized that the case illustrated the need for a comprehensive CNS workup in children with vocal cord paralysis, even in the absence of other neurological signs.

MRI may also prove useful for identifing neuroanatomical correlates of developmental contributions to different types of speech disorders, including dysfluencies. While some researchers have reported anatomically normal brains viewed with MRI in individuals with a history of stuttering (e.g., Watson et al., 1991, Ingham et al., 1995), it should be noted that in these studies, the criteria for normality were based on guidelines developed in clinical neurology. A focus on finer details than those required to identify frank neural lesions may be more relevant.

For example, measures of cerebral asymmetries developed for assessing neural correlates of disorders such as dyslexia (Galaburda et al., 1990, Schultz et al., 1994) and Specific Language Impairment (SLI -- Plante et al., 1991) may also be useful in studies of developmental stuttering. MRI in combination with several other tests in the Coordinated Noninvasive Studies (CNS) Project (Lauter, 1990) was used to evaluate an adult male with a history of stuttering. The MRI protocols were identical to those developed by Plante for her studies of SLI, and are designed to quantify left-right volume asymmetries in perisylvian cortex (Plante et al., 1989). The individual with a history of stuttering proved to have volume *symmetry* in these regions -- the same characteristic that has been associated with SLI and other disorders affecting communication, such as central auditory processing disorder (Lauter, 1991). Since these hemispheric volume proportions are established before birth, this finding might point to a *prenatal etiology in some types of stuttering*. Physiological correlates of this atypical anatomical sign studied in this same subject will be noted in appropriate sections below.

BRAIN PHYSIOLOGY

Overview of methods

Techniques currently available for studying physiological aspects of brain function can be subdivided into three categories according to the feature of the brain which they access: 1) electrophysiology, 2) blood flow, and 3) metabolism -- e.g., oxygen and glucose utilization, or distribution of chemicals such as neurotransmitters. With minor modifications of testing protocols, most of the same devices employed for blood flow studies can also be used to examine aspects of brain metabolism.

Methods based on *electrophysiology* include: evoked potentials (EPs), quantitative electroencephalography (qEEG), and magnetoencephalography (MEG). In addition, two techniques for *stimulating* the brain depend on electrophysiological properties: 1) direct electrical stimulation (e.g., via subdural or intracranial electrodes, as may be employed in management of epilepsy or chronic pain), and 2) transcranial magnetic stimulation (TMS), representing a type of "MEG in reverse," in which magnetic field fluxes are applied at the surface of the scalp, as a means of inducing electrical currents within the underlying brain.

Techniques which make it possible to study *blood flow* within the brain include: Doppler ultrasonography, single-photon-emission computed tomography (SPECT), positron-emission tomography (PET), and functional magnetic resonance imaging (fMRI). As noted above, by means of certain modifications in testing and analysis protocols, the last three may also be applied for studying aspects of *brain metabolism* and neurochemistry related to brain function. An example related to speech motor control is the use of PET and SPECT to image the atypical distribution of dopamine in patients with Parkinson's Disease.

I. Methods for monitoring brain electrical activity

Evoked potentials (EPs)

Properly termed averaged evoked potentials, these are responses called up from the nervous system by repeated sensory or motor stimulation in which each stimulus event is followed by measurement of electrical responses time-locked to some aspect of the stimulus. Measurement requires electrodes (surface, dermal, or at depth), and response averaging by a computer. EPs may be done with motor activation, or in any sensory modality, and provide a way to analyze responses from point to point along a neural pathway, accomplished by electrode placement combined with manipulation of test parameters such as measurement-time window, amplifier gain, and response filters.

For scalp recordings, subject preparation involves placement of electrodes, for which skin at each site is rubbed clean, and the electrode is attached with a drop of gel and a short strip of tape. If many electrodes are used, a cap may be employed, which encloses ring electrodes in small plastic cylinders. During testing, motor activity near each electrode site (for example, in temporalis muscle under scalp electrodes overlying motor cortex) must be kept at a minimum, since electrical potentials associated with muscle activity can overwhelm the much smaller signals traversing the skull and scalp from the brain.

Evoked potentials can be recorded with as few as three electrodes: an active, a reference, and a ground. If at least 32 electrodes are placed at different locations on the scalp, it is possible to do topographic mapping of responses, and newer systems with arrays of 128 electrodes provide additional capabilities for "Electrical Source Imaging" (ESI), to localize response generators not only within cortex, but also in subcortical regions of the brain. Analysis options for any type of evoked-potential waveform range from simple "peak-picking," for identifying amplitude and latency characteristics of different waveform features, to spectral analysis based on the same mathematics used to analyze sound waveforms, to topographic mapping displaying temporal or spectral features of the EPs.

Evoked potentials associated with brain *motor* commands have been used to study brain activity associated with speech and nonspeech gestures. For instance, Wohlert (1993) compared long-latency evoked potentials (Event Related Potentials, ERPs) recorded at the top of the head ("vertex") and at mirror-image locations over left and right sensorimotor cortex, while subjects performed lip rounding, lip pursing, and production of a single word. Results indicated that of these tasks, word production gave rise to the most negative amplitude at the vertex site, and that none of the tasks evoked asymmetrical responses. The latter finding was also reported by Fujimaki and co-workers (Fujimaki et al., 1994) in an ERP study of *silent speech*. They found activity centers over occipital cortex (response to a visual cue) and over frontal (motor) cortex, focused at the midline.

These results of *symmetrical electrophysiological activation during silent speech* are in agreement with findings of an earlier unpublished study (Lauter, 1989), in which *symmetrical activation* over left- and right-side motor cortex, as measured with qEEG, was observed during silent speech, which contrasted with a strongly left-side-dominant response produced during nonspeech movement of the tongue in the vertical plane (see below, under qEEG). Note that due to the possibility of artifactual confounds between muscle activity (temporalis, etc.) and brain potentials, recordings of either EPs or EEG during time-varying speech gestures may be difficult to interpret. Measures taken before or after actual movements, or observed during sub-vocal performance, may be more useful for analyzing the "mental set" involved in speech, without reflecting electrical interference from muscle potentials.

Testing with *sensory* evoked potentials has also been applied in assessments of general CNS organization in individuals with speech-motor and fluency disorders, from cortex (Zimmerman & Knott, 1974) to brainstem (Decker et al., 1982, Finitzo-Hieber et al., 1982). For example, Dietrich et al. (1995) compared auditory middle-latency responses (MLRs) in

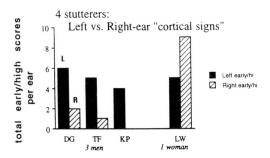

Figure 2. Abnormal physiological signs in four individuals with a history of stuttering, based on testing with the Repeated Evoked Potentials version of the Auditory Brainstem Response (REPs/ABR). The REPs scoring procedure classifies departures from normal in terms of two categories: 1) "early/high scores," in which absolute latency is earlier than normal, or peak amplitude, latency stability, or amplitude stability is higher than normal; and 2) "late/low scores," in which absolute latency is later than normal, or the other three measures are lower than normal. The preponderance of early/high signs in these four subjects is interpreted as indicative of a failure in *top-down modulation* by cortex on the brainstem, leading to these sensory versions of "Jacksonian release signs." Abnormalities appearing primarily during right-ear stimulation in the three men point to left-side cortical dysfunction, while the woman's data suggest that both sides of the cortex may be involved, perhaps via abnormal interhemispheric coordination. (Adapted from Lauter, 1993, unpublished report.)

two groups of males, one with and one without a history of stuttering. They found that the latency of one component of the MLR was earlier in the group who stuttered. This finding may be related to the "Jacksonian release" phenomena demonstrated in another group of stutterers by means of our Repeated Evoked Potentials (REPs) technique, which makes it possible to quantify the repeatability of EP waveform parameters such as peak latency and amplitude.

The REPs technique was designed as a way to derive more information from these least expensive "windows" on brain function. For example, the REPs version of the Auditory Brainstem Response (REPs/ABR) was used to document that four individuals with a history of stuttering (including the one patient whose MRI data were described above) showed abnormal "release signs" in the brainstem, interpreted as pointing to asymmetric dysfunction at the cortical level (Figure 2). In addition, the data suggested possible gender differences regarding the pattern of cortical/brainstem interaction (Lauter, 1993).

Similar REPs/ABR testing in individuals with *spasmodic dysphonia* (SD) suggested that they too may have dysfunction affecting areas above the brainstem, signalled by a "released" brainstem response which, in the case of SD, may fluctuate in severity over time in parallel with clinical signs (Lauter et al., 1992).

This suggestion of cortical dysfunction in SD is in line with the work reported by Watson and colleagues (1991), based on use of cortical auditory evoked potentials (cAEPs) to examine electrophysiological function at the level of the cortex. In the cited study, patients were examined with a battery including MRI (to "confirm" normal cortical and subcortical anatomy), an acoustic laryngeal reaction-time task, discourse analysis, and cortical AEPs monitored at several sites on the scalp. Findings grouped subtle linguistic difficulties with both longer reaction times and abnormal AEPs over the anterior left hemisphere. Were REPs/ABR also done in such patients, it might be possible to link cortical abnormalities with "top-down" effects on responsivity of the brainstem, with obvious implications for assessing physiological modulation on brainstem centers important for laryngeal motor control.

Quantitative electroencephalography (qEEG)

This is the favored generic term for any type of computer-based EEG which provides capabilities for *spectral analysis* of EEG waveforms, based on "narrative EEG," i.e., not averaged via time-locking to a regularly repeated stimulus. The attractions of qEEG are that it may be recorded during "ecologically valid" behavior, while several different areas of the brain are monitored simultaneously. In this way it is similar to the blood-flow techniques to be discussed below, with the advantage to qEEG of a relatively innocuous subject interface -- scalp electrodes -- instead of the radioactivity required by SPECT and PET, or the claustrophobic surround involved in fMRI. Following data collection, spectral analysis is generally performed offline, and the results are reported in terms of power according to each of several bandwidths, at each electrode location. A measure unique to qEEG of the methods described here is *coherence,* which indexes the degree of correlation between electrical activity observed at two electrode sites. Coherence makes it possible to evaluate the way in which different brain regions are either coordinated or act independently under different testing conditions, and is particularly useful for studies of hemispheric interactions such as those related to bilaterally coordinated motor control.

Subject preparation is similar to that described for EPs above, with the same options of few to many electrode sites. While there are many issues related to brain function in speech motor control which might best be addressed only with large electrode arrays, there are also many which require only a few sites in order to yield novel findings. As long as spectral and coherence results are available, information from even a few sites can be put to original use. As mentioned above for EPs, recordings from EEG sites over motor cortex can represent combinations of activity in underlying muscles such as temporalis, along with neural responses. Thus careful within-subject designs must be utilized in order to dissociate electricity originating in muscle from neural sources, and/or task conditions need to be configured to assure that muscle potentials do not swamp the much smaller signals from cortex. In general, EEG recordings cannot be done during dynamic speech that involves extensive jaw movements; however, it should yield useful information contrasting static postures such as sustained phonation vs. silence, rounded vs. unrounded lips, or movements of the tongue, etc. within a fixed-jaw vocal-tract space.

Within-subject studies based on sequences of test conditions may readily be done using qEEG, with patterns of activity compared with initial and spaced resting conditions. This can be a powerful way to study the topography of brain electrical potentials related to speech

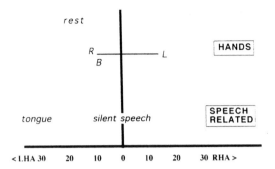

Figure 3. Asymmetries in beta power (13 - 20 Hz) measured with qEEG over frontal cortex locations (F7 vs. F8) in a single subject during a resting control condition ("Rest"), and five types of activation related to motor control: 1) right-hand flexion at a rate of 1 Hz ("R"); 2) left-hand flexion ("L"); 3) flexion of both hands ("B"); 4) "silent speech" consisting of internal rehearsing of memorized poetry and texts, with speech-like manipulation of the lower (sub-laryngeal) but not the upper (larynx and above) airway; and 5) rhythmic movement of the "tongue" up and down in the vertical plane, at a rate of approximately 1 Hz. The abscissa is an axis of asymmetry in beta power calculated as a percent difference between F7 vs. F8, with values favoring the right side plotted on the right side of the space ("Right Hemisphere Advantage, RHA"), and vice versa. Note that while the very speech-like control of older structures evokes no asymmetry in this part of the brain, the non-speech-related movements of the tongue are associated with a striking left-hemisphere advantage (LHA) in beta power. (Adapted from Lauter, 1990, unpublished report.)

motor control. For example, qEEG can show distinctions in the degree of asymmetry observed in motor cortex during non-speech tongue movement, as compared with subvocal speech involving only movements in the lower respiratory tract (diaphragm and intercostal-muscle manipulation: Lauter, 1989, cf. Figure 3). In this experiment, the observed difference was attributed to a possible distinction in the *degree of control laterality,* with a lower degree of laterality posited for older portions of the speech motor-control system (respiratory components), contrasted with highly lateralized control of newer components (larynx through upper vocal tract, including the tongue).

Also, monitoring qEEG during resting conditions in the CNS-Project patient with a history of stuttering referred to above, revealed *very low levels* of cortical activity in the beta band bilaterally, a finding in agreement with the "released" brainstem responses observed in this individual, and also with reports by Finitzo et al. (1991) of abnormally low cortical activity observed with qEEG in a group of developmental stutterers.

The *symmetry* of qEEG activity in the same CNS-Project patient was in agreement with findings reported earlier by Wells and Moore (1990), where analyses of EEG asymmetries in the alpha band (8-13 Hz) revealing symmetrical activity during resting and speaking conditions, contrasted with marked left-side dominance during speaking in non-stuttering controls.

While many clinical neurologists continue to depend on visual examination of EEG waveforms for evaluating their patients, a number of researchers have championed the promise of qEEG for yielding new insights into the neurological bases of behaviors such as reading (Duffy & McAnulty, 1990) and general cognitive functions (Gevins & Schaffer, 1980). Some studies depended on a crude form of qEEG to study speech motor performance, the old measure of "alpha blocking," to index activation (Boberg et al., 1983, Moore, 1984; Moore & Haynes, 1980), but more recent qEEG research has exploited the multi-channel, multi-band capabilities provided by newer computer systems. Foremost among proponents of utilizing qEEG to study disorders of speech motor control are the collaborative team from Dallas. For instance, in their pioneering qEEG study of aphasia (Finitzo et al., 1991), these authors concluded that the spatial and temporal detail available from qEEG means that for evaluation of individuals with acquired speech problems, "objective electrophysiologic methods ... [may] rival the reliability of the language examination."

This same collaborative team gave an overview of applications of qEEG in the study of motor-control disorders of speech to the first conference in this series (Pool et al., 1987), and at the next meeting, reported an update of findings specifically addressing developmental stutterers, tested with cortical AEPs, qEEG, and SPECT (Finitzo et al., 1991). The authors concluded that the convergent results from the three types of testing provided evidence of a neurogenic basis for stuttering.

Magnetoencephalography (MEG)

MEG is a technology based on the use of sensors called Superconducting Quantum Interference Devices (SQUIDs), which must be bathed in liquid helium to ensure their sensitivity. These sensors can detect fluctuations in magnetic fields created by electrical currents within the body and brain, with a high degree of temporal and spatial resolution. For example, source generators can be localized to within 1 mm, more than an order of magnitude finer grain than is possible with qEEG, at least for qEEG systems which do not include the large arrays of electrodes used in Electrical Source Imaging (ESI). Until approximately 1990, MEG testing was very laborious, since systems included fewer than eight sensors; newer MEG systems provide arrays of as many as 128 detectors, which make Magnetic Source Imaging (MSI) possible, for localizing subcortical as well as cortical sources.

Neither radioactivity nor electrodes are required for MEG -- the SQUID sensors (and their liquid-helium bath) are enclosed in a cylinder or helmet which fits snugly against the subject's head. Data collection and analysis are modelled on EPs and qEEG, with the possibility for observing either resting activity or activation, analyzed via spectral analysis of "narrative MEG," or by means of time-locked averaging of magnetic "Evoked Fields" (EFs).

Perhaps the most exciting application of MEG in studies of motor control involves a type of "reversed MEG," in which magnetic field fluctuations are applied at the surface of the scalp, in order to evoke electrical currents within the underlying brain. This is referred to as Transcranial (or Transdermal, if done peripherally) Magnetic Stimulation (TMS), and developments in technology and methods have given rise to a burgeoning literature (cf. Cohen et al., 1990, Amassian et al., 1990, Levy et al., 1991).

The possibilities for research with MEG related to speech motor control can be considered in three categories: 1) "narrative MEG" and evoked-field studies of basic aspects of neural organization, similar in design to those in EEG and EPs mentioned above; 2) studies of motor control in general, examined via MEG or TMS; and 3) experiments involving MEG or TMS assessments directly related to speech control.

To our knowledge, there have been no reports of MEG, and only a few of TMS, to study aspects of speech production or performance of related nonspeech gestures. The TMS studies will be considered below, together with other examples of MEG/TMS applications to issues of motor control in humans.

The high spatial resolution of MEG technology has made it possible for researchers to map regions of sensorimotor cortex specific to the movement of single fingers (Okada et al., 1982), and to observe TMS effects in individual muscles of the hand (Hess et al., 1987). Measures have not only revealed activation in primary cortex related to motor control, but also signs of planning in cases where subjects are cued as to the nature of a future response.

For example, the MEG version of a Contingent Negative Variation (CNV) paradigm was used to study brain activity related to finger movements in response to auditory cues (Ioannides et al., 1994). In two right-handed subjects, there were clear patterns including "priming" in related areas following cue and preceding actual movement. There were also marked individual differences in the two subjects as to areas activated, timing and extent of activation, and asymmetrical responses related to whether movement involved the preferred or non-preferred hand (Figure 4.).

Another group of researchers considered the effects of motor learning on activity in sensorimotor cortex (Elbert et al., 1995). Two groups of subjects, with and without extensive experience as violin players, were measured with MEG to assess areas of response to somatosensory stimulation of the fingers. The findings indicated that in individuals with longer experience playing the violin, there was a relatively larger amount of cortex devoted to responding to left-hand stimulation. The authors interpreted this as a "use-dependent" effect.

Studies using TMS have been reported for some time -- for principles and applications, cf. reviews and reports in Chokroverty (1990). The intensity of the applied magnetic fields (MFs) can be related to differential effects. For example, MFs of very low intensity have been reported to have *beneficial effects* on perceptual organization and drawing in Parkinson's patients (Sandyk 1993), and to facilitate muscular action (Nielsen et al., 1993), while high-intensity MFs can produce analgesia for chronic pain (Ellis, 1993), evoke epileptic activity for diagnostic purposes in epilepsy (Jennum & Winkel, 1994), and inhibit evoked responses (and ongoing behavior) in subjects who are performing visual (Amassian et al., 1989) and linguistic (Coslett & Monsul, 1994) tasks. TMS stimulation has also been reported to change affective tone (Richards et al., 1993). The level of detail available from TMS is such that it may be used to identify changes in the level of tonic arousal provided from the cerebellum

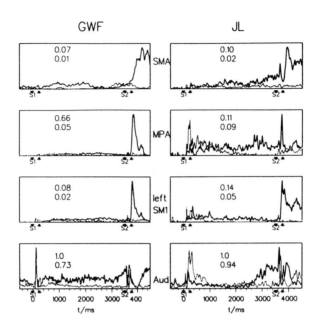

Figure 4. Temporal plots of activity measured with MEG over four areas of cortex in two subjects (GWF, JL) during a CNV-type paradigm. In each panel, activity is plotted as an amplitude-like measure against an abscissa of time marked in ms. In this task, subjects heard an initial "warning" tone (S1), the pitch of which signalled whether at a second "command" tone (S2), they would either flex the right index finger ("Go" condition, heavy tracings) or keep the finger still ("NoGo" condition, lighter tracings). Areas sampled (reading panels top to bottom) were: Supplementary Motor Area (SMA), a middle-parietal area (MPA), left sensorimotor cortex (left SM1), left auditory cortex (Aud). Salient aspects of these plots related to issues of motor control include: 1) persistence of activity in some areas long after movement has ceased, particularly notable in SMA for both subjects; 2)"sensory priming" in auditory cortex leading up to the command tone in the Go but not the NoGo condition; and 3) spread of sensory response such that it is visible even in non-auditory areas (cf. the marked response in JL's auditory cortex to the NoGo condition, which is also visible in a reduced form in left SM1). (Reprinted with permission from Ioannides et al., 1994.)

acting on motor cortex (Lazzaro et al., 1994).

Applications to non-speech-related motor function have included examination of responses in brain following TMS to peripheral nerves (Kunesch et al., 1993), and assessments of responses seen in muscle following cortical TMS (Awiszus and Feistner, 1994, Terao et al., 1994). Some studies have also reported speech arrest coincident with TMS applied over areas of motor cortex purportedly involved in laryngeal motor control (Amassian et al., 1988, Day et al., 1989, Pascual-Leone et al., 1991, Wasserman et al., 1991).

TMS has been also used peripherally to evoke responses in laryngeal musculature, in order to assess function and evaluate status or recovery following injury to the recurrent laryngeal nerve. However, for confident applications in "neurolaryngology," Ludlow et al.

(1994) have suggested that quantitative studies of the *natural variation* of laryngeal responses to TMS must be done before its usefulness for assessing the integrity of laryngeal innervation can be established.

II. Methods based on imaging brain blood flow

Single-photon-emission computed tomography (SPECT)

As its name implies, SPECT depends on radioisotopes which decay by emitting photons (gamma rays). These substances are administered to a subject via injection or inhalation, and the resulting radiation products are sufficiently powerful to be detectable outside the skull. As imaged by the computer, the distribution of radioisotope reflects a distribution of cerebral blood flow (CBF), which in turn is interpreted as a topography of brain activity, since neurons require a constant supply of raw materials via the bloodstream to continue working.

Because of the design of the scanning hardware, SPECT must employ isotopes with longer half-lives than those which can be used with PET (see below); as a result, SPECT scanning inherently exposes subjects to relatively higher levels of radiation than PET. Thus SPECT is less commonly used in subjects free of neurological disorder, and does not support multiple scans in the same individual (typically no more than two conditions are done per subject). Its most frequent use is to image the resting brain in patients with brain damage, or to assess differences during a single activation condition compared with the same brain at rest, also for clinical purposes.

With regard to studies of speech motor control, SPECT has been used to study children who are labelled dysphasic (Denays et al., 1989, Billard et al., 1988, Lou et al., 1984), and several groups of individuals with a history of stuttering (Pool et al., 1991; Watson et al., 1992, 1994).

The usefulness of SPECT for studies of patients with frank brain damage has been illustrated many times; for a review of several clinical applications, cf. Devous (1995). One example recounted in this review involved several patients with nonfluent aphasia who were studied using SPECT, with an initial assessment within 30 days post-onset, and again at 3 months post. Initially, regions of abnormally low blood flow, both cortical and subcortical, could be identified in all of these patients. Blood flow changes were observed in all monitored areas over time, but it was only those increases in flow seen in inferior frontal areas which were correlated with improvements in speech fluency. In four of the five patients who continued to have difficulties 3 months post-insult, inferior frontal regions were still hypoperfused; however, in eight of the nine individuals who showed good recovery of speech fluency, increased ability for speech production was accompanied by a return of inferior-frontal blood flow to normal levels.

Positron-emission tomography (PET)

Current PET technology makes it possible to complete a scan of the entire cranial nervous system in as short a time as 40 sec, with approximately 5 mm spatial resolution. The scan time and experimental design both depend on the isotopes used; as with SPECT, PET depends on introducing radiopharmaceuticals into the bloodstream, either via injection or inhalation, and then detecting the radiation products from outside the body. With long-half-life isotopes, such as flourine-18 used to label glucose, scan times can be as long as 45 min, resulting in high exposure to the subject and thus the inability to do repeated conditions in the same individual; in contrast, isotopes such as oxygen-15 (O-15), with a half life of about 2 min, make it possible to have short scans, thereby reducing exposure and providing a basis for multiple conditions per subject. It is oxygen-15 that has been employed for most of the activation studies done with PET, in normals as well as in disordered populations.

Although some researchers have decided that PET requires averaging results over subjects (cf. Petersen et al., 1988), experimental results can be reported on a within-subject basis, if care is taken to maximize responses in individuals, and thereby exploit the sensitivity which PET shows to patterns of activation in individual brains. This approach to PET scanning is particularly well illustrated in the functional mapping procedures reported by some neurosurgical groups, where O-15 PET is used in combination with sodium amytal testing to assess localization of brain activity during the performance of specific movements, particularly with regard to speech production, in order to guide planning for neurosurgery (Leblanc et al., 1992, Martin et al., 1992).

Recent PET studies related to speech motor control range from basic research on reading (Ingvar et al., 1994), word repetition/monitoring (Demonet et al., 1994; Herholz et al., 1994), and bilingual speech production (Klein et al., 1994), to assessments of resting blood flow in stuttering (Wu et al., 1995) and aphasia (Tamas et al., 1993). Methodological points which need to be made regarding PET protocols include: 1) "persistence" phenomena involving brain activity left-over from previous conditions, may interfere with meaningful interpretation of "onion-layer" task designs where each of a succession of conditions is used as the control for the following task (Lauter et al., 1990; Lauter, 1992); 2) activation conditions may enhance diagnostic symptoms over their appearance in resting states (Bromfield et al., 1991); and 3) when MRIs are obtained for each subject, individually-specific details of PET-measured changes in CBF topography can be studied and interpreted.

For example, Herholz and colleagues (Herholz et al., 1994) used three-dimensional MRI to obtain "customized brain atlases" for six right-handed normal subjects, who were then examined for glucose metabolism using PET while they repeated words. The authors found that several cortical regions were activated consistently in all subjects, while cerebellar activation, though it did occur, was quite variable from individual to individual. They concluded that "in contrast to previous blood flow activation studies with averaging across subjects, the new technique permits the anatomical localization and quantitation of activation areas in each individual" (see Figure 5).

Functional magnetic resonance imaging (fMRI)

A growing number of functional studies using modified MRI technology has been reported since the first experiment described by Belliveau and colleagues in 1991 (Belliveau

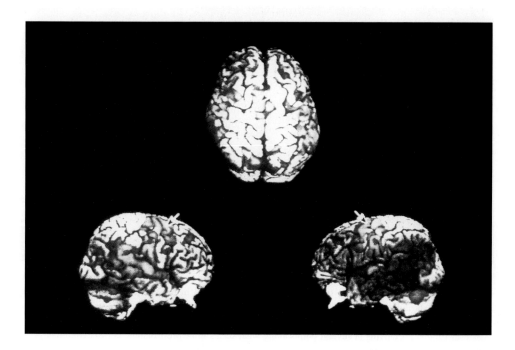

Figure 5. Images of PET blood-flow images superimposed on MRI anatomical images for one right-handed non-aphasic man, tested during repetition of each item in a list of words read by an experimenter. The PET scanning was based on labelled glucose, and thus required control testing be done on one day, and activation delayed to a session held on a different day, with a total scan time on each occasion of 30 min. Note the variety of areas activated, including the supplementary motor area (SMA) which can be visualized at some depth when reconstructed on a coronal MRI slice (top image), but which is invisible on MRI images of the cortical surface (SMA location indicated by arrows on the lower two images). (Reprinted with permission from Herholz et al., 1994.)

et al., 1991). This method depends on the fact that, as noted above, MR is actually a form of chemical analysis. While anatomical MRI depends on producing a "map" of the distribution of *hydrogen* atoms as they appear in different tissues, functional MRI in most reports to date is based on identifying changes in the *oxygen* content of the blood around a target area of the brain.

Applications have already been made in a number of areas, including psychiatry, as well as normal visual, auditory, and motor function (for a brief overview, cf. Le Bihan et al., 1995). For instance, fMRI images obtained during finger tapping and movements of the lower face in a woman being assessed for epilepsy surgery, yielded localization which was subsequently confirmed by recordings through implanted subdural electrodes, suggesting that fMRI (like individualized PET, discussed by Herholz et al., 1994, above) has the potential as a noninvasive tool for presurgical functional mapping.

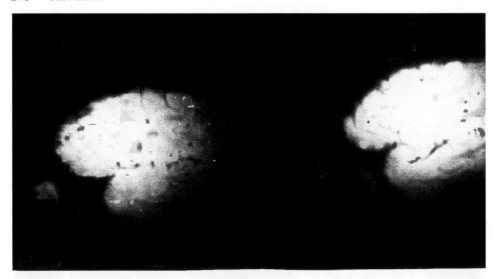

Figure 6. Blood-flow changes measured with fMRI, superimposed on anatomical MR images (left hemisphere on the left, right hemisphere on the right), observed in one subject. The images compare activation seen during a control condition (e.g., visualizing a night sky filled with stars) vs. a test condition (silently generating as many words as possible beginning with a given letter). Note positive-change responses (orange) occurring at several points along what seems to be pre-Rolandic cortex, combined with some negative changes (green) in other locations. There is clearly more positive activation in the left hemisphere than in the right, during this silent word-generation task. The marked negative change at the extreme far left of this figure is shown superimposed on the eye, and represents a lower level of eye movements occurring during the test condition, perhaps reflecting the change in task demands from a primarily visual mental operation ("imagining a night sky") to a primarily word-oriented one. (Reprinted with permission from Le Bihan et al., 1995.)

Other aspects of motor control have also been used to "calibrate" fMRI as an imaging technique, such as laterality (Kim et al., 1993), comparisons of actual movement vs. ideation (Fieldman et al., 1993, Tyszka et al., 1994), and activation of cortex both in and outside of primary motor areas (Schad et al., 1993, Rao et al., 1993, Schad et al., 1994).

Cortical activation related to speech has also been studied with fMRI, primarily during "covert" word generation to avoid movement artifacts (McCarthy et al., 1993, Hinke et al., 1993, Rueckert et al., 1994). These studies found activation in Broca's area, even though overt production was not involved (Figure 6). Other regions activated were inconsistent from subject to subject; Rueckert has observed (Le Bihan et al., 1995) that the individually-specific patterns of activation seen with fMRI should not be surprising simply because they contrast with the results typically reported with PET -- she notes that "some rarely activated regions might disappear in PET studies when results from participants are averaged together."

EXPERIMENTAL DESIGN

The unprecedented spatial and temporal resolution of these new methods make it possible to address questions of speech motor control and fluency which have never been answered. By combining such technological features with sophisticated experimental design, students of speech production have the opportunity to study speech and nonspeech motor control in normal subjects of all ages, individuals with developmental disorders, and those who have speech problems subsequent to acquired injuries.

The need for sophisticated experimental design is crucial; it is not possible to forego careful consideration of stimulus and task components, simply because the brain is being imaged. In fact, since most of the uncertainty is in the imaging procedure (what will the brain look like under this modality?), it becomes even more important to bring as many aspects of the testing situation as possible under rigorous experimental control.

Thus, all of the testing techniques which are traditional in speech science and clinical speech research represent invaluable adjuncts to brain-imaging studies of production and fluency. If subjects are to be imaged during resting conditions, then complete information on each subject acquired via clinical and behavioral testing batteries provides the requisite context within which to interpret the patterns of organization seen during imaging.

For activation studies, it is difficult to assess the results of brain monitoring during speech production or the performance of other motor tasks if concomitant measures of that performance are not taken, whether via video documentation or other analyses of movements, including appropriate quantitative assessments of parameters of speech and voice. With the exception of MEG and fMRI, the imaging methods reviewed here are not hampered by the presence and operation of traditional speech- and voice-measurement tools, such as acoustical recording, electroglottography (EGG), electromyography (EMG), and devices for assessing airway dynamics. Thus for advanced imaging studies of speech production, the results of performance should be recorded and measured simultaneously with imaging.

Experimental design should also take advantage of the incredible quality of detail offered by the imaging methods regarding individually-specific patterns of activity and response. From CT through fMRI, the first and foremost feature revealed by every imaging/monitoring technique is the *individuality* of the brain. Only by careful documentation of the range of individual variation, in patients and in normal subjects, will we be able to appreciate the "repertoire" of ways in which brain structure and function give rise to behaviors, and to comprehend the variety of ways in which failure of nervous-system operation is expressed in the symptoms of dysfunction.

The "neurological fingerprints" of individuals which can be described using these techniques (Lauter, 1994) promise to provide us with new insights into diagnostic signs and classifications, novel concepts for therapeutic management, and guidelines for outcome assessment tailored to the expression of a disorder in a single individual. For constructing such "fingerprints," it is crucial to depend on a combination of imaging/monitoring methods, ideally in the form of a *coordinated test battery*.

COORDINATING METHODS

Of course, test-battery approaches are the rule in speech and hearing practice -- we teach our students that no one test can alone provide a definitive diagnostic profile of an individual client. The case is the same for brain-imaging techniques, where the brain features provided by each method are only one view of brain/behavior correlates, much like the report of one of the seven blind men looking at an elephant. Considering the complementary nature of the different "windows on the brain," it is clear that *the only way to obtain the complete picture is to integrate details across several methods.*

As we have seen, this is the model utilized by the group from Dallas in their studies of speech motor control; this team routinely test subjects with batteries including CT/MRI, EPs, qEEG, SPECT, and a rich variety of behavioral instruments. The unique advantages of a "hybrid" approach are also described at length by a team of researchers working in California, on protocols for clinical neurosurgery. A review of their methods focusing on "the language areas, particularly the motor systems," outlines a combination of MRI, EPs, qEEG, "superselective angiography" with local Amytal injection, and PET (Martin et al., 1992). Illustrated with case histories, these descriptions demonstrate how information based on the different degrees of spatial and temporal resolution of the various methods can be combined to identify the exact localization of functional areas to be avoided in surgical procedures. Of course, in neurosurgery, the individuality of brain functional organization is of crucial importance, and these workers emphasize the *"tremendous interindividual variability* in the location of essential (productive and expressive) language areas" [italics added].

The same respect for the striking degree of individual specificity of brain/behavior correlates is basic to the design of the Coordinated Noninvasive Studies (CNS) Project (Lauter, 1988, 1990, 1995). This research program combines methods in an aggressively coordinated way for basic studies of functional organization in normal brains, as well for clinical assessments in individuals whose conditions are "neurologically silent," such as some types of speech disorder including stuttering and spasmodic dysphonia, central auditory problems, dyslexia, attention deficit, and chronic pain. More than two decades of work based on this approach have given rise to new concepts of brain organization, describing dynamic "handshaking" relations among neural centers and pathways considered along all three vectors of body/brain orientation (Lauter, in preparation). The "Handshaking Model" posits that these graded and highly interactive relations provide mechanisms enabling different parts of the brain to coordinate like members of a theatrical "repertory company," for accomplishing the "performances" of everyday behavior (Lauter, in Press).

CONCLUSIONS AND IMPLICATIONS

As we learn to make use of the advantages of the new imaging techniques for revealing the organization of individual brains, we should begin to appreciate the basic importance of *systemic organization* -- that brains do not accomplish their work "phrenologically," one area at a time, but by means of coordinated, interrelated teams of centers and pathways. As Pool et al. (1991) said of their multi-test studies of spasmodic dysphonia, "The view emerging is . . . of *systems of neurons* rather than single anatomical sites" [italics added].

A systems-level approach can provide new conceptual frameworks for considering and comparing different types of speech motor control disorders. For example, if we utilize Hughlings Jackson's categories of damage, based on a systems-level formulation of CNS function, we might characterize Broca's aphasia as a "loss symptom," where injury to association motor cortex is followed by a loss of the ability to control fluent, complexly coordinated gestures of the larynx and upper vocal tract.

Along the same lines, the style of speech production common in patients with more posterior damage, as in Wernicke's aphasia, may be referred to as a "release symptom," based on the supposition that the posterior regions exert a normal level of executive control forward onto motor regions, which when lost as a result of post-Rolandic damage, results in a kind of "over-production" by the motor cortex. Given some of the recent work on low-level magnetic stimulation with TMS cited above, it is therefore possible to consider focal stimulation of Wernicke's area in such patients, to attempt to recruit marginally functional neurons to exert more control over the logorrheic frontal cortex.

A Jacksonian approach modernized via the Handshaking Model (Lauter, in preparation) also suggests that spasmodic dysphonia, along with some other dystonias, might be types of release signs associated with damage to upper motor neurons of the extrapyramidal system. Even the neurological correlates of stuttering could be modelled according to these formulations, as dysfunctional coordinative relations between left- and right-hemisphere areas responsible for overseeing the control of midline structures for vocal production. Several types of evidence, from anecdotal observations to details from brain studies reviewed here, are consistent with such an approach. Not least among these is the fact that the myelination of the corpus callosum, crucial for the formation of efficient linkages between left- and right-side neocortex, occurs over the same period in early childhood development (2-5 years of age) during which the majority of cases of developmental (and even "normal") stuttering emerge.

It is a sobering thought that 100 years after Freud and other clinicians of the 19th century deplored the reductionist, simplistic notions about brain function espoused by the "map makers," much of the research in human neuroscience, particularly that utilizing the most expensive machines, is still concerned with "single anatomical sites." Given the amount of experimental and philosophical work during the second half of this century that has focused on the dynamic network nature of the brain, it is amazing that these new imaging devices -- which allow us to watch the *whole brain* in action in *almost simultaneous,* sometimes *near-real-time* detail -- are not being employed to study systems-level organization, but are still for the most part being used to look for a "center for hearing," a "center for seeing," and in disorders, to search for hypothetical "holes in the brain."

For example, the terms of discussion used in some very recent PET studies on stuttering reveal the continuing presence of what we might call the "lesion fallacy" -- the underlying assumption that there is a "center for stuttering." The alternative, which seems to be suggested and even demanded by virtually all of the experimental and clinical evidence on this puzzling speech disorder, is that stuttering, along with many other types of speech disorders, can be meaningfully studied *only at the systems level.* The 19th-century neurological giants on whose shoulders we stand might not be surprised that the map-makers are still with us, but they would probably be dismayed to find that they are still so vocal.

There are many new details to be seen through the new "windows on the brain," and of course as with all new information, we may find that they challenge long-established notions regarding brain function. But like the mountains on the moon shown by Galileo's telescope, the details are after all the test of the imaging device -- if a new method of observation and measurement did not show us details we had never seen before, of what value would it be? We must learn to look, and measure, and try to comprehend, if our "brain cosmology" is ever to move beyond the primitive limitations of its lesion-oriented beginnings.

The Copernican revolution in astronomy depended in part on realizing that the descriptive solution to the seemingly bewildering details of planetary motion was not to invent models consisting of ever more circles within circles, but to take a fresh new approach -- departing from the underlying assumption that motion *had to be circular.* In order to revolutionize our concepts of the brain, we may find that the asssumption to be discarded is that human brains are more alike than they are different. If we can make that intellectual leap, the new imaging methods will come into their own as the ideal tools for our new philosophy.

Then, instead of employing statistical methods which act to degrade their powers of resolution, we may learn to optimize the access the noninvasive techniques provide to details of *individual structure and function.* The more we know about those details, the more sophisticated formulations we can make regarding the variety of ways in which these details combine to create systems-level organization in human brains. The Copernican revolution of human neuroscience still awaits us, with implications for our vision of the brain and of ourselves -- but we will achieve that revolution only when we come to understand and functionalize in our research protocols, that the brain works not as a collection of isolated, independent parts, but as a set of dynamic systems, coordinatively integrated over space and time.

REFERENCES

Amassian, V.E., Anziska, B.J., Cracco, J.B., Cracco, R.Q., & Maccabee, P.J. (1988). Focal magnetic coil excitation of frontal cortex activates laryngeal muscles in man. *Journal of Physiology, 298,* 41P.

Amassian, V.E., Cracco, R.Q., Maccabee, P.J., Cracco, J.B., Rudell, A., & Eberle, L. (1989). Magnetic stimulation of human occipital cortex suppresses visual perception. *Electroencephalography and clinical Neurophysiology, 74,* 458-462.

Amassian, V.E., Maccabee, P.J., Cracco, R.Q., & Cracco, J.B. (1990). Basic mechanisms of magnetic coil excitation of nervous system in humans and monkeys: Application in focal stimulation of different cortical areas in humans. In S. Chrokoverty (Ed.), *Magnetic stimulation in clinical neurophysiology* (pp. 73-111). Boston: Butterworths.

Awiszus, F., & Feistner, H. (1994). Correlations between size parameters and the amplitude of the excitatory postsynaptic potential evoked by magnetic brain stimulation in human hand muscle motoneurons. *Experimental Brain Research, 98,* 128-134.

Belliveau, J.W., Kennedy, D.N., McKinstry, R.C., Buchbinder, B.R., Weisskoff, R.F., Cohen, M.S., et al. (1991). Functional mapping of the human visual cortex by magnetic resonance imaging." *Science, 254,* 716-719.

Billard, C., Dulac, O., & Raynaurd, C. (1988). Brain SPECT imaging in developmental childhood dysphasia. *Journal of Nuclear Medicine, 29,* 792.

Boberg, E., Yeudall, L., Schopflocher, D., & Bo-Lassen, P. (1983). The effects of an intensive behavioral program on the distribution of EEG alpha power in stutterers during the processing of verbal and visuospatial information. *Journal of Fluency Disorders, 8,* 245-263.

Boey, H.P., Cunningham, M.J., & Weber, A.L. (1995). Central nervous system imaging in the evaluation of children with true vocal cord paralysis. *Annals of Otology, Rhinology, and Laryngology, 104,* 76-77.

Bromfield, E.B., Ludlow, C.L., Sedory, S., Leiderman, D.B., & Theodore, W.H. (1991). Cerebral activation during speech discrimination in temporal lobe epilepsy. *Epilepsy Research, 9,* 49-58.

Chokroverty, S. (Ed.) (1990). *Magnetic stimulation in clinical neurophysiology.* Boston: Butterworths.

Cohen, L.G., Hallett, M., & Lelli, S. (1990). Noninvasive mapping of human motor cortex with transcranial magnetic stimulation. In S. Chokroverty (Ed.), *Magnetic Stimulation in Clinical Neurophysiology* (pp. 113-119). Boston: Butterworths.

Coslett, H.B. & Monsul, N. (1994). Reading with the right hemisphere: Evidence from transcranial magnetic stimulation. *Brain and Language, 46,* 198-211.

Day, B.L., Rothwell, P.D., & Thompson, P.D. (1989). Delay in the execution of voluntary movements by electrical or magnetic brain stimulation in intact man: Evidence for storage of motor programs in the brain. *Brain, 112,* 649-663.

Decker, T.N., Healy, E. & Howe, S. (1982). Brainstem auditory characteristics of stutterers and non-stutterers: A preliminary report. *Journal of Fluency Disorders, 7,* 385-389.

Demonet, J.-F., Price, C., Wise, R., & Frackowiak, R.S.J. (1994). Differential activation of right and left posterior sylvian regions by semantic and phonological tasks: A positron-emission tomography study in normal human subjects. *Neuroscience Letters, 182,* 25-28.

Denays, R., Tondeur, M., Foulon, M., Verstraeten, F., Ham, H., Piepsz, A., & Noel, P. (1989). Regional brain blood flow in congenital dysphasia: Studies with Technetium-99m HM-PAO SPECT. *Journal of Nuclear Medicine, 30,* 1825-1829.

Devous, M.D.S. (1995). SPECT functional brain imaging. In E.L. Kramer, & J.J. Sanger (Eds.), *Clinical SPECT imaging* (pp. 97-128). New York: Raven.

Dietrich, S., Barry, S.J., & Parker, D.E. (1995). Middle latency auditory responses in males who stutter. *Journal of Speech and Hearing Research, 38,* 5-17.

Duffy, F.H. & McAnulty, G. (1990). Neurophysiological heterogeneity and the definition of dyslexia: Preliminary evidence for plasticity. *Neuropsychologica, 28,* 555-571.

Elbert, T., Pantev, C., Wienbruch, C., Rockstroh, B., & Taub, E. (1995). Increased cortical representation of the fingers of the left hand in string players. *Science, 270,* 305-307.

Ellis, W.V. (1993). Pain control using high-intensity pulsed magnetic stimulation. *Bioelectromagnetics, 14,* 553-556.

Fieldman, J.B., Cohen, L.G., Jezzard, P., Pons, T., Sadato, R., & Turner, R. (1993). "Functional neuroimaging with echoplanar imaging in humans during execution and mental rehearsal of a simple motor task." [recounted in Le Bihan, D., Jezzard, P., Haxby, J., Sadato, N., Rueckert, L., & Mattay, V. (1995) Functional magnetic resonance imaging of the brain. *Annals of Internal Medicine,*

122, 296-303.

Finger, S. (1994). *Origins of Neuroscience; A history of explorations into brain function.* New York: Oxford University Press.

Finitzo, T., Pool, K.D., & Chapman, S.D. (1991). Quantitative electroencephalography and anatomoclinical principles of aphasia. *Annals of the New York Academy of Sciences, 620,* 57-72.

Finitzo, T., Pool, K.D., Freeman, F.J., Cannito, M.P., Schaefer, S.D., Ross, E.D., & Devous, M.D. (1987). Spasmodic dysphonia subsequent to head trauma. *Archives of Otolaryngology and Head and Neck Surgery, 113,* 1107-1110.

Finitzo, T., Pool, K.D., Freeman, F.J., Devous, M.D., & Watson, B.C. (1991). Cortical dysfunction in developmental stutterers. In H.F.M. Peters, W. Hulstijn, & C.W. Starkweather (Eds.), *Speech motor control and stuttering*(pp. 251-261). Amsterdam: Elsevier Science Publishers.

Finitzo-Hieber, T., Freeman, F.J., Gerling, I.J., Dobson, L., & Schaefer, S.D. (1982). Auditory brainstem response abnormalities in adductor spasmodic dysphonia. *American Journal of Otolaryngology, 3,* 26-30.

Fujimaki, N., Takeuchi, F., Kobayashi, T., Kuriki, S., & Hasuo, S. (1994). Event-related potentials in silent speech. *Brain Topography, 6,* 259-267.

Galaburda, A.M., Rosen, G.D., & Sherman, G.F. (1990). Individual variability in cortical organization: Its relationship to brain laterality and implications to function. *Neuropsychologia, 28,* 529-546.

Gevins, A.S. & Schaffer, R.E. (1980). A critical review of electroencephalographic (EEG) correlates of higher cortical functions. *CRC Critical Reviews in Bioengineering, 4,* 113-164.

Herholz, K., Pietrzyk, U., Karbe, H., Wurker, M., Wienhard, K., & Heiss, W.D. (1994). Individual metabolic anatomy of repeating words demonstrated by MRI-guided positron emission tomography. *Neuroscience Letters, 182,* 47-50.

Hess, C.W., Mills, K.R., & Murray, N.M.F. (1987). Responses in small hand muscles from magnetic stimulation of the human brain. *Journal of Physiology, 388,* 397-419.

Hinke, R.M., Hu, X., Stillman, A.E., Kim, S.G., Merkle, H., & Salmi, R. (1993). Functional magnetic resonance imaging of Broca's area during internal speech. *Neuroreport, 4,* 675-678.

Ingham, R.J., Fox, P.T., & Ingham, J.C. (1995). A report on a functional-activation and functional-lesion PET study of stuttering in adults. Presented to American Speech/Language/Hearing/Association, Orlando FL.

Ingvar, M., Eriksson, L., Greitz, T., Stone-Elander, S., Dahlbom, M., & Rosenqvist, G. (1994). Methodological aspects of brain activation studies: Cerebral blood flow determined with [15O] butanol and positron emission tomography. *Journal of Cerebral Blood Flow and Metabolism, 14,* 628-638.

Ioannides, A.A., Fenwick, P.B.C., Lumsden, J., Liu, M.J., Bamidis, P.D., Squires, K.C., Lawson, D., & Fenton, G.W. (1994). Activation sequence of discrete brain areas during cognitive processes: Results from magnetic field tomography. *Electroencephalography and Clinical Neurophysiology, 91,* 399-402.

Jennum, P., & Winkel, H. (1994). Transcranial magnetic stimulation: Its role in the evaluation of patients with partial epilepsy. *Acta Neurological Scandinavica, 152,* 93-96.

Kim, S.G., Ashe, J., Hendrich, K., Ellermann, J.M., Merkle, H., Ugurbil, K., & Georgopoulous, A.P. (1993). Functional magnetic resonance imaging of motor cortex: Hemispheric asymmetry and handedness. *Science, 261,* 615-617.

Klein, D., Zatorre, R.J., Milner, B., Meyer, E., & Evans, A.C. (1994). Left putaminal activation when speaking a second language: Evidence from PET. *Neuroreport, 5,* 2295-2297.

Kunesch, E., Knecht, S., Classen, J., Roick, H., Tyercha, C., & Benecke, R. (1993). Somatosensory evoked potentials (SEPs) elicited by magnetic nerve stimulation. *Electroencephalography and Clinical*

Neurophysiology, 88, 459-467.

Lauter, J.L. (1988). Functional asymmetries in normal humans studied with quantitative EEG (qEEG): First tests in the CNS Project. *Journal of the Acoustical Society of America, 84,* S57.

Lauter, J.L. (1989). Asymmetries in frontal cortex measured with qEEG during silent speech and non-speech tongue gestures: A single-subject study. *Unpublished report.*

Lauter, J.L. (1990). The Coordinated Noninvasive Studies (CNS) Project. Presented to Society for Neuroscience, St. Louis MO.

Lauter, J L. (1991). Central auditory dysfunction: qEEG and MRI correlates of individual differences in ear advantages and REP/ABR results. *Journal of the Acoustical Society of America, 90,* 2292.

Lauter, J.L. (1992). Processing asymmetries for complex sounds: Comparisons between behavioral ear advantages and electrophysiological asymmetries based on quantitative electroencephalography (qEEG). *Brain and Cognition, 19,* 1-20.

Lauter, J.L. (1993). REPs/ABR in four individuals with a history of stuttering: Brainstem evidence for abnormal cortical function, with suggestions of gender differences. *Unpublished report.*

Lauter, J.L. (1994). Keynote Address -- Windows on the Brain: Imaging the face of human communication, a tutorial. *Presented to Conference on Research Frontiers in Brain Imaging, 4th Annual ASHA Research Conference,* New Orleans LA.

Lauter, J.L. (1995). Visions of speech and language: New noninvasive imaging techniques and their applications to the study of human communication. In H. Winitz (Ed.), *Human Communication and its Disorders, Volume IV* (pp. 277-390). Timonium, MD: York Press.

Lauter, J.L. (In Press). The auditory system as repertory company: A new approach to the neurobiology of speech perception. In W. Ainsworth and S. Greenberg (Eds.), *The auditory perception of speech: Proceedings of the ECSA Conference in Keele, England.*

Lauter, J.L. (In Press). Envisioning how we hear and keep our balance: Images of human auditory and vestibular processing. In T. Gallagher, & J.L. Lauter (Eds.), *Brain imaging tools for communication neuroscience.* Lawrence Erlbaum.

Lauter, J.L. (In Press). Imaging the face of human communication: New techniques and their implications for communication sciences. In T. Gallagher, & J.L. Lauter (Eds.),*Brain imaging tools for communication neuroscience.* Lawrence Erlbaum.

Lauter, J.L. (In preparation). The handshaking model of brain organization: Notes toward a theory.

Lauter, J.L., Hawkins, L.K., Fisher, K., & Owen, A. (1992). Stability of brainstem responses in spasmodic dysphonia measured using the REPs/ABR protocol. *Presented to Voice Foundation,* Philadelphia PA.

Lauter, J.L., Tucker, F., & Hubner, K. (1990). Quantitative demonstration using positron emission tomography, of regional activation, response asymmetries, and residual effects of hand flexion in the normal human brain. *Unpublished report.*

Lazzaro, V.D., Restuccia, D., Molinari, M., Leggio, M.G., Nardone, R., Fogli, D., & Tonali, P. (1994). Excitability of the motor cortex to magnetic stimulation in patients with cerebellar lesions. *Journal of Neurology, Neurosurgery, and Neuropsychiatry, 57,* 108-110.

Le Bihan, D., Jezzard, P., Haxby, J., Sadato, N., Rueckert, L., & Mattay, V. (1995). Functional magnetic resonance imaging of the brain. *Annals of Internal Medicine, 122,* 296-303.

Leblanc, R., Meyer, E., Bub, D., Zatorre, R.J., & Evans, A.C. (1992). Language localization with activation positron emission tomography scanning. *Neurosurgery, 31,* 369-373.

Levy, W.J., Cracco, R.Q., Barker, A.T., & Rothwell, J.C. (Eds.) (1991). *Magnetic motor stimulation: Basic principles and clinical experience. Electroencephalography and Clinical Neurophysiology,* Supp. 43.

Lou, H.C., Henriksen, L., & Bruhn, P. (1984). Focal cerebral hypoperfusion in children with dysphasia and/or attention deficit disorder. *Archives of Neurology, 41,* 825-829.

Ludlow, C., Yeh, J., Cohen, L.G., Van Pelt, F., Rhew, K., & Hallett, M. (1994). Limitations of electromyography and magnetic stimulation for assessing laryngeal muscle control. *Annals of Otology, Rhinology and Laryngology, 103,* 16-27.

Martin, N., Grafton, S., Vinuela, F., Dion, J., Duckwiler, G., Mazziotta, J., Lufkin, R., & Becker, D. (1992). Imaging techniques for cortical functional localization. *Clinical Neurosurgery, 38,* 132-165.

McCarthy, G., Blamire, A.M., Rothman, D.L., Gruetter, R., & Shulman, R.B. (1993). Echo-planar magnetic reonance imaging studies of frontal cortex activation during word generation in humans. *Proceedings of the National Academy of Sciences, U.S.A., 90,* 4952-4956.

Moore, W.H., Jr. (1984). Hemispheric alpha asymetries during an electromyographic biofeedback procedure for stuttering: A single-subject experimental design. *Journal of Fluency Disorders, 17,* 143-162.

Moore, W.H., Jr., & Haynes, W.O. (1980). Alpha hemispheric asymmetry and stuttering: Some support for a segmentation dysfunction hypothesis. *Journal of Speech and Hearing Research, 23,* 229-247.

Nielsen, J., Petersen, N., Deuschl, G., & Ballegaard, M. (1993). Task-related changes in the effects of magnetic brain stimulation on spinal neurones in man. *Journal of Physiology, 471,* 223-243.

Okada, Y. C., Williamson, S.J., & Kaufman, L. (1982). Magnetic field of the human sensorimotor cortex. *International Journal of Neuroscience, 17,* 33-38.

Pascual-Leone, A., Gates, J.R., & Dhuna, A. (1991). Induction of speech arrest and counting errors with rapid-rate transcranial magnetic stimulation. *Neurology, 41,* 697-702.

Petersen, S.E., Fox, P.T., Posner, M.I., Mintun, M., & Raichle, M.E. (1988). Positron emission tomographic studies of the cortical anatomy of single-word processing. *Nature, 331,* 585-589.

Plante, E., Swisher, L., & Vance, R. (1989). Anatomical correlates of normal and impaired language in a set of dizygotic twins. *Brain and Language, 37,* 643-655.

Plante, E., Swisher, L., Vance, R., & Rapcsak, S. (1991). MRI findings in boys with Specific Language Impairment. *Brain and Language, 41,* 52-66.

Pool, K.D., Freeman, F.J., & Finitzo, T. (1987). Brain electrical activity mapping: applications to vocal motor control disorders. In H.F.M. Peters, & W. Hulstijn (Eds.), *Speech Motor Dynamics in Stuttering* (pp. 151-160). Vienna: Springer-Verlag.

Pool, K.D., Devous, M.D., Freeman, F.J., Watson, B.C., & Finitzo, T. (1991). Regional cerebral blood flow in developmental stutterers. *Archives of Neurology, 48,* 509-512.

Rao, S.M., Binder, J.R., Bandettini, P.A., Hammeke, T.A., Yetkin, F.Z., & Jesmanowicz, A. (1993). Functional magnetic resonance imaging of complex human movements. *Neurology, 43,* 2311-2318.

Richards, P.M., Persinger, M.A., & Koren, S.A. (1993). Modification of activation and evaluation properties of narratives by weak complex magnetic field patterns that simulate limbic burst firing. *International Journal of Neuroscience, 71,* 71-85.

Rueckert, L., Appollonio, I., Grafman, J., Jezzard, P., Johnson, R., Jr., & LeBihan, D. (1994). Magnetic resonance imaging functional activation of left frontal cortex during covert word production. *Journal of Neuroimaging, 4,* 67-70.

Sandyk, R. (1993). The effects of picoTesla range magnetic fields on perceptual organization and visual memory in Parkinsonism. *International Journal of Neuroscience, 73,* 207-219.

Schad, L.R., Trost, U., Knopp, M.V., Muller, E., & Lorenz, W.J. (1993). Motor cortex stimulation measured by magnetic resonance imaging on a standard 1.5 T clinical scanner. *Magnetic Resonance Imaging, 11,* 461-464.

Schad, L.R., Wenz, F., Knopp, M.V., Baudendistel, K., Muller, E., & Lorenz, W.J. (1994). Functional

2D and 3D magnetic resonance imaging of motor cortex stimulated at high spatial resolution using standard 1.5 T imager. *Magnetic Resonance Imaging, 12,* 9-15.

Schultz, R.T., Cho, N.K., Staib, L.H., Kier, L.E., Fletcher, J.M., Shaywitz, S.E., Shankweiler, D.P., et al. (1994). Brain morphology in normal and dyslexic children: The influence of sex and age. *Annals of Neurology, 35,* 732-742.

Tamas, L.B., Shibasaki, T., Horikoshi, S., & Ohye, C. (1993). General activation of cerebral metabolism with speech: A PET study. *International Journal of Psychophysiology, 14,* 199-208.

Terao, Y., Ugawa, Y., Sakai, K., Uesaka, Y., Kohara, N., & Kanasawa, I. (1994). Transcranial stimulation of the leg area of the motor cortex in humans. *Acta Neurological Scandinavica, 89,* 378-383.

Tyszka, J.M., Grafton, S.T., Chew, W., Woods, R.P., & Colletti, P.M. (1994). Parceling of mesial frontal motor areas during ideation and movement using functional magnetic resonance imaging at 1.5 Tesla. *Annals of Neurology, 35,* 746-749.

Wasserman, E.M., Fuhr, P., Cohen, L.G., & Hallett, M. (1991). Effects of transcranial magnetic stimulation on ipsilateral muscles. *Neurology, 41,* 1795-1799.

Watson, B.C., Freeman, F.J., Devous, M.D., Chapman, S.B., Finitzo, T., & Pool, K.D. (1994). Linguistic performance and regional cerebral blood flow in persons who stutter. *Journal of Speech and Hearing Research, 37,* 1221-1228.

Watson, B.C., Freeman, F.J., Pool, K.D., Finitzo, T., Chapman, S.B., & Mendelsohn, D. (1991). Laryngeal reaction time profiles in spasmodic dysphonia: Relationship to cortical electrophysiologic abnormality. *Journal of Speech and Hearing Research, 34,* 269-278.

Watson, B.C., Pool, K.D., et al. (1992). Brain blood flow related to acoustic laryngeal reaction time in adult developmental stutterers. *Journal of Speech and Hearing Research, 35,* 555-561.

Wells, B.G., & Moore, W.H. Jr. (1990). EEG alpha asymmetries in stutterers and non-stutterers: Effects of linguistic variables on hemispheric processing and fluency. *Neuropsychologia, 28,* 1295-1305.

Wohlert, A.B. (1993). Event-related brain potentials preceding speech and nonspeech oral movements of varying complexity. *Journal of Speech and Hearing Research, 36,* 897-905.

Wu, J.C., & Maguire, G., et al. (1995). A positron emission tomography [18F] deoxyglucose study of developmental stuttering. *Neuroreport, 6,* 501-505.

Zimmerman, G., & Knott, J. (1974). Slow potentials of the brain related to speech processing in normal speakers and stutterers. *Electroencephalography and Clinical Neurophysiology, 37,* 599-607.

Speech Production: Motor Control, Brain Research and Fluency Disorders
W. Hulstijn, H.F.M. Peters and P.H.H.M. Van Lieshout, editors

Chapter 21

MULTI-PERSPECTIVE APPROACHES TO THE CORTICAL REPRESENTATION OF SPEECH PERCEPTION AND PRODUCTION: ELECTRICAL CORTICAL STIMULATION AND ELECTRICAL CORTICAL RECORDING

Barry Gordon, Dana Boatman, Nathan E. Crone, Ronald P. Lesser

The relationship between speech perception and production was investigated at the cortical level of the human system by using the clinical techniques of direct cortical electrical interference and direct cortical recording. This testing was performed as part of a routine clinical protocol to map speech and language functions in nine epilepsy patients prior to focal resection surgery. Relatively localized and temporary disruptions in cortical processing generated by the electrical interference technique identified a single site on the lateral posterior cortical surface of each patient where speech perception, as measured by syllable discrimination, and speech production, measured by oral word reading and naming, were both impaired. These results were corroborated by direct cortical electrical recordings obtained when the same perception and production tasks were performed without electrical interference. Our preliminary data suggest that speech perception and production share in common certain neural, and perhaps also functional, resources.

ISSUES AND TRADITIONAL APPROACHES

Whether and how speech production is linked to speech perception has long been debated in psycholinguistics and cognitive neuroscience. At one extreme in this debate is the position that the two are totally distinct, functionally as well as anatomically. At the other extreme is the claim that the two are fundamentally identical processes, and depend upon the same neural structures and mechanisms.

Most of the neurobiologic evidence that has been brought to bear on these theories has, until recently, come from patients who had suffered accidental brain injuries, typically ischemic strokes. For the most part, this evidence had been interpreted as clearly showing functional and anatomic differences between speech perception and speech production. Patients could be found with speech comprehension deficits (typically, but not always, occurring as part of a syndrome of Wernicke's aphasia), often with impairments in lower-level auditory functions, such as consonants discrimination (*pat versus* bat). Yet these patients did not have comparable speech production impairments. Conversely, there were patients with marked impairments in speech production (usually occurring as part of the syndrome of

Broca's aphasia), yet no apparent difficulties with speech comprehension or with lower-level speech perceptual functions. Speech perceptual difficulties and Wernicke's aphasia were strongly associated with lesions of the dominant (left), posterior temporal lobe and inferior parietal regions; speech production difficulties and Broca's aphasia, with lesions of the dominant, posterior inferior frontal lobe. The evidence for a functional as well as neuroanatomic separation between speech perception and speech production seemed clear.

However, later functional and neuroanatomic studies showed that this dissociation was less clearly defined than originally supposed. It was found that both Broca's and Wernicke's aphasics had difficulty discriminating fine phonetic feature differences between consonants such as voicing and place-of-articulation (Basso et al., 1977; Blumstein et al., 1977; Blumstein et al., 1984; Miceli et al., 1978, 1980); vowel discrimination, however, remained relatively intact. These subtle perceptual deficits may not have been apparent in the earlier studies, which relied primarily on assessing patients' understanding of conversational speech. The presence of perceptual impairments in both Wernicke's and Broca's aphasics suggested that the cortical representations of speech perception and production were less distinct than was originally assumed.

Although studies of patients with accidental focal lesions have proven very valuable, certain inevitable methodological limitations have recently become clearer. For example, the perceptual deficits observed in aphasic patients may have existed premorbidly, as a result of age-related hearing loss (presbycusis) or other acquired hearing problems. Consonant discriminations is particularly sensitive to age-related hearing loss.

A second concern with aphasia studies was that it became apparent that the clinical syndromes of Broca's and Wernicke's aphasia actually had overlapping neuroanatomies, in some cases. At the very least, the lesions responsible for persistent syndromes were relatively large, often greater than 5 cm^2 (Selnes et al., 1984). Therefore, any combination of perceptual and production deficits could have been the accidental result of simultaneous damage to functionally distinct cortical regions. Lastly, it began to become clearer that the mind and brain were not inert after lesioning ; recovery strategies and mechanisms occurred which may not have been operating in the normal system (Gordon et al., 1994), and which therefore may make it problematic to infer the normal mechanisms from chronic, post-lesion performance.

Recently, techniques have been developed which allow assessment of regional cerebral blood flow *in vivo*. PET and functional MRI therefore permit studies of normal individuals, an immense advantage. PET and functional MRI also allow the entire brain to be examined, another immense advantage over relying on the accidental location of natural lesions. However, studies that use either PET and functional MRI must rely on a different logic than do studies using lesions; they must infer how cognitive functions are related to regional changes from correlations, rather than from more definitive alterations in the cognitive functions. This logic has been well developed (Sarter et al., 1996), but it is more complicated and less definitive than lesion logic. In addition, both PET and functional MRI use changes in blood flow or blood oxygenation as their markers, which makes them insensitive to the time scales thought to be important for on-line processing of speech perceptual contrasts (which are on the order of 10s of milliseconds).

Recent developments in clinical brain mapping at our institution, and at others, have produced a pair of techniques that when combined can circumvent many of the problems of these other approaches. The two techniques are direct cortical electrical interference and direct cortical electrical recording. Direct cortical electrical interference, which we describe first, is based on the lesion-deficit approach but involves functional, as opposed to structural, lesioning.

DIRECT CORTICAL ELECTRICAL INTERFERENCE

Direct cortical electrical interference has been used intraoperatively and, more recently, extraoperatively, to identify regions in the language dominant (usually left) hemisphere that are associated with specific language functions; such information is needed for planning focal resection surgery for intractable left temporal lobe epilepsy (Penfield & Roberts, 1959; Fried et al., 1981; Lesser et al., 1987; Creützfeldt et al., 1989). Extraoperative electrical interference testing is made possible by surgically implanted, subdural electrode arrays that remain indwelling for periods of days to weeks (Lesser et al., 1987, 1994; Hart et al., 1992). This approach typically permits more extensive investigation than intraoperative testing (Lesser et al., 1987, 1994). By applying direct cortical electrical interference to closely spaced electrodes implanted on the cortical surface, it is possible to induce relatively localized (~ 1 cm^2), temporary aphasic deficits in patients who otherwise perform within normal limits.

We have studied the effects of extraoperative electrical interference testing on speech perception and production in nine patients, who were selected from a larger pool of patients who were candidates for focal resection surgery. All nine were under the age of 40 (21-39 years) and were selected on the basis of stringent criteria developed to approximate the normally functioning system. Selection criteria included: no history of hearing or speech disorders, normal pure tone hearing thresholds, IQ scores within normal limits, no evidence of structural abnormality on MRI, and left hemisphere dominance for language confirmed by intracarotid sodium amobarbital testing. In all cases, in these and subsequently described studies, subjects had given full informed consent for both the clinical and the research activities, as approved by Johns Hopkins' Joint Committee on Clinical Investigation.

All patients underwent surgical implantation of electrode arrays in the subdural space over the lateral left cortical surface. A 6x8 electrode array was surgically placed in the subdural space over the lateral left cortical surface of each patient, according to pre-established clinical protocols (Uematsu et al., 1990; Lesser et al., 1994). The electrode array covered the temporal and inferior parietal regions. Portions of the pre-central motor area, inferior frontal and occipital lobes also received electrodes, with the extent and location of this coverage determined by the specifics of each patient's clinical circumstances. Additional electrode coverage was provided by implantation of one or more strips of electrodes in three of the five patients. Electrodes were composed of platinum iridium disks that were 3 millimeters in diameter, with 2.3 millimeters exposed surface. Electrodes were spaced 10 millimeters apart (center-to-center) and embedded in medical-grade silastic. Electrode locations were determined from intraoperative photographs, CT scans, and from three-dimensional MRI reconstructions of each patient's brain. Electrode positions were normalized across patients by using a standard brain atlas (Talairach & Tournoux, 1988) and referencing the Sylvian fissure and the anterior-posterior dimensions of the superior temporal lobe.

The electrical interference testing procedures have been described elsewhere (Lesser et al., 1994; Uematsu et al., 1990). Briefly, electrical interference was produced by 300-microsecond square-wave pulses, of alternating polarity, at a rate of 50 pulses per second, for 5-second intervals. The electrical current was generated between adjacent electrode pairs. Prior to testing, a threshold current for sensorimotor effects or afterdischarges (if any) was established by gradual (0.5-1.0 mA) increases in stimulus intensity. If no sensorimotor effects or afterdischarges were present, the current was set to a maximal level of 15 milliamps. In the event of afterdischarges, testing was conducted at the next lowest current level that did not produce afterdischarges. No language testing was performed at sites where sensory or motor effects were obtained.

We will focus here on the results of testing speech discrimination, reading, and repetition at all electrodes covering each patient's lateral left cortex. Speech discrimination testing is conducted by computer using digitized (44 kHz) natural speech tokens. Patients make judgments regarding the acoustic similarity or difference of 80 consonant-vowel (CV) stimulus pairs (e.g., /pa-ba/) presented in AB format. Stimulus pairs were contrasted by either their consonants or their vowels. Consonantal contrasts were based on classic phonetic feature differences that included: voicing (e.g., *pa-ba*), place-of-articulation (e.g., *pa-ta*), and manner-of-articulation (e.g., *pa-ma*). Vocalic contrasts were by vowel height and relative fronting-backing. Responses were made by pressing one of two color-coded buttons. The oral reading test used orthographic (written) versions ($N=50$) of the same stimuli. Patients were asked to read each stimulus aloud. Their responses are recorded onto audio tape. The repetition task used single tokens ($N=50$) of the auditory speech discrimination stimuli (e.g., un-paired). Patients were asked to repeat exactly what was heard. All auditory stimuli were presented binaurally through insert earphones. Patients' responses were scored as correct or incorrect. Responses occurring after the 5-second stimulation period were scored as incorrect.

Data Analysis Issues

Analysis of patients' baseline (without electrical interference) and electrical interference data raised a number of statistical issues. One issue is that all of our patients basically perform at ceiling without electrical interference. Therefore, conventional distribution-based parametric statistical inferences could not be used. Instead, paired comparisons between each patient's baseline and electrical interference performance were performed with the non-parametric McNemar's test (Armitage & Berry, 1994).

Second, conventional analysis of variance (ANOVA) procedures, such as the two-sample *t*-test procedures, were not suitable for analyzing patients' speech discrimination performance by phonetic feature (e.g., voicing, place-of-articulation, vowel height) because ANOVA procedures assume a continuous dependent variable and require that the variance of the dependent variable be the same for all trials. In our studies, proportions correct were discrete measures, and that discreteness was important because of the small numbers of trials in each comparison. For the proportion correct, the variance depends on the probability of a correct answer. This is also important for comparisons in which the probability of a correct answer differs between the tasks compared, especially when one of the tasks has a very low or very high probability. Unlike the first issue, this cannot be alleviated by large numbers of trials. For these reasons, analysis of our patients' speech discrimination performance was accomplished by directly estimating and analyzing relative odds (odds ratios). In addition to computing odds ratios, within-patient comparisons were performed with Mantel-Haenszel Chi Square Tests to ensure that our sample size did not affect our results. The Mantel-Haenszel Test is based on conditional likelihood functions and, therefore, is less sensitive to the problematic effects of small sample sizes (Armitage & Berry, 1994).

PRELIMINARY RESULTS

Speech discrimination deficits were associated with one, and only one electrode site per patient, the location of which was on the lateral left posterior superior temporal gyrus (Boatman et al. 1995). Analyses of patients' discrimination errors revealed significantly more consonant errors than vowel discrimination errors (Boatman et al., in press). In other words, the odds ratio confidence intervals were greater than 1.0 in all cases (and $p < 0.04$, Mantel-Haenszel Chi Square test). Of particular interest was the finding that *none* of the consonant phonetic feature comparisons tested (voice, place, manner) yielded significant differences (Boatman et al., 1994). Additional testing confirmed that patients were able to extract appropriate acoustic cues for phonetic feature mapping (e.g., formant frequency transitions).

Oral reading and repetition were both impaired at the same site where speech discrimination deficits were elicited in all patients. Production impairments were characterized primarily by speech arrest. For all within patient comparisons, odds ratios differed significantly from 1.0 at the 0.05 alpha level (odds ratios ≥ 2.47). In other words, the odds of observing repetition or oral reading errors were at least 2.5 times greater if syllable discrimination errors were also elicited at the same electrode site. At immediately adjacent electrode sites, oral reading, repetition, and speech discrimination remained relatively intact in all patients tested.

CORTICAL ELECTRICAL RECORDING

We have recently coupled the localization data obtained through cortical stimulation with maps of brain activation generated by Electrocorticographic Spectral Analysis (ESA). This technique utilizes direct electrocorticographic recordings through the same indwelling electrode arrays used for cortical stimulation. By analyzing changes in the power spectrum of cortical electrical activity during syllable discrimination, it is possible to map the spatial distribution of task related cortical activation. While multiple frequency bands were analyzed, we will focus here on spectral changes in the alpha frequency band (8-13 Hz).

Three of the nine patients who participated in the electrical interference studies were tested. We used the same CV syllable discrimination task (AB format) used in the electrical interference studies, but with two modifications for the format of ESA testing: 1) the number of trials was increased to 200, which was accomplished by re-duplicating the original stimulus set; and 2) we maintained a consonant syllable duration of 300 msec. The first modification was necessary in order to obtain a sufficient number of trials for averaging in the power spectrum analysis. The second modification was made in order to maximize the homogeneity of the stimuli's temporal envelopes across trials, so that averages of the ESA power spectrum across trials could be made with a consistent relationship between functional and brain activation. The oral word reading and repetition tasks and stimuli were identical to those of the electrical interference studies.

Electrocorticographic signals were digitally recorded (1 kHz sampling rate) from all electrodes in and around the surface of perisylvian cortex. We then filtered these signals and used the Fast Fourier Transform to calculate the spectral power for a series of frequency bands from 5 to 100 Hz--including alpha (8-13 Hz)--during consecutive 200 msec time segments. These spectral power measurements were compared across time segments using one-way analysis of variance in order to identify statistically significant ($p < 0.0001$) changes from the average baseline condition (1 second pre-stimulus). Significant changes were identified using paired t-tests (correcting for multiple comparisons) to identify those particular post-stimulus time segments during which significant changes took place. Spatiotemporal maps of the magnitude of brain activation were then generated using the percentage change in average (alpha) power.

Initial results of the speech discrimination data indicate that the initial source of electrocortical change (first 200 msec) occurs at the same electrode site where speech perception was impaired with electrical interference in the same patients. This same electrode site was implicated during the patterns of electrocortical change for oral word reading and repetition. Indeed for repetition, the initial source of the electrocortical change (first 200 msec) was localized to the exact same electrode site.

GENERAL DISCUSSION

Our preliminary electrical interference results suggest that speech discrimination is critically dependent on a relatively circumscribed region of the lateral left posterior superior temporal gyrus when language is lateralized to the left hemisphere. This speech discrimination region is located within the traditional Wernicke's area, thereby corroborating claims in the aphasia literature that the posterior perisylvian cortex is particularly crucial for auditory speech processing (Wernicke, 1874; Geschwind, 1979). The dissociation between our patients' consonant and vowel discrimination performance also concurs with previous reports in the aphasia literature, and suggests that consonant processing may have different neural, and by extension functional, requirements than vowel processing.

Syllable discrimination and oral reading and repetition errors co-occurred at a single posterior superior temporal lobe electrode site in each patient. This finding challenges the classical two-center view that speech perception and production are subserved by entirely distinct cortical resources. Our data suggest instead that speech perception and production share particular neural, and by extension, functional resources.

Our findings differ in two respects from those reported in the aphasia literature. One difference is that we did not elicit phonetic feature effects. In other words, our patients did not perform worse when asked to discriminate consonant pairs that differed by a particular phonetic feature (e.g., voicing, place, manner). A second difference is that speech discrimination deficits were not obtained with electrical interference testing in Broca's area.

The lack of phonetic feature effect with cortical interference testing points to an important difference between the spatial resolution of structural *versus* functional lesions. Phonetic feature effects have been reported for patients with structural lesions (e.g., strokes), which frequently involve subcortical structures in addition to cortex (Tallal & Newcombe, 1978; Blumstein et al., 1977; Miceli et al., 1978). Conversely, electrical interference generates relatively circumscribed functional lesions that are localized primarily to cortex (Nathan et al. 1994). An important caveat is that the lack of phonetic feature dissociation is predicated upon the anatomic resolution of the cortical stimulation, approximately 1 cm^2. We cannot exclude the possibility that a finer level of cortical resolution would result in the separability of feature type. It is the case, however, that these electrical interference data help to establish upper boundaries on the extent to which potential feature dissociations can be obtained.

Our results also fail to corroborate previous reports that speech discrimination is associated with Broca's area as well as more posterior cortical regions. The cortical coupling between perception and production in our patients appears to occur in posterior temporal lobe, but not the inferior frontal lobe. It may be argued again that naturally occurring structural lesions tend to be relatively large, potentially involving more than one functionally distinct cortical region (e.g. anterior and posterior). It may also be the case that speech perception and production are coupled at different functional levels. For example, we frequently find auditory comprehension deficits during electrical interference testing in Broca's area. Moreover, preliminary data suggest that phonological encoding, as measured by phoneme identification, may also be associated with Broca's area (Boatman & Gordon, in preparation). Thus, while syllable discrimination and production appear to share the neural resources of a relatively circumscribed area of the left posterior superior temporal lobe, other aspects of speech perception and production may be coupled with the support of different cortical resources, including Broca's area.

Our functional lesion-deficit studies provide evidence that syllable discrimination and production are not subserved by entirely distinct cortical systems, but rather appear to share neural, and by extension functional, resources. Application of stringent inclusion criteria combined with patients' high level of baseline (no electrical interference) accuracy, also helped to ensure closer approximation to the normal speech processing system than has typically been possible in studies of patients with fixed, relatively large structural lesions.

The same pattern of results was obtained when a subset of the same patients were re-tested using a different methodological approach, namely electrical recording. The convergence of these data further corroborate our findings. Moreover, the electrical recording data provided crucial information on the time-course of speech perception at the cortex, information that cannot be obtained using only the lesion-deficit approaches.

How generalizable are our results to the normally functioning system? It is important to ask this question because our data are elicited largely from patient populations. A clear advantage of functional activation techniques such as PET over lesion-deficit studies is that they can provide repeated measures data on normal subjects. To help address this question, we have been conducting a series of PET studies looking at changes in cerebral blood flow associated with the uptake of oxygen labeled water (O^{15}) during speech discrimination in normal right-handed volunteers. Initial analyses of data from 6 subjects (3 male, 3 female) showed activation of the posterior superior temporal gyrus of both hemispheres during speech discrimination, with greater activation in the left temporal gyrus. This area is considered part of the traditional Wernicke's area and is the same region that when damaged by stroke leads to receptive (auditory) aphasia. Interestingly, we did not find activation of Broca's area during speech discrimination as might have been predicted from the structural lesion-deficit studies described earlier. Whether this is because of limits of the respective techniques, or whether a more unitary explanation can be devised, cannot be determined from our data so far.

Although functional activation techniques such as PET help to identify cortical regions that are activated in association with speech and language in the normally functioning system, they cannot tell us to what extent those regions are *critical* for speech and language. Information on the relative importance of different cortical sites identified by functional activation techniques continues to be best determined by the lesion-deficit approach. Functional deficits associated with lesions to a particular region of cortex help to identify cortical areas that are either themselves crucial for language processing, or that support connections (i.e. white matter fibers) that are crucial for language processing.

By coupling cortical electrical interference and cortical electrical recording we obtain, in some sense, the best of both the lesion-deficit and functional activation methodological approaches. Our preliminary findings suggest that a multi-perspective approach to studying the same functions in the same subjects can offer some unique perspectives on complex issues such as the relationship between speech perception and production. Additional research is clearly needed to further explore the potential advantages of multi-technique approaches to the study of speech and language in the brain.

NOTES

[1]   This chapter is based, in part, on presentations at the 1995 Meeting of the Academy of Aphasia and at the 1996 3rd International Conference on Speech Motor Production and

Fluency Disorders in Nijmegen.

[2] This work was supported by grants from The National Institute of Neurological Disorders and Stroke (RO1-NS26553, RO1-29973, K08 NS01821), The National Institute on Deafness and Other Communication Disorders (R03-DC01881), the Seaver Foundation, the Johns Hopkins Center for Speech Processing, The Pew Charitable Trust, and the McDonnell-Pew Program in Cognitive Neuroscience. We thank Dr. John Hart (supported by NIDCD's K08 DC00099) for providing the electrode location data.

REFERENCES

Armitage, P. & Berry, G. (1994). *Statistical Methods in Medical Research*. Oxford: Blackwell Scientific Publications.

Basso, A., Casati, G., & Vignolo, L. A. (1977). Phonemic identification defect in aphasia. *Cortex, 13*, 84-95.

Boatman, D.F., Lesser, R.P., Hall, C.B., & Gordon, B. (1994). Auditory perception of segmental features: A functional-neuroanatomic study. *Journal of Neurolinguistics, 8*, 225-234.

Boatman, D., Lesser, R.P., & Gordon, B. (1995). Auditory speech processing in the left temporal lobe: An electrical interference study. *Brain and Language, 51*, 269-290.

Boatman, D., Hall, C., Goldstein, M.H., Lesser, R., & Gordon, B. (in press). Neuroperceptual differences in consonant and vowel discrimination: As revealed by direct cortical electrical interference. *Cortex*.

Boatman, D. & Gordon, B. (In preparation). The cortical coupling of speech perception and production: As revealed by direct cortical electrical interference.

Blumstein, S.E., Tartter, V.C., Nigro, G., & Statlender, S. (1984). Acoustic cues for the perception of articulation in aphasia. *Brain and Language, 22*, 128-149.

Blumstein, S.E., Cooper, W.E., Zurif, E.B., & Caramazza, A. (1977). The perception and production of voice-onset time in aphasia. *Neuropsychologia, 15*, 371-383.

Creutzfeldt, O., Ojemann, G., & Lettich, E. (1989). Neuronal activity in human lateral temporal lobe: I. Responses to speech. *Experimental Brain Research, 77*, 476-489.

Fried, M., Ojemann, G.A., & Fetz, E. (1981). Language related potential specific to human language cortex. *Science, 212*, 353-356.

Geschwind, N. (1979). Specializations of the human brain. *The Brain*. San Francisco: W.H. Freeman.

Gordon, B., Hart, J., Lesser, R.P., & Selnes, O.A. (1994). Recovery and its implications for cognitive neuroscience. *Brain and Language, 47*, 521-524.

Hart, J., Jr. & Gordon, B. (1992). Neural subsystems of object knowledge. *Nature, 359*, 60-64.

Lesser, R.P., Lueders, H., Klem, G., Dinner, D.S., Morris, H.H., Hahn, J.F., & Wyllie, E. (1987). Extraoperative cortical functional localization in patients with epilepsy. *Journal of Clinical Neurophysiology, 4*, 27-53.

Lesser, R., Gordon, B., & Uematsu, S. (1994). Electrical stimulation and language. *Journal of Clinical Neurophysiology, 11*, 191-204.

Miceli, G., Gainotti, G., Caltagirone, C., & Masullo, C. (1980). Some aspects of phonological impairment in aphasia. *Brain and Language, 11*, 159-169.

Miceli, G., Caltagirone, C., Gainotti, G., & Payer-Rigo, P. (1978). Discrimination of voice versus place contrasts in aphasia. *Brain and Language, 6*, 47-51.

Nathan, S.S., Sinha, S.R., Gordon, B., Lesser, R.P., & Thakor, N.V. (1993). Determination of current density distributions generated by electrical stimulation of the human cerebral cortex. *Electrocephalography and Clinical Neurophysiology, 86*, 183-192.

Penfield, W. & Roberts, L. (1959). In *Speech and Brain Mechanisms*. Princeton, NJ: Princeton University Press.

Sarter, M., Bernston, G., & Cacioppo, J. (1996). Brain imaging and cognitive neuroscience: Toward strong inference in attributing function to structure. *American Psychologist, 51*, 13-21.

Selnes, O.A., Niccum, N., Knopman, D., & Rubens, A.B. (1984). Recovery of single word comprehension: CT-scan correlates. *Brain and Language, 21*, 72-84.

Talairach, J., & Tournoux, P. (1988). *Co-Planar Stereotactic Atlas of the Human Brain*. New York: Thieme.

Tallal, P., & Newcombe, F. (1978). Impairment of auditory perception and language comprehension in dysphasia. *Brain and Language, 5*, 13-34.

Uematsu, S., Lesser, R.P., Fisher, R.S., Krauss, G.L., Hart, J., Vining, E.P., Freeman, J., & Gordon, B. (1990). Tailored resection of epileptogenic cerebral tissue with aid of a subdural grid-electrode. *Second International Cleveland Clinic Symposium.*

Wernicke, C. (1874). The aphasic symptom complex: A psychological study on a neurological basis. Cohen & Wartofsky (Eds.) *Boston Studies in the Philosophy of Science, 4*, Boston: Reidel.

Speech Production: Motor Control, Brain Research and Fluency Disorders
W. Hulstijn, H.F.M. Peters and P.H.H.M. Van Lieshout, editors

Chapter 22

PET RESEARCH IN LANGUAGE PRODUCTION

Peter Indefrey

The aim of this paper is to discuss an inherent difficulty of PET (and fMRI) research in language production. On the one hand, language production presupposes some degree of freedom for the subject, on the other hand, interpretability of results presupposes restrictions of this freedom. This difficulty is reflected in the existing PET literature in some neglect of the general principle to design experiments in such a way that the results do not allow for alternative interpretations. It is argued that by narrowing down the scope of experiments a gain in interpretability can be achieved.

INTRODUCTION

If asked whether there are specific areas in the human brain which subserve language production, most people would have the feeling that this question is too vague. It cannot be readily answered because the processing of written or spoken natural language not only involves different *levels*, such as a word level and a sentence level, but also different *kinds of processing*, such as phonological, lexical, syntactic, and semantic processing. It is highly probable that different neural populations subserve these different aspects of language production. Therefore, it does not seem to be a good idea to run a PET or fMRI study simply scanning subjects while they speak. Nonetheless, it has been done. In a PET study by Tamas et al. (1993), subjects were instructed to report how they spent the previous day. As might have been expected, the resulting brain activations comprise a widespread array of left and right areas of all cortical lobes and the cerebellum. One may call this the neural correlate of 'speech-from-memory', as the authors do, but any further interpretation can only be done in a circular way, such as ascribing memory functions to the observed hippocampal activations, because previous work has shown a relation between hippocampal activation and memory. This may be plausible, but the plausibility does not stem from the study at hand, which hasn't added anything to our knowledge. While it is true that to some extent the interpretation of every brain imaging study relies on the synopsis of results from the whole field for mutual validation and the generation of hypotheses, it is also true that this could not work, if not some study by its design had forced a certain interpretation without recurring to previous results. Obviously, the questions about language production that can be addressed successfully in this sense must be more restricted. For this reason, to date, most studies have focussed on language production on the word level, thereby avoiding the additional processing components involved in sentence (or even discourse) level processing.

GENERATING VERBS

Probably the most widely used word level production paradigm in PET and fMRI research is the Verb Generation Paradigm. It was introduced by Petersen et al. (1988), and in the form described here, first used in 1991 by Richard Wise and colleagues from the Hammersmith group in London. In this paradigm, subjects are auditorily presented with a common noun, such as CAKE and asked to produce subvocally as many appropriate verbs, such as 'bake' or 'eat', as they can think of before they hear the next noun. The paradigm today comes in a number of variations, such as presenting nouns visually or asking the subjects to respond aloud, the core of the task, however, has remained unchanged. The task is considered to involve an externally (by choice of the nouns and their presentation frequency) controlled 'semantic generation', that is, a semantically driven lexical search the result of which is the production of the verb. Since also in natural language the expression of a certain concept requires the search for a lexical item, it can be said that the Verb Generation Task must activate brain areas supporting this component of natural language production.

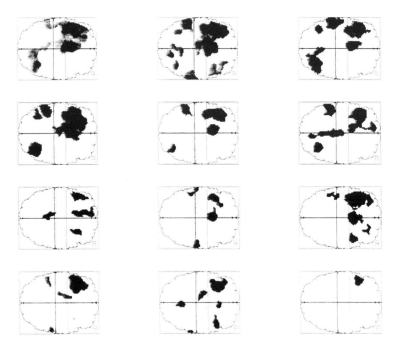

Figure 1. Individual center SPM analyses of a European multicenter PET experiment on verb generation. The subtraction images show transverse views of the significant (p < 0.20, corrected) regional cerebral blood flow (rCBF) increases during verb generation when compared with rest condition. (adapted from Poline et al., 1996)

In addition to that, it will activate brain areas supporting the subsequent retrieval of the lexically stored phonological word form and probably also secondary motor areas subserving the necessary preparation for spoken output.

The task has proven to be reliable in a recent European multi center study (Poline et al., 1996), for which the stimulus material was translated in seven different languages and subject pretraining, instructions and behavioral assessment were standarized. All data were submitted to a metaanalysis using the statistical parametric mapping (SPM) procedure. Figure 1 shows the high degree of between-center-reliability with respect to the locations of activated regions (centers with small-field-of-view PET cameras in the bottom row).

A further aim of this study was to raise the statistical power by running a pooled analysis over more than 60 subjects in order to reduce the number of false negatives, that is, to assess the number and extent of activated regions that in single center studies fail to become significant. As can be seen in Figure 2, this task does not only activate small specific areas of the brain, but most of the left frontal lobe along with some homologue areas of the right frontal lobe and large parts of the temporal lobes. While it is possible that all these areas indeed subserve the assumed processes, it is also reasonable to ask whether this task did not, after all, comprise additional cognitive components that may have been overlooked. When we look at some of the responses we obtained during the training session from one of the subjects whose data the Nijmegen/Duesseldorf/Juelich center contributed to the European multi center study (see Table 1), it becomes clear that the range of associated verbs cannot be accounted for by assuming a semantically guided search alone. While some of the produced verbs have a 'narrow' semantic relation to the presented noun (BANANA 'peel', TRUMPET 'blow'), many others have a more indirect relation in that they apply to objects in general ('put away').

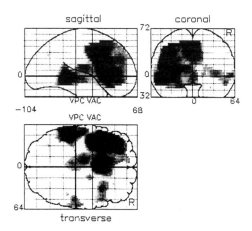

Figure 2. Pooled SPM analysis of the same experiment as in Figure 1 using data of nine centers with a large-field-of-view PET camera. Significant (p < 0.05, corrected) rCBF increases are displayed in three orthogonal views. (adapted from Poline et al. 1996)

Table 1. Responses to the Verb Generation Task

BANANA	peel, slip on, eat up, plant
TROUSERS	put on, wash, mend, buy, warm
CHAIR	sit, build, nail, sell, work, learn
GLASSES	clean, put on, step on, buy, see
TRUMPET	blow, make music, put away, hear, play
PENCIL	sharpen, break, put away, draw
BUTTON	tear off, close, open
BIRD	fly, eat up, sing
EAR	hear, pinch
DOOR	open, close, kick against

It is particularly problematic that the verbs are not mutually independent, but that they are produced in coherent sequences like 'blow, make music, put away' for TRUMPET or 'build, nail, sell' for CHAIR. These seem to be instances of small scenes that are either recalled from episodic memory or created ad hoc by the subject. In both cases additional processing components would be involved that might contribute to the observed extent of cortical activations. It seems, therefore, as if even a seemingly simple task like verb generation may at closer inspection contain a number of task components that are uncontrolled for. In this situation, it is impossible to attribute specific activation sites to isolated task components on the basis of the task design. It should be added that these problems are shared by a variation of the Verb Generation Paradigm where subjects only produce one verb to every given noun. Of course the episodic nature of verbal associations can then no longer be as easily detected because thematically linked verb sequences do not occur. The problems are also shared by another frequently used task, the Verbal Fluency Task, which is considered to consist in a 'phonologically' driven lexical search. Subjects are asked to produce as many nouns with a given letter as they can think of. While in this task subjects probably are less prone to use some episodic association strategy, they remain nonetheless unrestricted as to how they search for lexical items that meet the condition. Given the letter 'a', for example, some might go for a semantic strategy, producing 'ant, ape, antelope, ...', others might continue to follow the alphabetic route searching for words starting with 'ab...' then 'ac...' and so forth. Thus it remains unclear which additional cognitive processes may be involved in this task. In sum, language production tasks on the word level, although being much more restricted than a "What did You do yesterday?" task, in many cases are still to unrestricted to cope with the flexibility of human speakers on the conceptual level preceding language production.

GENERATING PHONOLOGICAL OUTPUT TO GRAPHEMIC INPUT

It has become clear that the question in functional imaging research is not so much "Can we *activate* certain cortical regions that are related to a specific cognitive task?" It is rather "Can we *isolate* those cortical regions that subserve the processing component we are interested in?" To give a positive answer to this question, we have to find control conditions that ideally allow for a unique interpretation of the resulting cortical activations. This will often mean that it is better to obtain interpretable results for a small processing component, for which it is possible to design adequate control conditions, than to obtain vague results which, because of a lack of adequate control, can only be interpreted speculatively or in a circular manner.

The processing component for which we tried to isolate the neural correlates in a PET experiment (Indefrey et al., 1995; Hagoort et al., in preparation) is grapheme-to-phoneme conversion. This process is one of two alternative routes to find the appropriate pronunciation for a given written input, the other one being lexical access to a stored phonological representation via a visual input lexicon. The functional distinction between the two pathways is supported by clinical findings (Figure 3 presents the visual-presentation pathways of the model of Patterson and Shewell (1987), which is based on clinical data), as well as by experimental data (see Carr & Pollatsek, 1985 for an overview). Grapheme-to-phoneme conversion relies on the fact that written language, at least in alphabetic and syllabic writing systems, has a non-arbitrary relation to spoken language. This means that it is possible to predict the pronunciation of a word from its spelling. The degree to which this prediction will be correct differs between languages (see Table 2). For languages with a high grapheme-to-phoneme correspondence, like Turkish, knowledge of the conversion rules suffices to pronounce every word correctly even without understanding the language, because there are practically no exceptions to those rules. English, on the other hand, is notorious for its very low grapheme-to-phoneme correspondence, making the pronunciation of an unknown word a risky thing. Just consider the four different pronunciations of the word-final letter string o-u-g-h in the words 'rough, plough, though, cough' or the idiosyncratic pronunciations of 'colonel' and 'gauge'. German, which was used in our PET experiment, lies somewhere between those extremes: correspondence rules will mostly generate the correct pronunciation, but there are exceptional words. Except for languages like Turkish where the writing is almost a phonetic transcription of the spoken language, the term 'grapheme-to-phoneme correspondence rule' is slightly misleading, because these rules are

Table 2. Grapheme-to-Phoneme Correspondence

	Language	Exceptional words
high		
↑	Turkish	none
	German	Agonie [agoˈniː], Begonie [beˈgoːnj]
		Kabel [ˈkɑːbl], Hotel [hoːˈtɛl]
↓	English	rough, plough, though, cough
low		shave, brave, have

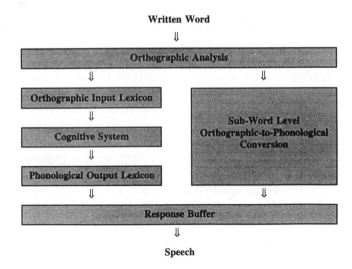

Figure 3. Dual pathway model for the pronunciation of written words. The model is based on clinical data. (adapted from Patterson & Shewell, 1987)

not simple one-to-one mappings of graphemes to phonemes, but rather a set of complex context-sensitive rules. This means that in order to predict the phonemic representation of a certain grapheme one has to inspect the preceding and following grapheme strings. Of course, we are not really dealing with conscious 'prediction' but with tacit linguistic knowledge. The intuitions of speakers of different languages about how to pronounce pseudowords demonstrate the operation of conversion rules (see Table 3). English and German share a rule which states that the quality of a vowel changes depending on whether the following consonant is written as a single or double letter. Exactly in which way the vowel changes, however, is different in the two languages. For Finnish speakers, on the other hand, single or double consonant letters do not indicate the vowel quality but whether the consonant itself has to be spoken short or long.

Grapheme-to-phoneme conversion seems to be an automatic process that is not only active when unknown written words have to be pronounced, but also in silent reading of known words.

Table 3. Pseudoword Pronunciation

	German	English	Finnish
pratte	[-at]	[-æti]	[-at:ɛ]
prate	[- :t]	[-eit]	[-atɛ]

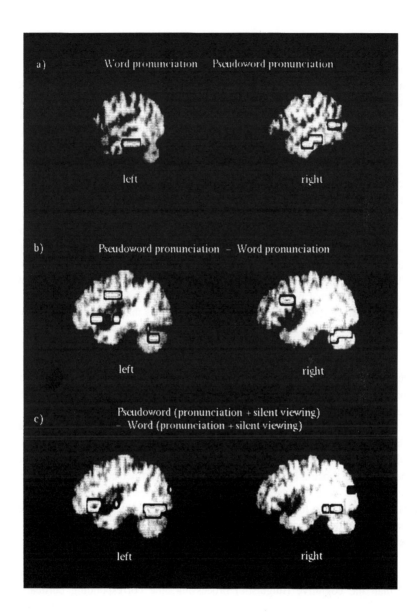

Figure 4. Subtraction images of a PET experiment on the reading of words and pseudowords. Significant (p < 0.05) rCBF increases in sagittal slices are projected onto corresponding slices of a standardized anatomical MR image. (From Hagoort et al., in preparation)

Thus, subjects need more time to reject visually wrong written sentences that are phonologically correct (e.g. "*He ran threw the streets.*" Baron, 1973; Doctor & Coltheart,

1980).

The crucial point for choosing grapheme-to-phoneme conversion as a processing component that can be successfully isolated in a PET experiment is that it clearly dissociates words and pseudowords. While the production of a phoneme code for words from written input can follow both the lexical and the conversion route, phoneme codes for pseudowords can only be generated through grapheme-to-phoneme conversion. Any additional cortical activation observed for pseudowords must be related to an enhanced recruitment of this process if visual and articulatory complexity are kept constant. In the PET experiment, we directly compared the activations for the conditions (1) Pronunciation of words and (2) Pronunciation of pseudowords. Figure 4 shows the significant activation differences for the subtractions (a) Pronunciation of words - pronunciation of pseudowords and (b) Pronunciation of pseudowords - pronunciation of words. The main finding in (a) is that the pronunciation of words results in a stronger bilateral activation of the middle and inferior temporal gyri than the pronunciation of pseudowords. This confirms previously reported data from other groups (Howard et al., 1992; Price et al., 1994,1996). According to the logic outlined above, however, it does not allow for a unique interpretation, because words have more than one additional property as compared to pseudowords. The observed activations may reflect lexical retrieval of a phoneme code as well as that of a meaning. They may even reflect cognitive processes subsequent to the lexical retrieval. This is different for the main finding in (b), an increase in activation of the left ventral pars triangularis of the inferior frontal gyrus (Broca's area) for pseudoword pronunciation as compared to word pronunciation. Since the only additional property of pseudowords is that their pronunciation relies on grapheme-to-phoneme conversion, the observed activation can be interpreted as being related to this process.

Admittedly, this is an idealized argumentation. The significant motor, premotor and cerebellar activations observed in (b) suggest that pseudowords were also articulatorily more demanding. It is possible to differentiate this motor output-related aspect of pseudowords from the linguistic process by taking into account two further conditions of the experiment, in which subjects read words and pseudowords without overt pronunciation. Although subjects did not speak in these conditions, there was some activation of motor areas relative to a baseline condition in which they silently viewed a fixation cross. This finding suggests that with word-like stimuli the subjects prepared pronunciation to a certain extent without actually executing it, which implies that they also produced a phonemic representation. If we assume that in the silent-reading conditions the motor output processing is more strongly reduced than the cognitive (linguistic) processing, the corresponding cortical activations should be relatively weaker in mean images combining the silent reading and the pronunciation conditions. On the other hand, cortical activations related to grapheme-to-phoneme conversion, which takes place in both conditions, should appear enhanced, due to an improved signal-to-noise ratio. Subtracting the mean image for words from that for pseudowords (c) reveals that the differential activation of Broca's area appears as clearly as before (now together with a bilateral activation of the fusiform gyri which probably reflects some aspect of the visual processing of word-like stimuli which is stronger for pseudowords in both the silent and the pronunciation conditions). Motor, premotor and cerebellar activations, however, no longer reach the significance level. This suggests that they are indeed related to some aspect of articulatory planning that is stronger for pseudowords. There are several possibilities what this aspect might be. A simple explanation might be based on residual segment level differences in the stimulus materials, such as a higher proportion of long as opposed to short vowels in the pseudoword stimuli. It is also possible (and, if true, unavoidable) that the mere fact that a word was novel motivated subjects to articulate it more distinctly. A third, and most interesting explanation would be the following: if motor programs were not only stored for single phonemes but also for syllables (see Levelt, 1989), then the novel words we used in our experiment would not only differ from the known ones in that they required the assembly of a phonemic representation by grapheme-to-phoneme conversion. They would also differ in that they required the assembly of syllable motor programs, because the pseudowords contained a certain proportion of pseudosyllables (all monosyllabic pseudowords, for instance, were by definition at the same time pseudosyllables), which could not possibly have been listed in a memory store. It seems plausible that such an assembly of syllable motor programs might recruit neurons in or near cortical areas known to be involved in motor planning. Interesting as it is, the hypothesis of a memory store for syllable motor programs cannot be confirmed (or rejected) on the basis of the evidence provided by the experiment at hand, simply because the experiment was not planned to confirm it. It nonetheless provides a nice endpoint for this paper, for it is another example of a problem a well designed PET experiment could successfully address, since pseudowords composed out of known syllables and pseudowords composed out of pseudosyllables would differ in just the relevant aspect.

One may object that PET experiments are too invasive, expensive, and time consuming to be devoted to such rather specialized questions. The answer to that is that only PET research on specialized and theoretically well motivated questions provides a chance to slowly create something like a firm ground of knowledge about the neural correlates of cognition.

REFERENCES

Baron, J. (1973) Phonemic stage not necessary for reading. *Quarterly Journal of Experimental Psychology*, 25, 241-246

Carr, T.H., & Pollatsek A. (1985) Recognizing Printed Words: A Look at Current Models. In Besner, D., Waller, T.G., & MacKinnon, G.E. (Eds.) *Reading Research: Advances in Theory and Practice, Vol.5* (pp. 1-81). New York, Academic Press

Doctor, E., & Coltheart, M. (1980) Children's use of phonological encoding when reading for meaning. *Memory and Cognition*, 8, 195-209

Hagoort, P., Indefrey, P., Brown, C., Herzog, H., & Seitz, R.J. (in preparation) The Reading of Words and Legal Nonwords: A [^{15}O]-Butanol PET Study.

Howard, D., Patterson, K., Wise, R., Brown, W.D., Friston, K., Weiller, C., & Frackowiak, R. (1992)

The Cortical Localization of the Lexicons. *Brain, 115,* 1769-1782

Indefrey, P., Hagoort, P., Brown, C., Law, I., Herzog, H., Steinmetz, H., & Seitz, R.J. (1995) The Reading of Words and Legal Nonwords: A [^{15}O]-Butanol PET Study. *Human Brain Mapping,* Suppl. *1,* 220.

Levelt, W.J.M. (1989) *Speaking. From Intention to Articulation.* (pp. 326-329) Cambridge (MA), London, MIT Press

Patterson, K., & Shewell, C. (1987) Speak and spell: dissociations and word class effects. In M. Coltheart, G. Sartori, & R. Job (Eds.), *The cognitive neuropsychology of language.* (pp. 273-294) London, Erlbaum

Petersen, S.E., Fox, P.T., Posner, M.I., Minton, M., & Raichle, M.E. (1988) Positron emission tomographic studies of the cortical anatomy of single-word processing. *Nature, 331,* 585-589

Poline, J-B., Vandenberghe, R., Holmes, A.P., Friston, K.J., & Frackowiak, R.S.J. (1996) Reproducibility of PET Activation Studies: Lessons from a Multi-Center European Experiment. *NeuroImage, 4,* 34-54

Price, C.J., Wise, R.J.S., Watson, J.D.G., Patterson, K., Howard, D., & Frackowiak, R.S.J. (1994) Brain activity during reading. The effects of exposure duration and task. *Brain, 117,* 1255-1269

Price, C.J., Wise, R.J.S., & Frackowiak, R.S.J. (1996) Demonstrating the Implicit Processing of Visually Presented Words and Pseudowords. *Cerebral Cortex, 6,* 62-70.

Tamas, L.B., Shibasaki, T., Horikoshi, S., & Ohye, C. (1993) General activation of cerebral metabolism with speech: a PET study. *International Journal of Psychophysiology, 14,* 199-208

Wise, R., Chollet, F., Hadar, U., Friston, K., Hoffner, E., & Frackowiak, R. (1991) Distribution of Cortical Neural Networks Involved in Word Comprehension and Word Retrieval. *Brain, 114,* 1803-1817

1997 Elsevier Science B.V.
Speech Production: Motor Control, Brain Research and Fluency Disorders
W. Hulstijn, H.F.M. Peters and P.H.H.M. Van Lieshout, editors

Chapter 23

A TYPICAL LATERALIZATION OF HEMISPHERAL ACTIVITY IN DEVELOPMENTAL STUTTERING: AN $H_2{}^{15}O$ POSITRON EMISSION TOMOGRAPHY STUDY.

A.R. Braun, M. Varga, S. Stager, G. Schulz, S. Selbie, J.M. Maisog, R.E. Carson, C.L. Ludlow

Cerebral blood flow was measured with $H_2{}^{15}O$ and positron emission tomography (PET) in order to assess dynamic brain function in adults who had stuttered since childhood. PET scans were performed during oral motor control tasks and speech tasks designed to evoke stuttering. Speech samples were acquired simultaneously and quantitatively compared with the PET images. Stuttering subjects differed markedly in the formulation and expression of language, failing to demonstrate left hemispheric lateralization typically observed in controls; instead, regional responses were either absent, bilateral, or lateralized to the right hemisphere. Covariance analyses indicated that activation of left hemispheric regions may be related to the production of stuttered speech, while activation of right hemispheric regions may represent compensatory processes associated with the production of fluent speech.

INTRODUCTION

A number of causative factors have been proposed for developmental stuttering. Pathophysiological theories have implicated abnormalities in language development (Bates, 1976), dysfunctional auditory monitoring of speech output (Rosenfeld & Jerger, 1984), speech planning or programming difficulties (McKay, 1982), and sequelae of psychological trauma (Wyatt, 1969). The concept that incomplete or abnormal patterns of cerebral hemispheric dominance characterize this disorder was first advanced in the 1920's (Orton, 1928; Travis, 1931). Since that time evidence for altered lateralization patterns - in particular, greater right hemispheric activation - has accumulated in a number of studies utilizing a variety of techniques (Moore, 1990), but the categorical nature of these findings has remained uncertain: increased activity in the right hemisphere, for example, could represent either functional competition with intact or compensation for dysfunctional left hemispheric mechanisms. The issue has never been resolved. In spite of a wealth of data, the pathophysiology of stuttering, and the brain mechanisms which may underlie it, remain an enigma.

Imaging using $H_2{}^{15}O$ and PET provides a means of examining the activity of brain areas in both hemispheres during symptom production. The H$_2$^{15}O technique furthermore permits individuals to be scanned while performing several different types of tasks. Subtraction of a task of interest from an appropriately chosen control task highlights the activity of those areas of the brain which differ between the two conditions. Of interest to the question of hemispheric function in stuttering, we chose to compare an oral motor task devoid of linguistic content with a spontaneous narrative task in order to highlight areas that may be active during language formulation. A comparison between persons who do and persons who do not stutter would pinpoint any differences between the groups in brain regions activated during language formulation, allowing us to identify atypical patterns of hemispheric lateralization should these exist.

A second way of examining the question of hemispheric activity is to determine if the level of activity in a subset of brain regions is correlated with the degree of symptom production within persons who stutter. That is, we can determine which brain regions are more activate when speech is dysfluent and which are active as compare these with areas in which increased activity is correlated with the production of fluent speech. Atypical patterns of hemispheric lateralization should also be apparent using this approach.

METHODS

Subjects

Informed consent was obtained from all subjects after the risks, hazards and discomfort associated with these studies were explained. Control subjects included 8 females [36 $\pm$ 10 years of age (Mean 1 SD), range 24-50 years] and 12 males [33 $\pm$ 8, range 23-47 years]. Developmental stuttering subjects included 8 females [34 $\pm$ 11, range 23-51 years] and 10 males [37 $\pm$ 10, range 23-50 years]. Each subject performed all skilled manual functions (writing, throwing a ball, combing, using scissors or other tools, etc.) with the right hand. All subjects were free of medical or neuropsychiatric illnesses which might affect brain function on the basis of history and physical examination, baseline laboratory evaluation and magnetic resonance brain imaging. The diagnosis of developmental stuttering conformed to DSM-IV criteria; symptom intensity during the scans ranged from mild to severe.

Scanning Methods

PET scans were performed on a Scanditronix PC2048-15B tomograph (Uppsala, Sweden) which has an axial and in-plane resolution of 6.5 mm. 15 planes, offset by 6.5 mm (center to center), were acquired simultaneously. Subjects' eyes were patched, and head motion was restricted during the scans by the use of a thermoplastic mask. 30 mCi of H$_2$^{15}O were injected intravenously for each scan. Speech tasks were begun 30 seconds prior to the injection of radiotracer and continued throughout the scanning period. Emission data were corrected for attenuation by means of a transmission scan. Arterial blood was sampled automatically during this period, and PET scans and arterial time-activity data were used to calculate cerebral blood flow (CBF) images with a rapid least squares method (Koeppe et al., 1985).

Speech and Language Tasks

Tasks were presented in a counterbalanced order and consisted of a motor control condition (non-linguistic oromotor-laryngeal movements) and two dysfluency-evoking language tasks. Prior to the PET study, all subjects underwent at least one hour of training and practice in the performance of these tasks. The motor control task was designed to produce laryngeal and oral articulatory movements and associated sounds utilizing all of the muscle groups activated during speech, but was devoid of linguistic content. Subjects produced vocal fold vibrations periodically interrupted by glottal stops at a rate consistent with speech production (about 5 Hz), varying pitch throughout a range that approximated the prosody of spoken English. At the same time subjects moved the lips, tongue and mandible at a rate and range of movement which were qualitatively similar to those produced during speech. Subjects were instructed not to produce movements that are not typically seen during speech, such as lateral movements of the tongue or jaw, clenching of the teeth, protrusion of the tongue or hyperextension of the jaw. Dysfluency evoking conditions included narrative speech and sentence construction tasks. In the narrative speech task, subjects were instructed to spontaneously recount an event or series of events from memory, using normal speech rate, rhythm and intonation. In this task, semantic content was typically rich in visual episodic detail. In the sentence construction task, subjects were instructed to produce a series of novel sentences using a verb that was assigned shortly before the onset of the scan. Speech rate, rhythm and intonation were normal while semantic content was typically constrained (compared to that produced during the narrative task). During execution of the language tasks, subjects were instructed to avoid using any behaviors (circumlocution, word substitution) which might prevent the expression of stuttering symptoms.

Speech Recording and Analysis

Subjects' speech output was recorded during each scan on one channel of an instrumentation tape recorder and a computer generated signal, identifying the start of scan, was recorded on a second channel. The acoustic signal stream (from 20 sec before to 40 sec following the start of the scan) was digitized, acoustically monitored and visually marked to identify the presence or absence of dysfluent symptoms in 2 second epochs. This information on the timing of dysfluency episodes during each scan was used to derive weighted dysfluency scores which quantified the probable contribution of speech symptoms to each PET image. Our approach, which is conceptually similar to that previously described by Silbersweig et al. (1994), is based on the hypothesis that transient dysfluent episodes would be associated with transient changes in local CBF in the involved brain areas. Because of the tracer kinetic behavior of $H_2^{15}O$ in brain tissue, the observed change in the PET signal depends upon when during data acquisition the dysfluencies occur. We therefore calculated a weighting function which describes these changes in the PET signal. It was derived by a) solving the Kety flow model (Kety, 1951) for predicted tissue activity in the case of changing flow; b) calculating the sensitivity (derivative) of the predicted PET tissue activity to the flow at each second during the scan; and c) normalizing the resultant sensitivity curve to an integral of 1.0. The sensitivity curves from 20 independently derived $H_2{}^{15}O$ scans were averaged to generate the final weighting function, which was then shifted -5 sec from the start of scan to account for the approximate hemodynamic response time. Subjects' scores during each scan were determined by summing the sensitivity values (dysfluency scores x the associated weights at each point throughout the scan), such that if a subject were symptomatic during the entire scan, the score would be 1.0.

PET DATA ANALYSIS

Image averaging and spatial normalization

PET scans were registered, stereotaxically averaged, normalized for differences in global blood flow and analyzed using statistical parametric mapping (SPM) software [MRC Cyclotron Unit, Hammersmith Hospital, London, UK]. Images were smoothed with a Gaussian filter (20 x 20 x 12 mm in the x, y and z axes) in order to accommodate intersubject differences in anatomy, and stereotaxically normalized using a nonlinear transformation to produce images of 26 planes parallel to the anterior-posterior commissural line in a common stereotaxic space (Friston et al., 1989) cross-referenced with a standard anatomical atlas (Talairach & Tournoux, 1988). Differences in global activity were removed by analysis of covariance with measured global flow as the covariate, permitting calculation of an adjusted error variance associated with mean flow in each voxel (Friston et al., 1990)

Hierarchical task contrasts

Paired comparisons were carried out both within- and between-groups; that is, task contrasts were performed within each group individually, as well between patient and control groups. The results of the individual contrasts were then compared. Using SPM activation was evaluated using the t statistic calculated for all voxels in parallel (Friston et al., 1991). The resulting set of values, transformed to z-scores, constitutes a statistical parametric map (SPM {z}). Both within and between group contrasts generated such maps. For within-group comparisons, the profile of significant rCBF increases or activations was defined as the subset of voxels with z-scores > 3 (approximately p=.001, one-tailed). Between-group differences were evaluated only for brain regions in which significant differences were detected in at least one of the within-group comparisons. That is, differences between patient and control groups are reported only for regions which showed significant activation in at least one of the groups when this contrast was evaluated independently in patients and controls. This restriction was applied to limit type I error.

For between-group comparisons, voxels with z-scores greater than 2 in absolute value are reported. This z-score threshold results in a conjoint significance level of $p < .0005$.

Covariance Analyses

PET images which had been registered, interpolated, stereotaxically normalized and smoothed according to methods outlined above were utilized prior to ANCOVA correction. Global flow rates were calculated by averaging within-brain pixel values, and the global rate was used to normalize each image, generating reference ratios (regional/global CBF) on a pixel by pixel basis. The resulting normalized rCBF images were correlated with individuals' dysfluency scores utilizing a modification of the SPM software (Horwitz et al., 1993; Horwitz & McIntosh, 1994). The results of correlations carried out across all 18 subjects included a Pearson product-moment correlation coefficient assigned to each pixel in the image. Correlation coefficients were arbitrarily thresholded at a level of .5 (equivalent to a pairwise value of $p < .025$, $n = 18$). These uncorrected values, although not in themselves significant, can be treated as discrete, dichotomous variables and their distribution evaluated using non-parametric methods. The proportions of positive and negative correlations in right and left hemispheres were evaluated using the chi square statistic.

RESULTS

Task contrasts

The spontaneous narrative - motor task contrast was designed to determine how stuttering subjects differ from controls in the formulation and expression of *language* under conditions in which they are dysfluent. The differences identified (Figure 1, Table 1) bear a potential relationship to stuttering behavior.

During the narrative task, regional cerebral blood flow in control subjects was consistently lateralized to the left hemisphere. Significant differences were detected in stuttering subjects and included the following:

In the frontal association cortices: The dorsolateral prefrontal cortex, in which activation was confined to the left hemisphere in controls, was bilaterally activated in stuttering subjects. Unlike controls, stuttering subjects did not activate the inferior portion of the anterior operculum.

In the cingulate cortex: rCBF responses were increased in stuttering subjects in both dorsal and ventral portions of the anterior cingulate cortex. Activation of the dorsal ACC was lateralized to the left in controls, but was bilaterally active in stuttering subjects. During the narrative task control subjects activated the caudal portion of the posterior cingulate cortex at the level of Wernicke's area; stuttering subjects did not, but instead activated more dorsal regions, adjacent to the medial SPL.

In occipital, temporal and parietal sensory cortices: Unlike controls, stuttering subjects failed to activate the central portion of Wernicke's area in the left posterior

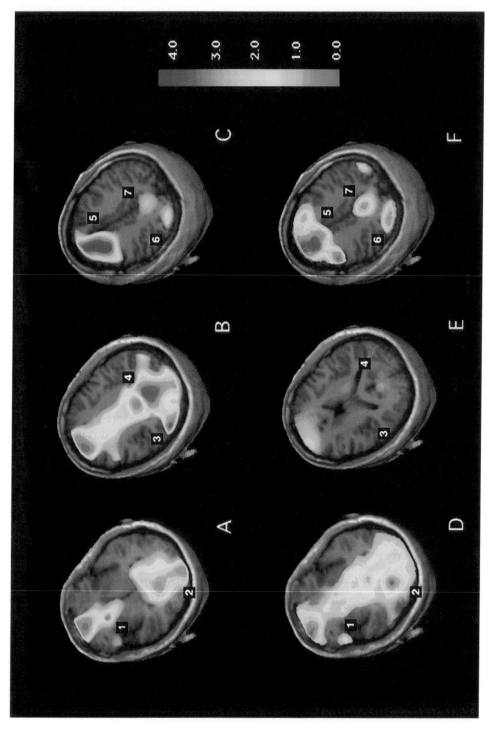

Figure 1. Focal rCBF activations during the formulation and expression of language in stuttering subjects and controls. For both groups, statistical parametric (SPM {z}) maps, comparing a task in which stuttering subjects were dysfluent, narrative speech, with a non-linguistic oral motor task, are displayed on a standardized MRI scan. The MR image, acquired in a control subject, was transformed linearly into the same stereotaxic (Talairach) space as the SPM {z} data. Using Voxel View Ultra (Vital Images, Fairfield, Iowa), SPM and MR data were volume-rendered into a single 3-dimensional image for each group. The volume sets are truncated and displayed at selected planes of interest. Data for control subjects are displayed in the upper row, for stuttering subjects in the lower row. Planes of section, relative to the anterior commissural - posterior commissural line, are located at 0 mm (A and D), +20 mm (B and E) and +40 mm (C and F). Values are z-scores representing the significance level of focal activations in each voxel; the range of scores is coded in the color table. Selected regional CBF responses showing differences between stuttering subjects and controls are numbered (see text for details): caudate nuclei (to the right of [1]); lateral occipital cortex, (to the right of [2]) and fusiform gyrus, (anterior to [2]); Wernicke's area (posterior STG and inferior angular gyrus, posterior to [3]); posterior cingulate cortex (to the left of [4]); dorsolateral prefrontal and dorsal anterior cingulate cortices [5]; dorsal portion of the inferior parietal lobule (posterior to [6]); and the medial portion of the superior parietal lobule (to the left of [7]).

superior temporal gyrus (STG). Nor did stuttering subjects activate the portion of the left inferior angular gyrus adjacent to the STG. Instead, individuals who stutter activated a dorsal region of the angular gyrus, adjacent to the superior parietal lobule (SPL) as well as somatosensory association cortices in the SPL, while control subjects did not. Unlike controls, stuttering subjects did not activate the left middle temporal gyrus (Brodman 21), and during the narrative task - in which events were recounted from visual memory - control subjects consistently activated primary and secondary visual association areas in the left occipital cortex, while activity in stuttering subjects failed to reach statistical significance.

In subcortical regions: stuttering subjects activated the right but not the left caudate nucleus during the narrative task. In addition, the mesencephalic periaqueductal grey was activated in stuttering subjects but not in controls, and stuttering subjects activated the cerebellar vermis rather than the cerebellar hemisphere; rCBF responses in this midline cerebellar region exceeded those of controls.

Correlational analyses

Correlations between dysfluency scores and regional cerebral blood flow were used to characterize the functional anatomical substrates of the speech disruptions - blocks, prolongations and repetitions - themselves.

Dysfluency scores associated with the sentence construction task had the widest dynamic range, making it more appropriate for the use of correlational techniques and this task was selected for analysis. The hemispheric distribution of positive and negative correlation coefficients exceeding 1.5 was non-random ($X^2 = 7.67$, 1df, p < .01).

Dysfluency scores were positively correlated with regional cerebral activity principally located on the *left* side of the brain, in anterior brain regions - subcortical motor areas, frontal association cortices and related (archicortical) paralimbic regions (Figure 2). Higher dysfluency scores were associated with increased regional CBF rates in the left posterior putamen, ventral thalamus, medial and dorsolateral prefrontal cortices. Dysfluency scores were also positively correlated with rCBF in inferior (left hemisphere) and superior anterior cingulate cortices (in both right and left hemispheres). Significant correlations were in each case associated with anterior regions of the ACC (Brodman's

Table 1. Results of within-group contrasts in control and stuttering subjects. Spontaneous narrative speech is contrasted with the oral motor task as baseline. Regions in which rCBF responses differ from baseline are tabulated along with z-scores (representing local maxima or minima), followed by magnitude of rCBF differences (ml/100g/min normalized to a mean of 50) and associated Talaraich coordinates. Instances in which rCBF responses in stutterers and controls differed in between-group contrasts are identified by asterisks, indicating the higher values (conjoint significance of p < .0005 in each case).

Regions	Brod No.	Control Subjects Left					Control Subjects Right					Stuttering Subjects Left					Stuttering Subjects Right				
		Zscore	Mag.	X	Y	Z	Zscore	Mag.	X	Y	Z	Zscore	Mag.	X	Y	Z	Zscore	Mag.	X	Y	Z
Subcortical																					
Caudate Nucleus	-	3.47	1.97	-10	18	0	-	-	-	-	-	-	-	-	-	-	4.00	3.33	8	10	-4 *
Cerebellar Hemisphere	-	-	-	-	-	-	3.33	3.78	20	-82	-20	-	-	-	-	-	-	-	-	-	-
Midline Cerebellum	-	-	-	-	-	-	-	-	-	-	-	4.36	3.33	-6	-72	-12 *	3.45	3.38	2	-44	-8
Periaqueductal Grey	-	-	-	-	-	-	-	-	-	-	-	4.00	3.04	-4	-32	-4 *	3.13	3.14	-2	-34	-8 *
Frontal																					
Dorsolateral Prefrontal Cortex	8, 9	4.53	4.09	-20	30	40	-	-	-	-	-	4.40	3.33	-22	30	40	3.13	2.94	26	30	40 *
Inferior Anterior Frontal Operculum	47	3.19	2.63	-38	26	-8	-	-	-	-	-	-	-	-	-	-	-	-	-	-	-
Cingulate																					
Inferior Anterior Cingulate Cortex	-	-	-	-	-	-	-	-	-	-	-	4.52	4.10	-2	32	-8 *	4.68	3.91	2	34	-8 *
Superior Anterior Cingulate Cortex	-	4.76	4.24	-16	24	36	-	-	-	-	-	4.52	3.28	-14	26	36	3.45	3.33	2	22	36 *
Unimodal Sensory																					
Lateral Occipital Cortex	17, 18	3.10	2.34	-16	-90	20	-	-	-	-	-	-	-	-	-	-	-	-	-	-	-
Posterior Superior Temporal Gyrus	22	4.02	3.03	-46	-54	20 *	-	-	-	-	-	-	-	-	-	-	-	-	-	-	-
Medial Superior Parietal Lobule	-	-	-	-	-	-	-	-	-	-	-	3.29	2.31	-38	-62	36	-	-	-	-	-
Heteromodal Sensory																					
Middle Temporal Gyrus/STS	21	3.56	2.68	-54	-12	-12 *	-	-	-	-	-	-	-	-	-	-	-	-	-	-	-
Inferior Angular Gyrus	39	3.32	3.23	-44	-54	24	-	-	-	-	-	-	-	-	-	-	-	-	-	-	-
Superior Angular Gyrus	-	-	-	-	-	-	-	-	-	-	-	3.77	3.04	-6	-52	32	-	-	-	-	-

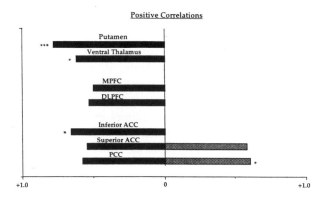

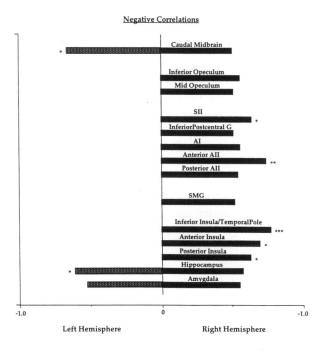

Figure 2. Correlations between weighted measures of dysfluency and normalized regional cerebral blood flow rates (see methods for details). Bars illustrate the magnitude of positive (top) and negative (bottom) correlation coefficients for regions in left (projecting left) and right hemispheres (projecting right). Values represent local minima and maxima. Asterisks indicate associated significance levels: *p < .01, **p < .001, ***p < .0001, otherwise P, .025. [MPFC, medial prefrontal cortex; DLPFC, dorsolateral prefrontal cortex; ACC, anterior cingulate cortex; PCC, posterior cingulate cortex; SII, second somatosensory area; AI, primary auditory cortex; AII, secondary auditory association cortices; SMG, supramarginal gyrus].

area 32/24), and maxima were located deep within the cingulate sulcus. Dysfluency scores were also positively correlated with rCBF in the posterior cingulate cortex (in both left and right hemispheres).

Dysfluency scores were *negatively* correlated with regional cerebral activity principally located on the right side of the brain, in posterior and perisylvian regions including unimodal sensory areas, parietal association cortices, and related (paleocortical) paralimbic regions (Figure 2). *Lower* dysfluency scores were associated with increased regional CBF rates in primary auditory and auditory association cortices, somatosensory areas and supramarginal gyrus. Dysfluency was also negatively correlated with activity in the right insular and temporal polar cortices, in the right frontal operculum (pars opercularis and triangularis) as well as the caudal brainstem and limbic regions of the mesial temporal cortex (in both right and left hemispheres).

DISCUSSION

The notion of altered hemispheric dominance and possible differences in the roles played by left and right hemispheres in the pathophysiology of developmental stuttering have been the subject controversy since the concept was first advanced early in the 20th century (Orton, 1928; Travis, 1931). As outlined above, while increased activity in the right hemisphere has been documented in developmental stutterers (Moore, 1990), it has never been clear whether this activity might be interfering with normal left hemispheric processing or compensating for left hemispheric dysfunction. The present results suggest a tentative resolution, underscoring the likelihood of left hemispheric dysfunction in developmental stuttering.

Hierarchical task contrasts indicate that during the formulation and expression of language, stuttering subjects do not activate regions or networks of regions in the left hemisphere as do controls. During language formulation, cerebral activity in control subjects was markedly asymmetrical, consistently lateralizing to the left hemisphere. Stuttering subjects, on the other hand, failed to activate left hemispheric regions in this fashion: rCBF responses were absent, bilateral or, as in the case of the caudate nucleus, lateralized to the right.

These differences were conspicuous in the neocortical regions constituting the central elements of the classical Wernicke-Geschwind model of language processing (Geschwind, 1979; Geschwind, 1965) - in both anterior (or expressive), as well as posterior (or receptive) areas. During the performance of tasks in which they were dysfluent, stuttering subjects failed to activate left temporoparietal regions which traditionally constitute Wernicke's area and showed reduced activation of the left anterior frontal operculum - areas which are conventionally held to be instrumental in the formulation and expression of spoken language (Penfield & Roberts, 1959; Ojemann et al., 1989).

In previous PET studies in normal subjects (Petersen et al., 1988; Wise et al., 1991; Dimonet et al., 1992; Zatorre et al., 1992) it has been shown that Wernicke's area and contiguous portions of the temporal and parietal lobes appear to be involved in both phonological and semantic processing of speech and language. Thus, our results suggest that when they are dysfluent, stuttering subjects may not be monitoring speech-language output in the same fashion as controls. Perhaps an inability to effectively monitor rapid, spontaneous speech output may be related, at some level, to the production of stuttered speech.

Altered lateralization patterns in stuttering subjects were evident not only in classical neocortical language areas, but also in association areas - dorsolateral prefrontal cortices, middle temporal gyrus, anterior cingulate cortex - which are also thought to play a significant role in language processing, but for which precise linguistic functions are less well characterized. (Frith et al., 1991a; Yetkin et al., 1995; Mazoyer et al., 1993). In the present study, left lateralized activation of these regions was evident in controls but not in stuttering subjects. Lateralized activation was also evident in controls, but not in stuttering subjects, in visual association areas which may be involved in the processing of visual imagery during discourse formulation (Sakai & Miyashita, 1993).

Thus, in summary, under conditions which precipitate dysfluent speech, stuttering subjects show a striking distortion of the normal pattern of left hemispheral dominance for language, either not activating left hemisphere neocortical areas which are normally engaged in language processing or activating these regions bilaterally.

However, a closer look at our results indicates that dysfluent speech production may be associated not only with distorted lateralization patterns, but with alterations in the intrahemispheric relationships between brain regions as well: In our stuttering subjects, failure to activate left hemispheral regions *entirely* is seen in post-rolandic sensory areas and related paleocortical paralimbic regions of the brain - regions which play a role in perception and decoding of sensory information. On the other hand, bilateral activation was more common in anterior forebrain regions and associated archicortical paralimbic areas - regions which play a role in the regulation of motor function.

Taken together, these results suggest a tentative hypothesis: that dysfluent speech production may be associated with a functional imbalance between anterior forebrain regions which mediate the organization, initiation, and regulation of motor activity and post-rolandic regions involved in reception and decoding of sensory information. It is possible that the posterior regions fail to provide integrated sensory input upon which anterior regions depend in order to effectively regulate motor function. Such a dissociation may underlie the production of stuttering symptoms.

As a corollary, stuttering subjects exhibit atypical sensory activation patterns which appear to extend across modalities. That is, while they did not activate auditory association areas - i.e. posterior superior temporal gyrus and contiguous portions of the inferior angular gyrus - stuttering subjects, unlike controls, activated regions more closely associated with somatosensory information processing. These included a dorsal region of the angular gyrus, adjacent to the superior parietal lobule, as well as somatosensory association cortices in the medial SPL itself. Stuttering subjects may be more effectively processing somatosensory rather than auditory information during conditions in which they are dysfluent. Whether such activity is compensatory or antagonistic is unclear in the present contrast.

The covariance method, which makes no assumptions about the additivity of hierarchically organized task conditions, may represent the more robust approach in a patient population with variable levels of symptom severity. Results of this analysis suggest that limbic and paralimbic structures, including hippocampus, amygdala and anterior insula, may be involved in the generation of stuttering symptoms - a finding which is not unexpected in a disorder in which symptoms are frequently coupled to stress or other emotional features.

However, the covariance and task contrast analyses converge in a broader and potentially more significant fashion. Both support the concept of left hemisphere dysfunction in this disorder, indicating that activation of regions within the left hemisphere may be responsible for the generation of dysfluent speech. Furthermore, results of the correlation analyses indicate that activation of regions in the *right* hemisphere might represent compensatory processes which may alleviate the symptoms of stuttering.

Regions in which rCBF rates were positively coupled to the production of dysfluent speech - orbital, cingulate, opercular as well as dorsolateral prefrontal cortices, striatum and ventral thalamus - were located almost exclusively within the left hemisphere. Activity in these regions increased, in our subjects, as speech became more dysfluent. Even in the dorsolateral prefrontal cortices - where *bilateral* increases over baseline motor activity were evident during dysfluent language tasks - correlational analyses indicate that activity in the left hemisphere is exclusively related to stuttering.

On the other hand, rCBF rates in regions located almost exclusively in the right hemisphere were negatively correlated with stuttering symptoms, that is activity in these regions increased, in our subjects, as speech became more fluent. Many of these regions - AI, AII, insula and SMG -function at elementary levels of auditory processing, which may be carried out more effectively by stuttering subjects under fluency evoking conditions. However, these regions also constitute the elements of a more widespread perisylvian system, centered upon the posterior insula and extending along the anterior and posterior banks of the sylvian fissure. All of the elements of this distributed system - insular, auditory, somatosensory, and opercular cortices - were increasingly active in our stuttering subjects as their speech became more fluent.

The interconnections of these regions suggest a mechanism by which their activation may bring about such an effect: Auditory and somatosensory cortices project directly to the posterior insula, which may function as a parallel waystation for the integration of acoustic and somesthetic information (Mesulam & Mufson, 1982; Mufson & Mesulam, 1982; Pandya et al., 1969). From there, projections carry information frontal association regions of the brain (Mesulam & Mufson, 1982); one such projection, to the frontal operculum, may provide an alternative neural relay between the posterior-temporoparietal and anterior-opercular language areas (Mesulam & Mufson, 1986), perhaps subserving the role which the insula appears to play in language processing (Augustine, 1985; Vignolo & Mazzocchi, 1979) and the initiation of speech (Shuren, 1993).

It is possible that, in individuals who stutter, these right hemispheric perisylvian regions constitute an auxiliary system which integrates auditory and orolingual-laryngeal somesthetic information and provides an alternative relay to anterior forebrain areas. If, as suggested above, stuttering symptoms are predicated on a dissociation of anterior motor and posterior sensory mechanisms, this system may effectively couple anterior and posterior regions within the *right* hemisphere during - perhaps enabling - the production of fluent speech.

REFERENCES

Augustine, J.R. (1985). The insular lobe in primates including humans. *Neurological Research, 7(1),* 2-10.

Bates, E. (1976). Normal and Deficient Child Language. In D. Moorehead, & A. Moorehead (Eds.), Baltimore: University Park Press.

Dimonet, J.F., Chollet, F., Ramsay, S., Cardebat, D., Nespoulous, J.L., Wise, R., Rascol, A., & Frackowiak, R. (1992). The anatomy of phonological and semantic processing in normal subjects. *Brain, 115,* 1753-1768.

Friston, K.J., Passingham, R.E., Nutt, J.G., Heather, J.D., Sawle, G.V., & Frackowiak, R.S. (1989). Localisation in PET images: direct fitting of the intercomissural (AC-PC) line. *Journal of Cerebral Blood Flow Metabolism, 9,* 690-695.

Friston, K.J., Frith, C.D., Liddle, P.F., Dolan, R.J., Lammertsma, A.A., & Frackowiak, R.S. (1990). The relationship between global and local changes in PET scans. *Journal of Cerebral Blood Flow Metabolism, 10,* 458-466.

Friston, K.J., Frith, C.D., Liddle, P.F., & Frackowiak RS. (1991) Comparing functional (PET) images: the assesment of significant change. *Journal of Cerebral Blood Flow Metabolism, 11,* 690-699.

Frith, C.D., Friston, K.J., Liddle, P.F., & Frackowiak, R.S.J. (1991a). Willed action and the prefrontal cortex in man: a study with PET. *Proceedings of the Royal Society of London B, 244,* 241-246.

Geschwind, N. (1965). Disconnexion syndromes in animals and man. *Brain, 88,* 237-294.

Geschwind, N. (1979) Specializations of the human brain. In The Brain. San Francisco, W.H. Freeman.

Horwitz, B., Maisog, J., Krischner, P., Mentis, M., Friston, K., & McIntosh, A.R. (1993). A computerized system for determining pixel-by-pixel correlations of functional activity measured by positron emission tomography (PET). *Society of Neuroscience Abstracts, 19,* 1604.

Horwitz, B., & McIntosh, A.R. (1994). Quantification of Brain Function. In K. Uemura, N.A. Lassen, T. Jones & I. Kanno (Eds.), Amsterdam, Excerpta Medica, 589-596.

Kety, S.S. (1951). The theory and applications of the exchange of inert gas at the lungs and tissues. *Pharmacological Review, 3,* 1-41.

Koeppe, R.A., Holden, J.E., & Ip, W.R. (1985). Performance comparison of parameter estimation techniques for the quantitation of local cerebral blood flow by dynamic positron computed tomography. *Journal of Cerebral Blood Flow Metabolism, 5,* 224-234.

Mazoyer, B.M., Tzourio, N., Frak, V., Syrota, A., Murayama, N., Levrier, O., et al. (1993). The

Cortical Representation of Speech. *Journal of Cognitive Neuroscience, 5(4),* 467-479.

McKay, D.G. (1982). The problems of flexibility, fluency, and speech-accuracy trade-off in skilled behavior. *Psychological Review, 89,* 483-506.

Mesulam, M.-M., & Mufson, E. (1982). Insula of the old World Monkey. III: Efferent Cortical Output and Comments on Function. *Journal of Comp Neurology, 212,* 38-52.

Mesulam, M.-M., & Mufson, E.J. (1986). The Insula of Reil in Man and Monkey. In A. Peters, & E.G. Jones (Eds.), *Cerebral Cortex* Vol.4. New York, Plenum, 179-226.

Moore, W.H. Jr. (1990). Research Needs in Stuttering: Roadblocks and Future Directions. In J. Cooper (Ed.), ASHA Reports 18. Rockville, Maryland, *American Speech-Language-Hearing Association,* 72-81.

Mufson, E., & Mesulam, M.-M. (1982). Insula of the Old World Monkey. II: Afferent cortical Input and Comments on the Claustrum. *Journal of Comp Neurology, 212,* 23-37.

Ojemann, G., Ojemann, J., Lettich, E., & Berger, M. (1989). Cortical language localisation in left, dominant hemisphere. An electrical stimulation mapping investigation in 117 patients. *J Neurosurg, 71,* 316-326.

Orton, S.T. (1928). A physiological theory of reading disability and stuttering in children. *The New England Journal of Medicine, 199,* 1046-1052.

Pandya, D.N., Hallett, M., & Kmukherjee, S.K. (1969). Intra- and interhemispheric connections of the neocortical auditory system in the rhesus monkey. *Brain Research, 14(1),* 49-65.

Penfield, W., & Roberts, L. (1959). Speech and Brain Mechanisms New Jersey: Princeton Univ Press.

Petersen, S.E., Fox, P.T., Posner, M.I., Mintun, M., & Raichle, M.E. (1988). Positron emission tomographic studies of the cortical anatomy of single-word processing. *Nature, 331,* 585-589.

Rosenfeld, D.B., & Jerger, J. (1984). Nature and Treatment of Stuttering. In R.F. Curlee, & W.F. Perkins (Eds.), San Diego, College-Hill Press, 73-87.

Sakai, K., & Miyashita, Y. (1993). Memory and imagery in the temporal lobe. *Current Opinions in Neurobiology, 3,* 166-170.

Shuren, J. (1993). Insula and aphasia. *Journal of Neurology, 240(4),* 216-218.

Silbersweig, D.A., Stern, E., Schnorr, L., Frith, C.D., Ashburner, J., Cahill, C. et al. 1994). Imaging transient, randomly occurring neuropsychological events in single subjects with positron emission tomography: an event-related count rate correlational analysis. *Journal of Cerebral Blood Flow Metabolism, 14,* 771-782.

Talairach, J., & Tournoux, P. (1988). Co-planar stereotaxic atlas of the human brain. New York, Thieme.

Travis, L.A. (1931). Speech Pathology. New York, Appleton.

Vignolo, L.A., & Mazzocchi, F. (1979). Localisation of lesions in aphasia: clinical-CT scan correlations in stroke patients. *Cortex, 15,* 627-654.

Wise, R., Chollet, F., Hadar, U., Friston, K., Hoffner, E., & Frackowiak, R. (1991) Distribution of cortical neural networks involved in word comprehension and word retrieval. *Brain, 114,* 1803-1817.

Wyatt, G. (1969). Language learning and communication disorders in children. New York, Free Press.

Yetkin, F.Z., Hammeke, T.A., Swanson, S.J., Morris, G.L., Mueller, W.M., McAuliffe, T.L., et al. (1995). A comparison of functional MR activation patterns during silentand audible language tasks. AJNR *American Journal of Neuroradiology, 16(5),* 1087-1092.

Zatorre, R.J., Evans, A.C., Meyer, E., & Gjedde, A. (1992). Lateralization of phonetic and pitch discrimination in speech processing. *Science, 256,* 846-849.

Speech Production: Motor Control, Brain Research and Fluency Disorders
W. Hulstijn, H.F.M. Peters and P.H.H.M. Van Lieshout, editors

Chapter 24

A H$_2$^{15}O POSITRON EMISSION TOMOGRAPHY (PET) STUDY ON ADULTS WHO STUTTER: FINDINGS AND IMPLICATIONS.

Roger J. Ingham, Peter T. Fox, Janis C. Ingham.

Using H$_2$O^{15} PET to measure cerebral blood flow, we report the results of a *functional activation study* with 10 right-handed adult males stutterers and 10 matched controls. Counterbalanced scanning conditions (eyes closed rest, oral and chorus reading) identified neural activation contrasts between stuttered and nonstuttered speech. During oral reading stutterers showed right lateralized overactivations within the motor system. They did not show the normal activations of left-sided phonological input systems, but did show consistent deactivations in the auditory region (an activated region during oral reading by the controls). Chorus reading lessened or eliminated the overactivity in most motor areas and largely reversed the deactivations. The *functional lesion study* utilized rest condition data from the activation study, supplemented by data from 9 other controls who participated in similar studies. PET images were analyzed sampling 74 regions of interest, 37 per hemisphere. Highly significant between-region and between-hemisphere effects were found for both groups, as have been previously reported for normal subjects. However, no significant between-group differences were found in regional CBF values. This suggests that adult stutterers likely have an essentially normal functional brain at rest.

INTRODUCTION

Currently, the dominant general hypothesis governing stuttering research and theory is that developmental stuttering is a product of central nervous system dysfunction, possibly with genetic origins. The strength of this hypothesis is reflected in a plethora of recent studies into the neurophysiology and physiology of stuttering (see Bloodstein, 1995; Boberg, 1993; Cooper, 1990; Peters et al., 1991) and the influence of theories postulating hemispheric laterality and/or motor-system dysfunction (Webster, 1993; Zimmermann, 1980). There is some recognition (see, for example, Rosenfield & Nudelman, 1987; Smith, 1990) that stuttering must also be affect- and environmentally-sensitive, but this view still concedes primacy to a neurologic disorder hypothesis. The most favored view appears to be that the core problem is either a neural dysfunction or deficiency that is expressed most obviously in stuttering behavior, but equally significantly through a variety of relative deficiencies in speech-motor skills of persons who stutter (see Peters et al., 1991), albeit mainly among adults. Until recently researchers have largely relied on electromyography and reaction-time tasks to infer signs of unusual neural activity among persons who stutterer during speech-related tasks (see Caruso, 1991; Moore, 1990; Peters et al., 1991-many chapters; Webster, 1993). Brain imaging now offers far more direct methods for studying neural structure and function (Posner & Raichle, 1994), methods which are being used to investigate stuttering.

This paper overviews the results of an $H_2^{15}O$ positron emission tomography (PET) functional activation (Fox et al., 1996) and functional lesion (Ingham et al., 1996) brain imaging study of stuttering.

THE FUNCTIONAL ACTIVATION STUDY.

The functional activation study was conducted with 10 right-handed adult males who were independently diagnosed as chronic developmental stutterers (mean age, 32 years), who were rated from mild to severe, and 10 right-handed, adult male, normally fluent controls (also with a mean age of 32 years). In the course of this study it was also possible to conduct a study within a study; that is, a functional lesion study using the eyes-closed rest data. The findings of this latter study will be only briefly reported.

All PET data were collected using a GE 4096 scanner which simultaneously acquires 15 parallel image slices of the brain with a center-to-center interslice distance of 6.5 mm. MRI data were also obtained for image referencing using a 3-dimensional, fast spin echo, T-1 weighted sequence. The PET and MR images for each subject were spatially normalized, relative to the Talairach and Tournoux (1988) brain atlas, using software devised by Lancaster et al. (1996). All dimensions were obtained from the subjects MR image and applied to both the MR and PET images. They were then transformed into 3-dimensional, spatially-normalized, images using 2 x 2 x 2mm voxels.

Each subject completed 9 scans under 3 different conditions during a 2-3 hour session.

Table 1. This table shows the scanning order and task conditions followed by the 10 adult stutterers and 10 controls in the functional activation study (Fox et al., 1996). Half of the subjects in each group followed Order 1 and half followed Order 2.

ORDER 1	ORDER 2
1. REST	1. REST
2. SOLO READING	2. CHORUS READING
3. CHORUS READING	3. SOLO READING
4. REST	4. REST
5. CHORUS READING	5. SOLO READING
6. SOLO READING	6. CHORUS READING
7. REST	7. REST
8. SOLO READING	8. CHORUS READING
9. CHORUS READING	9. SOLO READING

These scanning conditions were 3 eyes-closed rest (hereafter labeled *Rest*), 3 oral readings alone (hereafter labeled *Solo*), and 3 chorus readings (hereafter labeled *Chorus*). These conditions were presented in 1 of 2 counterbalanced sequences (see Table 1). In the Solo and Chorus conditions subjects read aloud the same specially selected passage (from Abbey, 1975), with potential adaptation effects (Van Riper & Hull, 1955) controlled by a 15-min interval between scans that was occupied with casual conversation.

Subjects were in a supine position within the scanner and read the passage from a video terminal located above them. The subjects oral reading was audio recorded from a microphone positioned 3 inches from the chin. During Chorus conditions subjects read aloud to the accompaniment of an audio-recording of a normally fluent speaker reading the same passage and at a rate selected as most comfortable by each subject. The recorded passage was presented via an earphone inserted in the subjects left ear (Ingham & Packman, 1979). The blood flow data were collected during a 40 second scanning period following the intravenous injection of a $H_2^{15}O$ tracer.

Speech performance data.

The speech performance data were the number of 4 second intervals during the 40 second scan that were judged to contain stuttering (that is, the number out of 10) (Ingham, Cordes, & Finn, 1993), the number of syllables read aloud, and the mean rating of speech naturalness on a scale of 1 to 9 (Martin et al., 1984) per 40 s scan. These data were derived from counts made separately by two independent judges who had no knowledge of the recording conditions. The results are summarized in Table 2. During Solo the stutterers averaged 6.2 stuttered intervals (range 1-10) and 113 syllables. During Chorus reading no stuttering was

Table 2: Mean number of 4-s stuttered intervals, syllables spoken per 40-s scan, and speech naturalness rating (1 = highly natural sounding; 9 = highly unnatural sounding) during Solo and Chorus reading conditions. Range shown in parentheses.

GROUP	SOLO	CHORUS
Stutterers (n=10)		
Stuttered Intervals	6.2 (1-10)	0.0
Syllables Spoken	113 (82-154)*	143.7 (121-173)
Speech Naturalness	5.46 (3-9)	2.50 (1-4)
Controls (n=10)		
Stuttered Intervals	0.0	0.0
Syllables Spoken	146.8 (124-188)	145.6 (121-181)
Speech Naturalness	2.40 (1-4)	2.53 (1-4)

* Stutterers' mean speech rate for *nonstuttered only* intervals was 132.6 syllables per 40-s scan. This was not significantly slower than the mean 143.7 syllables produced during Chorus reading.

judged to have occurred and mean total syllables spoken increased to 143.7. Controls did not stutter in either condition and produced means of 146.8 and 145.6 syllables in Solo and Chorus, respectively. The speech naturalness ratings from both groups differed predictably during Solo, but were virtually identical for both groups during Chorus conditions.

Data for reliability were collected for stuttered and nonstuttered intervals and for syllable counts by an independent clinician from another university. Across subjects, interval-by-interval agreement regarding presence or absence of stuttering ranged from 85.0 to 100%, with 100% agreement that each person who stuttered did not stutter during the Chorus conditions. Total percent agreement for syllables ranged from 97.9 to 99.7. Speech naturalness rating agreement was within + or - 1 for 20/20 individual samples. There was no evidence of either an order- or stuttering-adaptation effect among these data.

Cerebral blood flow data

The cerebral blood flow data are presented as speech induced *changes* in cerebral blood flow for each group. That is, for each subject in each group the Solo and Chorus condition data were compared to the Rest condition data. This made it possible to identify significant cerebral blood flow increases (activations) and decreases (deactivations) in all voxels with respect to a nonspeaking condition. The data were initially averaged across subjects for group and within-condition analyses. Clusters of adjoining and significantly activated or deactivated voxels were then identified. These were composed of voxels that showed speech task-induced increases or decreases with Z score probability levels of less than .01.

The results are displayed as logical images within figures and bar graphs. In other words, Boolean logic was employed in order to identify regions of the brain that were significantly activated during Solo *as well as* during Chorus, during Solo but *not* during Chorus, and during Chorus but *not* during Solo. The logical images are color coded as shown in Table 3. Those effects that were common to Solo *and* Chorus reading conditions can be seen in Cyan or aqua blue within the images. The effects that occurred in Solo but *not* in Chorus are shown in red. Recall that this distinguishes the condition where the subjects who stuttered displayed *stuttering*, while the controls read normally. And the Chorus but *not* in Solo effects are shown in dark blue. These effects are distinctive to the condition where the speakers who stutter and the controls were *stutter-free* during oral reading.

Table 3: Table shows logical image and color coding employed in brain image figures

Logical Image	Color	Identifies reading condions where....
(1) Solo and Chorus	Cyan (aqua)	...there were common activations across conditions.
(2) Solo but *not* Chorus	Red	...stutterers *stuttered*, controls *stutter-free*.
(3) Chorus but *not* Solo	Dark blue	...stutterers and controls *stutter-free*.

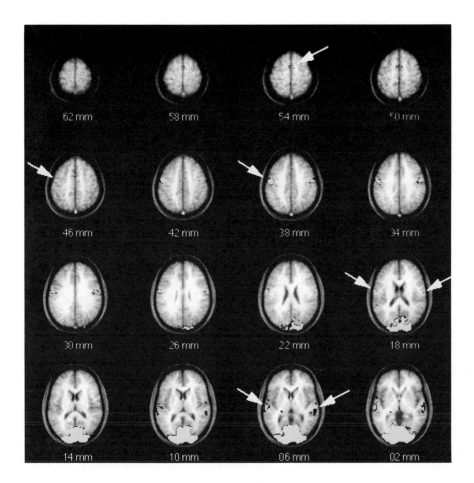

Figure 1. PET activation regions for controles (n = 10)

The following figures display the averaged horizontal sliced images of the brains (that is, looking down from the top of the head) of the controls and the stutterers at different z coordinate levels. These are levels, in this case, superior to the Anterior-Posterior Commissure, or AC-PC, line as referenced in Talairach and Tournoux (1988). In all figures left is the left side of the brain and right is the right side.

Normally fluent controls

Figure 1 shows the regional *activations* for the Controls within 16 horizontal slices that begin at the top of the brain and progress downward. The arrows highlight most of the areas that will be refered to in the following account of the results. Firstly, the prominent aqua coloring throughout this figure reflects the fact that there was very little difference between the Solo and Chorus reading cerebral blood flow data. Solo reading did significantly activate Supplementary Motor Area (SMA, medial BA6), Superior Lateral Premotor Cortex (SLPrM), Primary Motor Cortex for mouth (primarily on the left [M1, BA 4]), Inferior Lateral Premotor Cortex (ILPrM, BA6/44) or Brocaś Area, Anterior-Temporal Extraprimary Auditory Cortex (A2, BA22/21), the visual system, and Cerebellum (which is not shown). The activations were either left lateralized or bilateral. These activations are very similar to those reported in studies of single-word reading (Peterson et al., 1989; Pardo & Fox, 1993), but in the present *paragraph* reading data SMA was relatively *less* activated while anterior temporal cortex (A2) was relatively *more* activated. It is speculated that the much greater activation in the auditory region likely reflects a self-monitoring process necessary during continuous speech (Fairbanks, 1954). Lesser activation of SMA, despite the high complexity of the task and the much greater motor output, may have occurred because oral reading is a broadly coordinated motor process, rather than a series of discrete motor acts that might be expected to strongly activate SMA (Foxet al., 1985; Grafton, 1994).

Regional *deactivations* (relative to rest), which are rarely included in brain-imaging reports, were largely consistent across tasks. During Solo reading by the controls, deactivations were located in the *motor system* (insula, putamen, and premotor cortex [BA9]), the *memory system* (left hippocampal gyrus [BA34] and Right Lateral Prefrontal Cortex [BA47]), and the *attentional system* (multiple regions of deactivation throughout the cingulate gyrus [BA7,10,24,31,34]). Deactivations during Chorus reading were also largely identical to those that were produced during Solo reading. In other words, the chorus condition per se did not alter the normal areas of activation and deactivation produced during oral reading

Speakers who stutter

Figure 2 shows the results for the subjects who stuttered. Firstly, in Solo reading, when stuttering was present, the neural system activations proved to be strikingly and significantly different from those of the controls during Solo reading. These differences, which were largely in the motor and auditory systems, are shown in red and are as follows: SMA was far more active than in the controls, with two large, discrete foci. One focus was similar in location to the controls' SMA, but it was much larger and more intense - it was activated in both reading conditions so it is shown in aqua. A second focus was very extensive and more than 1 cm superior to the normally located focus, but activated only during Solo (red). Superior lateral premotor cortex (SLPrM; lateral BA6), which was minimally activated in the controls, was strongly activated and strongly right lateralized in the stutterers. M1 was similar to the controls with respect to the extent and intensity of activation, but the most intense activations were right lateralized. Cerebellar activations (not shown) were very prominent - more than double the extent of activation found in the controls - and this was the case in the Solo *and* Chorus reading conditions. Interestingly, ILPrM (Brocaś area) was the only motor region that activated in a "normal" manner in the stutterers; it was left-lateralized and similar in intensity and extent to the controls. Besides SMA and SLPrM, there were other motor system activations in the stutterers that were not seen in the controls.

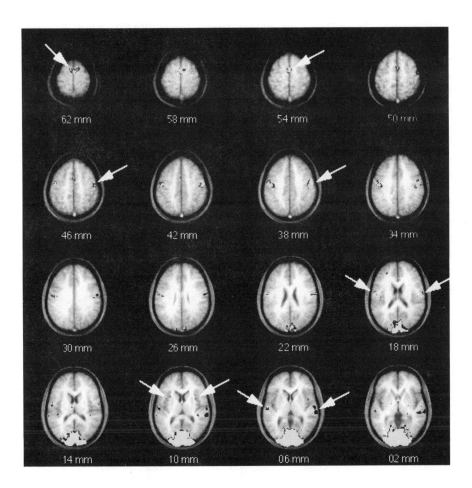

Figure 2. PET activation regions for stutterers (n=10)

These included the insula (bilaterally) and, also not shown here, claustrum (left), lateral thalamus (left), and globus pallidus (left). Thus, stuttering was characterized by extensive hyperactivity of the motor system, with right lateralization of primary and extraprimary motor cortices. Most noteworthy was the finding that the primary auditory area (left superior temporal cortex) activations, which were so prominent in the controls, were essentially *absent* during stuttering (notice - no red). This was a surprising finding and may mean that stutterers do not employ auditory monitoring to the same extent as nonstutterers during oral reading.

There were also areas where cerebral blood flow was significantly deactivated. These areas were particularly distinctive in the auditory systems of the subjects who stuttered during Solo or stuttered reading. In fact, not only did left superior temporal cortex fail to activate, but left posterior temporal cortex (BA22) also showed significant deactivations that did not occur in the controls. In addition, left inferior frontal cortex (BA47), which has been implicated in verbal comprehension (Peterson et al., 1989; Posner et al., 1988) and in verbal production (Frith et al., 1991; Wise et al., 1991) was focally deactivated. The deactivations in left posterior temporal and left inferior frontal cortex strongly suggest that a frontal-temporal system, which has been reported necessary for verbal production, is not normally activated among adults who stutter.

The effects of the Chorus reading are considered by referring to Figure 3 which directly compares the groups with respect to the *volume* of activated voxels that clustered in crucial regions. It should be noted that this figure does not necessarily reflect the intensity of these activations. The figure displays the volume of the clusters in most of the previously mentioned regions of the brain during Solo conditions in the left section of the figure, and then for Chorus reading conditions in the figures' right section. For each region the subjects who stutter are graphed (in hatching) in the upper bar and the controls in the lower bar. The Solo section of the figure shows, for example, the prominent left and right hemisphere activations among the subjects who stutter in SMA during Solo and immediately beneath the much less prominent left sided SMA activations in the Controls. The cluster volume sizes for the stutterers and controls are shown for SLPrM, M1, ILPrM (on the left is Broca's area),

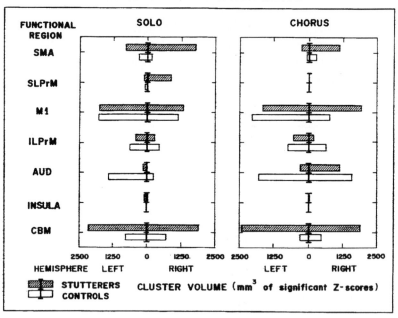

Figure 3. Shows the volume of activated voxels that clustered in regions of the brain during Solo and Chorus conditions.

Auditory areas, Insula and Cerebellum. It can be seen that Chorus reading reduced many of the differences between the normal speakers and the speakers who stuttered and certainly diminished the abnormalities seen in SMA, SLPrM and Insula for the subjects who stuttered. The effect of the chorus reading condition is shown most prominently in the motor systems of the subjects who stuttered, where the right lateralizations in SMA and SLPrM are either reduced or normalized. At the same time it is clear that the subjects who stuttered continue to show dramatically larger activations in cerebellum, possibly because of the greater motor effort that they probably expended during speech production. The Chorus condition did produce more normally intense activations in the auditory region of the subjects who stuttered, though this is only partly reflected in these volumetric data; the right sided prominence in both groups during Chorus was expected because the chorus reading stimulus was delivered via the left ear.

Incidentally, it might be argued that the differences in levels of activation by the persons who stutter in Chorus could be explained as due to their somewhat faster speech rate in Chorus relative to Solo reading (see Table 2). However, these findings are entirely contrary to what would be expected if that were the case. The fact is that one of the most well established brain imaging findings is that increases in motor activity produce increases in activation (Blinkenberg et al., 1995; Sabatini et al., 1993; Schlaug et al., 1995; Wexler et al., 1995). In this study the chorus condition actually produced mainly *decreases* in activation in the motor system.

The regional activations and deactivations observed during stuttering also showed remarkable intersubject agreement. Such information, incidentally, is rarely included within brain-imaging studies. Each individual's significant and nonsignificant Z voxel values to a binary value in order to calculate the percentage of subjects who were represented at each activated voxel. This provides the level of intersubject agreement among the regional activations. The resulting agreement values tended to range from 60% to 90%. The stuttering-specific activations in SMA, SLPrM, and insula, for instance, were present in 70-100% of subjects. This intersubject consistency is exceptionally interesting in view of the well known variability among persons who stutter. In this study, for example, the experimental group's severity of stuttering ranged from relatively mild to extremely severe.

FUNCTIONAL LESION STUDY

As mentioned earlier, this study also made it possible to derive a functional lesion study (Ingham et al., 1996) from the rest condition data in the present study and other studies conducted in the same laboratory. Functional lesion PET studies seek to identify regional physiological abnormalities that are disorder specific, but not due to gross structural abnormalities. The rest state regional cerebral blood flow data made it possible to determine if the subjects who stuttered in the present study showed any evidence of abnormalities of brain physiology. This study was prompted in part by Pool et al. (1991) SPECT study on 20 speakers who stutter and 78 controls. Their rest state findings suggested that persons who stutter showed abnormal neural asymmetries (right > left) in anterior cingulate gyrus, superior temporal gyrus, and middle temporal gyrus.

In the present rest state PET study it was possible to augment the control group to 19. Data were available from 9 additional right-handed male controls who had completed 3 eyes-closed rest state conditions in another PET study. A detailed account of the entire rest state study may be found in Ingham et al. (1996). It included the sampling of 74 regions of interest throughout the brain. This sampling was guided by the physiologically activated areas identified in the previously-described study, anatomical areas outside of those, and areas referred to in the Pool et al.(1991) study. The region of interest sampling placements (3 x 3 x 3 voxels, 216 cubic mm; or 5 x 5 x 5 voxels, 1000 cubic mm) were positioned by reference to Talairach and Tournoux (1988) and confirmed *for each subject* by use of a coregistered, high resolution MRI. The data were analyzed by an ANOVA across the 3 rest trials, the 2 hemispheres, the 74 brain regions and the 2 groups.

The results can be summarized quite simply: there were literally *no* differences between the experimental and control groups for any of the regional cerebral blood flow values. The expected between-Region and between-Hemisphere effects were obtained for both groups, but there were *no* significant differences between the groups. Moreover, the considerable statistical power available in this very large ANOVA made it possible to affirm these conclusions with some confidence. For instance, there were less than 6 chances in 1000 that there was any significant Region x Hemisphere x Group interaction. Equally interesting was the finding that there was no Trial x Region interaction and that a power analysis showed there was less than 1 chance in 10000 that this was a Type 2 error. In other words, there is every reason to believe that the eyes-closed rest state provided an extraordinarily stable neural state - thereby refuting a frequently heard concern about the stability of the eyes-closed rest state data in PET studies. In short, these findings do not support the suggestion that developmental stuttering is associated with abnormalities of brain blood flow at rest. In other words, their brain physiology is normal absent speech.

CONCLUSIONS

In summary, this study has mapped the neural systems of normal continuous speech, both activations and deactivations, and the neural systems of stuttering. As Table 4 indicates, those neural systems appear to include: 1) diffuse over-activity throughout the cerebral and cerebellar motor systems; 2) right dominance of the cerebral motor system; 3) lack of normal activation of the auditory system and, 4) deactivation of a verbal production circuit between left frontal (BA47) and temporal (BA22) cortex that has been previously identified in normal speakers. Current theories of stuttering each emphasize one or another individual component of what we seem to have identified as a dysfunctional *system or systems*. In fact, these results seem to give comfort to several prominent theories of stuttering (for example, Moore & Haynes, 1980; Travis, 1978; Webster, 1993), but they strongly suggest the need for a unifying theory sufficient to accommodate the full complexity of these observed neural system

Table 4. Table shows a summary of the principal findings of the functional activation study (Fox et al., 1996)

(1) Diffuse overactivity of the cerebral and cerebellar motor systems
(2) Right dominance of the cerebral motor system
(3) Lack of normal activation of the auditory system
(4) Deactivation of a verbal production circuit between left frontal (BA 47) and temporal (BA 22) cortex

actions and interactions. At the same time, it should be recognized that the subjects for this study were carefully selected to be chorus reading responders. It is quite possible that the pattern of neural actions observed in this population might differ in some important ways from the pattern that might be obtained among those who *do not* respond to chorus reading, but who do respond to some other fluency-inducing procedure. And of course it is also unclear whether the effects reported here are a cause or consequence of stuttering. Suffice it to say that this issue will be pursued in later studies. Perhaps the most profitable direction to pursue in this area will be to begin to systematically identify the circuits or pathways of neural activation that will characterize and may cause stuttering. At that point it might be possible to understand how these circuits are most profitably controlled and modified.

ACKNOWLEDGMENTS

Preparation of this chapter was supported, in part, by research grant number 5 RO1 DC 00060 from the U.S. National Institute of Deafness and Other Communication Disorders, National Institutes of Health.

REFERENCES

Abbey, E. (1975). *The monkey wrench gang.* New York: Avon Books.
Blinkenberg, M., Bonde, C., Paulson, O. B., Svarer, C., & Law, I. (1995). Rate dependence of cerebral activation during performance of a repetitive motor task. *Human Brain Mapping, S1,* 280.
Bloodstein, O. (1995). *A handbook on stuttering.* San Diego: Singular Publishing Company.
Boberg, E. (Ed.) (1993). *The neuropsychology of stuttering.* Edmonton: University of Alberta Press.
Caruso, A.J. (1991). Neuromotor processes underlying stuttering. In H.F.M. Peters, W. Hulstijn, & C.W. Starkweather, (Eds.), *Speech motor control and stuttering.* (pp. 101-116). Amsterdam: Excerpta Medica.
Cooper, J.A. (1990). Research needs in stuttering: Roadblocks and future directions. *ASHA Reports, 18.*
Fairbanks, G. (1954). Systematic research in experimental phonetics: 1. A theory of the speech mechanism as a servosystem. *Journal of Speech and Hearing Disorders, 19,* 133-139.
Fox, P.T., Fox, J.M., Raichle, M.E., & Burde, R.M. (1985). The role of cerebral cortex in the generation of saccadic eye movements: A positron emission tomographic study. *Journal of Neurophysiology, 52,* 348-368.

Fox, P.T., Ingham, R.J., Ingham, J.C., Hirsch, T., Downs, J.H., Martin, C., Jerabek, P., Glass, T., & Lancaster, J.L. (1996). A PET study of the neural systems of stuttering. *Nature, 382,* 158-162.

Frith, C.D., Friston, K.J., Liddle, P.F., & Frackowiak, R.S.J. (1991). A PET study of word finding. *Neuropsychologia, 29,* 1137-1148.

Grafton, S.T. (1994). Cortical control of movement. *Annals of Neurology, 36,* 3-4.

Ingham, R.J., Cordes, A.K., & Finn, P. (1993). Time-interval measurement of stuttering: Systematic replication of Ingham, Cordes, and Gow (1993). *Journal of Speech and Hearing Research, 36,* 1168-1176.

Ingham, R.J., Fox, P.T., & Ingham, J.C. (1994) Brain image investigation of the speech of stutterers and nonstutterers. Paper read to the Annual Convention of the American Speech-Language-Hearing Association, New Orleans, Lousiana, November 20.

Ingham, R.J., Fox, P.T., Ingham, J.C., Zamarripa, F., Martin, C., Jerabek, P., & Cotton, J. (1996). A functional-lesion investigation of developmental stuttering with positron emission tomography. *Journal of Speech and Hearing Research, 39,* 1208-1227.

Ingham, R.J., & Packman, A. (1979). A further evaluation of the speech of stutterers during chorus- and nonchorus-reading conditions. *Journal of Speech and Hearing Research, 22,* 784-793.

Lancaster, J.L., Glass, T.G., Lankapilli, B.R., Downs, H., Mayberg, H., & Fox, P. T. (1996). A modality-independent approach to spatial normalization of tomographic images of the human brain. *Human Brain Mapping, 3,* 209-223.

Martin, R.R., Haroldson, S.K., & Triden K.A. (1984). Stuttering and speech naturalness. *Journal of Speech and Hearing Disorders, 49,* 53-58.

Moore, W.H. Jr. (1990). Pathophysiology of stuttering: Cerebral activation differences in stutterers vs nonstutterers. *ASHA Reports, 18,* 72-80.

Moore, W.H., Jr., & Haynes, W.O. (1980). Alpha hemispheric asymmetry and stuttering: Some support for a segmentation dysfunction hypothesis. *Journal of Speech and Hearing Research, 23,* 229-247.

Pardo, J.V., & Fox, P.T., (1993). Preoperative assessment of the cerebral hemispheric dominance for language with CBF PET. *Human Brain Mapping, 1,* 57-68.

Peters, H.F.M., Hulstijn, W., & Starkweather, C.W. (1991). *Speech motor control and stuttering.* Amsterdam: Exerpta Medica.

Petersen, S.E., Fox, P.T., Posner, M.I., Mintun, M., & Raichle, M.E. (1989). Positron emission tomographic studies of the processing of single words. *Journal of Cognitive Neuroscience, 1,* 153-170.

Pool, K.D., Devous, M.D., Freeman, F.J., Watson, B.C., & Finitzo, T. (1991). Regional cerebral blood flow in developmental stutterers. *Archives of Neurology, 48,* 509-512.

Posner, M.I., Petersen, S.E., Fox, P.T., & Raichle, M.E. (1988). Localization of cognitive operations in the human brain. *Science, 240,* 1627-1631.

Posner, M.I., & Raichle, M.E. (1994). *Images of mind.* New York: Scientific American Library Rosenfield, D.B., & Nudelman, H.B. (1987). Neuropsychological models of speech dysfluency. In L. Rustin, H. Purser, & D. Rowley, (Eds.), *Progress in the treatment of fluency disorders* (pp. 3-42). London: Taylor & Francis.

Sabatini, U., Chollet, F., Rascol, O., Celsis, P., Rascol, A., Lenzi, G. L., & Marc-Vergnes, J-P. (1993). Effect of side and rate of stimulation on cerebral blood flow changes in motor areas during finger movements in humans. *Journal of Cerebral Blood Flow and Metabolism, 13,* 639-645.

Schlaug, G., Sanes, J.N., Seitz, R.J., Thangaraj, V., Knorr, U., Darby, D., Herzog, H., Edelman, R.R., & Warach, S. (1995). Pattern and magnitude of cerebral blood flow changes are determined by movement rate. *Human Brain Mapping, S1,* 296.

Smith, A. (1990). Toward a comprehensive theory of stuttering: A commentary. *Journal of Speech and Hearing Disorders, 55,* 398-401.

Talairach, J, & Tournoux, P, (1988). *Co-planar stereotaxic atlas of the human brain.* Verlag: Thieme Medical Publishers.

Travis, L.E. (1978). The cerebral dominance theory of stuttering: 1931-1978. *Journal of Speech and Hearing Disorders, 43,* 278-281.

Van Riper, C., & Hull, C.J. (1955). The quantitative measurement of the effect of certain situations on stuttering. In W. Johnson, & R.R. Leutenegger, (Eds.), *Stuttering in children and adults.* (pp. 199-206) Minneapolis: University of Minnesota Press.

Webster, W.G. (1993). Hurried hands and tangled tongues. In E. Boberg (Ed.), *Neuropsychology of stuttering.* (pp. 73 - 127) Edmonton: The University of Alberta Press.

Wexler, B.E., Fulbright, R.K., Skudlarski, P., Constable, R.T., & Gore, J.C. (1995). An fMRI study of motor system response to increasing rate and force of movement. *Human Brain Mapping, S1,* 297.

Wise, R., Chollet, F., Hadar, U., Friston, K., & Frackowiak, R. (1991). Distribution of cortical neural networks involved in word comprehension and word retrieval. *Brain, 114,* 1803-1817.

Zimmermann, G. (1980). Stuttering: A disorder of movement. *Journal of Speech and Hearing Research, 23,* 122-136.

Speech Production: Motor Control, Brain Research and Fluency Disorders
W. Hulstijn, H.F.M. Peters and P.H.H.M. Van Lieshout, editors

Chapter 25

A POSITRON EMISSION TOMOGRAPHY INVESTIGATION OF POST-TREATMENT BRAIN ACTIVATION IN STUTTERERS

Robert M. Kroll, Luc F. De Nil, S. Kapur, S. Houle

Using positron emission tomography scanning techniques with untreated, adult stutterers, De Nil and Kroll (1995) reported that stutterers demonstrate increased activation in primarily right temporal, motor and frontal regions, whereas a similarly matched nonstuttering group demonstrated a primarily left pattern of brain activation when reading a list of single words aloud. During a silent reading condition, the authors reported increased activation in the left anterior cingulate cortex of the stuttering group but not in the matched controls, a finding interpreted as a reflection of covert anticipation of stuttering in the experimental group.

The purpose of the present research was to further investigate regional cerebral blood flow in stutterers and to determine whether any changes in activation patterns could be observed immediately following intensive fluency shaping therapy. The subjects for the study included five right handed stuttering adult males who completed a three week intensive speech treatment program not more than two weeks prior to undergoing PET scanning. Data from this group were compared to those obtained from the untreated stutterers tested by De Nil and Kroll (1995).

Results obtained from the silent reading task indicated that treated stutterers did not show increased activation in the anterior cingulate cortex. When compared with the untreated stutterers on the oral reading task, the subjects having received treatment showed increased activation in the left motor cortex, while maintaining large areas of activity in the right hemisphere. It is concluded that increased fluency immediately post-treatment is associated with decreased covert anticipation of stuttering during silent reading, and increased activation of left motor cortex during oral reading, as the subject employs concious and deliberate fluency skills.

INTRODUCTION

Several investigators have reported evidence of atypical cortical activation patterns in stuttering individuals during speech and non-speech tasks, including abnormal electro-encephalogram measures (Fritzell, et al, 1965; Okasha, et al, 1974, Sayles, 1971) and patterns of alpha wave suppression (Boberg et al., 1983; Moore, 1986; Moore & Lang, 1977; Moore & Haynes, 1980; Moore & Lorendo, 1980; Moore et al., 1982). The latter studies, in particular, have shown that alpha wave suppression in stutterers during speech and language tasks is more pronounced over the right than the left hemisphere, indicating greater activation in the right hemisphere, while the reverse is true in nonstutterers. More indirect studies of brain lateralization in stuttering and nonstuttering subjects also have provided evidence of greater right hemisphere activation during processing of speech and language stimuli in stutterers. The majority of dichotic listening studies with stuttering and nonstuttering speakers have reported differences in ear advantage between the two groups, with the stutterers showing either a left-ear (right hemisphere) advantage, or no clear left or right ear advantage, while nonstutterers almost always showed a clear right-ear (left hemisphere) advantage (Blood & Blood, 1989; Cimorel-Strong et al., 1983). As Moore (1984) has pointed out, while results are not always consistent, the nature of the linguistic stimuli used in these studies is an important consideration. All studies in which meaningful stimuli were used have shown similar differences in ear preference between stutterers and nonstutterers. Increased right hemisphere processing of linguistic stimuli also have been reported for visual tachistoscopic studies (Hand & Haynes, 1983; Plakosh, 1978; Victor & Johannsen, 1984), and for studies of averaged evoked potentials (Ponsford et al., 1975; Zimmerman & Knott, 1974).

Moore (1984) has formulated the Segmental Disfunction Model in an attempt to account for these and related findings. This model is based on the fact that the right and left hemispheres differ in the way they process information, with the right hemisphere using a more holistic, nonsequential, time-independent process, while the left hemisphere processes information in a more analytical sequential manner. Stuttering, according to the segmental disfunction model, is associated with increased utilization of the nonsegmental processing functions of the right hemisphere for encoding segmental information at a linguistic-motor planning level (Moore et al., 1982). Such right hemisphere bias for language formulation may lead to "a disruption of the temporal-sequential relationships of language at major points of segmentation during speech production" (p. 220).

An alternative view has been put forward by Webster (Webster, 1989, 1990; Forster & Webster, 1991). Based primarily on dual-task interference studies, he has proposed an Attentional Lability Hypothesis to account for the atypical cerebral lateralization observed in stutterers. The basic tenet of this hypothesis is that while both nonstutterers and stutterers control linguistic processing with the left hemisphere, the stutterers inappropriately and ineffectively engage the right hemisphere during such processing. Based on studies showing different interference patterns between the left and right hand during fingertapping tasks (Webster, 1990a), writing tasks (Webster, 1990b), and concurrent upper and lower limb movements (Forster & Webster, 1991), Webster suggested that stutterers have a dissociation of hemispheric activation or attention from hemispheric specialization (Peters, 1995).

With the advent of modern functional brain imaging techniques, a number of researchers have reinvestigated previous hypotheses of atypical brain lateralization in stuttering individuals. In one of the first such studies, Wood et al. (1980) obtained rCBF measurements in two stutterers during stuttering and after administration of Haloperidol, which resulted in increased fluency. Asymmetrical blood flow was observed in Broca's area (right > left) and Wernicke's area (left > right) during stuttering, and a reversal of the blood flow pattern in

Broca's area during fluent speech (left > right), but not in Wernicke's area. They interpreted their findings as showing inadequate left cerebral dominance for speech production, but not for speech perception. However, the use of medication to increase fluency and the absence of a control group of nonstutterers make these findings hard to interpret. More recently, Pool et al. (1991) used SPECT to study adult stutterers during rest (eyes closed). They found a significant blood flow asymmetry (right > left) in temporal and anterior cingulate regions in these disfluent speakers, although for the temporal region the pattern was opposite to that reported by Wood et al. (1980). In addition, they found a significant correlation between the degree of blood flow asymmetry in the temporal regions and the stuttering subjects' laryngeal reaction times (Watson et al., 1992). Flow measures below the group median were associated with increased reaction times. They speculated that the temporal regions may be part of a cortical and subcortical fluency-generating system.

In contrast to SPECT, measuring rCBF with PET, using [^{15}O]H$_2$O as a tracer, provides researchers the opportunity to measure cerebral activation repeatedly during the same or different tasks in a single experimental session. As a result, this latter technique has quickly become the method of choice for the study of cognitive and other processes in humans, including speech and language (Wise et al., 1991; Petersen & Fiez, 1993; Chadwick & Whelan, 1991). In a study of solo and choral reading, Fox et al. (1996) reported extensive hyperactivity of the motor system, with right lateralization of primary and extraprimary motor cortices, and an absence of temporal activation during stuttered speech compared to fluent speech in the nonstuttering speakers. Fluent speech under choral reading in the stutterers resulted in a more normalized activation of motor regions, in particular in the supplementary motor area, superior lateral premotor area, and temporal regions. Stutterers continued to show increased cerebellar activation, which the authors suggested could be related to stutterers' greater motor effort during choral reading. Wu et al. (1995) also reported decreased neural activation, measured as glucose uptake using F-18 deoxyglucose as tracer, in the fluent speech of stuttering individuals during choral reading. Decreased activation was observed in Broca's and Wernicke's areas, as well as deep frontal orbital areas, in the left hemisphere and right cerebellum, and bilaterally in the superior frontal lobe and posterior cingulate cortex areas. Braun and Ludlow (1995), comparing stuttering and nonstuttering adult males on a variety of simple oral motor tasks, observed left hemisphere lateralization of activation in the nonstutterers, contrasted with primarily right lateralization in the stutterers. When the subjects were involved in language tasks, the nonstutterers again showed lateralized activation of left hemisphere regions, while the stutterers failed to show such lateralization.

A positron emission tomography study of silent and oral reading in stuttering and nonstuttering subjects

In our laboratory, we have used silent and oral single word reading tasks to compare the distribution of areas of increased activation between 10 stuttering and 10 matched nonstuttering English-speaking righthanded adults (De Nil et al., 1995). Subjects performed three different tasks: (1) a nonspeech baseline task which consisted of passively viewing a string of X's; (2) silent reading of a list of single words; and (3) oral reading of a list of words similar to (2). Scans of [^{15}O]H$_2$O distribution for each of the control and experimental tasks were averaged across all subjects within each group and analyzed by means of statistical parametric mapping (Friston et al., 1995). The most important findings of this study can be summarized in the following way. During silent reading, the stuttering subjects, but not the nonstuttering controls, showed a significant increase in activation in the anterior cingulate gyrus. Anterior cingulate activation in previous studies on normal speaking subjects, when observed, generally has been associated with tasks requiring cognitive processing of more complex language stimuli like the ones used in the Stroop paradigm. Using the Stroop paradigm, Pardo et al. (1990) suggested that the anterior cingulate cortex may be part of an inner articulatory loop which is active during such more complex tasks. For others, activation in the anterior cingulate during complex tasks may be related to selection for action (Petersen et al., 1989). It is well known that most adult stutterers have a strong tendency to scan the phonetic and orthographic structure of words for signs of potential fluency problems, even during tasks not requiring overt speech. It seems likely, therefore, that the silent reading task may have represented a cognitively more complex task for the stuttering than the nonstuttering subjects resulting in anterior cingulate activation in the former, but not the latter subjects. The localization of the neural activity peak (12 mm lateral to the midline) seems to suggest a significant involvement of neurons in the anterior cingulate sulcus, an area known to have extensive connections to the lateral cortical motor regions (Dum & Strick, 1993). This suggests to us that the increased anterior cingulate activation in stutterers observed in this study may be related primarily to silent articulatory rehearsal of the words in anticipation of stuttering, although influence of an action selection process can not be excluded based on the present data.

Analysis of the between-group differences during the oral reading tasks showed a pattern of largely unilateral left hemisphere activation in the nonstutterers, including occipital, temporal, frontal, premotor and motor cortex, which corresponds well to the regions identified in the model proposed by Petersen et al. (1988). The stuttering subjects also showed increased activation in the occipital, frontal, premotor, and motor cortex, but this activation clearly was right-lateralized. In contrast to Fox et al. (1996), increased activation in our study was observed in the stutterers also at the level of the middle temporal gyrus (BA 21) and the inferior parietal lobe (BA 40). In addition, higher activation levels in the stuttering subjects were found subcortically at the level of the globus pallidus. Interestingly, therapeutic stimulation of this area following implantation of electrodes has been observed to result in stuttering-like symptoms (Lozano, personal communication). These initial results provide support for the hypothesis that stuttering is associated with increased right hemisphere activation during speech. Importantly, increased activation was seen not only in traditional motor cortex, but also involved frontal (BA 9) and temporal cortex, which have been associated with semantic and phonological processing during language formulation. Interestingly, no right hemisphere lateralization was observed during silent reading. This finding can be interpreted as suggesting that the right hemisphere lateralization during oral speech is a direct consequence of the presence of stuttering. Alternatively, it is possible that the simple passive word reading task used in the present experiment may have failed to activate the semantic and phonological processes sufficiently to reach threshold. The hypothesis that the observed right-hemisphere activation reflects more than just the presence of stuttering finds some support in the observation that cortical regions traditionally hypothesized to be involved in other than motor tasks also showed right lateralization.

STUDY

A positron emission tomography study of post-treatment brain activation is stutterers

In contrast to Braun and Ludlow (1995) and Fox et al. (1996), our study did not include a fluency inducing speech condition. Instead, our subjects were instructed to speak in a normal manner and no specific instructions were given to reduce stuttering. The question thus remains to what extent the observed right hemisphere activation pattern in the stuttering subjects in our study reflects a fundamental difference in brain lateralization for language processing or is a direct consequence of the presence of stuttering during the task. The present preliminary study is an attempt to provide some answers to this question using PET to investigate brain activation patterns in stuttering subjects who have acquired high levels of speech fluency immediately following intensive speech treatment.

SUBJECTS

In our study, PET scan images were obtained from five stuttering male adults, ranging in age from 20-45 years. The subjects had completed an intensive course of speech therapy at the Clarke Institute of Psychiatry no more than two weeks prior to the experimental scanning session. All subjects were predominately right-handed, native speakers of English. Handedness was assessed via the Edinburgh Handedness Inventory. Because of the higher incidence of bilateral and right hemisphere lateralization for language in left handed individuals (Peters, 1995), only those subjects who obtained a score of 80 or above (right-handed) were asked to participate. Subjects were screened for histories of relevant neurological or other medical problems as well as histories of medical and recreational drug usage. Subjects were selected for the study only if reporting a negative history of speech, language or hearing problems other than the presenting stuttering problem. All subjects underwent a full speech and language assessment by a apeech-language pathologist, certified by the College of Speech Language Pathologists and Audiologists of Ontario. In addition, subjects were videotaped while reading a standard 150 word passage and answering a series of standard questions. Videotape sessions were conducted just prior to the treatment program and again at the conclusion of the treatment program. Stuttering severity ranged from moderate to severe, with four of the five subjects in the moderate range. No subject displayed more than three percent disfluency following the treatment program, and there were no instances of disfluency observed during the experimental scanning sessions from any of the subjects. It should be noted that only male subjects were recruited for the study because of the presenting caseload of patients at the Clarke Institute and also to eliminate any potentially confounding variables due to differences in language lateralization between females and males (Shaywitz et al., 1995)

TREATMENT PROGRAM

The treatment program at the Clarke Institute was first introduced by Kroll in 1975 and is based on the Precision Fluency Shaping Program (Webster, 1974) This intensive, three week treatment is based upon the premise that stutterers' speech responses can be modified to produce easier, fluent speech patterns by systematically modifying such behaviours as speech rate, respiration, voice onset and articulation. Incorporated within the program is a series of exercises and procedures that focus on the establishment of new speech patterns within the clinical setting. These newly acquired speech skills are then gradually and systematically transferred to everyday, naturalistic settings. Also incorporated within the program is a series of group and individual therapy sessions focusing on self talk or covert thinking as it pertains to effective mental preparation for communication. Patients are encouraged to employ both the fluency skills as well as the proper mental or cognitive set as they set out to transfer their newly acquired speech patterns. Post-treatment and long-term outcome data pertaining to the efficacy of this intensive fluency management program have been reported by Kroll (1991), Leibovitz and Kroll (1980) and De Nil and Kroll (1995).

PET SCANNING

Positron Emission Tomography scans were obtained using a GEMS-Scanditronix PC 2048-15B head scanner locate at the PET Centre of the Clarke Institute of Psychiatry. Subjects were scanned lying down with a custom-fitted thermoplastic mask for head stabilization, but which did not in any way interfere with speech movements. Emission scans were done using 30mCi of $[^{15}O]H_2O$ injected as a bolus into a forearm vein at the beginning of each task by a qualified technician. Scans were acquired for 60 seconds during each experimental task. Multiple injections within a scanning session were separated by a ten minute interval. PET scans were reconstructed using a Hanning filter and attenuation correction which was measured for each subject individually at the beginning of each scanning session.

DATA ANALYSIS

PET scans were analyzed using statistical parametric mapping (SPM). Within this method, between- and within-subject variations in global bloodflow across the scans is accounted for by co-varying the global flow as the independent variable (Friston et al., 1990). The SPM analysis involves the following steps: (1) stereotactic reorientation of the images along the AC-PC line; (2) plastic transformation of these images using a non-linear resampling technique to correct for anatomical variance across subjects; and (3) spatial filtering to enhance the signal in the presence of the noise introduced by anatomical and functional heterogeneity across subjects. All data were smoothed using a 12 mm filter in the x, y, and z directions. In SPM, the scans of different tasks are compared with each other on a pixel by pixel basis using an ANOVA design, and the statistical significance of each difference is assessed by comparing the magnitude of the difference at a pixel with the error variance at that particular pixel. The resulting map of the t-statistic at each pixel constitutes the SPM (Friston et al., 1995). Type 1 errors are minimized by comparing the total number of pixels where the t-statistic is significant at $p < 0.005$ to the number of such pixels expected by chance, using a χ^2 distribution, and reporting differences only if the χ^2 statistic is significant at $p < 0.05$. Brain regions of significant differential activation, obtained using the subtraction method, were interpreted with reference to Talaraich and Tournoux coordinates (1988).

EXPERIMENTAL TASKS

All subjects performed three different tasks identical to those used by De Nil et al. (1995). These tasks consisted of a nonspeech control task, a silent reading task, and an oral reading task Each task lasted approximately ninety seconds. During the control task, subjects were instructed to view passively a series of strings of X's on a computer screen suspended in front of them so as to allow for comfortable viewing. The strings of X's were randomly varied in length within the range of the words used in the other two tasks. A total of twenty individual character strings were presented with an interstimulus interval ranging from 1.5 to 2 seconds. Presentations of individual character strings were separated by a single x in the middle of the monitor screen. During the silent reading task, subjects were presented with a series of three-syllable, low imagery wordswhich were presented in a manner similar to the control task. They were instructed to read the words silently, without mouthing, but engaging in the cognitive activity of employing their learned fluency skills during the silent reading, a process referred to as covert practice during the treatment program. During the oral reading task, a list of similar but different three-syllable words was presented in a similar way and subjects were asked to read the words out loud while employing their fluency skills or speech targets which they had learnrned during the intensive treatment program.

The order of the oral reading and silent reading tasks was counterbalanced across the subjects. Each task was presented twice during the experimental session for a total of six tasks, with the two control tasks always the first and last during each experimental session. Each of the word lists for the two silent and the two oral reading tasks consisted of similar but different words. Interstimulus intervals ranged randomly from 1.5 to 2 seconds.

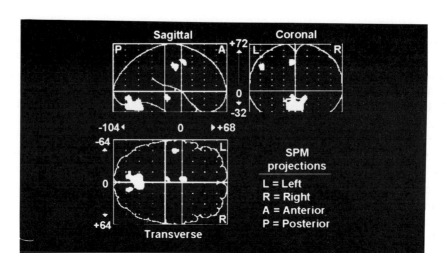

Figure 1. Increases in rCBF during silent reading minus baseline for 5 treated stuttering subjects.

RESULTS

Figure 1 shows differences in brain activation between silent reading and baseline activity for the group of five stuttering subjects post-treatment. As expected, the silent reading condition showed significantly increased bilateral activation in the occipital region, as well as in the cerebellar and left motor regions compared to the baseline condition. These findings essentially replicate those found in the study reported by De Nil et al. (1995) with untreated stutterers. The main difference in the observed activation patterns between the untreated and treated groups of subjects is the absence of the anterior cingulate area activation. A likely interpretation of this finding is that the stuttering subjects, post-treatment, were engaging in a very different cognitive activity during the silent reading task. Recall that they were asked to specifically focus covertly on their fluency facilitating speech targets. It is possible then, that, in contrast to the stuttering subjects in our first study (De Nil et al., 1995), the treatment enabled the subjects in this study to eliminate the cognitive scanning behaviour for potentially troublesome sounds and words during the silent reading task. This may account for the absence of the increased anterior cingulate activation in the present study.

Figure 2 shows the differences in brain activity patterns between the oral reading and silent reading tasks for the group of the five treated stutterers. This pattern is essentially similar to that reported by De Nil et al. (1995) for a group of untreated stutterers. Contrary to pre-post treatment data reported by Boberg et al. (1983), no significant shift to left hemisphere activation was found despite the fact that the stuttering subjects were now deliberately using fluency targets (stretched syllables, gentle onsets, light articulatory contacts and slow, diaphragmatic breathing) and no stuttering was observed for any of the subjects

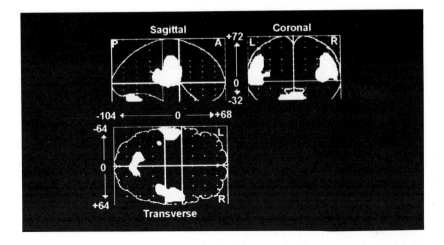

Figure 2. Increases in rCBF during oral reading minus silent reading for 5 treated stuttering subjects.

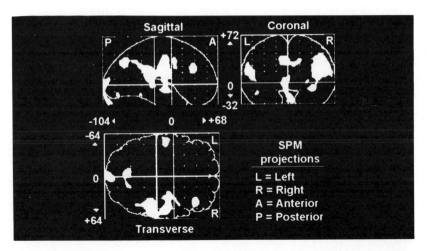

Figure 3. Increases in rCBF (oral reading minus silent reading) in 5 treated stuttering subjects vs. 10 control non-stutterers.

during the oral reading tasks.

Figure 3 compares the differences in brain activity patterns between silent and oral reading for the treated stuttering group in the present study against the control group used in our first study (De Nil et al., 1995). As was the case with the untreated stutterers, it is readily apparent that the post-treatment stuttering group shows primarily right hemisphere activation, even when effectively employing learned speech targets and exhibiting essentially controlled fluency during the course of the experiment.

316   R.M. Kroll, L.F. de Nil, S. Kapur, S. Houle

The data shown in Figures 2 and 3 do not corroborate previous reports of hemispheric activation shifts in adult stutterers, as measured electrophysiologically, from pre- to posttreatment (Boberg et al., 1983). It should also be noted that the subjects in the present study were using highly controlled and deliberate speech production characterized by an emphasis on sequential sound production and timing. According to the Segmental Disfunction Model, suggested by Moore (1984), such a speech pattern should reflect primarily left hemisphere brain activity. Clearly, such a dramatic shift from right to left hemisphere activation was not observed in our post-treatment subjects (figure 3).

While Figures 2 and 3 suggest that the activation patterns post-treatment are largely similar to those obtained in our initial study (De Nil et al., 1995), some differences between the untreated and treated stutterers became apparent when subtracting silent reading from oral reading scans (figure 4). The post-treatment subjects showed a slight increase in cortical activation in the left sensorimotor cortex. It is hypothesized that this increased activation reflects the deliberate application of the learned speech motor skills during task production.

CONCLUSIONS

The conclusions from this study must remain preliminary as data are presented on only five subjects who had undergone intensive fluency shaping treatment for stuttering. Based upon our initial findings however, our preliminary interpretations are as follows:
1. Stuttering subjects who have undergone fluency shaping treatment adopt a different cognitive or mental set during silent reading of single words. It appears that less anticipatory scanning is going on as the subjects are engaged in the covert rehearsal of their fluency producing targets.

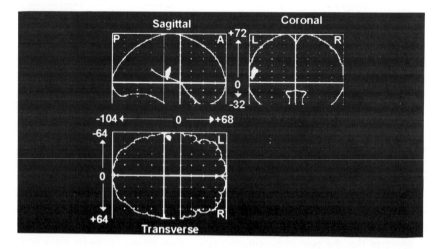

Figure 4. Increases in rCBF (oral reading minus silent reading) in 5 treated stuttering subjects vs. 10 untreated stuttering subjects.

The cogntive demands of the task are thus perceived differently because the subjects have been trained in the use of efficient reading and speaking production. This is reflected in the obvious lack of anterior cingulate activation post-treatment. 2. The similar pattern of right hemisphere activation during oral reading in both the untreated and treated stuttering subjects, despite significant differences in their overt speech behaviour, suggests that this right hemisphere activation is not merely a direct consequence of the presence or absence of stuttering, but is reflective of an inherent or acquired, but stable, characteristic of the speech and language processing system in individuals who stutter.

REFERENCES

Blood, G.W., & Blood, I.W. (1989). Laterality preferences in adult female and male stutterers. *Journal of Fluency Disorders, 14,* 1-10.

Boberg, E, Yeudall, L.T., Schopflocher, D., & Bo-Lassen, P. (1983). The effect of an intensive behavioral program on the distribution of EEG alpha power in stutterers during the processing of verbal and visuospatial information. *Journal of Fluency Disorders, 8,* 245-263.

Braun, H.G., & Ludlow, C. (1995). Advances in stuttering research using positron emission tomography brain imaging. *ASHA, 37,* 89

Chadwick, D.J., & Whelan, J. (Eds.) (1991) *Exploring brain functional anatomy with positron tomography.* New York: Wiley.

Cimorell-Strong, J.M., Gilbert, H.R., & Frick, J.V. (1983). Dichotic speech perception: A comparison between stuttering and nonstuttering children. *Journal of Fluency Disorders, 8,* 77-91.

Corbetta, M., Miezin, F.M., Dobmeyer, S., Shulman, G.L., & Petersen, S.E. (1991). Selective attention modulates extrastriate visual regions in humans during visual feature discrimination and attention. Exploring Brain Functional Anatomy with Positron Emission Tomography. *Ciba Foundation Symposium, 163,* 165-180.

De Nil, L.F., & Kroll, R.M. (1995). The relationship between locus of control and long-term treatment outcome in adults who stutter. *Journal of Fluency Disorders, 20,* 345-364.

De Nil, L.F., Kroll, R.M., Houle, S., Ludlow, C.L., Braun, A., Ingham, R.J., et al (1995). Advances in stuttering research using positron emission tomography brain imaging. *ASHA, 37,* 89 (Abstract)

Dum, R. and Strick, P. (1993). Cingulate motor areas. In: *Neurobiology of cingulate cortex and the limbic thalamus.* B. Vogt & M. Gabriel (Ed.), Boston: Berkhauser.

Forster, D.C. & Webster, W.G. (1991). Concurrent task interference in stutterers: dissociating hemispheric specialization and activation. *Canadian Journal of Psychology, 45,* 321-335.

Fox, P.T., Ingham, R.J., Ingham, J.C., Hirsh, T.B., Down, J.H., Martin, C., Jerabek, P., Glass, T., & Lancaster, J.L. (1996). A PET study of the neural systems of stuttering. *Nature, 382,* 158-162.

Friston, K.J., Frith, C.D., Liddle, P.F., Dolan, R.J., Lammertsma, A.A. & Fackowiak, R.S. (1990). The relationship between global and local changes in PET scans. *Journal of Cerebral Blood Flow and Metabolism, 10,* 458-466.

Friston, K.J., Holmes, A.P., et al. (1995). Statistical parametric maps in functional imaging: A general linear approach. *Human Brain Mapping, 2,* 189-210.

Frith, C.D., Friston, K., Liddle, P.F., & Frackowiak, R.S. (1991). A PET study of word finding. *Neuropsychologia, 29,* 1-12.

Fritzell, B., Petersen, I., & Sellden, U. (1965). *An EEG study of stuttering and nonstuttering school children.* XIII Congress of the International Society of Logopedics and Phoniatrics, 1.

Hand, C.R., & Haynes, W.O. (1983). Linguistic processing and reaction time differences in stutterers and nonstutterers. *Journal of Speech and Hearing Research, 26,* 181-185.

Kroll, R.M. (1991). *Manual of fluency maintenance, a guide for ongoing practice.* Toronto: Clarke Institute of Psychiatry.

Leibowitz, S., & Kroll, R.M. (1980). Intensive stuttering therapy: retrospective data and current maintenance considerations. *ASHA,* 89.

Moore, W.H. (1984). Central nervous system characteristics of Stutterers. *Nature and Treatment of Stuttering: New Directions.* In R.F. Curlee & W.H. Perkins (Eds.), San Diego: College-Hill.

Moore, W.H. (1986). Hemisperic alpha asymmetries of stutterers and nonstutterers for the recall and recognition of words and connected reading passages: Some relationships to severity of stuttering. *Journal of Fluency Disorders, 11,* 71-89.

Moore, W.H., & Lorendo, L.C. (1980). Hemispheric alpha asymmetries of stuttering males and nonstuttering males and females for words of high and low imagery. *Journal of Fluency Disorders, 5,* 11-26.

Moore, W.H., Craven, D.C., & Faber, M.M. (1982). Hemispheric alpha asymmetries of words with positive, negative, and neutral arousal values preceding tasks of recall and recognition: Electrophysiological and behavioral results from stuttering males and nonstuttering males and females. *Brain and Language, 17,* 211-224.

Moore, W.H., & Haynes, W.O. (1980). Alpha hemisperic asymmetry and stuttering: Some support for a segmentation dysfunction hypothesis. *Journal of Speech and Hearing Research, 23,* 229-247.

Moore, W.H., & Lang, M.K. (1977). Alpha asymmetry over the right and left hemisperes of stutterers and control subjects preceding massed oral readings: A preliminary investigation. *Perceptual and Motor Skills, 44,* 223-230.

Okasha, A, Moneim, S.A., Bishry, Z., Kamel, M., & Moustafa, M. (1974). Electroencephalographic study of stammering. *British Journal of Psychiatry, 124,* 534-535.

Pardo, J.V., Pardo, P.J., Janer, K.W., & Raichle, M.E. (1990). The anterior cingulate cortex mediates processing selection in the Stroop attentional conflict paradigm. *Proceedings of the National Academy of Sciences in the USA, 87,* 256-259.

Peters, M. (1995). Handedness and its relation to other indices of cerebral lateralization. In R.J. Davidson & K. Hugdahl (Eds.), *Brain Asymmetry.* Cambridge: MIT Press.

Petersen, S.E., & Fiez, J.A. (1993). The processing of single words studied with positron emission tomography. *Annual Revue of Neuroscience, 16,* 509-530.

Petersen, S.E., Fox, P.T., Posner, M.I., Mintun, M.,, & Raichle, M.E. (1988). Positron emission tomographic studies of the cortical anatomy of single-word processing. *Nature, 331,* 585-589.

Petersen, S.E., Fox, P.T., Posner, M.I., Mintun, M., & Raichle, M.E. (1989). Positron emission tomographic studies of the processing of single words. *Journal of Cognitive Neuroscience, 1,* 153-170.

Plakosh, P. (1978). The functional asymmetry of the brain: Hemispheric specialization in stutterers for processing of visually presented linguistic and spatial stimuli. Unpublished doctoral dissertation. Palo Alto School of Professional Psychology [referenced in Moore, W.H. (1984). Central nervous system characteristics of Stutterers. *Nature and Treatment of Stuttering: New Directions.* In R.F. Curlee & W.H. Perkins (Eds.), San Diego: College-Hill]

Ponsford, R.E., Brown,W.S., Marsh, J.T., & Travis, L.E. (1975). Evoked potential correlates of cerebral dominance for speech perception in stutterers and nonstutterers. *Electroencephalogr Clinical Neurophysiology, 39,* 434 (Abstract)

Pool, K.D., Devous, M.D., Freeman, F.J., Watson, B.C., & Finitzo, T. (1991). Regional cerebral blood flow in developmental stutterers. *Archives of Neurology, 48,* 509-512.

Sayles, D.G. (1971). Cortical excitability, perseveration, and stuttering. *Journal of Speech and Hearing Research, 14,* 462-475.

Shaywitz, B.A., Shaywitz, S.E., Pugh, K.R., Constable, R.T., Skudlarski, P., Fulbright, R.K., et al (1995). Sex differences in the functional organization of the brain for language. *Nature, 373,* 607-609.

Talairach, J., & Tournoux, P. (1988). *Co-planar stereotaxic atlas of the human brain: 3-dimensional proportional system: An approach to cerebral imaging.* Stuttgart: Thieme Verlag.

Victor, C. & Johannsen, H.S. (1984). Untersuchung zur zerebralen Dominanz fur Sprache bei Stotterer mittels Tachistoskopie. *Sprache-Stimme-Gehor, 8,* 74-77.

Watson, B.C., Pool, K.D., Devous, M.D., Freeman, F.J., & Finitzo, T. (1992). Brain blood flow related to acoustic laryngeal reaction time in adult developmental stutterers. *Journal of Speech and Hearing Research, 35,* 555-561.

Webster, R.L (1974). A behavioral analysis of stuttering: Treatment and theory. In K.S. Calhoun, H.E. Adams & K.M. Mitchell (Eds.). *Innovative Treatment Methods in Psychopathology.* New York: Wiley.

Webster, W.G. (1989). Sequence initiation performance by stutterers under conditions of response competition. *Brain and Language, 36,* 286-300.

Webster, W.G. (1990a). Evidence in bimanual finger-tapping of an attentional component to stuttering. *Behavioural and Brain Research, 37,* 93-100.

Webster, W.G. (1990b). Concurrent cognitive processing and letter sequence transcription deficits in stutterers. *Canadian Journal of Psychology, 44,* 1-13.

Wise, R., Chollet, F., Hadar, U., Fiston, K., Hoffner, E., & Frackowiak, R. (1991). Distribution of cortical neural networks involved in word comprehension and word retrieval. *Brain, 114,* 1803-1817.

Wood, F., Stump, D., McKeehan, A., Sheldon, S., & Proctor, J. (1980). Patterns of regional cerebral blood flow during attempted reading aloud by stutterers both on and off haloperidol medication: Evidence for inadequate left frontal activation during stuttering. *Brain and Language, 9,* 141-144.

Wu, J.C., Maguire ,G., Riley, G., Fallon, J., Lacasse, L., Chin, S., et al (1995). A positron emission tomography [18F]deoxyglucose study of developmental stuttering. *Neuroreport, 6,* 501-505.

Zimmermann, G.N., & Knott, J.R. (1974). Slow potentials of the brain related to speech processing in normal speakers and stutterers. *Electroencephalography and Clinical Neurophysiology, 37,* 599-607.

Speech Production: Motor Control, Brain Research and Fluency Disorders
W. Hulstijn, H.F.M. Peters and P.H.H.M. Van Lieshout, editors

Chapter 26

PET SCAN EVIDENCE OF PARALLEL CEREBRAL SYSTEMS RELATED TO TREATMENT EFFECTS

Glyndon D. Riley, Joseph C. Wu, Gerald Maguire

Goldberg (1985) described two cerebral systems, lateral and medial, that operate in parallel to accommodate speech production; our model adds the dopamine 2 system. In this model the lateral system has special functions related to language processing and production and the medial system specializes in speech motor planning. The dopamine 2 system is insufficiently controlled so that too much dopamine reaches the striatum in the medial system and reduces speech motor planning effectiveness. Treatments that require fluency monitoring at the language level seem to target the lateral system and work "top-down" to influence the medial system. Treatments that reduce the amount of dopamine 2 that reaches the striatum or that target speech motor planning directly seem to use a "bottom-up" strategy. This model, although oversimplified, may have the potential to describe neurological correlates related to observed treatment effects.

INTRODUCTION

This research report is organized into three parts. First, we describe three parallel cerebral systems and suggest that they form the basis for a partial explanatory model and also suggest some treatment effects predicted from the systems interactions. Second, (Wu et al., this volume, chapter 27), we present PET scan evidence from FDG (glucose uptake) and FDOPA (dopamine uptake) scanning procedures. Third (Maguire et al., this volume, chapter 32), we present some preliminary data that seems to explain one mechanism by which a class of medications, D-2 blockers, reduces stuttering.

OVERVIEW OF SYSTEMS

The three systems that operate in parallel and are proposed to form an interactive model are labeled: Lateral, Medial, and D2 (dopamine 2). Figure 1 illustrates the relation of these systems. The concept of lateral and medial systems is not new. Goldberg (1985) has described them in detail. The same or similar concepts are incorporated into reviews by Caruso (1991), Gracco (1991, 1994), McClean (1990), Nudelman et al., (1991), and Watson and Freeman (1997) among others.

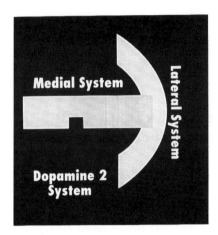

Figure 1. Schema of three parallel systems proposed to relate to stuttering and to treatment effects.

Lateral System

The lateral system is depicted at the top because it includes the classical, cortical areas associated with language reception (decoding) and production (encoding). The major cortices include Wernicke's area and Broca's area; there are of course many more. Part II of this report (Wu et al., this volume) describes additional cortical regions included in the PET data. The lateral system is where we live; "kindergarten learning" takes place at this level; we know that we are learning language and speech. This system interprets phonemes and words and produces linguistically accurate sentences. It uses *feedback* information to respond to external and internal conditions and make on-line adjustments.

Medial System

The medial system includes the striatum with special reference to the caudate and putamen as well as other brain regions described in part II of this report. The Medial system is not cognitively available to the speaker. It processes lots of information including hundreds of neural impulses per second. It is hard for the speaker to even conceive of it's functions much less access it in a conscious way. Note the comparison and contrast of Feedback vs Feed-forward depicted in Table 1.

Feed-forward refers to predictive control based on stored stereotypic patterns that are less modified by external reactions (Goldberg, 1985; Caruso et al., 1988; Wiesendanger & Wiesendanger, 1984). Since it doesn't need to wait for feedback, it can function much faster. The SMA along with the basal ganglia (including the striatum) are active during planning and initiating learned motor movements using feed-forward, predictive control (Goldberg, 1985; Webster, 1993; Gracco, 1991).

Table 1. Characteristics of the Proposed "Lateral" and "Medial" Systems.

LATERAL	MEDIAL
Cortical	Subcortical
* speech motor execution	* speech motor planning
* lateral motor cortex	* basal ganglia and SMA
Feedback	Feed Forward
* on-line revisions	* predictive control
* responds to external	* stored stereotypic
conditions	patterns
	* less on-line modification

The medial system is important to investigate because speech motor commands seem to originate at this level. These commands eventually control timing and sequencing of muscle movements that produce fluent or stuttered speech.

D2 System

The D2 system modulates dopamine effects on the brain. It includes the substantia nigra and its circuit to the striatum (nigro-striatal circuit). It has been described in detail using rat brains and is reasonably well understood in humans who have dopamine driven disorders such as Tourette's syndrome (Mercuri et al., 1994; Wolf et al., 1996; Wu et al., submitted). It is typically referred to as the nigro-striatal circuit. The dopamine processing begins in the substantia-nigra and eventually influences the striatum and other parts of the brain. We hypothesize that in people who stutter excess dopamine is allowed to reach the striatum and other speech motor planning regions and reduce their activation rendering them less effective.

Limitations of the Model

Our model is admittedly incomplete. Other systems must exist to account for observed features of stuttering such as social, environmental, communication disruptors, and emotional factors that may impact the limbic system, etc. For example, the lateral system may need to be divided into separate systems to accommodate reception, association, and production. Some entirely different model may be better than the one we present here. Therefore, these three systems represent a beginning step; hopefully in the right direction.

Along with other brain imaging labs, we are trying to provide some neurological description of any differences between stuttering and fluency; and between people who stutter and people who do not stutter (Wood et al. 1980; Ludlow et al., 1987: Pool et al., 1991; Watson et al., 1992, 1994; Wu et al., 1995, In Press, b, 1996; Fox ct al. 1996). We are a long way from relating our preliminary observations to any statement of etiology. We are not arguing that any of these differences represent causes of stuttering.

Table 2. Functions of the Dopamine 2 System in the Proposed Model.

DOPAMINE 2 SYSTEM
* Is responsible for modulation of dopamine 2.
* Referred to as the nigro-striatal circuit.
* If ineffective permits excess dopamine to interfere with striatal activation.
* The striatum is therefore less efficient in speech motor planning.

Our hypothesis that some people who stutter (PWS) have excess dopamine must await further support before it can qualify as a risk factor for stuttering. The experiences associated with stuttering may interact in as yet unknown ways to create these describable neurological differences.

We are suggesting that, if our initial impressions are correct, stuttering in some adults may fit into a category with other dopamine related disorders such as Tourette's syndrome.

RELATION OF THESE SYSTEMS TO TREATMENT EFFECTS

We will present some findings from several different studies including FDG (glucose uptake) PET studies, FDOPA (dopamine uptake) studies, and effects of a medication that blocks dopamine uptake. The preliminary results, based on a few subjects, indicate that these systems interact in a describable way. Since they do form a consistent pattern we thought it worthwhile to present a beginning model of parallel systems interacting with each other to modify stuttering behaviors.

The model predicts that "Top-down" treatment, which requires monitoring at the cognitive level, will increase activation in the lateral system. This lateral improvement may then influence the medial system indirectly. "Bottom-up" treatment, which employs overlearned motor patterns, should increase activation of the medial system and indirectly in the lateral system. Also, medications may be able to improve function in one or both systems.

We think that relating these systems to treatment changes or to fluency induced changes has some benefits. For one thing it provides data for testing the hypotheses. Researchers can try a given treatment and determine if changes predicted by this or some later model actually take place and then revise the model as indicated. Also it might be helpful from a clinicians point of view to think in terms of modifying certain neural patterns. A parallel exist in treatment of aphasia; we think of using melody or rhythm to take advantage of right hemisphere strengths.

Observed Effects

In the part II of this report (Wu et al., chapter 27), we present the results of FDG scans on 4 males who stutter and 7 controls.

Table 3. Predicted and Observed Treatment Effects that can be Assessed by Functional Brain Imaging

PREDICTED TREATMENT EFFECTS	
Top-down (e.g., monitor each syllable or occurance of stuttering)	Is predicted to improve lateral system functioning.
Bottom-up (e.g., speech motor training)	Is predicted to improve medial system functioning.
OBSERVED TREATMENT EFFECTS	
Choral reading	Increased lateral system (cortical) activation.
	Did not increase medial (subcortical) activation.
Risperidone, D2 blocking agent	Reduced stuttering (N = 4). Speculate that it decreased dopamine 2 effects on the striatum.

We found that the lateral systems of PWS were less activated than controls during solo reading (stuttering) but actually more activated than controls during the choral condition (fluency). So choral reading (fluency) "normalized" this system. However, the Medial system (striatum) of the PWS had reduced activation during stuttering and this reduction did not normalize during fluency. So the medial system was *under*-activated during both fluency and stuttering for the PWS in this study.

We have not run subjects to measure levels of dopamine before and after medication but we have run FDOPA scans to measure dopamine uptake in three stutterers and 8 controls. Details of the results of these scans are presented by Wu et al. (chapter 27). They show that during a resting condition the D2 system, which makes dopamine, is much more active in several brain regions including the striatum (caudate and putamen) in PWS than in people who do not stutter.

Preliminary results of an open trial of risperidone are presented in Part III of this report (Maguire et al., chapter 32). Frequency and duration of stuttering were reduced by 36 to 82 percent in four adults who stutter. All four requested to continue the medication after the study ended. Risperidone is assumed to reduce D2 effects on the medial system. Such an effect would be consistent with predictions based on the model under consideration.

Other treatments are predicted to influence brain activation based on the system that is targeted. Treatments that require monitoring each moment of stuttering or each syllable produced would seem to target the lateral system. Speech motor training would seem to target the medial system.

REFERENCES

Caruso, A.J. (1991). Neuromotor processes underlying stuttering. In H.F.M. Peters, W. Hulstijn & C.W. Starkweather (Eds.), *Speech motor control and stuttering*. Amsterdam: Elsevier Science Publishers.

Caruso, A.J., Abbs, J., & Gracco, V. (1988). Kinematic analysis of multiple movement coordination during speech in stutterers. *Brain, 111*, 439-455.

Fox, P.T., Ingham, R.J., Ingham, J.C., Hirsch, T.B., Downs, J.H., Martin, C., Jerabek, P., Glass, T., & Lancaster, J.L. (1996). A PET study of the neural systems of stuttering. *Nature, 382*, 158-162.

Goldberg, G. (1985). Supplementary motor area structure and function: Review and hypotheses. *The Behavioral and Brain Sciences, 8*, 567-616.

Gracco, V.L. (1991). Sensorimotor mechanisms in speech motor control. In H.F.M. Peters, W. Hulstijn, & C.W. Starkweather (Eds.), *Speech motor control and stuttering* (pp. 53-76). Amsterdam: Elsevier Science Publications.

Gracco, V.L. (1994). Some organizational characteristics of speech movement. *Journal of Speech and Hearing Research, 37*, 4-27.

Ludlow, C.L., Rosenberg, J., Salazar, A., Grafman, J., & Smutok, M. (1987). Site of penetrating brain lesions causing chronic acquired stuttering. *Annals of Neurology, 22*, 60-66.

Maguire, G.A., Riley, G.D., Wu, J.C., Franklin, D.L., & Potkin, S. (this volume). Pet scan evidence of parallel cerebral systems related to treatment effects, effects of Risperidone in the treatment of stuttering. In W. Hulstijn, H.F.M. Peters, & P.H.H.M. Van Lieshout (Eds.), *Speech production: motor control, brain research and fluency disorders*. Amsterdam: Elsevier Science.

McClean, M.D. (1990). Neuromotor aspects of stuttering: Levels of impairment and disability. In J.A. Cooper (Ed.), *Research needs in stuttering: Roadblocks and future directions*. ASHA Reports, Number 18. Rockville, MD: ASHA.

Mercuri, N.B., Bonci, A., Calabresi, P., Stratta, F., Stefani, A., & Bernardi, G. (1994). Effects of dihydropyridine calcium antagonists on rat midbrain dopaminergic neurones. *British Journal of Pharmacology, 113*, 831-838.

Nudelman, B.N., Herbrich, K.E., Hoyt, B.D., & Rosenfield, D.B. (1991). A neuroscience approach to stuttering. In H.F.M. Peters, W. Hulstijn & C.W. Starkweather (Eds.), *Speech motor control and stuttering*. Amsterdam: Elsevier Science Publishers.

Pool, K.D., Devous, M.D., Freeman, F.J., Watson, B.C., & Finitzo, T. (1991). Regional cerebral blood flow in developmental stutterers. *Archives of Neurology, 48*, 509-512.

Watson, B.C. & Freeman, F.J. (1997). Brain imaging contributions. In R.F. Curlee & G.M. Siegel (Eds.), *Nature and treatment of stuttering: New directions* (2nd ed.)(pp. 143-166). Boston: Allyn and Bacon.

Watson, B.C., Freeman, F.J., Devous, M.D., Chapman, S.B., Finitzo, T., & Pool, K.D. (1994). Linguistic performance and regional cerebral blood flow in persons who stutter. *Journal of Speech and Hearing Research, 37*, 1221-1228.

Watson, B.C., Pool, K.D., Devous, M.D., Freeman, F.J., & Finitzo, T. (1992). Brain blood flow related to acoustic laryngeal reaction time in adult developmental stutterers. *Journal of Speech and Hearing Research, 35*, 555-561.

Webster, W.G. (1993). Hurried hands and tangled tongues. In E. Boberg (Ed.), *Neuropsychology of stuttering*. Edmonton, Alberta: U. of Alberta Press.

Wiesendanger, M., & Wiesendanger, R. (1984). The supplementary motor area in light of recent investigations. *Experimental Brain Research, 9*, 382-392.

Wolf, S.S, Jones, D.W., Knable, M.B., Gesey, J.G., et al. (1996). Tourrettes syndrome prediction of phenotypic variation in monozygotic twins by caudate nucleus D2 receptor binding. *Science, 273*, 1225-1227.

Wood, F., Stump, D., McKeehan, A., Sheldon, S., & Proctor, J. (1980). Patterns of regional blood flow during attempted reading aloud by stutterers both on and off Haloperidol medication: Evidence for inadequate left frontal activation during stuttering. *Brain and Language, 9*, 141-144.

Wu, J.C., Bell, K., Najafi, A., Widmark, C., Keator, D., Tang, C., Klein, E., LaCasse, L., Fallon, J., & Bunney, W.E. (submitted). Decreasing striatal 6-FDOPA uptake with increasing duration of cocaine withdrawal.

Wu, J.C., Maguire, G., Riley, G., Fallon, J., LaCasse, L., Chin, S., Kleine, E., Tang, C., Cadwell, S., & Lottenberg, S. (1995). A positron emission tomography [18F] deoxyglucose study of developmental stuttering. *NeuroReport, 6*, 501-505.

Wu, J.C., Maguire, G., Riley, G., Lee, A., Keator, D., Tang, C., Fallon, J. & Najafi, A. (In Press). Increased dopamine activity associated with stuttering. *NeuroReport.*

Wu, J.C., Riley, G.D., & Maguire, G.A. (this volume). Pet scan evidence of parallel cerebral systems related to treatment effects, PART II: Preliminary FDG and FDOPA PET scan results. In W. Hulstijn, H.F.M. Peters, & P.H.H.M. Van Lieshout (Eds.), *Speech production: motor control, brain research and fluency disorders.* Amsterdam: Elsevier Science.

Speech Production: Motor Control, Brain Research and Fluency Disorders
W. Hulstijn, H.F.M. Peters and P.H.H.M. Van Lieshout, editors

Chapter 27

PET SCAN EVIDENCE OF PARALLEL CEREBRAL SYSTEMS RELATED TO TREATMENT EFFECTS: FDG AND FDOPA PET SCAN FINDINGS

Joseph C. Wu, Glyndon Riley, Gerald Maguire, Ahmad Najafi, Cheuk Tang

FDG PET scan studies during solo (dysfluent) vs. choral (fluent) reading were obtained for 4 males who stutter compared with 7 male normal controls. People who stutter show significant decrease in the medial system structures (striatum) compared to controls during both solo and choral reading conditions. People who stutter show significant decrease in the lateral system structures (medial prefrontal cortex, deep orbital cortex, insular cortex, parietal cortex) during solo reading compared to controls. During choral reading, people who stutter show significant increase in metabolism in lateral system structures (e.g. auditory cortex, homologous Broca's area) compared to controls. People who stutter also show significant increase in FDOPA uptake in striatal and mesocortical projections.

INTRODUCTION

We have previously presented absolute metabolic date from 4 people who stutter (3 men, 1 woman, mean age 41.5) and 4 controls (3 men, 1 woman, mean age = 29.5 years) during solo vs. choral reading for people who stutter compared with solo reading for controls (Wu et al., 1995). Our findings suggested the presence of a hypothetical two-part stuttering model with a medial and lateral systems component (see Riley et al., this volume, chapter 26). We hypothesize that there is a *trait-related metabolic decrease in medial system (e.g. striatum) which is present whether people who stutter are fluent or dysfluent.* We also hypothesize that there is a *state-dependent metabolic decrease in the lateral system (e.g. language areas, higher order association areas) during dysfluency and metabolic increases during fluency.*

In this chapter, we present relative metabolic data (normalized for absolute global metabolic differences) which may be more sensitive for identifying regional changes. This paper also draws upon a larger control pool and presents data comparing choral reading stutterers with choral reading controls.

Stuttering has been shown to be reduced by administration of dopamine blockers [e.g. haldol (Burns et al.,1978) or risperidone, (see Maguire et al., this volume, chapter 32) which raises the possibility that stuttering may be due to excess dopamine activity. Regional cerebral glucose metabolic rates also show decreases cortically and subcortically in stuttering subjects (Wu et al., 1995). This provides a second line of evidence that dopamine excessive activity may be present in stuttering subjects since amphetamine (Wolkin et al., 1987), a dopamine agonist, and cocaine, a dopamine reuptake inhibitor (London et al., 1990), have been found to be inhibitory to regional cerebral glucose metabolic activity. We were interested in testing this hypothesis *that excessive dopamine activity is present in people who stutter* by measuring FDOPA uptake using positron emission tomography. FDOPA PET scans have been shown to provide a noninvasive means of assessing presynaptic dopamine activity in vivo in humans. We report a preliminary finding in a small group of male stuttering subjects compared to male normal controls (Wu et al., in press).

METHODS

Subjects

For the FDG study, data from four males who stutter (age: 35.0 ± 16.6 years) who are dysfluent compared to seven male controls (age: 27.9 ± 16.2 years) were used. For the FDOPA study, data from three males who stutter (36.7 ± 16.6 years) and seven male controls (age: 39.6 ± 23.6 years) were used. All were free of major medical or psychiatric conditions and were not receiving psychotropic medications. All received full and informed consent in accordance with the institutional review board at the University of California, Irvine. Each stuttering subject had developmental stuttering with onset prior to five years of age and were of at least moderate severity as assessed by the Stuttering Severity Instrument-3 (SSI-3) (Riley, 1972). All subjects were right-handed. No one was excluded on the basis of gender or ethnic origin. The study took place at the Brain Imaging Center at the University of California, Irvine. All subjects had a medical history and a physical examination by a physician prior to the study.

FDG Procedure

Informed consent was obtained after the procedure was fully explained. During the uptake of FDG, the subjects received instructions in solo or choral reading; 3 min before injection of the FDG, the reading task was started. The subjects read aloud for 30 minutes in an acoustically attenuated room. The readings were from non-emotionally laden articles from news magazines. For solo reading, subjects read aloud to themselves. For choral reading, subjects read aloud in unison with another person. The solo and choral reading tasks were counterbalanced. Approximately 45 minutes following the injection of FDG, nine slice images were obtained on the NeuroECAT scanner (7.6 mm axial resolution, fwhm) in the Brain Imaging Center of the Department of Psychiatry, University of California, Irvine. Subjects were positioned in the scanner and held in a constant position during scanning with an individually molded plastic mask. The repositioning of the patients during the two studies is accurate to within 2 mm (Buchsbaum et al., 1992). The scan was transformed to glucose metabolic rate as described previously (Buchsbaum et al., 1992). Images were acquired with 600,000 to 1,000,000 counts, attenuation corrected and filtered as previously described (Buchsbaum et al., 1992). A dose calibrator served as the standard for gamma counting of blood samples and cylindrical phantom. PET scans were assigned to match the Matsui and Hirano atlas slice planes (Matsui & Hirano, 1978) and corresponding Talairach atlas slice plane (Talairach & Tournoux, 1988) by a technician who was blind to diagnosis and condition (Matsui & Hirano, 1978). Glucose utilization was calculated according to the Sokoloff method (Sokoloff, 1984). Kinetic constants and lumped constant from Phelps et al. (Phelps et al., 1979) were used. PET scans were normalized for size and then averaged pixel by pixel to arrive at the mean average PET scan for each condition. The data were analyzed as relative data (ratio of absolute metabolic rate for region of interest/absolute metabolic rate for whole brain). The relative metabolic data allow for more statistically powerful examination of local effects since global effects are removed. T-test images were generated. Only pixels which were significantly different ($p < .05$, 1-tailed) were displayed. Percent difference images were created by dividing the difference between two images by the first image. Monte Carlo resampling was used to define the minimum contiguous size of suprathreshold pixels required to occur at $p < .05$.

FDOPA procedure

Subjects were studied in a GE2048 scanner (full width half maximum resolution was equal to 4.5 mm in plane and 6.5 mm axially). Each subject was positioned with the aid of a vertical laser line. During the scanning procedure, subjects were lying supine with eyes open at rest. A custom molded thermoplastic head holder was used to minimize head movements. The canthomeatal line (CM-line) of the subject is marked on the mask for positioning purposes. Fifteen slices were obtained with the middle slice centered with the position (z-offset) of the striatum 40 mm above the CM-line. Subjects were administered 6-FDOPA, a positron tagged marker of presynaptic dopamine activiity (Barrio et al., 1990), intravenously (2-3.75 mCi) in forearm veins. 6-FDOPA was made using a "no-carrier added" synthesis resulting in high specific activity 6-FDOPA (Najafi, 1995). The left arm was used for injection and the right arm for sampling. Sixteen two-ml venous blood samples (approximately 32 ml total) were taken to determine kinetics of metabolism and uptake of 6-FDOPA. Twelve 10 minute sequential scans for 6-FDOPA uptake in striatum versus white matter (non striatum) were obtained. Radioactivity within the striatal ROI is assumed to consist of three components (Martin et al., 1989): Tissue and plasma activity are then analyzed graphically as described by Patlak and colleagues (Patlak & Blasberg, 1985; Patlak et al., 1983).

RESULTS

Between-group FDG differences during solo reading for people who stutter vs. controls

People who stutter show significantly lower metabolism in the medial system (caudate) as well as decreases in the lateral system (the frontal pole, Brodmann area 10), the medial prefrontal cortex (Brodmann area 32), deep orbital cortex (Brodmann area 11), parietal cortex and insular cortex compared to controls during the solo reading task. (see figure 3).

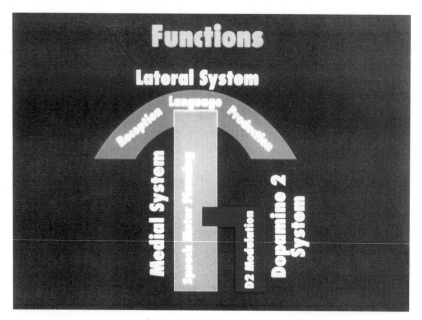

Figure 1.

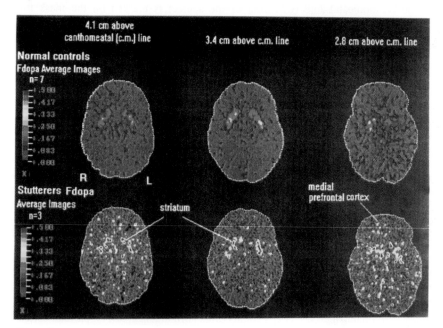

Figure 2.

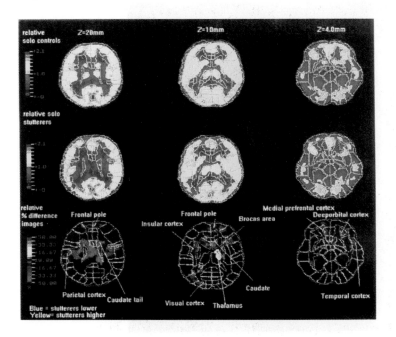

Figure 3.

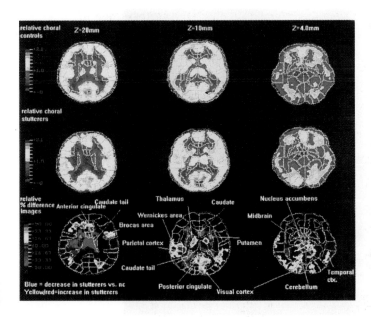

Figure 4.

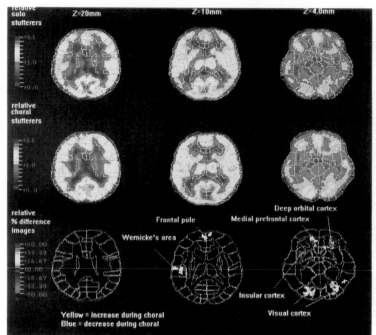

Figure 5.

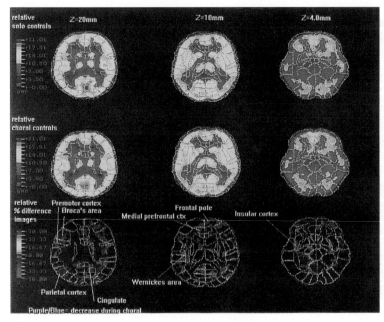

Figure 6.

The top row depicts averaged FDG brain maps at three different brain heights of controls during solo reading. The middle row depicts averaged FDG brain maps at three different brain heights of people who stutter during solo reading. The bottom row depicts percent difference images in regions which are significantly different. Blue regions depicts regions which are significantly lower in people who stutter during solo reading compared to normal controls. Yellow-red regions depicts regions which are significantly higher in people who stutter compared to controls.

Between-group FDG differences for choral reading for people who stutter vs. controls

Choral reading stutterers are lower in metabolism in the medial system structures (i.e. striatal regions such as caudate head, caudate tail, and putamen) compared to choral reading controls. Choral reading stutterers are higher metabolically in lateral system structures such as the left auditory cortex (BA22), right homologous Broca's area (BA44/45), visual association cortex (BA18), and posterior cingulate (BA23/31) than choral reading controls (see figure 4). Choral reading people who stutter also show increases metabolically in other structures such as thalamus, midbrain, and cerebellum. The top row depicts normal controls during choral reading. The middle row depicts people who stutter during choral reading. The bottom row depicts differences between people who stutter and normal controls. Blue regions depicts areas that are significantly lower in people who stutter compared to controls. The yellow-red regions depicts areas that are significantly higher in people who stutter.

Within-group FDG differences for people who stutter for solo vs. choral reading

People who stutter show significant increases in the metabolism of lateral system structure in medial prefrontal cortex, deep orbital cortex, Wernicke's area (Brodmann area 22), right-sided homologous Broca's area (BA45) and visual cortex (Brodmann area 18, 19, see figure 5). People who stutter also show a decrease in left insular cortex metabolism with choral reading. The top row depicts averaged FDG brain maps of people who stutter during solo reading when they are dysfluent. The second row depicts averaged FDG brain maps of people who stutter during choral reading when they are fluent. The bottom row depicts percent difference images in regions which are significantly different. The yellow-red regions depicts regions which are significantly higher during the fluent state. The blue regions depicts regions which are significantly lower during the dysfluent state.

Within-group FDG differences for solo vs. choral reading for controls

Normal controls show moderate decreases in brain metabolism during choral reading which is opposite to the direction of change in stutterers seen during choral reading. Areas that decrease in controls during choral reading are: premotor cortex (Brodmann area 6), Broca's area, parietal cortex, frontal pole, medial prefrontal cortex, cingulate, Wernicke's area (Brodmann area 22) and insular cortex (see figure 6). Little change is seen in striatal regions or thalamic regions with choral reading. The top row depicts normal controls during solo reading. The middle row depicts normal controls depicts normal controls during choral reading. The bottom row depicts differences seen between choral reading and solo reading. The blue regions indicates regions which show decreases during choral reading.

FDOPA results

Stuttering subjects showed an almost three fold increase in FDOPA uptake activity compared to normal in right ventral medial prefrontal cortex (BA32, see figure 2) and left caudate tail. FDOPA uptake in stuttering subjects compared to controls showed over 100% increase in limbic structures such as the left extended amygdala, left insular cortex, right deep orbital cortex, and caudate tail.

DISCUSSION

The increased metabolic rate in superior frontal (BA9), parietal regions (BA39/40), posterior cingulate (BA23), frontal pole (BA9) and midbrain which we reported in stutterers when they were fluent (during choral reading) compared to when they were dysfluent (during the solo reading task, see figure 5) can not be explained simply by choral reading since the changes seen in normal controls between choral reading and solo reading showed metabolic decreases during choral reading (see figure 6). The increased metabolism in stutterers during the choral reading task appears to be associated with an overnormalization of spoken language brain circuits which is inducible during the fluent state (see figure 4) compared with the underactivation of these regions during the dysfluent state (see figure 3). These changes in the lateral system appear to be state-dependent.

Even when the stutterers are fluent during the choral reading task, they continue to show decreased striatal metabolism compared to controls doing the exact same task (see figure 4). This is compatible with our conclusion of decreased striatal metabolism in stutterers from our earlier work that solo reading stutterers have decreased striatal metabolism compared to fluent controls doing a solo reading task which we have replicated with a larger group of controls (see figure 3). The lack of change of the striatal regions (as opposed to the cortical metabolic increases) seen in stutterers when compared under both solo and choral reading task suggested that the striatal region remains hypometabolic under both fluent and dysfluent state. This persistent trait of decreased activity seems to characterize the medial system in people who stutter.

Recently, Fox et al. (Fox et al., 1996) published a paper with findings similar to those we found in our first paper (Wu et al., 1995) and this paper. Both groups found that there was an underactivity of auditory system and speech production systems during dysfluency which were reversed by induced fluency. However, there are a number of differences between both groups. We find metabolic decreases in other cortical regions such as medial prefrontal cortex, bilateral frontal pole (BA10), and right homologous Broca's area (BA45) for people who stutter compared to controls during solo reading which are not reported by Fox et al. Most notably, we find metabolic decreases in striatum for people who stutter compared with controls during both solo reading and choral reading states which are not found by Fox et al. There are several methodological differences that could potentially account for some of these differences. First, Fox et al. used O-15 blood flow pet scans whereas we used FDG which is a measure of glucose metabolic rate. While O-15 blood flow and FDG pet scans generally show concordance, there are situations in which there are discrepancies. It is possible that FDG may be more sensitive at detecting differences than O-15 blood flow under certain circumstances (Gaillard et al., 1995). Second, Fox et al. used a different method of analysis which relied upon a rest minus task within group comparison and reported no direct between group statistics whereas the striatal differences that we find is present only for the between group comparisons. If people who stutter have decreased striatal metabolism at rest which is persistently low and does not change with task and if controls have increased striatal metabolism which is persistently high and does not change with task, then both groups would show no difference in striatal activation. Only a between group comparison would reveal that controls have a persistently high striatal metabolism compared to people who stutter who have a persistently low metabolism.

The increase in FDOPA uptake activity in the stuttering subjects (see figure 2) occurs predominantly in ventral limbic cortical regions, which have been hypothesized to be involved in a neural circuit for stuttering (Wu et al., 1995). Our finding of increased FDOPA uptake is compatible with our previous finding of decreased cerebral metabolic activity in many of these same regions since dopamine has an inhibitory effect on regional cerebral metabolism. These findings are also compatible with pharmacological studies which have reported that stuttering is improved by dopamine blockers (Burns et al., 1978).

There is an extensive dopaminergic innervation of medial prefrontal cortex (Bertolucci-D'Angio et al., 1990; Bunney & Aghajanian, 1977; Cenci et al., 1992; Chiodo et al., 1984; Tassin et al., 1977; Thierry et al., 1988; Weinberger et al., 1988). The medial prefrontal cortex is functionally connected to the supplementary motor area (Goldberg, 1985) and is also known as the vocalization center in primates. (Jurgens, 1986; Jurgens & Muller-Preuss, 1977; Jurgens & Pratt, 1979) The findings of significant differences in limbic cortical region suggest that the mesocortical dopamine tracts may be abnormally overactive in stutterers. In addition to the limbic cortex, dopaminergic innervation of temporal cortical regions (De Keyser et al., 1989) (to which the auditory cortex belongs) also exists. This study suggests that stuttering may be associated with increased dopamine activity.

The major limitations of this study is the small sample size of stutterers. Further research is needed on the relationship of regional cerebral glucose metabolic rate and FDOPA uptake activity within the same patients.

ACKNOWLEDGMENTS

We are grateful for the support of Dr. William Bunney, Dr. Siu wa Tang, the Brain Imaging Committee, and the National Stuttering Project.

REFERENCES

Barrio, J. R., Huang, S.C., Melega, W.P., Yu, D.C., Hoffman, J.M., Schneider, J.S., Satyamurthy, N., Mazziotta, J.C., & Phelps, M.E. (1990). 6-[18F]fluoro-L-dopa probes dopamine turnover rates in central dopaminergic structures. *Journal of Neuroscience Research, 27,* 487-493.

Bertolucci-D'Angio, M., Serrano, A., & Scatton, B. (1990). Mesocorticolimbic dopaminergic systems and emotional states. *Journal of Neuroscience Methods, 34,* 135-142.

Buchsbaum, M.S., Potkin, S.G., Siegel, B.V., Jr., Lohr, J., Katz, M., Gottschalk, L.A., Gulasekaram, B., Marshall, J.F., Lottenberg, S., Teng, C.Y., et al. (1992). Striatal metabolic rate and clinical response to neuroleptics in schizophrenia. *Archives of General Psychiatry, 49,* 966-974.

Bunney, B.S., & Aghajanian, G.K. (1977). Electrophysiological studies of dopamine- innervated cells in the frontal cortex. *Advences in Biochemical Psychopharmacology, 16,* 65-70.

Burns, D., Brady, J.P., & Kuruvilla, K. (1978). The acute effect of haloperidol and apomorphine on the severity of stuttering. *Biological Psychiatry, 13,* 255-264.

Cenci, M.A., Kalen, P., Mandel, R.J., & Bjorklund, A. (1992). Regional differences in the regulation of dopamine and noradrenaline release in medial frontal cortex, nucleus accumbens and caudate-putamen: a microdialysis study in the rat. *Brain Research, 581,* 217-228.

Chiodo, L.A., Bannon, M.J., Grace, A.A., Roth, R.H., & Bunney, B.S. (1984). Evidence for the absence of impulse-regulating somatodendritic and synthesis-modulating nerve terminal autoreceptors on subpopulations of mesocortical dopamine neurons. *Neuroscience., 12,* 1-16.

De Keyser, J., Ebinger, G., & Vauquelin, G. (1989). Evidence for a widespread dopaminergic innervation of the human cerebral neocortex. *Neuroscience Letters, 104,* 281-285.

Fox, P.T., Ingham, R.J., Ingham, J.C., Hirsch, T.B., Downs, J.H., Martin, C., Jerabek, P., Glass, T., & Lancaster, J.L. (1996). A PET study of the neural systems of stuttering. *Nature, 382,* 158-161.

Gaillard, W.D., Fazilat, S., White, S., Malow, B., Sato, S., Reeves, P., Herscovitch, P., & Theodore, W.H. (1995). Interictal metabolism and blood flow are uncoupled in temporal lobe cortex of patients with complex partial epilepsy. *Neurology, 45,* 1841-1847.

Goldberg, G. (1985). Supplementary motor area structure and function: Review and hypotheses. *Behavioral and Brain Sciences, 8,* 567-616.

Jurgens, U. (1986). The squirrel monkey as an experimental model in the study of cerebral organization of emotional vocal utterances. *European Archives of Psychiatry and Neurological Science, 236,* 40-43.

Jurgens, U., & Muller-Preuss, P. (1977). Convergent projections of different limbic vocalization areas in the squirrel monkey. *Experimental Brain Research, 29,* 75-83.

Jurgens, U., & Pratt, R. (1979). The cingular vocalization pathway in the squirrel monkey. *Experimental Brain Research, 34,* 499-510.

London, E.D., Cascella, N.G., Wong, D.F., Phillips, R.L., Dannals, R.F., Links, J.M., Herning, R., Grayson, R., Jaffe, J.H., & Wagner, H.N., Jr. (1990). Cocaine-induced reduction of glucose utilization in human brain. A study using positron emission tomography and [fluorine 18]-fluorodeoxyglucose. *Archives of General Psychiatry, 47,* 567-574.

Martin, W.R., Palmer, M.R., Patlak, C.S., & Calne, D.B. (1989). Nigrostriatal function in humans studied with positron emission tomography. *Annals of Neurology, 26,* 535-542.

Matsui, T., & Hirano, A. (1978). *An atlas of the human brain for computerized tomography.* Tokyo: Igaku-Shoin.

Najafi, A. (1995). Measures and pitfalls for successful preparation of "no carrier added" asymmetric 6-[18F]fluor-L-dopa from 18F-fluoride ion. *Nuclear Medicine and Biology, 22,* 395-397.

Patlak, C.S., & Blasberg, R.G. (1985). Graphical evaluation of blood-to-brain transfer constants from multiple-time uptake data. Generalizations. *Journal of Cerebral Bloodflow and Metabolism, 5,* 584-590.

Patlak, C.S., Blasberg, R.G., & Fenstermacher, J.D. (1983). Graphical evaluation of blood-to-brain transfer constants from multiple-time uptake data. *Journal of Cerebral Bloodflow and Metabolism, 3,* 1-7.

Phelps, M.E., Huang, S.C., Hoffman, E.J., Selin, C., Sokoloff, L., & Kuhl, D.E. (1979). Tomographic measurement of local cerebral glucose metabolic rate in humans with (F-18)2-fluoro-2-deoxy-D-glucose: validation of method. *Annals of Neurology, 6,* 371-388.

Riley, G.D. (1972). A stuttering severity instrument for children and adults. *Journal of Speech and Hearing Disorders, 37,* 314-322.

Sokoloff, L. (1984). Modeling metabolic processes in the brain in vivo. *Annals of Neurology, 15 Supplement,* S1-11.

Talairach, J., & Tournoux, P. (1988). *Co-planar stereotaxic atlas of the human brain.* Stuttgart: Thieme.

Tassin, J.P., Stinus, L., Simon, H., Blanc, G., Thierry, A.M., Le Moal, M., Cardo, B., & Glowinski, J. (1977). Distribution of dopaminergic terminals in rat cerebral cortex: role of dopaminergic mesocortical system in ventral tegmental area syndrome. *Advanced in Biochemical Psychopharmacology, 16,* 21-28.

Thierry, A.M., Mantz, J., Milla, C., & Glowinski, J. (1988). Influence of the mesocortical/prefrontal dopamine neurons on their target cells. *Annals of the New York Acaddemy of Science, 537,* 101-111.

Weinberger, D.R., Berman, K.F., & Chase, T.N. (1988). Mesocortical dopaminergic function and human cognition. *Annals of the New York Academy of Science, 537,* 330-338.

Wolkin, A., Angrist, B., Wolf, A., Brodie, J., Wolkin, B., Jaeger, J., Cancro, R., & Rotrosen, J. (1987). Effects of amphetamine on local cerebral metabolism in normal and schizophrenic subjects as determined by positron emission tomography. *Psychopharmacology (Berl.), 92,* 241-246.

Wu, J.C., Maguire, G., Riley, G., Fallon, J., LaCasse, L., Chin, S., Klein, E., Tang, C., Cadwell, S., & Lottenberg, S. (1995). A positron emission tomography [18F]deoxyglucose study of developmental stuttering. *Neuroreport, 6,* 501-505.

Wu, J.C., Maguire, G., Riley, A., Lee, A., Keator, D., Tang, C., Fallon, J., & Najafi, A. (in press). Increased dopamine activity associated with stuttering. *Neuroreport.*

Speech Production: Motor Control, Brain Research and Fluency Disorders
W. Hulstijn, H.F.M. Peters and P.H.H.M. Van Lieshout, editors

Chapter 28

NEUROPHYSIOLOGIC AND BEHAVIORAL EVIDENCE FOR A FLUENCY-GENERATING SYSTEM

Ben C. Watson, Frances J. Freeman

This chapter reviews our findings from structural (MRI) and functional (quantitative EEG and SPECT) brain imaging studies of 20 adults with developmental stuttering. MRI revealed no pattern of significant anatomical abnormalities across people who stutterer. However, we found evidence of altered CNS function. Furthermore, there was congruence among the two functional brain imaging technologies. We also examined the significance of altered CNS function in the identified regions (left anterior cingulate and temporal) in the context of behavioral measures of speech motor and language performance in a subset of these 20 subjects.

We propose a theory of fluency within which neurologic perspectives on stuttering can be framed. Central to this theory is the assumption that a neurophysiologic system integrates cognition, linguistic encoding, and speech motor processing for the production of oral/verbal fluency. The model predicts that disruption in one or more of cognitive, linguistic, or motor processes or of their integration can lead to fluency failure. In this context, stuttering is recognized as one of several possible forms of fluency failure. Parallel brain imaging and behavioral studies can elucidate the functional significance of CNS sites with respect to fluency production. Such studies will test the model and lead to improved differential diagnosis of stuttering.

Pool et al. (1987) presented a preliminary report of quantitative and topographic mapping of electroencephalographic data in three adults with developmental stuttering. That study revealed auditory evoked potential abnormalities over left frontal, bilateral temporal, and right parietal cortex and launched a series of studies of brain structure, brain function, and speech and language production in adults with developmental stuttering.

In the ensuing years, our research team investigated brain structure using magnetic resonance imaging (MRI) and brain function as revealed in cortical electrophysiologic methods (resting electroencephalography and auditory evoked potentials) (Finitzo et al., 1991) and regional cerebral blood flow, or rCBF, (using single photon emission computed tomography, SPECT) (Pool et al., 1991). We also examined resting rCBF findings for subgroups of these subjects in the context of speech motor (Dembowski & Watson, 1991; Watson et al., 1992), and linguistic (Watson et al., 1994) performance.

This report summarizes brain imaging findings that are corroborated by structural and functional imaging techniques and by behavioral data. Taken together, these findings provide evidence for a CNS-based fluency-generating system that underlies the production and dissolution of oral/verbal fluency. Finally, we share some thoughts regarding the design of future studies that seek to apply functional brain imaging technologies in stuttering research.

Neurophysiologic evidence for a fluency-generating system comes from contemporaneous structural and functional brain imaging studies. Methodological details of quantitative and topographic electroencephalographic (QTE) and SPECT rCBF studies are described in several published reports (Devous et al., 1986; Finitzo et al., 1991; Pool et al., 1991) and will not be described in detail herein. QTE findings for 20 adults with developmental stuttering were reported in Finitzo et al. (1991). People who stutter demonstrated significant global reduction in absolute Beta 1 amplitude and focal amplitude reductions over right posterior temporal and bi-occipital cortex. Amplitude reductions approached significance at adjacent paramedian central and parietal electrodes. Analysis of auditory evoked potentials (AEP) revealed significant amplitude reductions over left temporal and mesial frontal cortex.

SPECT rCBF data were analyzed both in terms of absolute and relative blood flow to anatomically defined regions of interest (ROIs) located in a tomographic transverse section oriented 6 cm above and parallel to the canthomeatal line. Absolute blood flow for the 20 people who stutter was reduced as compared to 43 age- and gender-matched people who do not stutter for 20 of 20 (10 in each hemisphere) ROIs. Relative rCBF ratios normalized to individual subject hemispheric flow (left ROI/left hemisphere – right ROI/right hemisphere) revealed blood flow asymmetries (left less than right) for the people who stutter in anterior cingulate, superior temporal, and middle temporal ROIs. A similar, but nonsignificant, asymmetry was noted for the inferior frontal ROI. Individual subject data revealed that all people who stutter showed relative flow asymmetries below the normal median for the left anterior cingulate or the left middle temporal ROIs. MRI scans for these 20 people who stutter revealed no significant vascular anomalies. It is likely that globally reduced absolute blood flow and focal reductions in relative blood flow reflect metabolic, or functional, rather than vascular anomalies in these subjects.

QTE and rCBF findings are noteworthy for their congruence. Reduced Beta 1 amplitude observed in resting EEG spectra is consistent with reduced blood flow noted on rCBF analyses. Sugar and Gerard (1938) and Lennox et al. (1938) described a correspondence between decreased Beta amplitude and reduced rCBF. AEP amplitude reduction over left temporal electrodes is consistent with rCBF asymmetries in temporal ROIs. Thus, similar patterns of altered resting brain function in these adults with developmental stuttering are confirmed by two different imaging technologies.

This ensemble of structural and functional brain imaging findings has several specific implications for a fluency-generating system. First, the finding of altered brain function in multiple regions implies that a fluency-generating system is diffusely represented in the CNS. Second, multiple regions of abnormality may result in multiple types of disruption of the system, and hence, of fluency. Involvement of inferior frontal, anterior cingulate, and temporal regions is of particular interest because these regions are hypothesized centers for speech motor control and for linguistic production. People who stutter who demonstrate deficits in speech motor and/or linguistic performance should also evidence distinct patterns of altered cortical activity.

We now consider sources of behavioral evidence for a fluency-generating system. This evidence comes from measures of speech motor and linguistic performance. The measure of speech motor performance was acoustic laryngeal reaction time (LRT) as a function of the complexity of the required response (i.e., sustained vowel, word, or sentence). Multiple measures of linguistic performance examined aspects of discourse production and comprehension. Both sets of performance measures were examined within the context of rCBF findings.

The rationale for the LRT studies arose, in part, from Goldberg's (1985) discussion of medial and lateral premotor systems. The medial system is hypothetically related to extended, spontaneous, propositional speech and has connections to cingulate cortex. The lateral system is hypothetically related to nonpropositional, repetitive speech or speech guided by auditory self monitoring. This system functions in a responsive mode to external stimuli and has connections to auditory association areas in temporal cortex classically related to language processing (Kent, 1984; Penfield & Roberts, 1976). The stimulus-dependent nature of the LRT task and manipulation of the linguistic complexity of the response should preferentially involve the lateral premotor system in Goldberg's model. That is, people who stutter and who have relative flow asymmetries (left < right) below the normal median in both left superior and middle temporal ROIs should show significantly longer LRT for the linguistically complex response than will normal speakers and people who stutter and who have relative flow asymmetries above the normal median value in at least one of these temporal ROIs. Goldberg's model predicts that asymmetric flows to the cingulate ROI should not affect LRT values.

LRT and rCBF were examined for the 16 people who stutter and who where native speakers of English. People who stutter were divided into two subgroups on the basis of comparison of their rCBF data to 78 people who do not stutter. The ten people who stutter in the first group had low relative blood flow to *both* superior and middle temporal ROIs. The six people who stutter in the second group had low relative blood flow to either the superior *or* the middle temporal ROIs.

Figure 1 shows LRT as a function of response complexity for the three groups. LRT differences between people who do not stutter and people who stutter and who have normal relative flow to at least one temporal ROI were not significant for any response. A significant LRT difference for the word and sentence responses was obtained between controls and people who stutter and who have reduced relative blood flow to both temporal ROIs. A significant LRT difference was also obtained for the sentence response between people who stutter and have normal relative blood flow to at least one left temporal ROI and people who stutter and have reduced relative blood flow to both left temporal ROIs. That is, only those people who stutter and who have asymmetric blood flow to *both* superior and middle temporal ROIs showed a pronounced response complexity effect on LRT values. Patterns of LRT as a function of response complexity did not change when reduced blood flow to the cingulate

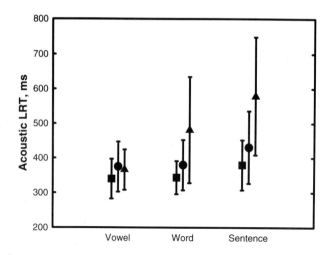

Figure 1. Acoustic LRT as a function of response complexity for nonstutterers (■), stutterers with reduced relative rCBF to left superior *or* middle temporal ROIs (●), and stutterers with reduced relative rCBF to left superior *and* middle temporal ROIs (▲). LRT values are shown as means and two (± 1) standard deviation dispersions.

ROI was considered in combination with temporal flow findings for the groups of people who stutter.

Relations between resting rCBF anomalies and speech motor performance deficits are consistent with predictions of Goldberg's (1985) model regarding defects in the lateral premotor system. While Goldberg's model has been invoked by others to explain stuttering behaviors (Caruso et al., 1988; Webster, 1988), they concluded that abnormality of the medial premotor system was the mechanism underlying stuttering. The discrepancy among these conclusions can be resolved if one considers the differential functions of the two premotor systems in Goldberg's model. The concept of functionally specific motor systems embodied in Goldberg's model suggests that the well-documented heterogeneity of the stuttering population may arise, in part, from differences in the presence, loci, and relative magnitude of neurophysiolgic abnormalities in multiple CNS regions that subserve speech motor control.

Watson et al. (1994) examined rCBF findings in the context of linguistic performance. Linguistic performance was evaluated using tasks that assess discourse production and comprehension. Discourse production was evaluated by an analysis of three subject-generated stories. Two stories were elicited using pictorial stimuli. The third, more complex story, was elicited by asking subjects to read a narrative silently and then to retell the story immediately. All stories were evaluated using a discourse grammar that models the core information components essential to story structure (Labov & Waletsky, 1967). Components include setting, complicating action, and resolution. Discourse comprehension was evaluated using two measures. One measure consisted of questions to probe comprehension of the complex story used in the production task. The second measure assessed subjects' ability to identify noun referents for pronouns within a different set of short stories read aloud by an examiner. Referents were major characters in the stories who were identifiable through the use of subtle linguistic cues within the text. A third task assessed subjects' ability to disambiguate grammatically or lexically ambiguous sentences (for example, "The duck is ready to eat.").

Linguistic performance and rCBF were examined for 16 people who stutter and 10 people who do not stutter. All were native speakers of English and completed both linguistic and SPECT rCBF testing. Each subject's number of errors across all linguistic assessments was transformed into a z score relative to the error mean and standard deviation of the 10 nonstutterers. Subjects whose z score was greater than 3.0 were classified as linguistically impaired. Analysis of z scores revealed that all 10 nonstutterers were classified as linguistically normal, 6 people who stutter were identified as linguistically normal, and 10 people who stutter were identified as linguistically impaired. Figure 2 summarizes the average number of errors ($\pm$ 1 standard deviation) exhibited by each subgroup.

Between-group comparisons of rCBF data were conducted for the superior and middle temporal, anterior cingulate, and inferior frontal ROIs. Comparisons between the 10 nonstutterers and 6 linguistically normal people who stutter revealed no significant differences in relative blood flow asymmetry for any of the four ROIs.

Comparisons between the 10 nonstutterers and 10 linguistically impaired people who stutter revealed significant differences in relative blood flow asymmetry (L<R) for the middle temporal ($p < 0.025$) and inferior frontal ($p < 0.025$) ROIs. The linguistically impaired people who stutter showed, on average, 10.95% lower rCBF in the left middle temporal ROI and 6.51% lower rCBF in the left inferior frontal ROI compared to the respective contralateral

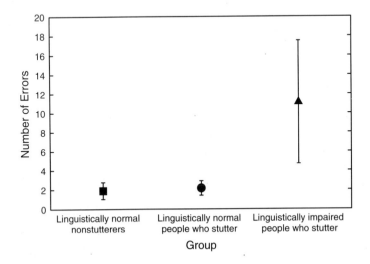

Figure 2. Average ($\pm$1 standard deviation) number of errors on linguistic assessments exhibited by nonstutterers (■), linguistically normal stutterers (●), and linguistically impaired stutterers (▲).

ROIs than did nonstutterers. Comparisons between the linguistically normal and linguistically impaired people who stutter revealed a significant difference in relative blood flow asymmetry (L < R) for the middle temporal ROI ($p < 0.025$). The linguistically impaired people who stutter showed, on average, 10.95% lower rCBF in the left middle temporal ROI compared to the contralateral ROI in than did linguistically normal people who stutter. The finding that linguistic performance deficits in these people who stutter are associated with asymmetric flows to the temporal region indicates that theories that attempt to explain fluency failures in people who stutter must extend beyond speech motor processing to include language processing.

The brain imaging studies reviewed here are preliminary and have generated controversy (Viswanath et al., 1992; Pool et al., 1992; Fox et al., 1993; Pool et al., 1993). By far, the greatest limitation with respect to the theoretical significance of their findings is the small number of subjects studied. This limitation is particularly important in light of the subgroups of people who stutter suggested by the findings. Because of the exploratory nature of these studies, our statistical analyses were biased toward Type 1 errors. This bias may have resulted in our failure to detect certain regions of abnormality in our QTE and rCBF studies.

With this caution in mind, it is worth noting that the design of these imaging studies strengthens the validity of their findings. First, subjects were studied using two different functional brain imaging technologies: one electrophysiologic and the other metabolic. The congruence of findings for the QTE and SPECT studies is striking. Second, imaging studies were combined with behavioral studies. The association between SPECT rCBF findings and behavioral findings with respect to speech and language performance for subgroups of people who stutter is consistent with classic anatamo-clinical principles of the cortical organization of speech and language.

When brain imaging findings are examined in the broader context of speech motor and language performance, they merge into a coherent picture of a neurophysiologic system that integrates linguistic, speech motor, and very likely, cognitive, processes for the production of fluency. Wingate (1988, p. 267) implied the existence of such a system when he stated, "Stuttering is not simply a problem of words per se, but of words as the pivotal elements in a system that can transduce ideas and thoughts into an audible code . . . ."

In keeping with a systems perspective, stuttering can be considered as one symptom of a defect in a fluent speech generating system that is diffusely represented in the central nervous system and that includes motor, linguistic, and cognitive processing. A similar conclusion was very recently expressed by Fox et al. (1996). This perspective motivates development of theories and models that go beyond stuttering/disfluency and seek a more global understanding of the processes and neural bases of fluency. A simple example of such a model is shown in Figure 3. The model includes cognitive, linguistic, and speech motor processes and candidate neuroanatomic sites at which processing may occur.

These component processes must be efficient, synchronized, and fully integrated to generate optimal fluency. Some degradation in fluency will result if a component process is delayed or if integration or synchrony among components is disrupted.

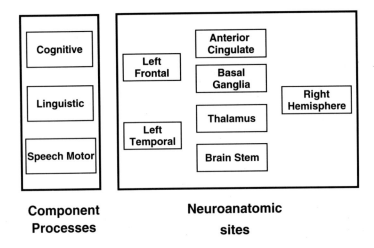

Component   Neuroanatomic
Processes   sites

Figure 3. Schematic model of component processes and neuroanatomic sites of a fluency-generating system.

Fluency can thus be viewed as a reflection of the functional integrity and coordination of the components of the system. Impaired fluency reflects inefficiency or dysfunction in some component process, disruption in the integration of components, or both. Disorders of fluency could manifest in different forms as a consequence of disruption at one or more processes within the system.

It is also useful to discuss fluency with reference to current models of normal speech and language production. For example, Levelt's (1989) model of the generation of fluent speech includes several "processing components" that are activated in the evolution from a speaker's communicative intent at the cognitive level to neuromuscular commands at the articulatory level. This model also includes error detection and correction components. Normal fluency occurs when operations within each processing component are accomplished successfully and efficiently. By implication, each processing component in Levelt's model is susceptible to disruption and is, therefore, a potential source of fluency failure. This implication is presented formally by Postma and Kolk (1993) as the covert repair hypothesis.

Our understanding of fluency can be expanded by empirical tests of models such as those presented by Levelt (1989) and Perkins et al. (1991). This brings us to the final point we wish to make concerning the design of future brain imaging studies in stuttering research. Regardless of the specific model under test, our experience, and that of others, provides guidance for the design of imaging studies.

We concur with Dr. Lauter (this volume) that the use of multiple, converging technologies is a stronger approach to understanding brain function associated with the generation of oral-verbal fluency than is exclusive reliance on a single technology. We believe that progress towards understanding mechanisms of fluency and its dissolution will advance more quickly if we stop treating stuttering as the only grouping variable. This population is nothing, if not heterogeneous. More to the point, this population is heterogeneous on dimensions that have very little to do with specific characteristics of stuttering behavior, per se; for example, resting brain function and linguistic performance. Our findings demonstrate that comparisons among subgroups of people who stutter and individual subject profiles are more informative than comparisons only between people who stutter and nonstutterers. Further, comparisons among different clinical populations (for example, stuttering, aphasia, and cognitive impairment) on the same measures of motoric, linguistic, and cognitive performance and of CNS structure and function may elucidate the processes underlying production of fluency and consequences of their failure. Finally, analyses should permit tests of models that assume distributed as well as localization models of the neural bases of fluency generation.

Insights into the production and dissolution of oral-verbal fluency will accrue through application of new analytic approaches to brain imaging data and new imaging techniques, but only if we avoid repeating methodological mistakes of the past as we apply technologies of the future.

ACKNOWLEDGMENTS

Research described herein was supported by National Institutes of Health grant NS 18276. Significant contributions to these studies were made by our co-investigators: M.D. Devous, Sr., PhD, K. Pool, MD, T. Finitzo, PhD, S. Chapman, PhD, and D. Mendelsohn, MD.

REFERENCES

Caruso, A.J., Abbs, J., & Gracco, V. (1988). Kinematic analysis of multiple movement coordination during speech in stutterers. *Brain, 111*, 439-455.

Dembowski, J. & Watson, B.C. (1991). Acoustic reaction time related to models of central nervous system function. In H.F.M. Peters, W. Hulstijn, & C.W. Starkweather (Eds.), *Speech motor control and stuttering.* (pp. 263-268) Amsterdam: Elsevier.

Devous, M.D., Sr., Stokely, E.M., Chehabi, H. H., & Bonte, F.J. (1986). Normal distribution of regional cerebral blood flow measured by dynamic single-photon emission tomography. *Journal of Cerebral Blood Flow and Metabolism, 6*, 95-104.

Finitzo, T., Pool, K.D., Freeman, F.J., Devous, M.D., Sr., & Watson, B.C. (1991). Cortical dysfunction in developmental stutterers. In H.F.M. Peters, W. Hulstijn, & C.W. Starkweather (Eds.), *Speech motor control and stuttering.* (pp. 251-262) Amsterdam: Elsevier.

Fox, P.T., Lancaster, J.L., & Ingham, R.J. (1993). On stuttering and global ischemia ___ letter to the Editor, *Archives of Neurology, 50*, 1287-1288.

Fox, P.T., Ingham, R.J., Ingham, J.C., Hirsch, T.B., Downs, J.H., Martin, C., Jerabek, P., Glass, T., & Lancaster, J.L. (1996). A PET study of the neural systems of stuttering. *Nature, 382*, 158-162.

Goldberg, G. (1985). Supplementary motor area structure and function: Review and hypotheses. *The Behavioral and Brain Sciences, 8*, 567-616.

Ingham, R.J., Fox, P.T., & Ingham, J.C. (1994). Brain image investigation of the speech of stutterers and nonstutterers. *ASHA, 36*, 188.

Kent, R. (1984). Stuttering as a temporal programming disorder. In R.F. Curlee & W.H. Perkins (Eds.), *Nature and treatment of Stuttering: New Directions* (pp. 283-301). San Diego: College Hill Press.

Labov, W. & Waletsky, J. (1967). Narrative analysis: Oral version of personal experience. In J. Helm (Ed.), *Essays on the verbal and visual arts.* (pp. 12-44). Seattle: University of Washington Press.

Lauter, J. (this volume).

Lennox, W.G., Gibbs, F.A., & Gibbs, E.L. (1938). The relationship in man of cerebral activity to blood flow and to blood constituents. *Journal of Neurology and Psychiatry, 1*, 211-225.

Levelt, W.J.M. (1989). *Speaking: From intention to articulation.* Cambridge: MIT Press.

Penfield, W., & Roberts, L. (1976). *Speech and Brain Mechanisms.* New York: Atheneum.

Perkins, W., Kent, R.D., & Curlee, R.F. (1991). A theory of neurolinguistic function in stuttering. *Journal of Speech and Hearing Research, 34*, 734-752.

Pool, K., Freeman, F.J., & Finitzo, T. (1985). Brain electrical activity mapping: applications to vocal motor control disorders. In H.F.M. Peters, & W. Hulstijn (Eds.) *Speech motor dynamics in stuttering.* (pp.151-160). Wien: Springer-Verlag.

Pool, K.D., Devous, M.D., Sr., Freeman, F.J., Watson, B.C., & Finitzo, T. (1991). Regional cerebral blood flow in developmental stutterers. *Archives of Neurology, 48*, 509-512.

Pool, K.D., Finitzo, T., Devous, M.D., Sr., Freeman, F.J., & Watson, B.C. (1992). Stutterers and cerebral blood flow ___ In Reply. *Archives of Neurology, 49*, 347-348.

Pool, K.D., Finitzo, T., Devous, M.D., Sr., Watson, B.C., & Freeman, F.J. (1993). On stuttering and global ischemia ___ in reply. *Archives of Neurology, 50*, 1289-1290.

Postma, A., & Kolk, H. (1993). The covert repair hypothesis: Prearticulatory repair processes in normal and stutterers disfluencies. *Journal of Speech and Hearing Research, 36*, 472-487.

Sugar, O., & Gerard, O.W. (1938). Anoxia and brain potentials. *Stroke, 1*, 558-572.

Viswanath, N.S., Rosenfield, D.B., & Nudelman, H.B. (1992). Stuttering and cerebral blood flow ___ letter to the Editor. *Archives of Neurology, 49*, 346-347.

Watson, B.C., Pool, K.D., Devous, M.D., Sr., Freeman, F.J., & Finitzo, T. (1992). Brain blood flow related to acoustic laryngeal reaction time in adult developmental stutterers. *Journal of Speech and Hearing Research, 35*, 555-561.

Watson, B.C., Freeman, F.J., Devous, M.D., Sr., Chapman, S.B., Finitzo, T., & Pool, K.D. (1994). Linguistic performance and regional cerebral blood flow in persons who stutter. *Journal of Speech and Hearing Research, 37*, 1221-1228.

Webster, W.G. (1988). Neural mechanisms underlying stuttering: Evidence from bimanual handwriting performance. *Brain and Language, 33*, 226-244.

Wingate, M.E. (1988). *The structure of stuttering: A psycholinguistic analysis.* New York: Springer-Verlag.

Speech Production: Motor Control, Brain Research and Fluency Disorders
W. Hulstijn, H.F.M. Peters and P.H.H.M. Van Lieshout, editors

Chapter 29

THE ELECTROPHYSIOLOGY OF SPEAKING: POSSIBILITIES OF EVENT-RELATED POTENTIAL RESEARCH ON SPEECH PRODUCTION

Peter Hagoort, Miranda van Turennout

In this chapter we discuss problems and possibilities of using electrophysiological recordings to study speaking. First we introduce the method of recording Event Related Potentials (ERPs). More in particular we discuss the so-called Readiness Potential (RP), an ERP component that precedes voluntary movements. We conclude that contamination of the EEG signal with EMG activity of the muscles involved in articulation and inconclusive results in earlier RP studies preclude strong conclusions on the basis of ERP recordings about the areas of the brain that supervise or dominate the articulation of speech. We argue that, rather than in localizing the brain regions involved in speaking, the importance of the electrophysiological recordings is related to the high temporal resolution of the ERP signal. This characteristic allows us to map out the time course of the retrieval of lexical information preceding overt articulation. We discuss an experimental paradigm that we used for estimating the time course of the retrieval of semantic, syntactic and phonological word information. On the basis of our results we present a rough estimate of the time course of the processes involved in lexical access during speaking. We conclude that, in principle, this experimental paradigm can be helpful in determining the locus of nonfluencies in speaking, provided that this locus precedes articulation.

INTRODUCTION

One way of recording brain activity related to language processing is by recording event-related brain potentials (ERPs). Human ERPs are recorded from a number of electrodes placed on the scalp. Scalp recording of ERPs provides a non-invasive technique for evaluating electrophysiological activity related to stimulus processing and response preparation.

As can be seen in Figure 1, ERPs are usually recorded time-locked to and averaged over a number of stimulus events. In the resulting averaged ERP waveform one can see a number of distinct ERP components emerge. These ERP components are often labeled on the basis of their polarity (P for positive, N for negative) and either their latency in milliseconds (e.g., P300) or their sequential number in the series of peaks (e.g., P3). For example, the P300 (or P3) is a late positive wave with a typical peak latency around 300 ms post-stimulus, that occurs when an infrequent target stimulus is detected in a series of frequent standard stimuli.

An example of a psycholinguistically more interesting ERP component is the N400.

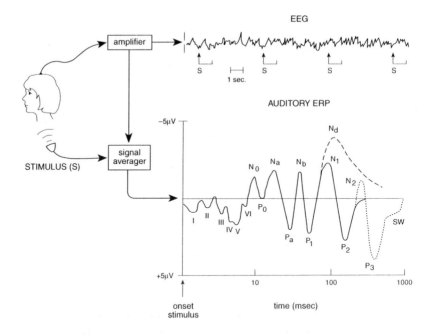

Figure 1 (after Hillyard & Kutas, 1983). Idealized waveform of a series of ERP components that become visible after averaging the EEG to repeated presentations of a short auditory stimulus. Usually, averaging over a number of stimulus tokens is required to get an adequate signal-to-noise ratio. Along the logarithmic time axis the early brainstem potentials (Waves I-VI), the midlatency components (No, Po, Na, Pa, Nb), the largely exogenous components (P1, N1, P2), and the endogenous, cognitive ERP components (Nd, N2, P300, Slow Wave) are shown. The components with a negative polarity are plotted upwards, the components with a positive polarity are plotted downwards.

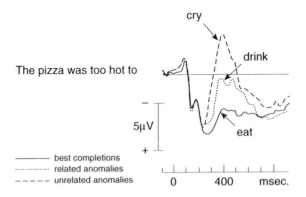

Figure 2 (after Kutas & Hillyard, 1980): ERP to the sentence-final words for visually presented sentences. The sentence-final semantic anomaly (i.c., *socks*) results in a substantial negative shift relative to the ERP elicited by the semantically expected ending (i.c., *butter*). This negative shift is known as the N400-effect.

This component can be elicited by a mismatch between the semantics of the sentence context and the lexical meaning of a particular word, as in the sentence "He spread his warm bread with *socks.*" (Kutas & Hillyard, 1980). Compared to the correct sentence-final word *butter*, these semantic anomalies elicit a large negative shift that onsets at about 250 ms after the semantic anomaly and reaches its maximal amplitude at about 400 ms.

The general advantage of ERPs over brain imaging techniques such as PET and fMRI is its millisecond temporal resolution. Especially for rapid, transient processes such as speaking or listening to language, this aspect of ERPs allows the investigation of a central aspect of language processing, namely its time course. However, a disadvantage of ERPs is that especially for the later components such as P300 and N400, the localization of the neural generators that contribute to the surface potentials recorded at the scalp is still problematic.

So far, we have discussed ERPs that are elicited by and follow the occurrence of a particular stimulus event, such as the presentation of tones or words. However, it is also possible to record ERPs that precede a response. The most well-known response related potential is the so-called Readiness Potential (or Bereitschaftspotential). This potential was first discovered by Kornhuber and Deecke (1965). These authors recorded brain potentials over the left and right motor cortex, before and during voluntary movement of the left hand. As can be seen in Figure 3, about 1 second before the actual hand movement can be registered in the EMG, a slow negative going potential appears in the EEG signal that reaches its maximum just after movement onset. Moreover, in the final phase before movement onset this negativity becomes larger for sites contralateral to the moving hand; that is, at sites over the motor cortex that are known to be involved in the initiation of the movement. Similar larger contralateral negativities have been obtained for arm and finger movements (Vaughan et al., 1968).

Readiness Potential and speech
 At first sight, the Readiness Potential (RP) seems to be appropriate for studying aspects

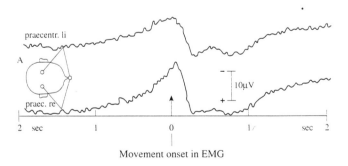

Movement onset in EMG

Figure 3 (after Kornhuber & Deecke, 1965). Readiness Potential or Bereitschaftspotential during voluntary movement of the left hand. The negative going potential during movement preparation is larger over the contralateral right hemisphere. Zero is the onset of movement in the electromyogram.

of the articulatory movements of speech, with potential applications for studying disorders of voluntary movement in for instance apraxia of speech and stuttering. However, the results of studies examining the RP in oral speech and non-speech gestures are less clear-cut (cf. Wohlert, 1993).

One serious problem that plagues ERP studies on speech production is the contamination of the ERP signal with the EMG activity of the muscles producing the articulatory gestures. Due to the proximity of the relevant orofacial muscles to the EEG recording sites, EMG activity is a much greater artifact source in the case of oral movements than in the case of finger or toe movements. Brooker and Donald (1980), for instance, observed that EEG recorded at inferior frontal lobe sites correlated with the EMG activity recorded from the masseter and temporalis muscles. Moreover, these and other muscles (e.g., the orbicularis oris) showed activity up to 500 ms before the vocalization trigger. Also it has been reported that tongue movements can contribute to scalp-recorded potentials (Szirtes & Vaughan, 1977).

The presence of major artifact sources in recording potentials related to speaking is clearly one of the main reasons why, compared to ERP studies on language comprehension, the number of ERP studies on speaking is very limited indeed.

An additional problem is that the few available studies do not provide an unequivocal pattern of results. Deecke, Engel, Lang, and Kornhuber (1986) examined the RP preceding the utterances of single words. To avoid the most problematic artifact sources, early facial EMG activity was chosen as the trigger for backwards averaging. This procedure is claimed to result in EEG activity not contaminated with articulatory EMG activity. In their study, Deecke et al. (1986) obtained an initial bilateral RP that lateralized over the left hemisphere during the last 100 msec preceding speech onset. They interpreted these results as suggesting that both motor cortices are involved in the initiation of articulation (the early bilateral RP), but that the final execution of the articulatory gestures was dominated by the left motor cortex (the lateralized component).

In contrast to the findings of Deecke and colleagues, no such lateralization of the RP was seen in a study by Wohlert (1993; see also Wohlert & Larson, 1991), who examined the RPs preceding three types of oral gestures: (i) a nonspeech gesture (lip press); (ii) a basic phonemic gesture (lip rounding, as in an unvoiced /u/; (iii) the production of the spoken word "pool". The EMG was recorded from the orbicularis oris superior, which is an important muscle for lip movements. For all three tasks, symmetrical activity in the RPs recorded over the left and right motor cortices was found. Interestingly, the greatest amplitude was seen over Cz, a midline site. Moreover, this midline effect was largest for the word task. Wohlert interpreted this finding as suggestive for a role of the Supplementary Motor Area (SMA) in rapid, continuous movements. In this interpretation the vertex RP for producing speech movements is largest, because the amount of sequenced muscle activity is greater in speaking than in the lip press and lip rounding movements (Wohlert, 1993).

In short, studies on the RP preceding overt speech activity have not resulted in consistent findings with respect to the brain areas that supervise or dominate the process of articulation in normal subjects.

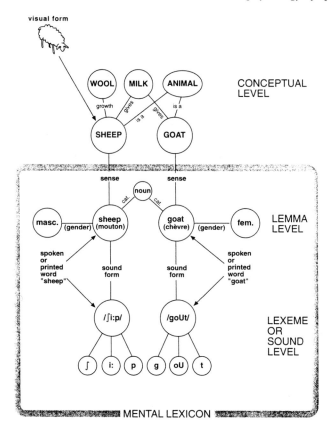

Figure 4. The Levelt and Roelofs model for speaking. Concept nodes (SHEEP) are activated on the basis of sensory and/or conceptual input. Activation from a concept node spreads to its lemma node (*sheep*) in the mental lexicon. Each concept node is linked to exactly one lemma in the lexicon. At the lemma level the syntactic word information is specified, such as grammatical gender and word class. For instance, in French the gender of the lemma *sheep* is male and the gender of the lemma *goat* is female. After the lemma has been selected, word form information is retrieved and prepared for articulation.

For the time being, this severely limits the possibilities of fruitfully using the RP in research on speech related movement disorders.

In the remainder we will discuss the approach that we developed to study the process of speaking (van Turennout et al., 1997). In our approach we were not so much interested in establishing the brain areas that are involved in speaking, but rather in using the superior temporal resolution of the ERP signal to examine the time course of speaking.

The issue: Lexical access in speech production

Figure 4 specifies the Levelt and Roelofs model for word production (cf. Levelt, 1989; Roelofs, 1992). According to this model the lexicon contains syntactic word nodes (lemmas) and word form nodes (lexemes). Lemmas are activated by the concepts that are part of the message that the speaker wants to utter. Before the articulators can be instructed to actually produce the speech sounds of the intended word, first a concept has to be activated, then its corresponding lemma has to be selected and finally the phonological form of the word has to be retrieved (for details of this latter process, see the contribution of Meyer). In fluent speech this whole cascade of activation and selection processes occurs extremely rapid. The precise temporal orchestration of these processes is, however, still a matter of debate.

In a series of ERP studies we have tried to track the time course of semantic activation, the retrieval of a word's syntactic specifications (lemma retrieval), and the phonological encoding of words. A crucial design aspect of these studies enabled us to record ERPs that could not be contaminated with speech related EMG activity. For this purpose we used one particular ERP effect, the so-called Lateralized Readiness Potential (LRP).

The Lateralized Readiness Potential (LRP).

It has been shown that the RP that we discussed above starts to lateralize as soon as the subject knows with which hand (s)he is supposed to react (Kutas & Donchin, 1980). Therefore, the lateralization of the RP can be used to detect and measure the preparation of a specific response (cf. Coles, 1989). This aspect of the RP is exploited for using and deriving the Lateralized Readiness Potential (LRP).

The LRP is derived from the RP which is recorded from C3' and C4', located above the left and right motor cortices. In our studies, subjects were asked to give left and right hand responses. The RP preceding hand movements is largest over the motor cortex contralateral to the corresponding hand. The LRP is derived as follows: First on each trial, the difference is obtained between the potentials recorded from C3' and C4'. These difference waveforms are averaged separately for trials in which the left versus the right hand is cued. Second, to cancel out lateralized potentials that are not specifically related to response preparation, the waveform obtained for the left-hand trials is subtracted from the waveform obtained for the right-hand trials. The resulting LRP reflects the average amount of lateralization occurring as a result of the preparation of the hand response (see Figure 5). The LRP deviates from the baseline in upward direction as soon as response preparation for the cued response hand occurs.

A finding in the LRP literature that is crucial for our purposes is that the LRP starts to develop as soon as relevant stimulus information is used for response preparation (Coles, 1989; De Jong et al., 1988; Miller & Hackley, 1992; Osman et al., 1992). This makes the LRP a real-time measure of the moments in time at which different kinds of information influence the preparation of a response.

The LRP and lexical access during speaking

We will illustrate the way in which we used this paradigm for testing an assumption in most models of language production, including the Levelt and Roelofs model. This assumption is that the meaning of a word is available before its phonological form can be

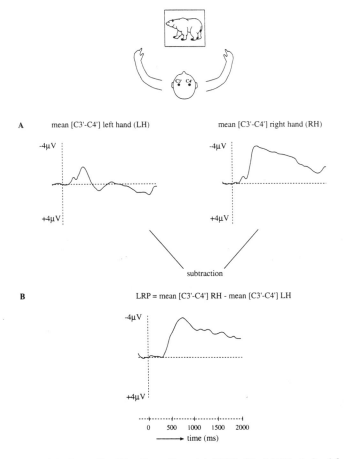

Figure 5. Derivation of the Lateralized Readiness Potential (LRP). The LRP is derived from the Readiness Potential (RP) which is recorded from C3' and C4', located above the left and right motor cortices. In this example subjects are presented with target pictures that either cue a left-hand or a right-hand response. The RP preceding hand movements is largest over the motor cortex contralateral to the corresponding hand. The LRP is derived as follows: First on each trial, the difference is obtained between the potentials recorded from C3' and C4'. These difference waveforms are averaged separately for trials in which the left versus the right hand is cued (a). Second, to cancel out lateralized potentials that are not specifically related to response preparation, the waveform obtained for the left-hand trials is subtracted from the waveform obtained for the right-hand trials (b). The resulting LRP reflects the average amount of lateralization occurring as a result of the preparation of the hand response. The LRP deviates from the baseline in upward direction as soon as response preparation for the cued response hand occurs.

retrieved. Tested in an LRP paradigm it implies that conceptual-semantic information should be transmitted earlier to the motor system than phonological information, provided that these sources of information are relevant for making a response.

The response relevance of both semantic and phonological information was guaranteed in the following way: We presented our subjects with a set of pictures that they had to name. However, the crucial task preceded the naming response. Half of the pictures depicted an animal, the other half an object (see Figure 6). Subjects were instructed to give a pushbutton reponse with one hand for animate picture referents, and with the other for inanimate picture referents. Since animacy is a basic semantic feature, this task requires the retrieval of conceptual-semantic information. Crucially, these left and right hand responses were made conditional on the nature of the phonological word form information. The materials shown in Figure 6 are from a study in which we instructed subjects to only give a pushbutton response if the word-final phoneme of the depicted animal or object ended with an /r/. A response should be withheld if the word-final phoneme was an /n/. In this way the task consisted of a conjunction of a go-nogo decision and a pushbutton response with the left or right hand.

Since the LRP is an index of response preparation, it starts to develop well before the actual pushbutton response is given. More interestingly, an LRP can even occur when no response is given at all. We were especially interested whether an LRP would develop on trials in which the subject decided not to respond on the basis of word form information (the nogo trials). The prediction of the Levelt and Roelofs model is that not only on go trials but also on nogo trials we should see an LRP, even in the absence of an overt response.

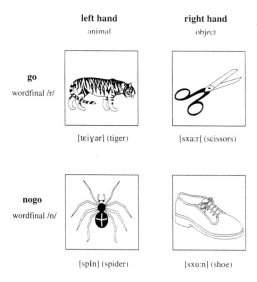

Figure 6 (after van Turennout et al., 1997). Examples of the pictures used in one of our LRP studies. In the figure, the Dutch picture names and their English translations are shown below the pictures. Dutch picture names are in the International Phonetic Alphabet. The four pictures depicted here represent separate trials for the four conditions in the experiment. In the example, an animal cues a left-hand response, and an object cues a right-hand response. The reponse has to be executed if the picture name ends with an /r/ (go-trials), but withheld if it ends with an /n/ (nogo-trials).

The logic behind this prediction is as follows: If during picture naming semantic information becomes available earlier than phonological information, the preparation of a hand response can start before phonological information informs the subject about whether or not to respond. This is exactly the pattern of results that we observed. An LRP developed not only for go trials, but initially also for nogo-trials, in the absence of an overt response.

The early availability of semantic information enabled response preparation, but when information about the word's phonological form became available, further response preparation was overruled on the nogo-trials (for details of design and results, see van Turennout et al., 1997).

In our studies we asked our subjects not only to determine their go-nogo decision on the word-final phoneme, but also on the word-initial phoneme. In addition we asked subjects not only to give a pushbutton response on the basis of a semantic component (i.e., animacy), but also on the basis of a syntactic feature of words (i.e., grammatical gender). Together the results of these studies allow the following conclusions:

(i) The retrieval of both semantic and syntactic word features precedes the retrieval of its phonological form.

(ii) The information about a word's phonological form is not available at once, but accrues in a left-to-right order. For the words in our study (on average 4.5 phonemes) it took an additional 80 ms to retrieve the full word form once the word-initial phoneme was available.

The results obtained with the LRP paradigm show that ERPs with their high temporal resolution can be used to observe the rapid mental processes that underly speaking, even before overt articulation is initiated. Clearly more research is needed before a temporally finegrained analysis of speaking will be completed. Nevertheless current ERP data already allow us to give a rough approximation of the time course from perception to articulation.

Let us assume that while walking in your back garden all of a sudden you stand eyes in eyes with a grizzly bear. Among all your behavioral options, the following two belong to the more probable ones. One reaction is to run away. An alternative one is to say: "A bear". For our purposes we are only interested in the second behavior. A recent ERP study suggests that it takes roughly 150 ms to perceive and categorize a picture as an animal (Thorpe et al., 1996). On the basis of this finding we think it is a reasonable guess that the activation of the concept BEAR on the basis of the visual input in your garden is less than 200 ms. On the basis of our own results we know that it takes about 600 ms before articulation of the word *bear* starts. The period in between (roughly 400 ms) has to do with the cascade of activation and selection processes of lemma and word form information. Our results indicate that the retrieval of the full phonological form of a word like *bear* takes in the order of 120 ms once the conceptual-semantic information has been activated. The remaining time is necessary for lemma selection and preparing the articulatory programme on the basis of the phonological information (for a comparable estimation and more details see Levelt et al., submitted).

Perspectives for further research

Clearly the LRP paradigm that we developed seems useful for tracking the time course of the processes of speaking that precede overt articulation. However, measuring the parameters of the actual execution of the articulatory gestures does not lend itself easily to a fruitful application of the ERP-technique. Until reliable algorithms become available for correcting EMG activity out of the EEG signal, the artifact problems seem too severe for investigating the speech motor production directly with the help of this technique. This, however, does not invalidate electrophysiological methods for studying nonfluencies in speech production. Since nonfluencies can arise and indeed are often claimed to arise at levels preceding overt articulation (Postma & Kolk, 1993; Wingate, 1988), in principle the LRP paradigm can be used to get a fairly precise estimation of the stages in speech production at which nonfluencies might arise. As such research on nonfluencies in speech production could benefit from exploiting the kind of paradigm that we discussed.

REFERENCES

Brooker, B.H., & Donald, M.W. (1980). Contribution of the speechmusculature to apparent human EEG asymmetries prior to vocalization. *Brain and Language, 9*, 256-266.

Coles, M.G.H. (1989). Modern mind-brain reading: Psychophysiology, physiology, and cognition. *Psychophysiology, 26*, 251-269.

Deecke, L., Engel, M., Lang, W., & Kornhuber, H.H. (1986).Bereitschaftspotential preceding speech after holding breath. *Experimental Brain Research, 65*, 219-223.

Hillyard, S.A., & Kutas, M. (1983). Electrophysiology of cognitive processing. *Annual Review of Psychology, 34*, 33-61.

Jong, de R., Wierda, M., Mulder, G., & Mulder, L.J.M. (1988). Use of partial information in responding. *Journal of Experimental Psychology: Human Perception and Performance, 14*, 682-692.

Kornhuber, H.H., & Deecke, L. (1965). Hirnpotentialänderungen bei Willkürbewegungen und passiven Bewegungen des Menschen: Bereitschaftspotential und reafferente Potentiale. *Pflüger's Archive, 284*, 1-17.

Kutas, M., & Donchin, E. (1980). Preparation to respond as manifested by movement-related brain potentials. *Brain Research, 202*, 95-115.

Kutas, M., & Hillyard, S.A. (1980). Reading senseless sentences: Brain potentials reflect semantic incongruity. *Science, 207*, 203-205.

Levelt, W.J.M. (1989). *Speaking: From intention to articulation.* Cambridge, MA: MIT Press.

Levelt, W.J.M, Roelofs, A., & Meyer, A.S. (submitted). A theory of lexical access in speech production

Miller, J., & Hackley, S.A. (1992). Electrophysiological evidence for temporal overlap among contingent mental processes. *Journal of Experimental Psychology: General, 121*, 195-209.

Osman, A., Bashore, T.R., Coles, M.G.H., Donchin, E., & Meyer, D.E. (1992). On the transmission of partial information: Inferences from movement-related brain potentials. *Journal of Experimental Psychology: Human Perception and Performance, 18*, 217-232.

Postma, A., & Kolk, H.H.J. (1993). The covert repair hypothesis: Prearticulatory repair processes in normal and stuttered disfluencies. *Journal of Speech and Hearing Research, 36*, 472-488

Roelofs, A. (1992). A spreading-activation theory of lemma retrieval in speaking. *Cognition, 42*, 107-142.

Szirtes, J., & Vaughan, H.G. (1977). Characteristics of cranial and facial potentials associated with speech production. In J.E. Desmedt (Ed.), *Language and hemispheric specialization in man: Cerebral ERPs* (pp. 112-126). Basel: Karger.

Thorpe, S., Fize, D., & Marlot, C. (1996). Speed of processing in the human visual system. *Nature, 381*, 520-522.

Turennout, van M., Hagoort, P., Brown, C.M. (1997). Electrophysiological evidence on the time course of semantic and phonological processes in speech production. *Journal of Experimental Psychology: Learning, Memory, and Cognition,* in press.

Vaughan, H.G., Costa, L.D., & Ritter, W. (1968). Topography of the human motor potential. *Electroencephalography and Clinical Neurophysiology, 25,* 1-10.

Wingate, M.E. (1988). *The structure of stuttering: A psycholinguistic analysis.* New York, NY: Springer-Verlag.

Wohlert, A.B. (1993). Event-related brain potentials preceding speech and nonspeech oral movements of varying complexity. *Journal of Speech and Hearing Research, 36,* 897-905.

Wohlert, A.B., & Larson, Ch.R. (1991). Cerebral averaged potentials preceding oral movement. *Journal of Speech and Hearing Research, 34,* 1387-1396.

© 1997 Elsevier Science B.V. All rights reserved.
Speech Production: Motor Control, Brain Research and Fluency Disorders
W. Hulstijn, H.F.M. Peters and P.H.H.M. Van Lieshout, editors

Chapter 30

EVENT-RELATED CORTICAL POTENTIALS PRECEDING PHONATION IN STUTTERERS AND NORMAL SPEAKERS: A PRELIMINARY REPORT

Lawrence F. Molt

Initial data from a study examining hemispheric amplitude and latency patterns of the readiness potential (RP) for phonatory activity (abrupt phonation of vowel) from seven adult persons who stutter (PWS) and matched normal speakers (NS) is presented. The RP is a slow cortical event-related brain potential occurring before movement onset, thought to reflect cortical preparation for movement. Once trained, subjects produced self-paced phonatory initiation (PI) activity. Electroencephalographic (EEG) recordings were made from 12 cortical sites with laryngeal area EMG activity used to halt and align EEG recordings for averaging. Both groups exhibited a typical RP slow negative shift waveform. Maximum amplitude preceding PI was obtained for nine subjects (six NS and three PWS) at Site CZ (central vertex) with all demonstrating similar patterns in latency & amplitude across electrode sites. The other four PWS and one NS demonstrated a lateralized pre-PI peak latency, generally to various right hemisphere sites.

INTRODUCTION

The current study presents pilot data from an ongoing project examining hemispheric amplitude and latency patterns of the readiness potential (RP) obtained for phonatory activity from persons who stutter (PWS) and normal speakers (NS). The RP is one of the movement-related cortical potentials (MRCPs). It is a slow cortical event-related brain potential occurring before movement onset and thought to reflect cortical preparation for movement. The RP is characterized by a slowly increasing negative amplitude wave, occurring at or near the pre-Rolandic fissure area. Activity begins approximately one second before voluntary movement and reaches maximum amplitude in the final milliseconds before movement onset.

The RP and other MRCPs has traditionally been recorded for movements of limb extremities, such as fingers and toes, where the EMG activity associated with the movement is far removed from the scalp surface cortical recording sites. These studies generally demonstrate maximum RP amplitude in the hemisphere contralateral to the limb/digit moved. Results for studies utilizing speech and nonspeech oral motor activity have had somewhat equivocal outcomes. McAdam and Whitaker (1971) and Levy (1977) reported lateralization of maximal RP amplitude to the left hemisphere for speech tasks. Deecke, Engel, Lang and Kornhuber (1986) reported an initial bilateral activation that showed a lateralized component over the left hemisphere during the final 100 msec prior to speech onset. Morrell and Huntington (1972) did not find clear evidence of lateralization. Wohlert (1993) reported successful RP recordings of muscle activity for facial areas associated with both non-speech lip movement and simple speech activity. Her results indicated that for a relatively easy single syllable automatic speech task, lateralization for motor control or language function was not seen (normal speaking subjects). Later studies (Deecke, et. al., 1986; Wohlert, 1993) stressed the importance of minimizing all extraneous movement, including strict control of respiration, to minimize artifacts during RP recordings. While limited information is currently available for describing RP activity during speech production, the RP recording technique appears to offer a noninvasive, time-sensitive, and relatively inexpensive method to analyze cortical processes associated with speech motor control.

There appears to be a strong possibility that PWS may exhibit deviant RP/MRCP patterns. Several studies using varying techniques to examine blood flow such as SPECT (Poole et al., 1991) and PET (Braun et al., chapter 23; Ingham et al., chapter 24; Kroll et al., chapter 25; Riley et al., chapter 26) have reported different patterns of hemispheric activation between PWS and NS for various speech tasks. The current study sought to determine if RP amplitude patterns differed between normal and stuttering speakers on a simple vocalization task.

METHODS

Subjects

Subjects consisted of seven adult PWS, and seven adult NS, matched on age (mean PWS age: 27.8; mean NS age: 25.2), sex (five males, two females), and handedness patterns (as assessed via the Edinburgh Handedness Inventory; Oldfield, 1971). A case history was taken to ascertain that no subjects had any known neurological disorders and to determine that all PWS reported a traditional developmental pattern to their stuttering. All stuttering subjects were identified as PWS by themselves and two speech-language pathologists familiar with stuttering. The SSI - 3 (Riley, 1994) was administered to all seven stuttering subjects. Overall scores ranged from 12 to 34, with the following resultant severity ratings: very mild (2), mild (1), moderate (2), and severe (2).

Procedures

Subjects were seated in a reclining armchair in a sound suite. All were instructed and trained to inhale and hold their breath (emphasizing diaphragmatic control) for approximately two seconds preceding initiation of phonation, and to maintain lips, lower jaw, tongue and facial muscles in a relaxed, neutral position during this period through to the initiation of phonation (abrupt phonation of / a /). Phonatory initiation (PI) was judged via laryngeal area surface EMG recordings, obtained via ECI Ag/AgCl miniature electrodes placed over the thyroid lamina at approximately the level of the base of the thyroid notch. Placement varied somewhat among subjects to meet the requirements of obtaining consistently high EMG readings, as the EMG signal was used to end each RP trial recording. It is important to note that the EMG methodology did not ensure measurement of intrinsic laryngeal muscular activity, although it did reflect laryngeal area activity associated with phonation. Each subject generally produced two-to-three vocalizations on a breath group, with 100 vocalizations produced overall. Artifact monitoring was done via visual inspection of EEG channel recordings.

Electroencephalographic (EEG) recordings were made from 15 monopolar cortical sites (using ECI Electro-Caps in International 10-20 System configuration) with frontal bone ground and nasal tip reference electrode (all impedances < 5 K). Ongoing EEG was recorded on a Neuro Scan Corporation 16 channel Syn-Amps system with SCAN software utilized to initially record and store continuous digitized EEG recordings. Digitized EEG/EMG records were later visually inspected and electronically marked at onset of each EMG activity period. At this time clearly artifacted trials were discarded. The remaining trials (no less than 61 for any subject) were aligned in time on the marked EMG onset and, using a window/epoch setting of 700 ms before EMG onset/PI, were computer-averaged to remove EEG activity extraneous to the movement task.

PWS subjects were instructed to report any phonatory initiation trials on which stuttering occurred. No stuttering behavior was reported by any subject, and none was observed in terms of EMG artifacts on any EEG channel nor visually by the researcher.

RESULTS

For purposes of the present study, amplitude values suggestive of lateralization were defined as an amplitude difference of greater than 0.5 microvolts between vertex/midline sites and hemispheric sites. At least two runs were completed for each subject, with similar waveform patterns seen across both data runs for all subjects. Both groups of subjects exhibited a typical RP slow negative shift waveform, however, there was considerable individual variation in waveform pattern across subjects. Table 1 presents the RP amplitude values (in microvolts) for each subject from left hemisphere (odd numbered), vertex ("Z"), and right hemisphere (even numbered) at the frontal lobe area "F" line (F3, FZ, F4) and central sulcus area "C" line (C3, CZ, C4) electrode sites.

A lack of lateralization (in terms of maximum amplitude preceding PI) was observed for nine subjects (three NS and six PWS). These nine subjects demonstrated maximal amplitude at Site CZ (central vertex). While maximal amplitude was obtained at CZ for these subjects, individual differences in rise rate of the negative shift, maximum amplitude, and hemispheric distribution across all electrode sites were readily apparent.

The other four PWS and one NS demonstrated a lateralized pre-PI peak latency, all to various right hemisphere sites. Two subjects (both PWS) displayed maximum amplitude at C4 (at/near primary motor strip), and 2 PWS and 1 NS exhibited maximum amplitude at F4

Table 1. Amplitude values (in microvolts) for the Readiness Potential taken at 30 ms preceding phonatory EMG initiation for each stuttering subject (SS) and normal speaking subject (NS) from left hemisphere (odd-numbered), vertex ("Z"), and right hemisphere (even- numbered) electrode sites. Measures shown are for frontal lobe area "F" line (F3, FZ, F4) and central sulcus area "C" line (C3, CZ, C4) sites, with site of highest amplitude indicated by *.

Subject Electrode Site (Type/Number)	F3	FZ	F4	C3	CZ	C4
SS1	3.2	3.6	4.7*	3.2	3.4	3.9
SS2	2.4	2.9	2.1	2.9	3.2*	2.7
SS3	3.6	3.4	2.9	2.9	3.9*	3.4
SS4	4.0	4.4	5.2*	3.7	4.1	4.7
SS5	3.8	4.9	4.5	4.2	5.7*	4.9
SS6	1.5	2.1	2.4	2.1	2.4	3.2*
SS7	2.9	3.1	3.9	2.4	3.4	4.2*
NS1	4.8	5.2	4.9	5.1	5.7*	5.4
NS2	3.7	3.9	4.4	4.1	6.8*	5.1
NS3	2.8	2.4	3.8*	2.2	2.7	2.9
NS4	3.4	3.4	3.1	3.4	3.9*	3.2
NS5	4.7	5.1	4.3	4.9	7.4*	5.5
NS6	2.1	2.2	2.6	2.4	3.8*	2.1
NS7	7.1	7.4	7.4	6.7	7.7*	7.4

(mid-frontal). A sample waveform map for a NS subject with maximum amplitude at CZ, and a similar plot for a PWS subject with lateralized maximal response at C4 are shown in Figure 1.

DISCUSSION

There were differences in patterns of cortical activity preceding phonatory initiation for several (4/7) of the stuttering subjects when compared to those of the majority (6/7) of normal speakers. These differences took the form of a lateralization of peak amplitude to the right hemisphere. Three of the seven PWS did not appear to differ from six of the seven normal speakers in maximal amplitude or latency patterns, indicating that cortical motor timing/activation patterns as measured by the RP procedure do not necessarily differ between normal speakers and some PWS, at least for a simplistic vocalization task as utilized in the present experiment. The lack of a dominant hemisphere (i.e., peak amplitude at midline rather than lateralized) for these nine subjects was similar to one other study that used a similar speech task. Wohlert (1993) reported similar results for oral motor movements (lip pursing) and simple single syllable word productions.

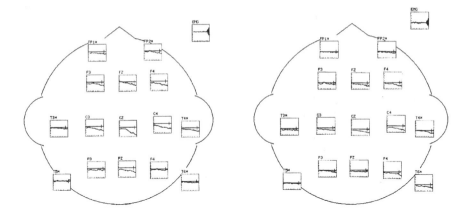

Figure 1: Averaged EEG activity (Readiness Potential waveform) at each cortical site for two subjects. Headplot on left is from a normal speaker, with greatest amplitude at site CZ (central vertex); plot on right is from a stutterer, with greatest amplitude at site C4 (right hemisphere). Window begins 700ms pre-EMG onset, extends 100 ms beyond.

The results for these nine differed, however, from results reported by Deecke et al. (1986) which reported a lateralized response in the final 100 msec preceding speech initiation. Subjects in that particular experiment were required to think of a new word to say in each of 128 trials in rapid sequence, a task which would require linguistic as well as motor activity.

Results from the other four PWS, however, indicate a preponderance of right hemisphere activity, similar to that reported in studies examining blood flow patterns during speech production. It is important to note that the current study utilized an extremely simplistic phonatory task, far removed from normal speech demands and patterns, and a much more simplistic task than utilized in the blood flow studies. There is no certainty that patterns observed during fluent productions of a simplistic phonation task will reflect activity preceding a more complex task or stuttered word. Indeed, research (Deecke et al., 1986) has indicated that increased task complexity has an effect on RP patterns, resulting in a lateralization effect. Use of more linguistically complex paradigms may further delineate differences between PWS and NS.

An alternative explanation for the existence of a different pattern for four of the seven stuttering subjects is that the results reflect patterns within a subgroup of PWS with a motor-related component. Expansion of the paradigm may also assist in identifying or delineating such a subgroup. It must also be mentioned that while extensive training was conducted to reduce EMG activity extraneous to the task and five subjects in the original PWS group were excluded from the study due to a lack of repeatability of waveform patterns, the possibility exists that despite the training and use of both on-line and off-line monitoring to reduce facial area EMG (especially lingual) from contributing to the response, the differences observed may be due to EMG, rather than cortical activity. Further research aimed at delineating EMG effects is warranted.

It should be noted that the differences occurred during production of fluent utterances. The differences apparently cannot be attributed to the occurrence of stuttering, at least on a conscious level. All PWS subjects reported fluent production of all recorded trials and subjects were monitored visually by the researcher. Off-line evaluation of digitized EEG activity did not show evidence of excessive EMG activity that might be associated with stuttering and which might alter the averaged RP waveform.

While the main purpose of the present study was to examine differences between the two groups, a second intent was to explore the utility of the RP technique in exploring cortical activity preceding speech production. The following characteristics were noted. The neuroelectric activity associated with the scalp recorded movement related brain potentials is of low amplitude (generally less than 5 - 10 microvolts). EMG activity associated with facial area muscle movement is 5 - 50 times greater and can easily mask the RP and other MRCPs. Speech related muscle activity must be significantly limited to prevent masking of the components. Subjects in the present study underwent extensive training to limit facial area movement during the task (phonation of a vowel). Several individuals selected for participation could not consistently control extraneous movement and could not be used.

While RP/MRCP recording techniques may prove to be a useful tool in examining cortical patterns reflecting neurologic activity for speech, many methodological questions remain unanswered. The high inter-subject variability may limit its utility in describing normal versus abnormal patterns. Much more research needs to be accomplished in defining RP patterns across tasks in unimpaired individuals. The realities of speech-related EMG activity may limit the usefulness of the technique to only simplistic utterances which may not be sensitive enough to identify differences between groups.

REFERENCES

Braun, A.R., Varga, M., Stager, S., Schultz, G., Selbie, S., Maisog, J.M., Carson, R.E., & Ludlow, C.L. (this volume). H_2O^{15} positron emission photography studies in developmental stuttering: Comparisons of brain activity during non-linguistic orolaryngeal motor activity, fluency- and dysfluency-evoking language conditionsIn H.F.M. Peters, P.H.H.M. Van Lieshout, & W. Hulstijn, (Eds.). Speech production: motor control, brain research and fluency disorders. Amsterdam: Elsevier Science, chapter 23.

Deecke, L., Engel, M., Lang, W., & Kornhuber, H.H. (1986). Bereitschaftspotential preceding speech after holding breath. *Experimental Brain Research*, *65*, 219-223.

Ingham, R., Fox, P.T., & Ingham, J.C. (this volume). An O^{15} Positron emission tomography (PET) study on adult stutterers: Findings and implications. In H.F.M. Peters, P.H.H.M. Van Lieshout, & W. Hulstijn, W. (Eds.). Speech production: motor control, brain research and fluency disorders. Amsterdam: Elsevier Science, chapter 24.

Kroll, R., De Nil, L., Kapur, S., & Houle, S. (this volume). A positron emission tomography investigation of post-treatment brain activation in stutterers. In H.F.M. Peters, P.H.H.M. Van Lieshout, & W. Hulstijn, (Eds.). Speech production: motor control, brain research and fluency disorders. Amsterdam: Elsevier Science.

Levy, R.S. (1977). The question of electrophysiological asymmetries preceding speech. In H. Whitaker, & H.A. Whitaker, (Eds.), *Studies in Neurolinguistics*. New York: Academic Press (287-318).

McAdam, D., & Whitaker, H. (1971). Electroencephalographic localization in the human brain. *Science*, *172*, 499-502.

Morrell, L.K., & Huntington, D. (1972). Cortical potentials time-locked to speech production: Evidence for probable cerebral origin. *Life Sciences*, *11*, 921-929.

Oldfield, R. (1971). The assessment and analysis of handedness: The Edinburgh Inventory. *Neuropsychologica*, *9*, 97-113.

Poole, K.D., Devous, M.D., Freeman, F.J., Watson, B.C., & Finitzo, T. (1991). Regional Cerebral blood flow in developmental stutterers. *Archives of Neurology, 48,* 509-512.

Riley, G. (1994). *Stuttering Severity Instrument for Children and Adults: Third edition*. Austin, TX: Pro-Ed.

Riley, G., Wu, J.C. & Maguire, G. (this volume). PET scan evidence of parallel cerebral systems related to treatment effects. In W. Hulstijn, H.F.M. Peters, & P.H.H.M. Van Lieshout, (Eds.). *Speech production: motor control, brain research and fluency disorders*. Amsterdam: Elsevier Science.

Wohlert, A. (1993). Event-related brain potentials preceding speech and nonspeech movements of varying complexity. *Journal of Speech and Hearing Research, 36,* 897-905.

1997 Elsevier Science B.V.
Speech Production: Motor Control, Brain Research and Fluency Disorders
W. Hulstijn, H.F.M. Peters and P.H.H.M. Van Lieshout, editors

Chapter 31

A DOUBLE-BLIND TRIAL OF PIMOZIDE AND PAROXETINE FOR STUTTERING

Sheila Stager, Karim Calis, Dale Grothe, Meir Bloch, Nannette Turcasso, Christy Ludlow, Allen Braun

A randomized double-blind, placebo-controlled crossover study was designed to examine the effects on fluency of a highly selective dopamine antagonist, pimozide, and a highly selective serotonin reuptake inhibitor, paroxetine, in adult persons who stutter. Eleven persons who stutter enrolled in this study but only a total of 6 individuals completed the pimozide phase, 6 the placebo phase, and 5 the paroxetine phase. This paper examined the following treatment outcome measures; self-perceptions of changes in fluency and factors to which they attributed these changes; comparison of self-ratings of fluency with objective measures of fluency; self-perceptions about changes in symptom severity, consistency of fluency, and measures of speech anxiety such as confidence in speaking, anxiety levels and satisfaction with speech; and reports from others noting fluency change. On pimozide, a positive clinical response was found for 4/6 individuals, and a negative clinical response for the other 2 individuals. Trends for significant differences between placebo and pimozide phases were found for percent of symptoms reported changed (p=0.03), percent of days where fluency change was attributed to medication (p=0.03); consistency of fluency (p=0.04); confidence in speaking (p=0.07), satisfaction with speech (p=0.08), anxiety while speaking (p=0.09) and level of fluency (p=0.1). Individuals randomized to the pimozide phase might have been more likely to report a change in fluency attributable to medication because they reported experiencing more side effects on pimozide than on paroxetine or placebo. No significant clinical response was found for paroxetine using any outcome measure, and significant side effects were experienced by 2 individuals while withdrawing from this medication.

INTRODUCTION

In the literature on pharmacological treatment for stuttering, three classes of medications have been shown to improve fluency in persons who stutter. The class of medications showing the most consistent improvement in fluency are the dopamine antagonists, such as haloperidol, (e.g. Prins et al., 1980), tiapride (Rothenberger et al., 1994), and risperidone (Maguire et al., this volume). Less consistent benefit has been demonstrated using calcium channel blockers such as verapamil (Brady et al., 1989) and nimodipine (Maguire et al., 1994). The third class includes medications that have serotonin reuptake inhibitor properties such as paroxetine (Costa & Kroll, 1995) and clomipramine (Stager et al., 1995).

The average improvement in fluency on clomipramine was 15-20% (Stager et al., 1995), but clomipramine is not a selective medication. It can also act as a dopamine antagonist, and it may be this action, or the combination of serotonin reuptake inhibition and dopamine antagonist action that is important to improving fluency. Therefore, a crossover study comparing a highly selective dopamine-D2 antagonist and a highly selective serotonin reuptake inhibitor would allow for the assessment of the roles that both dopamine antagonists and selective serotonin reuptake inhibitors might play a role in changing fluency. This study used pimozide as the selective dopamine (D2) antagonist, and paroxetine as the highly selective serotonin reuptake inhibitor.

Documenting outcome measures resulting from treatment has become an important part of the therapeutic process, but the nature of the disorder of stuttering makes this process complex. Objective measurement of changes in fluency is one level of outcome measure. However, one may see measurable changes in fluency that individuals may feel is attributable to factors such as periods of natural fluctuation in fluency behaviors (i. e., "good" or "bad" days) or periods of stress (i. e., bad day at work vs. day of relaxation). Another level of outcome measure is the opinion of the person receiving treatment. Understanding and being able to measure what variables may impact on individuals' decisions as to whether they felt their treatment was effective would be useful. This may be especially important in treatment involving medications, because depending on the specific medication, other aspects can be affected that may in turn influence fluency levels, such as changes in anxiety levels. For example, during previous placebo-controlled medication trials carried out at the National Institutes of Health, individuals on active medication anecdotally reported that they felt more confident and less anxious when speaking, that the effort level of their blocks had changed, and that they noticed their fluency levels became more consistent across time. These reports were not necessarily associated with measurable changes in fluency. A third level of outcome measure is whether others recognize and comment on a change in fluency.

To try and elucidate factors that may relate to perceived effectiveness of the medications, daily self-rating scales were designed to assess individual perceptions about the following: 1) symptom severity; 2) levels of fluency; 3) consistency of fluency; 4) speech anxiety measures such as confidence as a speaker, satisfaction with speech, and anxiety while speaking; and 5) possible internal and external factors that might contribute to fluency change. Changes in perceived levels of fluency were then correlated with objective measures of changes in fluency.

METHODS

Subject Selection

Individuals participated in this study only after giving their informed consent. All potential individuals were screened to exclude those with psychiatric disorders and any medical condition contraindicated by either of the medications (i.e. liver and cardiac disease).

Subjects were also excluded if they were concurrently enrolled in speech therapy.

Design

This study was a randomized, double-blind placebo-controlled crossover study of 18 weeks duration. The study consisted of 2 active medication phases (6 weeks each) and included a 6 week placebo washout phase in between the medication phases. The two active medications were pimozide (final dose range - 2 to 10 mg/day) and paroxetine (final dose range - 40 to 50 mg/day), and the medication given first was randomized across individuals. The sequence of medication/placebo/medication was not revealed to those participating. Individuals took five capsules in the morning and five in the evening during each phase. At the end of each phase, blood samples were taken to analyze for drug levels and thereby assess compliance.

Measures

Fluency was assessed every three weeks using a speaking task which involved individuals talking in front of an audience of 4 to 6 listeners. From this task, percent fluency was determined by subtracting the total duration of dysfluent speaking time from total duration of speaking time, dividing by total duration of speaking time and multiplying the result by 100.

Individuals were asked to complete a self-rating scale daily. The format was as follows. The rating scales began with a visual analogue scale (VAS) from 0 (worst it's ever been) to 100 (best it's ever been) where individuals marked their average level of fluency for that day. In relation to their perceived fluency levels, they were asked to check the appropriate box(es): one box if their blocks were not present that day; one of three boxes for whether their blocks were shorter, average or longer than usual in duration; one of three boxes for whether their blocks were fewer, same or greater in number; and one of three boxes for whether their blocks were less effortful, same effort or more effortful. Also in relation to their perceived level of fluency, they were asked to determine if they attributed their fluency levels to natural fluctuation of symptoms, stressful events or medication. If they felt that any of these factors had improved their fluency, they put a plus sign in the appropriate box. If they felt any of them had made their fluency worse, they put a minus sign in the box. If none of these factors influenced their fluency, then they put a 0 in the box. Next, the rating scales had a VAS from 0 (very variable) to 100 (very consistent) where individuals marked their average consistency of fluency that day. They were then asked to determine if their consistency was influenced by natural fluctuation of symptoms, stressful events or medication in the same manner that they attributed change to their fluency. Then, three more VAS were given, to examine level of confidence in speaking (0 = very fearful, 100 = very confident), level of satisfaction with fluency (0 = very unsatisfied, 100 = very satisfied) and level of anxiety when speaking (0 = very anxious, 100 = very relaxed). Finally, individuals were asked to check the appropriate box if others had told them they saw improvement in their speech, or thought their speech was worse, or if no one made any comment that day.

RESULTS

Ten male and one female persons who stutter between the ages of 23 and 48 years enrolled in this study. Their symptom severity ranged from mild to severe. The study was stopped after 2 individuals experienced previously unreported side effects (behavioral dyscontrol and suicide ideation) while withdrawing from paroxetine (Bloch et al., 1995). Three individuals were found noncompliant on one of their drug phases, so their data were not included. At the time the study was stopped, a total of 6 individuals completed the pimozide phase, 6 the placebo phase, and 5 the paroxetine phase (three individuals had completed all phases, 2 just the paroxetine phase, and 3 the pimozide and placebo phases).

To ensure that the effects were measured during the time that individuals were on medication, and the medication levels in the body had reached steady-state, the objective measurements of fluency were made on the last day of each 6 week phase, approximately 3 hours after the first daily dose of medication. This was considered the time when the medications would have reached their peak response. The subjective reports were based on an average of ratings made on the last seven days of each phase, and the dosage was not changed during that week.

The following measures were calculated: 1) for the objective measure of fluency, the difference in percent fluency between placebo and each phase; 2) for determining their perception of changes in the length, number and effort of their blocks, the percent of each of these symptoms that they reported changed (i. e. number of symptoms changing/21 (3 symptoms for 7 days) X 100) (a positive percent meant that the changes they reported were consistent with improved fluency (i. e. shorter blocks, fewer in number, and less effortful) and a negative percent meant that the changes were consistent with their fluency becoming worse (i. e. longer blocks, greater in number and more effortful)); 3) for determining their perception as to whether they attributed the change in fluency to medications, the percent of days that they reported change (i. e. number of days/7 X 100) (a positive percent was associated with improved fluency, and a negative percent with fluency becoming worse); 4) for determining their perceptions as to whether they attributed the change in fluency to factors other than medication, the percent of days that they reported change (i. e. number of days/7 X 100) (a positive percent was associated with improved fluency, and a negative percent with fluency becoming worse; and 5) for determining their perceptions of the consistency of their fluency, their level of fluency, their confidence as a speaker, their satisfaction with their speech, and their anxiety while speaking, the mean of VAS scores across the 7 days.

For purposes of comparison with the medication phases, Table 1 summarizes the individual data for the placebo phase.

On the placebo phase, 4 of 5 individuals did not report a large percentage of change in their symptoms, and if they did, they reported them as worse. Three individuals (S5, S7, S8) did not feel that the medication affected their fluency, while 2 (S3, S6) felt it made their fluency worse. All individuals reported that other factors were affecting their fluency during this phase. In spite of the factors they reported as changing their speech, 4 individuals (S5,

Table 1. Individual percent of change in symptoms ($\triangle$ SYMP), percent of days they attributed changes in fluency to medications (MEDS) or other factors (OTHER), and perceived levels of fluency (FLU), consistency (CONS), confidence in speaking (CONF), satisfaction with speech (SATIS) and anxiety while speaking (ANX) during placebo phase.

SUBJ	$\triangle$ SYMP	MEDS	OTHER	FLU	CONS	CONF	SATIS	ANX
S8	0	0	50	50	53	48	51	51
S5	-24	0	-57	47	49	43	49	52
S7	-33	0	-83	46	42	46	47	48
S6	-14	-100	-100	57	55	58	59	55
S3	-100	-100	-100	20	82	21	25	26

S6, S7, S8) reported their perceived levels of fluency, consistency, confidence in speaking, satisfaction with speech and anxiety while speaking as average (around 50).

Table 2 summarizes the individual data for the pimozide phase.

From Table 2, four individuals (S3, S5, S6, S7) reported that a large percentage of their symptoms had improved under pimozide, and their change in percent fluency ranged from 13 to 46%, indicating improved fluency. One individual (S4) reported all his symptoms had gotten worse, and one (S8) reported no change in symptoms. The change in percent fluency for these two ranged from -9 to -17%, indicating their fluency was worse. Only individuals who reported that their symptoms had improved attributed this improvement to the medication. This may be related to the fact that individuals reported many side effects on pimozide, so they were probably aware that they were on medication. The 4 individuals who reported improvements in symptoms also reported greater than average (greater than 50) scores on their VAS scales in perceived levels of fluency, consistency, confidence in speaking, satisfaction with speech and anxiety while speaking. These scores were also greater than their respective ratings under placebo (Table 1). It was interesting to note that S7 reported both improvement in symptoms due to the medication and a worsening of symptoms due to other factors, and this appeared to be reflected in the relatively small change in perceived fluency level from placebo compared to the change in others. The changes in objective measures of fluency as measured by percent fluency positively correlated with the changes in subjective levels of fluency as measured by the VAS ($r=0.801$). Significant correlations were found between changes in subjective level of fluency, and subjective levels of confidence ($r=0.953$), satisfaction, ($p=0.953$) and anxiety ($r=0.958$).

By comparing Table 1 with Table 2, differences between the pimozide and placebo phases were apparent in measures. For example, the mean differences in VAS scores between these two phases were: 22.2 for level of fluency, 12.4 for consistency of fluency, 25.4 for confidence in speaking, 20.8 for satisfaction with speech, and 25.8 for anxiety while speaking. To determine if the differences between phases were significant, Paired t-tests were computed. Trends for significant differences between phases (overall experimentwise: $p=0.05$, Bonferoni correction: $p=0.05/7=0.007$) were found for: percent of symptoms

Table 2. Individual percent of change in symptoms (△ SYMP), percent of days they attributed changes in fluency to medications (MEDS) or other factors (OTHER), and perceived levels of fluency (FLU), consistency (CONS), confidence in speaking (CONF), satisfaction with speech (SATIS) and anxiety while speaking (ANX) during pimozide phase.

SUBJ	△ SYMP	MEDS	OTHER	FLU	CONS	CONF	SATIS	ANX
S3	100	100	0	80	80	76	79	77
S5	100	100	0	75	72	68	72	70
S7	56	100	-50	59	55	51	51	51
S6	89	100	100	66	72	70	73	70
S4	-100	0	-100	19	23	19	18	16
S8	0	0	0	51	64	58	60	58

reported changed (p=0.03), percent of days where fluency change was attributed to medication (p=0.03), consistency of fluency (p=0.04), confidence in speaking (p=0.07), satisfaction with speech (p=0.08), anxiety while speaking (p=0.09), and level of fluency (p=0.1).

Table 3 summarizes the individual data for the paroxetine phase.

In contrast to the pimozide phase, 3 of 4 individuals (S1, S2, S5) did not report a very high percentage of their symptoms improved on paroxetine. The changes in percent fluency between baseline and paroxetine ranged from 0 to 12%. Only 1 individual (S2) attributed a majority of any change in perceived fluency to paroxetine, and the change in percent fluency for this individual was 0%. Patients on paroxetine reported fewer side effects (e.g. sedation) than on pimozide, so it is possible that patients might not have been aware that they were taking active medication on this phase. The perceived levels of fluency, consistency, confidence in speaking, satisfaction with speech and anxiety while speaking were close to average (50) for S1 and S5. The small improvement in symptoms for S2, attributed to both medication and other factors, resulted in an increase in perceived levels compared to average (50) for the other factors. The worsening of symptoms reported by S3, which was attributed to other factors, resulted in a decrease in perceived levels compared to the average (50) for

Table 3. Individual percent of change in symptoms (△ SYMP), percent of days they attributed changes in fluency to medications (MEDS) or other factors (OTHER), and perceived levels of fluency (FLU), consistency (CONS), confidence in speaking (CONF), satisfaction with speech (SATIS) and anxiety while speaking (ANX) during paroxetine phase.

SUBJ	△ SYMP	MEDS	OTHER	FLU	CONS	CONF	SATIS	ANX
S1	6	0	0	49	69	63	51	58
S2	22	83	83	70	68	70	68	68
S3	-100	0	-100	30	79	24	26	26
S5	5	14	0	54	51	53	55	56

the other factors.

Only 2 individuals completed both paroxetine and placebo phases, so measures from these phases could not be meaningfully compared.

Another level of outcome measure was whether someone else commented to an individual that they had noticed a change in his/her fluency. During the last 7 days of the 4 individuals whose fluency improved on pimozide, someone else reported an improvement on 35% of those days. During the last 7 days of the 2 individuals whose fluency became worse on pimozide, someone else reported that they also saw a decrease in fluency on 12% of the days. During the last 7 days, no individual reported any days that someone else saw improvement, or felt fluency got worse on either the placebo or paroxetine phases.

DISCUSSION

The purpose of this study was to examine treatment outcomes following 6 week trials of two medications, pimozide and paroxetine. Outcome measures included subjective reports of changes in symptoms, changes in perceived fluency levels, confidence in speaking, satisfaction with speech and anxiety while speaking, correlations with objective measures of fluency, as well as observations by others of changes in fluency. Results suggested agreement between all outcome measures that there was a positive clinical response on pimozide compared to placebo for 4 individuals, and a negative clinical response for the other 2 individuals. The significant correlations between the perceived levels of fluency, confidence in speaking, satisfaction with speech and anxiety while speaking suggest that these concepts are integrated with one another, such that a change in one would likely be reflected in all of them. Results from the objective measures of fluency on the paroxetine phase suggested that there was no clinical response. However, at least 1 individual felt his fluency had improved on paroxetine, although we could not document this improvement with our objective measures.

It did appear that individuals' perceptions of their fluency level were affected by changes which they attributed to both medications or other factors. Attributing changes to medications may be related to whether individuals experienced side effects, which would confirm for them that they were taking a medication.

These results are clearly preliminary, and need to be repeated with a larger sample of individuals. The fact that measures of fluency from these daily self-rating scales were highly correlated with objective measures of fluency for pimozide, the medication that improved fluency, suggests that these self-rating scales are potentially useful as outcome measures. However, this self-rating scale needs to be validated in order to use it as an outcome measure of the effects of medications, as well as other behavioral treatments, and to further understand day-to-day changes in fluency.

In terms of the value of these medications as treatment for stuttering, the sample size was too small to be able to make a positive recommendation about pimozide. However, the side effects of pimozide were such that individuals who saw improvement in their fluency did not want to continue on the medication. It was also clear that the use of paroxetine should not be considered as a treatment of choice for stuttering, as there was no apparent clinical response, and there was the possible occurrence of rather severe side effects when withdrawing from this medication.

REFERENCES

Bloch, M., Stager, S., Braun, A., & Rubinow, D., (1995). Severe psychiatric symptoms associated with paroxetine withdrawal. *Lancet, 346(8966),* 57.

Brady, J.P., Price, T.R., McAllister, T.W., & Dietrich, K., (1989). A trial of verapamil in the treatment of stuttering in adults. *Biological Psychiatry, 25(5),* 630-633.

Costa, D., & Kroll, R., (1995). Treatment of stuttering with paroxetine: A case study. In C. W. Starkweather & H. Peters (Eds.). *Stuttering: Proceedings of the first world congress on fluency disorders.* International Fluency Association: Nijmegen University Press.

Maguire, G., Riley, G., Hahn, R., & Plon, L., (1994). Nimodipine in the treatment of stuttering. *ASHA Journal, 36,* 51.

Maguire, G., Riley, G.D., Wu, J.C., Franklin, D.L., & Potkin S. (this volume). PET scan evidence of parallel cerebral systems related to treatment effects: effects of risperidone in the treatment of stuttering. In W. Hulstijn, H.F.M. Peters, & P.H.H.M. Van Lieshout, (Eds.), *Speech production: motor control, brain research and fluency disorders.* Amsterdam: Elsevier Science.

Prins, D., Mandelkorn, T., & Cerf, F.A., (1980). Principal and differential effects of haloperidol and placebo treatments upon speech disfluencies in stutterers. *Journal of Speech and Hearing Research, 23,* 614-629.

Rothenberger, A., Johannsen, H.S., Schulze, H., Amorosa, H., & Rommel, D., (1994). Use of tiapride on stuttering in children and adolescents. *Perceptual and Motor Skills, 79(3 Part 1),* 1163-70.

Stager, S.V., Ludlow, C.L., Gordon, C.T., Cotelingam, M., & Rapoport, J., (1995). Fluency changes in persons who stutter following a double-blind trial of clomipramine and desipramine. *Journal of Speech and Hearing Research, 38,* 516-525.

Speech Production: Motor Control, Brain Research and Fluency Disorders
W. Hulstijn, H.F.M. Peters and P.H.H.M. Van Lieshout, editors

Chapter 32

PET SCAN EVIDENCE OF PARALLEL CEREBRAL SYSTEMS RELATED TO TREATMENT EFFECTS: EFFECTS OF RISPERIDONE IN THE TREATMENT OF STUTTERING

Gerald A. Maguire, Glyndon D. Riley, Joseph C. Wu, David L. Franklin, Steven Potkin

Several medications have been studied for the treatment of stuttering. Only haloperidol has been shown in replicated double-blind placebo controlled studies to be effective, however it is poorly tolerated and not widely prescribed. Recent PET scan evidence suggest that risperidone which works similarly to haloperidol by blocking dopamine-2 receptors may be effective in the treatment of stuttering. Four adult males who stutter participated in an open clinical trial of risperidone 1 mg daily for four weeks. Each subject's fluency improved on average of %54 by stuttering frequency and %60 by duration. We conclude that further research be conducted to evaluate this potentially promising agent for the treatment of stuttering.

INTRODUCTION

Stuttering is a speech disorder characterized by involuntary, frequent repetitions and prolongations of sounds and words. Several medications have been studied as adjunctive therapy for the treatment of stuttering, however, none has proven to be effective and well tolerated. Brady (1991) reviewed pharmacologic treatment studies and concluded that in placebo controlled, double blind studies only haloperidol was effective in reducing some symptoms of stuttering.

Possible insights may be gained from comparing stuttering to Tourette's disorder because the two share many similarities in that both begin in childhood, follow a waxing-waning course, have a 4:1 male to female ratio, are worsened by stimulant medications (Burd, Kerbeshian, 1991), have striatal hypometabolism secondary to dopamine 2 activity (Wolf, et al., 1996; Wu et al., in press) and both respond to treatment with dopamine-2 receptor antagonists such as haloperidol. However, unlike in Tourette's disorder, haloperidol is not widely prescribed for stuttering because of its poor tolerability and its risk of tardive dyskinesia. Therefore, we hypothesize that risperidone which antagonizes dopamine-2 without intolerable side-effects may prove to be beneficial in the treatment of stuttering.

In an open, clinical trial, we prescribed risperidone to four individuals who stutter (ages

17-63). Severity was varied with one being severe, one moderate, and two mild. All were started on a low dose of 0.5 mg orally at night. After one week, all were increased to 1 mg total given all at night. Higher doses, as used in schizophrenia, were not prescribed for fear of sedation. All subjects tolerated the 1 mg dose well. Stuttering severity was measured pre-treatment and 4 weeks post-treatment utilizing objective fluency ratings of the percentage of syllables stuttered in conversation and reading, and the duration in seconds of the three longest stuttering events. Stuttering frequency during conversation was reduced an average of 54% (range 41 - 63); duration was reduced an average of 60% (range 44 - 68) (See table 1.)

Table 1. Differences in Percent Stuttered Syllables (%SS) During Conversation and Reading and Differences in Duration of the three Longest Stuttering Events Following Treatment with Risperidone.

Sub.	Age	Sex	Hand-edness	Stuttering variables	Pre	Post	Differences Reduced	Percent
1	20	M	right	Percent syl st				
				Conversation	9.6	5.7	3.9	40.6%
				Reading	19.1	8.0	11.1	58.1%
				Duration 3 L	6.5	2.1	4.4	67.7%
2	17	M	right	Percent syl st				
				Conversation	11.8	5.1	6.7	56.8%
				Reading	10.1	1.8	8.3	82.3%
				Duration 3 L	2.0	.5	1.5	75.0%
3	63	M	right	Percent syl st				
				Conversation	7.2	3.3	3.9	54.2%
				Reading	0.0	0.0	na	na
				Duration 3 L	2.5	1.4	1.1	44.0%
4	34	F	right	Percent syl st				
				Conversation	4.3	1.6	2.7	62.8%
				Reading	10.2	6.5	3.7	36.3%
				Duration 3 L	1.1	.5	.6	54.5%
				Percent syl st				
Overall Means				Conversation	8.2	3.9	4.3	53.6%
(Standard deviations)					(3.2)	(1.9)	(1.7)	(9.4)
				Reading	13.1	5.4	7.7	58.9%
					(5.2)	(3.2)	(3.7)	(23.0)
				Duration 3 L	3.0	1.1	1.9	60.3%
					(2.4)	(.8)	(1.7)	(13.8)

All four subjects subjectively noted improved fluency and wished to continue taking risperidone after the initial one month trial. Based on these preliminary, open trial data, risperidone holds some promise as a pharmacologic agent to reduce stuttering severity. An double-blind, placebo-controlled study is ongoing to further investigate the effects of risperidone.

Medications such as risperidone that block dopamine-2 receptors presynaptic have the effect of increasing striatal metabolism (Buchsbaum et al., 1991). In our pilot PET study (Wu et al., 1995) we found striatal metabolism to be decreased in stuttering. We hypothesize the mechanism of risperidone to be its ability to antagonize dopamine-2 receptors in the striatum thereby increasing striatal metabolism.

My colleagues report a companion pilot study of three adult males who stutter and seven adult male controls who received FDOPA positron emission tomography scans (Wu et al., chapter 27). These scans show the distribution of pre-synaptic dopamine activity during a resting condition. Subjects who stuttered had 50 to 200% more pre-synaptic dopamine uptake than controls in cortical regions associated with speech and language and 50 to 100% more in the striatum. Risperidone may exert its possible beneficial effect by antagonizing elevated dopamine activity seen in stuttering.

Based on these open-trial data and supporting PET scan evidence, risperidone holds promise as a potentially useful pharmacologic agent for the treatment of stuttering and further research is warranted.

REFERENCES

Brady, J.P. (1991). The pharmacology of stuttering: A critical review. *American Journal of Psychiatry*, *148*, 1309-1316.

Buchsbaum, M.S., Potkin, S.G., Siegel, B.V. Jr, Lohr, J., Katz, M., Gottschalk, L.A., Gulasekaram, B., Marshall, J.F., Lottenberg, S., & Tang, C.Y., et al. Striatal metabolic rate and clinical response to neuroleptics in schizophrenia. (1992). *Archives of General Psychiatry*, *49(12)*, 966-74.

Burd, L., & Kerbeshian, J. (1991). Stuttering and stimulants. *Journal of Clinical Psychopharmacology*, *11*, 72.

Riley, G. (1994). *Stuttering Severity Instrument - Third Edition*, Austin, TX: ProEd.

Rosenberger, P.B., Wheelden, J.A., & Kalotkin, M. (1976). The effect of haloperidol on stuttering. *American Journal of Psychiatry*, *133*, 331-334.

Riley, G.D., Wu, J.C., & Maguire, G.A. (this volume). Pet scan evidence of parallel cerebral systems related to treatment effects. In W. Hulstijn, H.F.M. Peters, & P.H.H.M. Van Lieshout (Eds.), *Speech production: motor control, brain research and fluency disorders*. Amsterdam: Elsevier Science.

Swift, W.J., Swift, E.W., & Arellano, M. (1975). Haloperidol as a treatment for adult stuttering. *Comparative Psychiatry*, *16*, 61-67.

Wells, P.G. (1975). Haloperidol in the treatment of stuttering. *British Journal of Psychiatry*, *126*, 491-492.

Wolf, S.S., Jones, D.W., Knable, M.B., Gorey, J.G., Lee, K.S., Hyde, R.C., & Weinberger, D.R. (1996). Tourette syndrome: Prediction of phenotypic variation in monozygotic twins by caudate nucleus D2 receptor binding. *Science*, *273*, 1225-27.

Wu, J.C., Maguire, G., Riley, G., Fallon, J., LaCasse, L., Chin, S., Klein, E., Tang, C., Cadwell, S., & Lottenberg, S. (1995). A positron emission tomography [18F] deoxyglucose study of developmental stuttering. *NeuroReport, 6,* 501-505.

Wu, J.C., Maguire, G., Riley, G., Lee, A., Keator., Tang, C., Fallon, J., & Najafi, A. (in press). Increased Dopamine Activity Associated with Stuttering. *NeuroReport.*

Wu, J.C., Riley, G.D., Maguire, G.A., Najafi, A., & Tang, C. (this volume). Pet scan evidence of parallel cerebral systems related to treatment effects: fdg and fdopa PET scan findings. In W. Hulstijn, H.F.M. Peters, & P.H.H.M. Van Lieshout (Eds.), *Speech production: motor control, brain research and fluency disorders.* Amsterdam: Elsevier Science.

Methods and measurements in pathological speech

Speech Production: Motor Control, Brain Research and Fluency Disorders
W. Hulstijn, H.F.M. Peters and P.H.H.M. Van Lieshout, editors

Chapter 33

THE CONCEPT OF SUBPERCEPTUAL STUTTERING: ANALYSIS AND INVESTIGATION

Anne K. Cordes, Roger J. Ingham

The existence of covert or subperceptual stuttering, or stuttering that exists in the absence of perceived stuttering, has been proposed by several previous authors. The arguments used to support the existence of subperceptual stuttering, however, lead to the illogical conclusion that any repetitive or prolonging pattern in physiological data could be diagnostic of a fluency problem, even if the speaker does not experience a fluency problem and observers do not hear or see a fluency problem. A weaker definition of subperceptual stuttering may also be recognized: that some stuttering may be imperceptible to an observer and still be perceived by the speaker. Two studies described in this paper were designed, in part, to address hypotheses related to the identification of stuttering by speakers and by observers. Data from these studies do not support the existence of stuttering that can be consistently recognized by the speaker and consistently imperceptible to an observer.

INTRODUCTION

Many current perspectives on stuttering view this disorder in terms of internal physiological or neurophysiological processes, rather than in terms of overt speech behaviors. For some researchers, the underlying assumption appears to be that the speech of a person who stutters will incorporate physiological abnormalities not only during a behavioral moment of stuttering, but perhaps also in the speech surrounding a stutter (e.g., Howell & Wingfield, 1990), or even as a general characteristic whether the speech happens to sound fluent or disfluent at the moment or not (e.g., Smith, 1990; Smith et al., 1996, footnote 2). It is only a small step from this perspective to the claim that the fundamentally different speech-motor system of the person who stutters may be interpreted as including "covert" stuttering or "subperceptual" stuttering, terms used by several authors to describe stuttering that exists in the absence of perceived stuttering. This paper will review the concept of subperceptual stuttering and its supporting logic, and then will present some data from two relevant studies of perceptual judgments of stuttered and normally disfluent speech.

SUBPERCEPTUAL STUTTERING: REVIEW OF THE CONCEPT

The existence of covert or subperceptual stuttering has been proposed by several previous authors. Alfonso argued, for example, that some utterances can be "dysfluent" without being perceptually disfluent; "that is, while a segment of a stutterer's speech may be judged 'fluent' by a group of listeners, the acoustic, and/or movement, and/or electromyographic signals underlying the perceptual segment may appear inappropriate or 'dysfluent'" (Alfonso, 1990, p. 18). Similarly, Adams et al. (1984) described data obtained by Freeman in 1977 as showing "physiological blocks," even though these were "too brief in duration to trigger listener perception of stuttering" (Adams et al., 1984, p. 110). Armson and Kalinowski (1994) provided a similar example, explaining that the reiterative respiratory and laryngeal gestures observed in one example from a study by Story (1990) may be "easily recognized as subperceptual stuttering" because they "closely correspond to. . . repeated articulatory gestures during part-word repetitions" (Armson & Kalinowski, 1994, p. 72). Freeman and Ushijima (1978) and Shapiro (1980) also reported finding unusual laryngeal activity during fluent periods of stutterers' speech, as did Alfonso, Watson, and Baer (1984; see Alfonso, 1990).

In his commentary on the *second* international conference on speech motor control and stuttering, Folkins suggested that it might be better to "reserve the concept of disfluency. . for the level of behavioral output. . . . Movements and muscles are not disfluent, behaviors are" (Folkins, 1991, p. 564). We would like to underscore this point. More strongly phrased, it does not strike us as useful or meaningful to interpret a repetitive pattern in a respiratory or other physiological trace as necessarily signaling a subperceptual stuttered repetition, or to interpret an imperceptible pause as a block. This reasoning would suggest that if the repetitive head movements or eyeblinks that sometimes co-occur with overt stuttering happen to be produced in the absence of stuttering then they should be classified as subperceptual stutterings. In fact, a strong form of this argument suggests that any repetitive or prolonging pattern in physiological data could be diagnostic of a fluency problem, even if the speaker does not experience a fluency problem and observers do not hear or see a fluency problem.

It is possible, of course, to recognize a weaker version of subperceptual stuttering. The essence of this argument is that some stuttering may be imperceptible to an observer and still be perceived by the speaker. The descriptions offered by Alfonso (1990) and by Starkweather (1990), for example, allow the possibility that subperceptual stuttering could be perceived by the speaker. This notion also forms the core of Perkins' (1983, 1990; Perkins et al., 1991) argument that stuttering can only be identified by a speaker's self-judged sensation of "loss of control." Despite the theoretical arguments raised around Perkins's definitions, however (see, e.g., Ingham, 1990; Smith, 1990), it has yet to be established whether the behaviors that persons who stutter identify as stuttering while speaking is the same as those that they would identify while observing themselves speaking. If those events identified by the speaker during speech, or in real time, are the same as those identified by the speaker observing a recording, then arguments about the special status of the self-judgments of stuttering made while talking are not supported. And if events identified by the speaker as stuttered are the same as those identified by other observers, then arguments about the possibility of stuttering that is perceived by the speaker but subperceptual to an observer are also not supported.

SELF-JUDGMENTS AND OBSERVER JUDGMENTS OF STUTTERING

The first study to be discussed, therefore, was designed to address the question of whether speakers and other observers perceive the same speech to include stuttering. Subjects included a total of 15 persons who stuttered, who served as speakers and judges, and 10 well-established and internationally recognized academic and clinical authorities on stuttering (see Cordes & Ingham, 1995). The full study included four different judgment tasks in three experiments (Ingham & Cordes, in press), but this paper will concentrate on just a portion of the larger study.

One task was a Real-time self-judgment task that required adults who stuttered to record their own perceptions of when they were stuttering. Each speaker sat alone and spoke in spontaneous monologue, recording his stuttering by pressing a computer mouse button during and throughout the times that he felt he was stuttering. Speakers were instructed to record their own perceptions of their stuttering, not simply to press the button because they had a repetition or some other stereotypical disfluency. Speakers practiced this task beginning with trials of 30 sec and increasing to 5 min, with increases contingent on the speaker's report that during two consecutive trials his button presses had remained accurate reflections of his perceptions.

Two other tasks, the Continuous task and the Interval task, required speakers to watch audiovisual recordings of their own speech. While they watched, they judged whether they perceived stuttering in the recording. Five speakers watched tapes that had been recorded during the Real-time task, thus providing both Real-time judgments and off-line judgments for those speech samples. The other speakers watched tapes of their own spontaneous speech from a simple monologue condition that had not included simultaneous judgments of stuttering. All recordings showed head and shoulders only, and it was verified in pilot work that there were no visual or auditory cues on the tapes that could reveal when button presses had occurred during the Real-time task. The Continuous task presented the recording as one continuous 5-min recording, and the speakers made judgments of the duration of each stuttering, as described for the Real-time task. The Interval condition presented the recording as a series of 60 5-sec intervals, each followed by a 3-sec silent pause, and the speaker judged each interval to either contain or not contain stuttering. Both tasks were repeated at least four times for each speaker, and until a stability criterion was met that required not more than 5% variation in self-agreement across consecutive pairs of trials.

A fourth condition involved all 15 speakers making judgments of each other's speech, and another involved the authorities making judgments of all speakers. These conditions used a Multispeaker videotape that included 24 5-sec intervals from each of the 15 speakers (360 intervals). The Multispeaker task was similar to the Interval task, in that isolated 5-sec intervals were presented and were judged to include or not include perceived stuttering. Each judge completed the entire Multispeaker task on two occasions, several weeks apart.

In the context of subperceptual stuttering, one of the most relevant findings from this large study was that speakers and observers who met an intrajudge stability criterion of 90%

(i.e., whose self-agreement was high enough that their judgments could be considered trustworthy) judged many of the same 5-sec intervals of speech to contain stuttering. Final comparisons across the many tasks and conditions were made using only those speakers and judges who met the 90% self-agreement criterion in the four interval-recording tasks: the speaker's repeated self-judgments in the Interval condition, the speaker's self-judgments within the Multispeaker task, judgments made by other judges who stutter within the Multispeaker task, and judgments by authorities within the Multispeaker task.

Figure 1 shows that 7 of the 15 speakers met these criteria and were included in these analyses. Of all intervals from these speakers judged in these conditions, 65.4% were agreed across all conditions to be either Stuttered or Nonstuttered, including in judgments made by the speaker, by others who stuttered, and by the academic authorities. Two of these speakers had participated in the Real-time task, and the results are the same if their Real-time judgments are included: That is, for the speakers who had participated in these five conditions, it was precisely the same intervals that were judged the same way across those five conditions or across the four off-line conditions.

Further analyses then assessed the 34.6% of intervals that were not judged consistently across all conditions. These intervals can be broken down into four sets. Approximately 35% of them (20/58) were judged Stuttered by the speakers in Interval and Multispeaker conditions, and by the authorities, but were Disagreed by the other judges who stuttered. Another 18% (10/58) were judged Nonstuttered by the speakers in Interval and Multispeaker conditions, and by the other judges who stuttered, but were Disagreed by the authorities, and 12% (7/58) were assigned a judgment of Nonstuttered by the speaker in all self-judgments

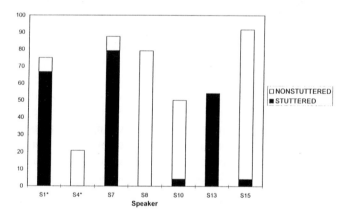

Figure 1. Percent of intervals judged the same way, stuttered or nonstuttered, in all four interval-recording tasks of a study comparing self-judgments and observer judgments of stuttering (see text). Speakers marked with an asterisk also participated in the Real-time judgment task; comparisons of the five conditions yielded the same results.

while both the other judges who stuttered and the authorities were disagreed.

The remaining intervals, another 35%, showed essentially no meaningful patterns across the conditions.

One of the most noteworthy results is that many of the intervals that drew disagreement from the authorities were consistently judged Nonstuttered by the speaker who had produced them. Zero intervals, including within the Other Patterns group, were consistently judged by the speaker to be stuttered and consistently judged by the two other judge groups to be nonstuttered. In fact, for the speakers who participated in the Real-time task and who met the intrajudge agreement criterion in their other tasks, there were no intervals that were judged stuttered by the speaker in the Real-time task and then agreed by the authorities to be Nonstuttered. In other words, there was no indication in these data that there were periods of speech that a speaker would consistently perceive as stuttering and that a listener would consistently be unable to identify as stuttered. These data showed many intervals that were judged the same way by the speaker and by other judges (Figure 1), and they showed no evidence of stuttering that was perceptible to the speaker but "subperceptual" to either other adults who stuttered or to academic and clinical authorities on stuttering.

PERCEPTUAL JUDGMENTS OF STUTTERING AND NORMAL DISFLUENCIES

A second study was designed to provide further perceptual information about the Disagreed intervals, the intervals that some authorities label stuttered and some label nonstuttered. This study involved perceptual judgment tasks with three kinds of stimulus intervals (see Table 1). The first were agreed Stuttered intervals from people who do stutter.

These intervals had been used in previous studies, including the study described above, and they were consistently categorized by the group of authorities as Stuttered (i.e., at least 80% of available judgments had been judgments of "stuttered"; see Cordes & Ingham, 1995, 1996). Second, there were Disagreed intervals, intervals that had been categorized as Disagreed because between 20% and 80% of judgments provided by the authorities had labeled them stuttered. The Disagreed intervals and the Stuttered intervals for this study were drawn in matched numbers from the same speakers, 4 each from each of 7 speakers. The third group of intervals used in this study was agreed normal disfluencies from normal speakers, or intervals of speech from a group of 7 speakers who do not stutter. These intervals were agreed to be disfluent, according to the same definition: At least 80% of judgments made by a group of 10 clinicians, on two occasions, in a pilot study of normal disfluencies, labeled these intervals as disfluent.

Eight stimulus videotapes were created by combining the three types of intervals in different ways. Four tapes combined the agreed Stuttered intervals, from persons who stutter, with the normally disfluent intervals, from persons who do not stutter. The other four combined the Disagreed intervals, from the same persons who stutter as were represented on the first tapes, with the same normally disfluent intervals that were on the first tapes.

Several groups of judges, in two universities, then completed two different judgment tasks.

Table 1. Percent of "stuttered" judgments from two occasions for Judgment of Interval task (Interval), and percent of "person who stutters" judgments from two occasions for Judgment of Speaker task (Speaker), for a total of 106 student clinician judges (see text). Preliminary results from 12 specialist clinicians judging the Disagreed intervals with the normally disfluent intervals are shown in parentheses.

TASK	INTERVALS FROM STUTTERERS	INTERVALS FROM NORMAL SPEAKERS
	AGREED STUTTERED INTERVALS	NORMAL DISFLUENCIES
Interval	76%	9%
Speaker	97%	24%
	DISAGREED INTERVALS	NORMAL DISFLUENCIES
Interval	33%	36%
Speaker	35%	22%
(Speaker)	(71%)	(29%)

The first task, Judgment of Interval, involved a total of 50 student clinicians as judges, 24 at one site and 26 at the other. This task presented each judge with one of the combinations of intervals, either agreed Stuttered intervals with normally disfluent intervals or Disagreed intervals with normally disfluent intervals. The intervals were in a random order for this task, and judges categorized each interval as containing stuttering or not containing stuttering. The second task, Judgment of Speaker, was completed by different student clinicians, a total of 56 in the two sites. The Judgment of Speaker task presented the tapes with the intervals grouped by speaker and required judges to determine, after seeing four 5-second intervals from the same speaker, if that person was perceived as a person who stutters or as a normal, or normally disfluent, speaker. In both tasks judges viewed the tape three times during each judgment session, once to familiarize themselves with the range of behaviors presented, once to be recording their judgments, and once to check, and potentially change, their responses. All judges repeated their task on a second occasion at least 2 weeks later, with their stimulus intervals in a different order.

Results from the first task, Judgment of Interval, are summarized in Table 1 by combining all judgments, from all student clinician judges on both occasions, and determining how many of those were judgments that the interval did contain stuttering. In the condition that combined normal disfluencies with the agreed Stuttered intervals, 76% of the judgments made for intervals that the authorities had previously agreed to be stuttered were stuttered judgments. At first glance, this result seems to represent an underidentification of stuttering, but two observations suggest that this may not be the case. First, the definition of "agreed" stuttered intervals used in these studies requires only that 80% of a group of judgments be stuttered judgments (see above). Second, inexperienced judges tend to identify less stuttering than experienced judges (see Cordes & Ingham, 1994). A finding of 76% stuttered judgments from a group of relatively inexperienced student clinicians, in other words, is actually quite consistent with earlier findings. In the other condition, judges saw the normal disfluencies with the Disagreed intervals. In 33% of the total judgment opportunities for the Disagreed intervals, judges categorized the interval as stuttered; in other words, intervals that had previously been labeled Disagreed because they received some judgments of stuttered and some of nonstuttered also received mixed judgments in this study.

The judgments of the normally disfluent intervals from the normal speakers were less predictable. In the context of the agreed Stuttered intervals, only 9% of the judgments made about the normal intervals were "stuttered" judgments. In the context of the Disagreed intervals, however, 36% of the judgments made about the *same* normal intervals were "stuttered" judgments. In other words, the judges who saw Stuttered intervals and normally disfluent intervals were generally able to distinguish between the two, and only 9% of the normal intervals were judged stuttered. The judges who saw the same normally disfluent intervals with the Disagreed intervals, however, do not appear to have been able to identify a clear perceptual boundary between the two: About one third of both sets were judged to contain stuttering.

Results from the Judgment of Speaker task are also shown in Table 1. Given all four of the agreed Stuttered intervals from a speaker who does stutter, the student judges decided on approximately 97% of opportunities that the speaker was a person who stutters. In the context of these agreed Stuttered intervals, but given the four normally disfluent intervals, 24% of judgments labeled a normal speaker as a person who stutters. The other combination, Disagreed intervals with the normal disfluencies, yielded 35% judgments of stutterer given four Disagreed intervals from a stutterer and 22% judgments of stutterer given four normal intervals from a normal speaker.

It appeared, overall, from both tasks, that the student clinicians made similar judgments for the Disagreed intervals and the normally disfluent intervals when these were presented on the same tape. Because of this negative result, the finding that judges could not distinguish between these two kinds of intervals, an ongoing investigation is replicating this study with specialist clinicians from several stuttering treatment centers who have extensive experience with stuttering and stutterers. At the time of this writing, 12 such specialist clinicians have completed judgments of the Disagreed intervals with the normal disfluencies on one occasion. Overall, their performance was only slightly better than the student clinicians' performance: The specialist clinicians made correct identifications that the person was one who stutters in only 71% of judgments of the Disagreed intervals, and they made false positive identifications of stutterer in almost 29% of their judgments of the normal disfluencies from normal speakers (Table 1).

CONCLUSIONS

In summary, it appears that normal disfluencies were labeled stuttered, and the people who produce them were labeled stutterers, in approximately the same proportion as the Disagreed intervals produced by stutterers were so labeled. It appears, in other words, that these Disagreed intervals may not be perceptually distinguishable from normal speech, or at least may not lead to functionally different judgments about the presence of stuttering or about the status of the speaker as one who stutters. The first study discussed above also showed that very few of the Disagreed intervals were judged consistently by the speaker who produced them to be stuttered. In fact, only two of the speakers who were represented in the second study had consistently judged any of their Disagreed intervals to be stuttered (Speaker GL from Figure 1, and one who did not meet the 90% intrajudge agreement criterion for the comparison of conditions and was not shown in Figure 1), and those two speakers were correctly and consistently identified as stutterers by both the student clinicians and the specialist clinicians. Once again, then, these investigations have uncovered no evidence of stuttering that can be consistently perceived by the speaker and consistently not perceived by an observer. One issue that these studies did not address directly is the clinical belief that some persons who stutter may complain of stuttering even when the resulting speech sounds nonstuttered to a listener, perhaps because they are using word-avoiding tactics or because they are using some other control over their speech. If this was the case in the current studies, then these behaviors were not entirely subperceptual: The observers were somehow also perceiving the speech to be stuttered.

The first section of this paper distinguished between a strong form and a weak form of the subperceptual stuttering argument. It is the weak form, the idea that stuttering might be perceived by the speaker but not by an observer, that the data presented have failed to support. The strong form of the definition, defining stuttering as an event that is only in a physiological trace, experienced neither by the speaker nor by the listener, is difficult to support even at a logical level; this idea ruptures the necessary link between a theoretic construct and the disorder it is supposed to describe. The theory that speech-motor physiology and overt behavioral stuttering are related simply because both include repeating and pausing, for example, does not connect the underlying physiological features with the speech behaviors. We are obviously working from the perspective that stuttering is a perceptible *speech* disorder that affects overt, observable, behavioral human communication. This perspective may not be the most common current perspective on stuttering; such a distinction arguably falls either to the neurophysiological perspectives or to a parent-child interaction model. No matter which theoretical perspective one chooses to adopt, however, it appears that an argument that stuttering can occur as a subperceptual phenomenon will be difficult to support either logically or empirically.

REFERENCES

Adams, M.R., Freeman, F.J., & Conture, E.G. (1984). Laryngeal dynamics of stutterers. In R.F. Curlee & W.H. Perkins (Eds.), *Nature and treatment of stuttering: New directions* (pp. 89-129). San Diego, CA: College-Hill.

Alfonso, P.J. (1990). Subject definition and selection criteria for stuttering research in adult subjects. *ASHA Reports, 18*, 15-24.

Alfonso, P.J., Watson, B.C., & Baer, T. (1984). Muscle, movement, and acoustic measurements of stutterers' larngeal reaction times. In M. Edwards (Ed.), *Proceedings of the 19th congress of the International Association of Logopedics and Phoniatrics, Vol. II*, (pp. 580-585). Perth, Scotland: Danscott Print Limited.

Armson, J., & Kalinowski, J. (1994). Interpreting results of the fluent speech paradigm in stuttering research: Difficulties in separating cause from effect. *Journal of Speech and Hearing Research, 37*, 69-82.

Bloodstein, O. (1995). *A handbook on stuttering.* (5th Ed.) San Diego: Singular Publishing Group.

Cooper, J.A. (1990). Research directions in stuttering: Consensus and conflict. *ASHA Reports, 18*, 98-100.

Cordes, A.K., & Ingham, R.J. (1994). The reliability of observational data: II. Issues in the identification and measurement of stuttering events. *Journal of Speech and Hearing Research, 37*, 279-294.

Cordes, A.K., & Ingham, R.J. (1995). Judgments of stuttered and nonstuttered intervals by recognized authorities in stuttering research. *Journal of Speech and Hearing Research, 38*, 33-41.

Cordes, A.K., & Ingham, R.J. (1996). Time-interval measurement of stuttering: Establishing and modifying judgment accuracy. *Journal of Speech and Hearing Research, 39*, 298-310.

Folkins, J.W. (1991). Stuttering from a speech motor control perspective. In H.F.M. Peters, W. Hulstijn, & C.W. Starkweather (Eds.), *Speech motor control and stuttering* (pp. 561-569). Amsterdam: Excerpta Medica.

Freeman, F., & Ushijima, T. (1978). Laryngeal muscle activity during stuttering. *Journal of Speech and Hearing Research, 21*, 358-362.

Howell, P., & Wingfield, T. (1990). Perceptual and acoustic evidence for reduced fluency in the vicinity of stuttering episodes. *Language and Speech, 33(1)*, 31-46.

Ingham, R.J. (1990). Commentary on Perkins (1990) and Moore and Perkins (1990): On the valid role of reliability in identifying "What is stuttering?" *Journal of Speech and Hearing Disorders, 55*, 394-397.

Ingham, R.J., & Cordes, A.K. (in press). Identifying the authoritative judgments of stuttering: Comparisons of self-judgments and observer judgments. *Journal of Speech and Hearing Research.*

Moore, W.H., Jr. (1990). Pathophysiology of stuttering: Cerebral activation differences in stutterers vs nonstutterers. *ASHA Reports, 18*, 72-80.

Perkins, W.H. (1983). Onset of stuttering: The case of the missing block. In D. Prins & R.J. Ingham (Eds.), *Treatment of stuttering in early childhood: Methods and issues* (pp. 1-20). San Diego: College-Hill Press.

Perkins, W.H. (1990). What is stuttering? *Journal of Speech and Hearing Disorders, 55*, 370-382.

Perkins, W.H., Kent, R.D., & Curlee, R.F. (1991). A theory of neuropsycholinguistic function in stuttering. *Journal of Speech and Hearing Research, 34*, 734-752.

Peters, H.F.M. (1990). Clinical application of speech measurement techniques in the assessment of stuttering. In J. Cooper (Ed.), *Assessment of speech and voice production: Research and clinical applications* (pp. 172-182). NIDCD conference proceedings. Bethesda, MD: U.S. Department of Health and Human Services.

Perkins, W.H. (1990). What is stuttering? *Journal of Speech and Hearing Disorders, 55*, 370-382.

Perkins, W.H., Kent, R.D., & Curlee, R.F. (1991). A theory of neuropsycholinguistic function in stuttering. *Journal of Speech and Hearing Research, 34*, 734-752.

Smith, A. (1990). Toward a comprehensive theory of stuttering: A commentary. *Journal of Speech and Hearing Disorders, 55*, 398-401.

Smith, A., Denny, M., Shaffer, L.A., Kelly, E.M., & Hirano, M. (1996). Activity of intrinsic laryngeal muscles in fluent and disfluent speech. *Journal of Speech and Hearing Research, 39*, 329-348.

Starkweather, C.W. (1990). The assessment of fluency. In J. Cooper (Ed.), *Assessment of speech and voice production: Research and clinical applications* (pp. 30-41) NIDCD conference proceedings. Bethesda, MD: U.S. Department of Health and Human Services.

Speech Production: Motor Control, Brain Research and Fluency Disorders
W. Hulstijn, H.F.M. Peters and P.H.H.M. Van Lieshout, editors

Chapter 34

AUTOMATIC STUTTERING FREQUENCY COUNTS

Peter Howell, Stevie Sackin, Kazan Glenn, James Au-Yeung

Stuttering frequency counts are time-consuming and difficult to make. Some preliminary results of our automatic stuttering frequency counts are reported here which would circumvent these difficulties. The approach has been to divide dysfluencies into two logically distinct categories (termed lexical and supralexical dysfluencies). Supralexical dysfluencies are removed by a parser. The software described locates word and part-word repetitions (as a single class) and prolongations. Training data are provided by a procedure which segments words and assigns them to a lexical dysfluency catgeory. The program also involves segmentation and classification stages. Assessment of the performance of the classification phase with word segments provided and the segmentation and classification phases automated are reported.

INTRODUCTION

Stuttered speech has episodes of dysfluency which are interspersed with stretches of fluent speech. A major source of information about stuttering is the frequency with which the episodes occur relative to the time the stutterer spends speaking (dysfluency counts). Wingate (1988) lists the types of dysfluent episodes that need to be counted as 1. interjections (extraneous sounds and words such as "uh" and "well"), 2. revisions (the change in content or grammatical structure of a phrase or pronunciation of a word as in "There was once a young dog, no, a young rat named Arthur"), 3. incomplete phrases (the content not completed), 4. phrase-, 5. word-, and 6. part-word-repetitions, 7. prolonged sounds (sounds judged to be unduly prolonged) and 8. broken words (words not completely pronounced).

The goal of the current programme of work is to assess the feasibility of an automated approach at locating stutterings in speech to provide dysfluency counts. The advantages of automation are (1) added objectivity and a standard benchmark for assessments and (2) assessments would be made quicker and easier. The system reported in this chapter works on a read text.

The dysfluency categories are divided into lexical and supralexical classes which will be dealt with in different ways by the system. Supralexical dysfluencies (SDs) include the first four types of dysfluency in the list. These have similarity with "repairs" which occur in fluent speech (Levelt, 1983). Levelt has shown how fluent speakers monitor their speech and, when they detect an error, what steps they take to repair the speech so that a listener can follow the speaker's intended meaning. So, in the revision illustrated above, a speaker needs to signal that he wanted to change "dog" for "rat". Levelt has investigated how the syntactic, semantic and prosodic aspects of speech are employed during repairs.

The work on the syntax of repairs has provided information which has been employed for automatic repair of fluent (Howell & Young, 1991) and stuttered speech (Howell et al., submitted). Repairs basically involve repeated, inserted and omitted words or sounds. Howell et al. (submitted) describe a system which compares a text stutterers were required to read with a transcription of the text the stutterer actually produces. The repairs are parsed in the manner Levelt describes and the repeated, inserted and omitted words located. The speech is then repaired (repeated and inserted words and phrases left out) to leave a version of the speech which is close to the original text insofar as it removes parts of repairs. This does well when compared to human judgments made about SDs in the passage. Besides providing an SD count, the repair step removes vestiges of SDs which means a text is left which only contains lexical dysfluencies (LDs).

Without this pre-parsing from the provided text, it is likely that all the words in the passage would need to be recognized in order to locate the SDs. It has to be admitted that this is a "fix" at present as it involves a human transcription. A possible way of by-passing the need for lexical recognition to locate SDs that will be explored in the future is to use prosodic changes which stutterers make in their vicinity (Howell & Young, 1991; Howell et al., 1990) since this would have the extra advantage that it could be applied to other than read text. Even if this was not possible, there is a lot of information that can be obtained about how stuttering is changing from repetitions and prolongations alone.

The main advantage removing Sds is that when dealing with LDs, generic rather than particular acoustic patterns can be spotted: In a repetition, alternation of energy and silence might be located rather than looking for a run of "k"s in a repetition such as in k..k..Katy. This means lexical or phonemic recognisers, which are currently not robust, are not necessary. Howell et al.'s (submitted) processing strategy for marking parts of SDs has been performed on the material employed below leaving material which contains only LDs. The focus in the remainder of this chapter is on the feasibility of using an artificial neural network (ANNs, Rumelhart & McClelland, 1986) for locating LDs in a read passage.

The types of LDs counted here differ from those given in Wingate (1988). Prolongations (pros) are defined as in Wingate (1988) but word and part-word repetitions are not differentiated but recognized as a single category (abbreviated "reps"). Second at present no attempt had been made to recognize "broken words". Wingate (1988) notes that this category is used to allocate all dysfluencies which do not fall within any of the other categories. This leads to these words being specified vaguely and the dysfluencies allotted to this category are more heterogeneous than those in the remaining categories.

ANNs are able to learn complex mappings between multiple inputs and desired outputs which need not be apparent to human observers. They learn from examples they are provided with. Here a set of acoustic parameters is extracted which will differentiate reps, pros and fluent words. Stuttered words can vary a lot in duration. Unfortunately, variation in duration is not easily dealt with by ANNs. It is usually solved by feeding information about the current behaviour of the network back into itself so the feedback can affect the ANN's subsequent behaviour (recurrence). The two main types of recurrent net differ with respect to whether feedback goes to the hidden units (Elman & Zipser, 1988) or back to the input (Jordan, 1986). Recurrence allows activity to be maintained so a long "ah" can be called the same category as a short "ah", it does not explicitly represent information about systematic differences between durations of different category outputs (e.g. fluent from stuttered word) to be employed.

Besides wanting to be able to provide duration information to help classify stuttered speech, a number of other parameters pertinent for classifying sounds as stuttered or not could be obtained if it was known where the words started and finished. These mainly depend on the fact that LDs occur almost exclusively at word, or syllable, onsets (Wingate, 1988). Our solution to enable us to use duration and word-position-dependent parameters is to segment the speech into words[1]. Each word is then processed for the desired parameters which are then input to the ANN classifier.

Evidence that the human perceptual system processes speech by first segmenting, then processing before classifying has been reported (Howell, 1978; Myers et al., 1975). Also, technical advances are providing improved segmentation procedures for use in speech recognition which promises well for future developments (Hunt, 1993; Kortekaas et al., 1996). Nevertheless, the idea about how segmentation could aid classification has not been explored in speech recognition previously. Undoubtedly it will be in the future since it offers a new solution for classifying events that vary in duration by allowing a fixed vector to be presented to an ANN irrespective of the length of the word. Also it permits use of temporal parameters that are lost in recurrent nets (here, for instance, word-positional information). Finally, it should be noted that including a principled segmentation of the speech makes this approach diametrically opposed to Ingham's time interval analysis procedure which takes fixed length intervals irrespective of what is occurring in the speech recording at that point in time. Consequently TI inputs alone preclude using word/syllable duration or a comparison of parameters in different parts of words.

Of course, this solution would be inappropriate if the difficulty has been shifted from one of categorizing to one of segmenting the speech. The main concern here is to demonstrate the viability of the approach. So, in the initial version, human labels are provided (which side steps this issue). Even so the input patterns have been developed to make them robust so they are not dependent on absolutely accurate detection of the start of a word. Results are reported with a crude (as it is applied here) segmentation algorithm based on dynamic time warping (DTW) algorithm (Deller et al., 1993).

TRAINING MATERIALS

The software described was developed on training material obtained from six stutterers readings of the "Arthur the rat" passage. Readings by a further six speakers were prepared in the same manner for test material and the results for all 12 speakers are given. Word boundary markers provided by two human judges were in close agreement whether the words were stuttered or not. Each word was heard and categorised as fluent (F) or containing an LD in the classes rep (R), pro (P) or broken word (O, for "other") by these same two judges. They also provided a rating on a five-point scale which indicated how smoothly flowing each word was. (A fuller description of the psychometric procedures applied to different materials is given in the chapter by Howell et al., chapter 49.) The confusion matrix for word categories by judge one against two is as follows:

| | | Judge 2 | | | |
		F	P	R	0
	F	3700	205	14	116
	P	8	82	2	3
Judge 1	R	2	13	181	20
	O	70	24	4	56

Agreement over all categories is 89.3%. However, it has to be noted that this figure is dominated by the high proportion of Fs which both judges agreed on. It is also of note that there is little confusion between dysfluency classes (1.46% of the words). Thus, the confusion matrix can be broken down to three separate ones (FxR, FxP and FxO) with the loss of very little () data:

	F	P			F	R			F	O
F	3700	205		F	3700	14		F	3700	116
P	8	82		R	2	181		O	70	56

These separate 2 x 2 confusion matrices show that there is little residual disagreement for Rs. For Ps and Os, there is somewhat more. It is difficult to pinpoint what the basis of the disagreement might be for the F x O matrix since the O category is so heterogeneous and no network is to be trained to recognize these. For the F x P matrix, it appears that the confusions are due to variability in judging whether a sound is prolonged sufficiently long to be called a pro. The overall durations for agreed F are 0.306 s, for agreed P 0.968 s, for F by judge 1 but P by judge 2 0.535 s, and for P by judge 1 but F by judge 2 0.672 s. In cases where there is disagreement, then, durations were intermediate between FF and PP. A further factor of note is that only 3/213 (1.4%) F x P confusions occurred for flow ratings of 4 and 5.

What lessons do these data teach us about selection of training data? First, notwithstanding the earlier comment about the high proportion of agreed Fs, overall agreement is good particularly for reps. Judges agreed about whether a word was repeated in virtually all cases (only 16 confusions in total between judges). If prolongations with flow ratings 4 and 5 are considered, once again there is very little confusion with F words. It is going to be necessary, then, to choose pros from these categories. The category responses and flow ratings given by judge 1 were employed and any words he had labelled as O were omitted from both training and testing. Even if only reps with flows of 4 and 5 are considered, there are still significantly more reps than pros. The same number of rep training examples with 4 and 5 flow ratings as for the pros was selected. The same number of fluent words with flow rating of 1 were also selected at random as training examples. This procedure cuts down on training exemplars particularly for fluent words. This is necessary otherwise the high number of fluent words would swamp the recognition process requiring lengthy training or producing poor recognition.

DESCRIPTION OF PARAMETERS TO REPRESENT REPS AND PROS

The general requirements for the input parameters to the ANN are that (1) generic reps and pro patterns are needed which (2) do not require the word boundaries to be located exactly and (3) they should be to some extent immune from noise since pathologists working in a clinic may not have quiet recording conditions available. The first step in obtaining the input parameters to the ANN was to define what characterizes reps and pros. Parameters are then obtained which provide an elemental pattern description of a rep or pro consistent with this definition.

Reps are usually longer than fluent words (*duration*). The repetitive sections have a pattern of alternating energy and silence referred to as *fragmentary pattern* which occurs specifically at the word onset (*position effect*, Wingate, 1988). Each rep emitted will tend to have a similar *spectral structure* to the extent that they are all representations of the first part of the same phonemic event. Each repeated spectral pattern may be dynamic (when, for instance, the repeated sound is consonantal with associated formant transitions) and if the repeated sections vary in duration the range of the transitional sections may vary. These are termed *transition and duration smearing effects*. The sections with similar spectral structure will alternate with periods of silence (if these are absolute silence, they will have no energy in any spectral region). Thus, in the repetitive portion, regions with similar spectral makeup (affected by transition and duration smearing) are separated by regions with different spectral properties.

Pros like reps tend to be long in comparison to fluent words and the prolonged section occurs at the start of the word. In ideal form, the prolonged section has a sustained spectral structure throughout the pro (the same sound is continued). Thus the sound is not fragmented by interposed silence and should show little, if any, transitional and durational smearing. However, amplitude modulations are observed (for instance of sustained low-energy fricatives like [f]s) which can lead to apparent fragmentation of the sustained spectral pattern. Thus, the fragmentation property may not be a clear cut factor for voiceless sounds. Voiced sounds particularly can modulate in amplitude and these modulations reflect attempted, but aborted, formant transitions to the subsequent sound in the word leading to transitional and duration smearing (if the various attempts vary in duration in the latter case). Thus, fragmentation, transition and duration smearing properties which at first sight appear to differentiate reps from pros, are not guaranteed to reveal the differences. It is probably fair to say that humans may not employ them in classifying sounds since we are not aware of any protocols for dealing with them.

The preceding definitions highlight the features to represent in ANN input. These concern three measurable aspects: Duration, fragmentation and spectral similarity. Each of these is described for the whole word and sub-divided for position in the word. The way the operationalized parameters were reasoned to work to separate rep, pro and fluent words is described. Though fragmentation and spectral comparison are logically distinct, it was found necessary to make the fragmentation measure robust to apparent break up into energy and silence in low energy fricatives by way of spectral comparison of these respective regions.

All measures were obtained either from oscillograms or from energy measured in the 19 frequency bands of Holmes' vocoder. The first measure taken on the whole word was its duration here obtained from the word position labels indicated by judge 1. Next, a measure of the fragmentation of the word was obtained. This was obtained from a procedure for calculating intensity peaks. A threshold was calculated for each frequency band based on a proportion of the maximum energy in that band. A second threshold was then applied which was based on the maximum number of bands above threshold for a time frame. Sections were located which were above (ATE) and below (BTE) this threshold energy. Higher order parameters representing the number of ATE sections, their average duration and sd were obtained (similar measures were obtained for BTE sections).

The preceding step provides separation into energy and supposed silence. This separation might be spurious if energy is low. One function of the spectral measures is to take care of this. The spectral measure also indicates the extent of stability in the spectrum. The measure of spectral stability has to be general rather than tied to specific frequency regions. The sections of ATE energy were taken and an averaged spectrum (averaged over each 20 ms frame) obtained. If these sections have the same spectral structure, this will be exaggerated by averaging. Looking across frequency bands, pro or rep sections will have a peaky structure, whereas if a word is fluent throughout, it will tend to have spectral movements which will make any spectral peaks diluted. Thus, when the word is fluent it will tend to have a flat spectrum whereas the spectrum will tend to be peaky in rep and pro cases. The sd of the energy values across frequency gives a measure of this peakiness - if there is little peakiness it will be low as all the values will be around the mean value, but large when there are noticeable peaks.

The BTE regions should be silent if the fragmentation measure has worked correctly. The same processing as applied to the ATE regions is applied to the BTE regions and should offer an indication whether these sections are truly silent. Finally, the difference between adjacent ATE and BTE sections were differentiated. If ATE and BTE regions have been correctly separated, (the BTEs are truly silent) the difference will be large. If there has been some inappropriate fragmentation, there will be little difference between the spectra. This information may or may not prove useful, all that is being presented is the logic behind why the parameters were included. It is up to network to learn to use this information if the parameters break down in the way supposed.

Employing the whole word does not allow information about where the stuttering is likely to be positioned in a word (i.e., at its start). Fragmentation and spectral stability are likely to be more prominent at the beginning of a word. To this end, the words were separated into first and second parts by cumulating the energy over the total word and taking the half energy point. The parameters of duration of the first and second parts and sd of energy in the first and second parts were obtained. Next, part-word fragmentation and spectral measures calculated as for whole word for first and second parts.

ANN ARCHITECTURE

The input parameters described previously were computed for each selected training word for the training set of speakers. All possible parameter combinations for the groups of parameters associated with 1. whole word duration, 2. whole word fragmentation measures, 3. whole word spectral measures, 4. part word durations, 5. part word energies, 6. first part fragmentation measures, 7. first part spectral measures, 8. second part fragmentation measures, 9. second part spectral measures, were tested (9! combinations). The networks attempted to associate the input parameters that have been described with one of the three category responses. Once the ANNs were trained the parameters were calculated for the test data and the ANNs assessed.

RESULTS WITH WORD BOUNDARIES SUPPLIED BY HUMAN LABELLERS

The majority of networks perform well. The one that performed best involved whole word fragmentation and spectral parameters and part word duration and energy. This separated out Ps and Rs and also did well with F words: It gets 95.07% of the F and 78.01% of the D words. Performance on Ps was 58.14% and on Rs 42.86%. The overall accuracy which reflects frequency imbalances between categories is a very respectable 92.0%. The principal limitation in this network is that it shows some confusion between Ps and Rs which was not seen in the human assessments. The reason for this is still unclear: The two most obvious possibilities are (1) that human observers are insensitive to variations that the ANNs pick up (e.g., amplitude fluctuations on pros that cause apparent fragmentation) and (2) that the input parameters to the ANNs need improving (principally the spectral similarity parameters).

RESULTS WITH COMPUTED WORD BOUNDARIES

Next word boundaries were computed, rather than being supplied by humans, using a

DTW algorithm. To do this, a fluent reading of the text was obtained from a non-stuttering boy who made no reading errors. This was used to create from the fluent speaker a version which was close to what each stutterer produced. The transcriptions employed earlier were used for this purpose which resulted in a list of pointers to the words the stutterer used and their order. The fluent version of what the stutterer said (the template speech) was aligned against the stutterer's version (the target speech) using DTW. DTW compresses and expands the target speech through time to produce an optimum fit with the template speech. The word-boundary positions are known for the template speech. Consequently after the target speech has been aligned with the template, the word boundary markers can be transferred to the corresponding point in the target speech. This results in a set of word boundary markers on the target speech.

DTW is not ideal for the current purposes: It requires a template for all the speech that is to be matched, it is usually used to match templates and target speech from the same speaker, it is most successful with short segments of speech and the alignment between the template and target speakers would not be as good for words spoken dysfluently as for those spoken fluently since both types of words are being matched against fluent templates. However, DTW has the advantage that it is relatively easy to implement and, therefore, is suitable for this point in development of the two-stage ANN recogniser where the feasibility of the approach is the principle concern. In the implementation the one-stage algorithm was used (Deller et al., 1993). The algorithm worked on 100 s-worth of the target speech at a time and these were abutted to create the alignments for the whole file.

Making comparison with the results when word boundaries were supplied is not straightforward: This is because the DTW words do not always align exactly with those supplied by human judges. When this happens, this raises the problem how to compare the categorisations given by the human judges with those given by the automatic ANN categorisation process. To give an approximate idea of how performance with DTW segmentation performs, the "correct" category response to any DTW word was taken as the category response given to the manually-located word whose onset was the nearest neighbour to the onset of the DTW word. Using this criterion, the ANN plus DTW segmenter located 89.18% of F words, 72.34% of D words. Performance on Ps and Rs was somewhat lower than that of D words (at 59.03% and 38.12% respectively) as occurred wirh the manually-supplied word markers. In subsequent work, the problem of comparing categorisation performance across non-aligned segments has been circumvented by employing automatically segmented syllables as the segments to be categorised. Human and ANN algorithms classify these same segments side-stepping this difficulty. An example file can be found on our web site which can either be replayed or down-loaded. Our web site address is http://www.speech.psychol.ucl.ac.uk/index.html.

ACKNOWLEDGEMENT

This research was supported by a grant from the Wellcome Trust.

NOTE

[1]   Most of the words in the passage used are monosyllabic so the procedure is de factor mainly being applied to syllables. It would require no modification other than provision of syllable rather than word indications, to implement a syllable-based ANN.

REFERENCES

Deller, J.R., Proakis, J.G., & Hansen, J.H.L. (1993). *Discrete-time processing of speech signals.* Englewood Cliffs: Macmillan.

Elman, J.L., & Zipser, D. (1988). Learning the hidden structure of speech. *Journal of the Acoustical Society of America, 83,* 1615-1626.

Howell, P. (1978). Syllabic and phonemic representations for short-term memory of speech stimuli. *Perception & Psychophysics, 24,* 496-500.

Howell, P., Kadi-Hanifi, K., & Young, K. (1990). Phrase repetitions in fluent and stuttering children. In H.F.M. Peters, W. Hulstijn, & C.W. Starkweather (Eds.), *Speech motor control and stuttering* (pp. 415-422). New York: Elsevier.

Howell, P. Kapoor, A., & Rustin, L. (this volume). The effects of formal and casual interview styles on stuttering incidence. In W. Hulstijn, H.F.M. Peters, & P.H.H.M. Van Lieshout (Eds.), *Speech production: motor control, brain research and fluency disorders.* Amsterdam: Elsevier Science.

Howell, P., & Young, K. (1991). The use of prosody in highlighting alterations in repairs from unrestricted speech. *Quarterly Journal of Experimental Psychology, 43A,* 733-758.

Howell, P., Au-Yeung, J., Sackin, S., & Glenn K. (submitted). Detection of supralexical dysfluencies in a text read by child stutterers.

Hunt, A. (1993). Recurrent neural networks for syllabification. *Speech Communication, 13,* 323-332.

Jordan, M.I. (1986). *Serial order: A Parallel Distributed Approach.* ICI Report 8604. Institute for Cognitive Science, University of California at San Diego.

Kortekaas, R.W.L., Hermes, D.J., & Meyer, G.F. (1996). Vowel-onset detection by vowel-strength measurement, cochlear-nucleus stimulation, and multilayer perceptrons. *Journal of the Acoustical Society of America, 99,* 1185-1198.

Levelt, W.J.M. (1983). Monitoring and self-repair in speech. *Cognition, 14,* 41-104.

Myers, T.F., Zhukova, L.A., Chistovich, I.A., & Mushnikov, V.N. (1975). Auditory analysis and the perception of speech. In G. Fant, & M.A.A. Tatham (Eds.), *Auditory analysis and the perception of speech* (pp.243-174). New York: Academic Press.

Rumelhart, F., & McClelland, J.L. (1986). *Parallel distributed processing: Explorations in the microstructure of cognition: Vol 1 Foundations.* MA: MIT Press.

Wingate, M.E. (1988). *The structure of stuttering: A psycholinguistic study.* New York: Springer-Verlag.

Speech Production: Motor Control, Brain Research and Fluency Disorders
W. Hulstijn, H.F.M. Peters and P.H.H.M. Van Lieshout, editors

Chapter 35

THE MEASUREMENT OF PHYSIOLOGIC AND ACOUSTIC CORRELATES OF VOICE ONSET ABRUPTNESS

Klaas Bakker, Roger Ingham, Ronald Netsell

Gentle voice onsets often are incorporated as part of stuttering treatments. However, there is little or no agreement today on what are the relevant physiologic and acoustic correlates of voice onset abruptness, let alone the most suitable methods for measurement and feedback in a clinical context.

Four subjects produced series of voice onsets that either increased, or decreased, in level of abruptness. Results indicated that intended, and subsequent listener perceived, levels of voice onset abruptness were strongly related features. In the physiologic domain, DC flow, and to some extent the accelerometric data, were related to intended abruptness. In the acoustic domain, only the peak-to-peak derived voice onset values revealed a consistent and moderate-to-strong relationship to intended level of abruptness. For the latter a moderate-to-strong relationship to perceptual abruptness also was evidenced.

Gentle voice onsets often are part of stuttering treatments that use modified phonation or prolonged speech related procedures. Some of popular fluency enhancement programs emphasize modified phonatory onsets as the primary means for establishing fluency in adult or adolescent persons who stutter (e. g., Webster, 1974). Nevertheless, there is little or no agreement today on what are the relevant physiologic and acoustic aspects of voice onset abruptness, let alone the most suitable methods of feedback, in a clinical context. Moreover, little is known about the relationship between these variables and perceptual judgments of voice onset abruptness.

A number of speech production parameters may be related to variations in perceived or experienced abruptness of phonatory onsets. Most workers operationally define voice onset abruptness in terms of rate of increase in acoustic energy (Koike, 1967; Webster et al., 1987; Peters et al., 1986; Bakker, 1994). Following one approach, the rate increase is calculated from peak amplitudes of glottal pulses (Koike, 1967; Webster et al., 1987). This obviously requires that peak values are identified and measured, which represents this method's chief limitation for widespread use in clinical applications. Such manual determinations of voice onset abruptness are labor intensive, and slow, and probably unacceptable for therapies that depend on frequent and immediate feedback on voice onset related performance. Computerized forms of this 'peak picking' strategy, although feasible when applied to isolated instances of phonation, run into exceptionally high computational demands when applied during running speech. Currently, there is no widely available system for the online measurement of voice onset abruptness that is dependent on peak values of the initial glottal pulses of phonation.

Voice onset abruptness may be determined from amplitude envelopes which outline, rather than fully describe, instances of phonation (e.g., Peters et al., 1986; Bakker, 1994). In order to accomplish this conversion, the individual bursts of acoustic energy associated with phonation are rectified, integrated and smoothed, thus producing a curve from which voice onsets may be easily identified and measured. Importantly, the conversion can be achieved through inexpensive electronic procedures which reduce the computational demands on computer hosts. Voice onset abruptness estimation from amplitude envelopes clearly makes real time voice onset evaluation a feasible option for clinicians, and perhaps has utility for applications that target running speech. There is one possible caveat, however. Amplitude envelopes, because of their data reducing nature, may introduce limitations of which the effects on voice onset evaluations are presently unknown. It may well be, then, that some of the necessary features for judging voice onset abruptness may be affected by the degree of integration and smoothing that is applied to the signal.

The procedures discussed so far were based on acoustic data. Because of this, the potential contributions of the transfer function to voice onset abruptness determination is presently undetermined and potentially a confounding source. That is, abruptness could depend, at least in part, on differences between vowels and types of consonantal valving that accompany instances of phonation. In order to obtain objective measures of voice onset abruptness, it may be necessary that such measures are from the laryngeal structure directly. This may be possible through the use of accelerometers, or contact microphones, positioned in close proximity to the larynx. The use of accelerometers for depicting voice onset abruptness, however, has not been empirically studied.

Electroglottography (EGG) also reveals glottal vibrations directly. Specifically, EGG reflects variations in area and duration of vocal fold contact throughout glottal cycles. As such, EGG has potential for revealing characteristics of the initial stages of phonation not available from the aforementioned measures. Though relatively insensitive to variations in intensity in general, EGG does reflect a gradual increase in vocal fold contact during the initial glottal cycles. It is unlikely that EGG signals are directly affected by the transfer function. Yet, little is known about the use of EGG for the clinical evaluation and feedback of voice onset abruptness.

Microphones, accelerometers and electroglottographs all produce signals that parallel the increments in vibratory energy characteristic of voice initiations. They do not necessarily reflect the volume or velocity of air that is expended during this behavior. Therefore, the measurement of air flow could present another ostensibly valid measure of voice onset abruptness. While ignoring the relatively quick variations in flow associated with individual glottal pulses (i.e., AC flow), measures of DC flow reflect the subject's overall usage of air in preparation for and during the execution of voice onsets.

At present there are no empirical data that compare the effectiveness of the aforementioned measures for identifying acoustic or physiologic correlates of perceived and intended voice onset abruptness. The clinical use value of these measures, then, is unknown and in need of investigation. The purpose of the present study was to systematically evaluate issues of validity of voice onset measures such as they may be derived from acoustic, electroglottographic, accelerometric, and air flow signals. Where available, comparison data will be provided for both peak, and amplitude envelope, dependent calculations of voice onset abruptness. Also, where possible this information will be analyzed with respect to both perceived and intended levels of voice onset abruptness.

METHOD

Subjects
      Four normal speakers, 2 males and 2 females, participated in this investigation. They varied in age from 23 to 58 years. Each subject was selected because of his or her experience with speech-language-pathology. The subject selection was restricted because of our prior experience that the experimental task is difficult for some naive subjects. None of those who participated had present or previous problems with speech or voice.

The Task
      Each subject produced 8 series of 10 consecutive voice onsets [^]. The first four series were recorded using physiological transducers and the remaining series were recorded acoustically. In each set of four, two series started at the subject's normal level of voice onset abruptness and became gradually more abrupt with each subsequent token. The remaining two series in each set also initiated at the subject's normal intensity level but gradually declined in abruptness. Each condition was modeled twice to the subject on audio tape, while up to ten practice trials were allowed for achieving productions that were judged satisfactory by one experimenter. The incremental abruptness task was used first in all cases because it was the easiest task for most subjects in a pilot investigation. The voice onset series were limited to ten at a time so that the respiratory capacities of the subjects would not be compromised, and to ensure that the voice onsets were produced from comparable respiratory conditions.

Data Collection and Analysis
      In the physiologic portion of this study, voice onsets were recorded using four different types of transduction. The acoustic signal was transduced with a head-mounted microphone (Sure, Model SM130; dynamic; omnidirectional) and used merely as a reference for identifying the physiologic tokens of interest. The microphone was positioned close to, but not touching upon, the lateral surface of a face mask. Laryngeal vibrations associated with the phonatory onsets were transduced through means of an acoustic piezzo resistive accelerometer (Penwalt, ACH10; linear in frequency response between 3Hz and 25kHz). It was positioned over the front of the neck slightly above the thyroid notch and kept in place

by a Velcro strap. The EGG signal was obtained with a Laryngograph (Kay Elemetrics). Its electrodes were positioned over the thyroid laminae and held in place by the same Velcro strap as used for the accelerometer. Finally, the DC flow signal was transduced with the face mask and pneumotachometer (Hans Rudolph). Its signal was amplified and filtered (DC to 50 Hz) to reflect the overall variations in flow associated with voice initiations. All signals were recorded with a Honeywell FM recorder (Model 5600E) for later processing employing an RC Electronics EGAA (version 3.2; digitization rate: 4KHz on all active channels).

The accelerometer and EGG signals were converted to intensity envelopes to make them comparable to the DC flow signal. After bandpass filtering (-24 dB/Octave; LP at 350Hz and HP at 80 Hz; Coulbourn Instruments, Model S75-34), the Accelerometer and EGG were led separately through a rectifier/integrator (Coulbourn Instruments, Model S76-01), to produce its respective contour-following envelope. The integration time was set at 20 ms in order to reduce the effect of the fundamental frequency of phonation.

Four additional sets of sequences of voice onsets were recorded during the acoustic portion of this investigation. Only acoustic and accelerometric signals were recorded and stored on tape using a TASCAM reel to reel recorder for later analysis with a CSL work station (Kay Elemetrics, Model 4300). A macro was developed for this purpose. It produced separate views (120 ms in duration) of a voice onset, based on the filtered acoustic and accelerometric signals (-24 dB/Octave; LP at 350Hz and HP at 80 Hz; Coulbourn Instruments, Model S75-34). Two additional views were available which presented the rectified/integrated forms of these onsets using specifications comparable to those employed in the physiologic part of this study. The peaks of initiating glottal pulses, that is those prior to 40, 50, or 60 ms following the acoustic onset of phonation, were separately recorded in order to determine the slopes of the best fitting linear regression lines for the peak values in the aforementioned time frames. The intensity envelopes used to determine the increments of the rectified/smoothed signal at 40, 50 and 60 ms following the voice onsets.

Finally, all acoustically recorded voice onset productions, which were digitized by the CSL workstation, were saved on disk in a randomized order in preparation for a perceptual abruptness evaluation by one of the experimenters (Judge 1). Abruptness ratings were expressed on a visual analog scale. Furthermore, twenty five percent of these onsets, again randomly selected, were used for independent determination of the respective levels of internal and external reliability. The limited selection of voice onsets were scored once more by Judge 1 for a determination of internal reliability, while these same tokens were analyzed by a second experimenter (Judge 2) for the determination of external reliability of the scaling procedure. *Table 1* demonstrates the coefficients of reliability which were obtained for the perceptual ratings of voice onset abruptness. As can be seen, both internal and external reliability were quite high ($r_{xy} > .91$). It is apparent that the perceptual rating procedure used in this experiment was not observer dependent.

Table 1. Coefficients of internal and external reliability for the perceptual abruptness ratings of voice onset tokens produced during the acoustic recordings (based on a random selection of 25% of the voice onsets across all subjects).

Internal reliability:	.911 *)	df=38
External reliability:	.920 *)	df=38

*) r statistically significant, at least at p<= .01.

Table 2. Correlations between the subjects' intended levels of voice onset abruptness and corresponding perceptual ratings by Judge 1.

Subject 1	.930 *)	df=38
Subject 2	.803 *)	df=38
Subject 3	.905 *)	df=38
Subject 4	.831 *)	df=38

*) r statistically significant at p< .01 level.

RESULTS

The relationship between the subjects' intended abruptness (i. e., the rank order in the voice onset series), and the corresponding perceptual ratings by Judge 1, are displayed in *Table 2*. Despite the possibility that the range of intended abruptness levels likely varied across the subjects, these correlations were quite strong and positive ($r_{xy} > .80$). It would appear that there was a good correspondence between the level of voice onset abruptness such as it was intended by the subjects and the way it was perceived by an independent listener. Moreover, the subjects were apparently successful in producing voice onsets which ranged systematically in abruptness.

One part of this study involved the potential usefulness of physiologic variables as indicators for voice onset abruptness. *Table 3* reveals how DC flow, EGG, and accelerometric signals were related to the subjects' intended abruptness. It is apparent that DC flow, and to a lesser extent the accelerometric measure, were positively related to intended abruptness. The correlations were not strong for all subjects, however. In contrast, the EGG signal was inconsistently related to the subjects' intention to produce voice onsets that systematically varied in abruptness.

The interrelationships between physiologic measures of voice onset abruptness are found in *Table 4*. From this table it is apparent that the DC flow and accelerometric measures are generally significantly and positively correlated. Nevertheless, the relationship between either DC flow or the accelerometric signal, and EGG was inconsistent across the subjects.

Table 3. Correlations between the physiologic abruptness characteristics of voice onsets (i. e. DC Flow, EGG and accelerometric) and the intended abruptness rankings, by subject.

| | Intended abruptness | | | |
	Sb1	Sb2	Sb3	Sb4
DC Flow:	.89 *)	.42 *)	.77 *)	.77 *)
EGG:	-.61 *)	.33 *)	.75 *)	.00 ns)
Accelerometer:	.85 *)	.70 *)	.55 *)	.26 ns)

*) r statistically significant, at least at $p < = .01$
ns) r not statistically significant

Table 4. Intercorrelations between DC Flow, accelerometric and EGG related signals, by subject.

DC Flow and accelerometric signals		
Subject 1:	.793 *)	df=38
Subject 2:	.598 *)	df=38
Subject 3:	.631 *)	df=36
Subject 4:	.537 *)	df=36
DC Flow and EGG related signals		
Subject 1:	-.477 *)	df=38
Subject 2:	.175 ns)	df=38
Subject 3:	.699 *)	df=36
Subject 4:	.268 ns)	df=36
Accelerometric and EGG related signals		
Subject 1:	-.475 *)	df=38
Subject 2:	.367 *)	df=38
Subject 3:	.798 *)	df=36
Subject 4:	.608 *)	df=36

*)   r statistically significant at least at .05
ns) r not statistically significant

Overall, then, it appears that DC Flow and a rectified/integrated accelerometric signal reflected the intended voice onset abruptness to a similar extent, while these signals were moderately interrelated as well.

An explanation for the inconsistency between EGG and the remaining two physiologic signals is not obvious. The current data do not permit one to conclude if such inconsistencies were due to (1) EGG as a recording technique, (2) individually different styles of voice onset production, or (3) qualitative differences between the individual voice onset tokens that varied in abruptness. Perhaps, some degree of breathiness, differentiated the individuals, while this qualities, in turn, could have varied with voice onset abruptness.

The final question in this study involved the potential relationships between either acoustic or accelerometric measures and intended, or listener judged, levels of voice onset abruptness. Interestingly, as can be seen in Table 5, both the intended and perceived abruptness measures demonstrated a tendency to be consistently and positively related to the abruptness measures that were derived from the individual peak amplitudes in the acoustic signal. Unfortunately, a similar relationship was not evident for the abruptness measures derived from the acoustic amplitude envelopes.

Table 5. Correlations between acoustic and accelerometric measures (peak and envelope rise values), and judged or intended levels of voice onset abruptness, by period (i. e., at 40, 50, and 60 ms following the onset).

Correlations with *judged level of voice onset abruptness*:

	Acoustic: Sb1 Sb2 Sb3 Sb4				Accelerometric: Sb1 Sb2 Sb3 Sb4			
Peaks								
at 40 ms	.71	.61	.79	.73	.34	.12	.72	-.58
at 50 ms	.76	.66	.80	.78	.28	.25	.78	-.63
at 60 ms	.79	.54	.80	.74	.35	.28	.81	-.70
Envelope rise values								
at 40 ms	-.07	-.01	.89	.53	.58	.36	.73	-.10
at 50 ms	.05	.04	.85	.53	.54	.40	.76	-.16
at 60 ms	.10	-.01	.84	.57	.50	.47	.69	-.20

Correlations with *intended level of voice onset abruptness*:

	Acoustic: Sb1 Sb2 Sb3 Sb4				Accelerometric: Sb1 Sb2 Sb3 Sb4			
Peaks								
at 40 ms	.72	.63	.74	.74	.30	.28	.64	-.47
at 50 ms	.78	.67	.76	.74	.23	.39	.70	-.56
at 60 ms	.81	.49	.76	.57	.30	.47	.73	-.59
Envelope rise values								
at 40 ms	.10	.15	.79	.40	.57	.52	.64	-.13
at 50 ms	.04	-.12	.77	.42	.55	.57	.66	-.19
at 60 ms	.14	-.16	.77	.48	.50	.57	.61	-.21

The pattern of relationships that evidenced for the accelerometric data differed from that of the acoustic data. That is, intended and perceived abruptness, here, were moderately related to the resulting amplitude envelopes for three of the subjects, while the peak dependent values failed to show a consistent relationship to either intended or perceived voice onset abruptness. It is apparent, then, that the acoustic and accelerometric signals of the recorded voice onsets differ and cannot be treated as similar ways for assessing voice onset abruptness. The relatively consistent relationship between the acoustic peak dependent abruptness measure and perception should not come as a surprise, however. After all, perception is based on this acoustic end product, rather than on activity at the laryngeal source itself.

DISCUSSION AND CONCLUSIONS

Although normal speakers apparently are successful in producing voice onsets that systematically vary in abruptness in the perceptual domain, the physio-acoustic reality of these behaviors as measured in the present study is neither consistent nor clear. Of course, it is possible that what is intended, and consequently perceived by the listener, as voice onset abruptness involves more than just a relatively sharp increase in acoustic, or physiologic, energy. Also, individuals may naturally differ in how they use their physiologic resources in order to bring about voice onsets that vary in abruptness.

At the very least, the present findings are suggestive for new research that is aimed at uncovering which aspects of gentle voice onsets are responsible for success in a number of currently popular approaches to the treatment of stuttering. Only with this information can we develop an optimal feedback signal to facilitate the desired therapeutic results.

REFERENCES

Bakker, K., (1994). Gentle voice onset feedback during running speech: its design and technical specifications. *Proceedings of the First World Congress of the International Fluency Association*, 396, Munich, Germany.

Koike, Y., (1967). Experimental studies on vocal attack. *Practica Otologica Kyoto*, 60, 663-688.

Koike, Y., Hirano, M, & von Leden, H., (1967). Vocal initiation: acoustic and aerodynamic investigations of normal subjects. *Folia Phoniatrica*, 19, 173-182.

Peters, H.F.M., Boves, L., & van Dielen, I.C.H., (1986). Perceptual Judgment of Abruptness of Voice Onset in Vowels as a Function of the Amplitude Envelope. *Journal of Speech and Hearing Disorders*, 51, 299-308.

Webster, R.L., Morgan, B.T., & Cannon, M.W., (1987). Voice Onset Abruptness in Stutterers Before and After Therapy. In H.F.M. Peters & W. Hulstijn (Eds.), *Speech Motor Dynamics in Stuttering*. Springer verlag, Wien, Austria.

Webster, R.L., (1974). *The Fluency Shaping Program: Speech reconstruction therapy for stutterers*. Roanoke, Virginia, Communications Development Corporation, Ltd.

Speech Production: Motor Control, Brain Research and Fluency Disorders
W. Hulstijn, H.F.M. Peters and P.H.H.M. Van Lieshout, editors

Chapter 36

ON-OFF VOICING ADJUSTMENTS IN STUTTERERS AND NORMAL SPEAKERS

George Wieneke, Peggy Janssen

It is suggested that stutterers tend to avoid on-off laryngeal adjustments. The present study was intended to test this hypothesis by counting the number of these transitions in stutterers and comparing these data to those of normal speakers. Voice transitions were counted across ten repetitions of a test sentence in three speech rate conditions. The variability in these numbers among the repetitions was also determined. The speech condition was varied by instructing the subjects to decrease or increase their speech rate with 20%. No significant differences were found between the stutterers and normal speakers, except for a higher variability of laryngeal transitions among the stuttering subjects. Similarities and differences with previous research and the implications for a demand model of stuttering are discussed.

INTRODUCTION

The precise coordination of the articulatory and laryngeal system is an important task in fluent speech that contributes to the complexity of the control of a speech movement. If motor complexity of speech movements plays a role in the interruption of fluency, stutterers may adapt their speech in order to simplify the speech motor control. Coordination can be simplified by reducing the number of speech subsystems included in a phoneme transition. The least complex situation is created when only one subsystem is moved. Reduction of the phonetically required speech movements in a phoneme transition will lead to an incorrect production of the phoneme. However, within the context of a sentence it is not necessary for intelligible speech to produce all phonetically defined features of the phonemes. For example, producing the voiceless consonant /s/ as a voiced speech sound /z/ will generally not lead to a misunderstanding of the meaning of a sentence. Stutterers may use the option of reducing the number of simultaneously moving speech subsystems in phoneme transitions in order to simplify speech motor control.

A link between the ability to quickly initiate or terminate phonation and stuttering was suggested by the studies of Adams and Reis (1971, 1974) and Runyan and Bonifant (1981). They found that stuttering was less severe when reading an all-voiced text than when reading a normal text. These and other investigations suggest that coordination of laryngeal and articulatory activation is difficult for many stutterers. Therefore, if stutterers use strategies to simplify coordination, one way to achieve this may be to decrease the number of times the phonation is turned on or off. Consequently, when stutterers read a text, a smaller number of voicing transitions is expected than when normal speakers read the same text. This effect will occur regardless of the rate at which the text is read. Moreover, it is expected that stutterers tend to use the smallest number of voicing transitions that is needed to maintain intelligibility. That is, stutterers will show relatively less variation in number of voicing transitions across repetitions of the same text than normal speakers. These expectations were investigated in this study.

METHOD

Subjects

Twenty six adult stutterers (22 males and 4 females) and 17 controls (13 males and 4 females) served as the subjects of this investigation. The control subjects were normal speakers who had never received speech therapy and were judged by the experimenters to be free of speech disorders. The mean age of the stutterers was 21.1 years (range 15 to 29 years) and that of the controls was 21.1 years (range 19 to 24 years). The stutterers were selected from those on a waiting list for therapy. None had received treatment for stuttering for at least two years prior to participation in the current project. According to the Riley Stuttering Severity Instrument (Riley, 1972), 12 of them were mild, 11 moderate and 3 severe.

Procedure

The subjects were required to emit ten fluent productions of the test sentence, "Zij studeert ook wijsbegeerte in Utrecht". This sentence contains 14 voicing transitions according to the phonetical rules. In the baseline condition subjects were instructed to read the sentence at their usual speech rate. In the two experimental conditions the subjects were instructed to modify their speech rate according to a model presented to them on audiotape. In one condition the speech rate of the model was 20% faster and in the other it was 20% slower than their own normal speech rate. The time from the start of the first period of glottal vibration to the end of the last period was used as a measure for speech rate. The vibrations of the subject's vocal folds were recorded by means of electroglottography (F-J Electronics EG 830) together with the speech signal. All recordings were carefully checked to determine if speech was fluent. More details about the experimental procedure can be found in Wieneke and Janssen (1991).

Analysis

In each subject voicing transitions (off-on and on-off) were counted across the ten repetitions of the test sentence, separately for normal, slow and fast speech rates. Differences in the number of voicing transitions between the normal and the fast or the slow speech rate condition were normalized by dividing the proportional change from the

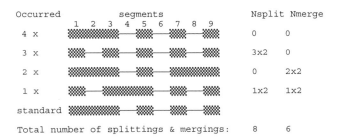

Figure 1. An example of segmental variability in ten repetitions of a sentence with 9 segments. ░░░░░ = voiced; ——— = unvoiced.

normal speech rate by the proportional change of the sentence duration.

In addition to the number of voicing transitions, also variation of these numbers within the ten repetitions was determined. In each repetition the voiced and voiceless segments were transcribed. When a segment was produced voiced or voiceless in the majority of the ten repetitions, this realization was considered to represent the standard for the subject. For each subject a standard voicing pattern was composed consisting of the sequence of these 'standard' segments. In a particular repetition, deviations from the standard voicing pattern could occur when three sequential segments merge to one or one segment split up into three segments (see figure 1). For each subject all cases of segment merging and segment splitting were counted. This number was used as a measure for the variability in the voicing pattern.

The number of voicing transitions and the log transformed segmental variability values were tested by an analysis of variance with groups as between subject factor and speech rate as within subject factor. Differences between groups in the ratio of the proportional change in number of voicing transitions and the proportional change in sentence duration were tested by means of a Mann-Whitney U-test.

RESULTS

Although the number of voicing transitions among the stutterers was somewhat lower than among the control speakers (table I), this difference was not significant $(F(1,41)=2.39; p=.13)$. On the other hand, significant differences were found for the effect of speech rate $(F(2,40)=46.8; p<.001)$. These differences are about the same in both groups with respect to the change from normal to a reduced speech rate. However, when speaking fast the stutterers reduced their number of voicing transitions to a greater degree than control speakers (table I). The last result may be influenced by the fact that the change in number of voicing transitions is slightly correlated with the actual change in sentence duration. Therefore, for each subject the ratio of the proportional changes in number of voicing transitions and sentence duration was computed. The median values are shown in table I.

Table I. The mean (Standard Deviation) of the number of voicing transitions in three speech rate conditions and differences between the conditions. Last two columns: the median (IQR) of the ratio of the proportional change in number of voicing transitions and sentence duration from the normal speech rate.

	Number of voicing transitions: mean (SD)				
				diff.from normal	
speech rate:	slow	normal	fast	to slow	to fast
stutterers	169 (25)	155 (33)	128 (29)	14 (27)	-27 (29)
control	175 (16)	159 (18)	147 (17)	15 (18)	-12 (20)
Ratio proportional differences from normal: median (IQR)					
speech rate:				to slow	to fast
stutterers				.53 (.99)	.62 (.93)
control				.43 (.71)	.31 (.55)

The values indicate that on the average the proportional change in voicing transitions is about half of the proportional change in sentence duration. Descriptively, the stutterers changed their number of voicing transitions more frequently than the control speakers, statistically there were no significant differences.

The variability in patterns of segmentation was defined as the number of voicing transitions that deviate from the subject's standard pattern across the ten repetitions. The number of voicing transitions increases (with 2) when a segment was split up into three segments and decreases (with 2) when three segments merges to one. The median values of the number of mergings and splittings are shown in figure 2. Although about 50% of the stutterers had values that fell within the range of the control speakers, on the average the stutterers show more variation in their segmental pattern than the control speakers (median values 14 and 10). Merging of three segments occurred more frequently than splitting one segment in three segments, particularly in the fast rate condition. An analysis of variance with logarithmically transformed values yielded a significant difference between the groups ($F(1,39)=11.79$, $p<0.001$) and between merging and splitting segments ($F(1,39)=14.56$, $p<0.001$). Other effects and the two-way interactions were not significant. The three-way interaction involving group, speech rate and type of variation was also significant ($F(2,38)=5.27$, $p<0.01$). This effect reflects the difference between stutterers and control speakers in strategies used when they were speaking at a slow rate.

DISCUSSION

Although the results indicate that stutterers tended to produce less voicing transitions than control speakers, the effect is clearly not significant. Therefore, it can be concluded, that the expectation put forward in the introduction was not confirmed. The coordination

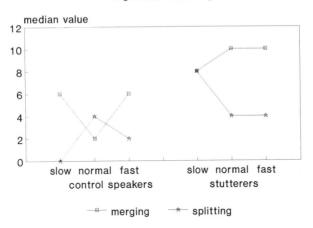

Figure 2. Median values of the segmental variation of control speakers (left) and stutterers (right) when speaking at a normal rate, slower rate and faster rate. Splittings = star, mergings = square.

of laryngeal adjustments and articulatory movements may still be a difficult task for the stutterer's motor system, but they do not seem to avoid it.

The most clear result of this study was the greater variability among stutterers in the pattern of segmentation. Increased variability in speech movements is a consistent finding for stutterers (Cooper & Allen, 1977; Janssen & Wieneke, 1987; Kalveram & Jäncke, 1989; DeNil & Brutten, 1991; Wieneke & Janssen, 1991; Jäncke, 1994.). The source of the instability within the speech production systems is still unclear. The neural mechanism responsible for the production of time intervals between events as well as the retrieval of features for the phomenes may play a role. There may be limits for the time interval between start of articulatory activation and activation of laryngeal adjustments. When the variability in the mechanism that produces time intervals for coordination is increased, the time intervals may sometimes exceed these limits. This may suppress laryngeal adjustments. However, we found no correlation between the subject's variability in segment duration and variability in segmentation. This suggest that there are two different mechanisms responsible for these experimental results. Alternative explanations based on the assumption that the theories of socalled neural networks are adequate to describe the retrieval of the features specifying the phonemes, may be less artificial. For example, errors in the retrieved patterns may occur more frequently when the connections are not yet stabilized due to an incomplete learning process. Since slowing down the rate of speech generally reduces the frequency of stuttering, the variability may be related to prolonged retrieval times due to an increased 'noise' level in the system.

REFERENCES

Adams, M.R., & Reis, R. (1971). The influence of the onset of phonation on the frequency of stuttering. *Journal of Speech and Hearing Research, 14*, 639-644.

Adams, M.R., & Reis, R. (1974). Influence of the onset of phonation on the frequency of stuttering: A replication and reevaluation. *Journal of Speech and Hearing Research, 17*, 752-754.

Cooper, M.H., & Allen, G.D. (1977). Timing control accuracy in normal speakers and stutterers. *Journal of Speech and Hearing Research, 20*, 55-71.

DeNil, L.F., & Brutten, G.J. (1991). Voice onset times of stuttering and nonstuttering children: The influence of externally and linguistically imposed time pressure. *Journal of Fluency Disorders, 16*, 143-158.

Jäncke, L. (1994). Variability and duration of voice onset time and phonation in stuttering and nonstuttering adults. *Journal of Fluency Disorders, 19*, 21-37.

Kalveram, K.T., & Jäncke, L. (1989). Vowel duration and voice onset time for stressed and nonstressed syllables in stutterers under delayed auditory feedback condition. *Folia Phoniatrica, 41*, 30-42.

Riley, A. (1972). A stuttering severity instrument for children and adults. *Journal of Speech and Hearing Disorders, 37*, 314-322.

Runyan,C.M., & Bonifant,D.C. (1981) A perceptual comparison: All-voiced versus typical reading passage read by children. *Journal of Fluency Disorders, 6*, 247-255.

Wieneke, G., & Janssen, P. (1991). Effect of speaking rate on speech timing variability. In H.F.M. Peters, W. Hulstijn, & C.W. Starkweather (Eds). *Speech Motor Control and Stuttering*. Amsterdam: Elsevier Science Publishers, pp. 325-331.

Speech Production: Motor Control, Brain Research and Fluency Disorders
W. Hulstijn, H.F.M. Peters and P.H.H.M. Van Lieshout, editors

Chapter 37

STUTTERING: WHERE AND WHYS OF TERMINATIONS OF ATTEMPTS DURING PART-WORD REPETITION

Nagalapura S. Viswanath, David B. Rosenfield

Part-word repetition (PWR) is a marker of stuttering. During a PWR, a stutter initiates, abruptly terminates and returns to the beginning of a word, one or more times, before producing the word fluently (resolution). Here, we report acoustic analyses of PWRs in adults and children to illuminate two issues: (1) *where* and *why* a stutterer terminates an attempt, (2) age differences with regard the Where-question. In adults and children, for words beginning with voiceless stops, terminations are likely to occur before voice onset (after release) producing fragments without vowel (Frg-V). For words beginning with voiced stops, terminations are likely to occur after voice onset producing fragments with vowel (Frg+V). In adults, subsegmental acoustic dynamics of Frg-V, Frg+SV (fragments with short vowel), Frg+LV(fragments with long vowel) - the latter two variants of Frg+V - differ uniquely when compared to resolution, thereby, suggesting different proximal causes for their terminations.

INTRODUCTION

The field of stuttering is replete with investigations and models of various kinds. There are innumerable studies on differences between stutterers and non-stutterers on kinematic, behavioral, perceptual and cognitive variables. Those studies that discover differences between stutterers and non-stutterers must ideally suggest a plausible link between the differences and certain *forms of fluency failures characteristic of stutterers (stuttering events)*. Similarly, general models must cogently explain how their central constructs link with the stuttering events. Achievement of this "linkage" presupposes at least one critical requirement - studies which examine stuttering events at multiple levels (perceptual, acoustic, articulatory and neuromuscular) of communication process. Such studies generate data and models important for constraining more general models of stuttering. The acoustic studies of part-word repetitions (PWR) followed by fluent production of the target word (resolution) in our laboratory were motivated by such considerations.

A comprehensive model of PWR and resolution must address several issues: (1) Why does a stutterer typically restart from the beginning of the word following an aborted attempt?, (2) Where does he terminate an attempt and is the point of termination of an attempt (PTA) shaped by the target word?, (3) What are the acoustic - articulatory dynamics immediately before terminations?, (4) Is there spectra-temporal pattern leading to resolution?, (5) Are there differences in articulatory and control processes in fast - and slow - resolving part-word repetitions?, (6) Is the factor that causes disruption endogenous or exogenous to the speech-language module, and, finally (7) why is the beginning of words primarily affected? We are developing answers to some of these questions. In this report we summarize and discuss the results of studies on PTAs in words beginning with English stops (/p/, /t/, /k/, /b/, /d/ and /g/) and acoustic dynamics immediately before terminations. To this end, we draw upon three strands of data from (1) Viswanath and Neel's (1995) study on adult stutterers, (2) Joullian's (1995) study on incipient stutterers, and (3) Viswanath and Joullian's study (1995) confirming hypotheses generated regarding PTA.

The conceptual framework for the studies is provided by several theoretical assumptions. These assumptions provide justification for the *initial within - subject, within - event* comparisons undertaken in the study. These assumptions have been thoroughly articulated elsewhere (Viswanath & Neel, 1995). Briefly, the core assumptions are: (1) the termination-restart cycles during PWRs are viewed as feedback mediated response to overcome the effects of disrupting influence to achieve the planned contextually adjusted acoustic shape of the word, (2) Resolution signals attainment of the planned acoustic shape of the word. Therefore, the measures of variables on resolutions is a reasonable estimate of what was planned.

METHOD

Six male adult stutterers (mean age = 45.5 yrs; range= 34-59) were recorded while answering a standard set of questions and reading passages in a sound treated room. Seven children (mean age 4.5 yrs., range= 3 to 10 yrs.) who were diagnosed to be stutterers with duration of problem less than one year (median= 8 mo., range=4 to 12 months) were similarly recorded. The children were recorded while they conversed and played with one of the investigators. PWRs and resolutions were carefully selected (adults: n= 142, Children: n= 46) for further analysis. Each instance of PWR and resolution and the adjacent words were digitized and analyzed in two stages on Computerized Speech Laboratory (model 4300). Two stages were:

(1) Identification of the basic fragment type defined by PTA

An aborted attempt was classified as fragment without vowel (Frg-V), if it was terminated following release and *before* voice onset; and classified as fragment with vowel (Frg+V), if it was terminated *after* voice onset. Further subtyping of Frg+V was undertaken. This subtyping was relativistic, i.e., it was based on the comparison of duration of each fragment vowel with fluent vowel in resolution. Thus, if a vowel was terminated before it attained fluent vowel duration it was classified as fragment with short vowel (Frg+SV). And, if a vowel was lengthened beyond the duration of fluent vowel before being terminated, it was classified as fragment with long vowel (Frg+LV). There are 169 Frg-Vs, 66 Frg+SVs and 33 Frg+LVs in the adult corpus and 52 Frg+Vs and 28 Frg-Vs in children corpus.

(2) Acoustic analysis of spectral and temporal variables immediately preceding points of termination

Gap durations and release burst spectral peak frequencies in Frg-Vs and resolutions were compared. Gap duration, release burst spectral peak frequencies and VOTs in Frg+V and resolutions were compared. In addition, multiple spectral slices were taken from fragment vowels and fluent vowels to extract F0, F1 and F2. Typically, three spectral slices (initial, medial and final) on Frg+SVs and two (Initial and medial) on Frg+LVs were made. The spectral slices on fluent vowel were taken at the same intervals as in the fragment vowel (Viswanath & Neel, 1995 for details). This part of analysis was confined to adult data.

RESULTS

The details of statistical analysis can be obtained from the original sources (Viswanath & Neel, 1995; Viswanath & Joullian, 1995; Joullian, 1995) A rejection probability of .05 or lower is reported as significant.

(1) Point of Termination

There are significantly more Frg+Vs than Frg-Vs when target words beginning with voiced stops are stuttered on ; the picture is reversed when target words begin with voiceless stops (Figure 1). Since voicing distinctions are made in terms of VOT (Lisker and Abramson, 1964), we correlated mean target VOT of each stop with percentage of Frg+V. There is high negative correlations between mean VOT and percentage of Frg+Vs (adults: $r = -0.97$; children : $r = -0.87$), which indicates that the relation between VOT and PTA is robust and is not affected by the age of the stutter (Figures 2 and 3).

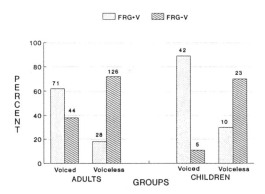

Figure 1. Percentage of Frg+V (fragments with vowel) and Frg-V (fragments without vowel) for stops categorized by voicing feature (voiced, voiceless) and the age groups (adults and children). Number of fragments in each category is shown on the bars.

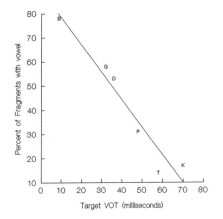

Figure 2. Plot of mean target VOT of the Stops (B, D, G, P, T and, K) and percent of Frg+V (fragments with vowel) in adults.

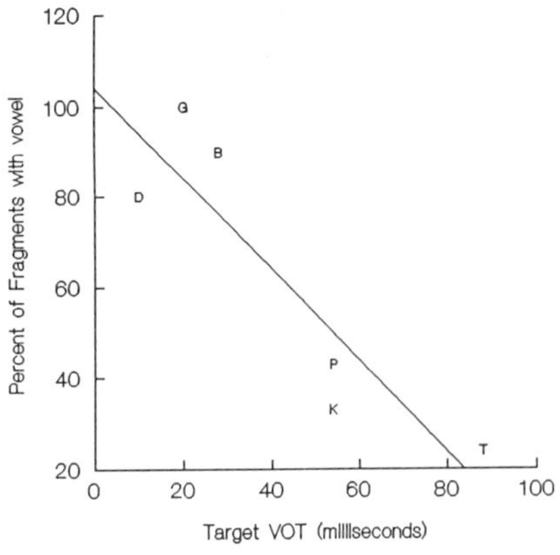

Figure 3. Plot of mean target VOT of Stops (B, D, G, P, T and K) and percent of Frg+V (fragments with vowel) in children.

The relation between VOT and PTA must hold if we evaluate data for each stop. The reasoning is as follows. A range of VOTs mediate a stop percept (Lisker & Abramson, 1964). As a consequence, a speaker has a range of values to "choose" from, albeit, constrained by factors such as rate and linguistic stress (Wayland et al., 1994; Viswanath & Rosenfield, 1991). Hence, if a stutterer repeats when these factors have constrained VOT to the lower end of the range, he is likely to terminate after the onset of voicing. In contrast, if he is constrained to upper end of the range, he is likely to terminate before voice onset. If this reasoning is correct we must find that, as a group, Frg+V must have lower mean target VOT than Frg-Vs for each stop. The adult data in Figure 4 bears out this prediction.

Similarly, the relation between target VOT and PTA must be sustained if we examine the data by place of articulation. VOT increases as place of articulation shifts from bilabial to alveloar to velar (Klatt, 1975). Therefore, we expected percentage of Frg+Vs to decrease as place of articulation shifts in the same direction. Fig 5 shows that VOT data are in accord with Klatt (1975) and the trend of percentage of Frg+Vs is as predicted.

(2) Acoustic Dynamics Before Termination

Fragments Without Vowel

Frg-Vs have significantly longer gap duration than resolutions (Speaking context: Fr -V mean = 185 msec., and Resolution mean = 135 msec.; Reading Context: Frg-V mean = 254 msec and Resolution mean = 162 msec.). The release burst spectral peak frequency did not differ in the fragments and resolutions. Thus, stutterers have longer than planned closure phase when they terminate an attempt before voice onset.

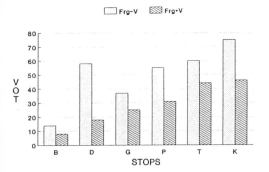

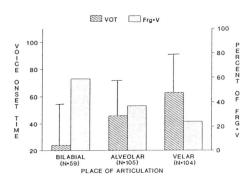

Figure 4. Mean target VOTs for Stops (B, D, G, P, T and K) grouped by Frg+V (fragments with vowel) and Frg-V (fragments without vowel) in adults.

Figure 5. The relation among percent of Frg+V (fragments with vowel), place of articulation and mean target VOT in adults.

This tendency is frequently present when target word begins with voiceless stops.

Fragments With Long Vowel

Frg+LVs are 30 msec longer than fluent vowel (Frg+LV mean = 98 msec. ; Resolution mean = 68 msec.). Duration of stop gap, VOT did not differ in Frg+LV and resolutions. Likewise, release burst peak frequency, F0, F1, F2 in fragment vowel and fluent vowel did not differ.

Fragments with Short Vowel

Fragment vowels collapsed across contexts are half as long as fluent vowels (Frg - V mean = 57 msec. ; Resolution mean = 105 msec.). Gap duration, release- burst peak frequency, VOT and F2 in fragments and resolutions do not significantly differ in both contexts. F1 is significantly lower at the selected points in fragment vowel than fluent vowel in both contexts (Figures 6 and 7).

F0 at the initial point is significantly lower in fragment vowel than fluent vowel in the speaking context (Figure 8).

DISCUSSION

Acoustic studies of PWRs have generally focused on the identity of fragment vowel while ignoring the other subsegmental phases in a stop+Vowel sequence (e.g., Howell & Williams, 1992). The studies summarized are unique in that they give a taxonomy of fragments based on points of termination and suggest a theoretically motivated comparison between fragments and resolutions to gain insight into proximal causes of terminations. Below, we will discuss the summarized results in general terms.

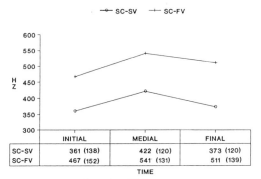

Figure 6. A graph of mean F1 at selected points for Short Vowels (SV) and Fluent Vowels (FV) in Speaking Context (SC). The table below graph shows means and standard deviations (in parentheses).

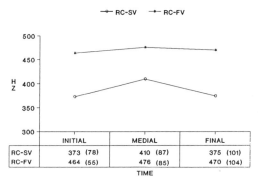

Figure 7. A graph of mean F1 at selected points for Short Vowels (SV) and Fluent Vowels (FV) in Reading Context (RC). The table below the graph shows means and standard deviations (in parentheses).

The details of some of the more involved arguments can be obtained from original articles (Viswanath & Neel, 1995; Joullian, 1995; Viswanath & Joullian, 1995).

With regard to the first issue, we have found that target VOT strongly constrains PTA. Three findings highlight this relationship : (a) relation between percentage of Frg+V and mean target VOT, (b) distribution of Frg+V and Frg-V within a stop range, and (3) relation between percentage of Frg+V and place of articulation.

Stuttering and associated behaviors change over time. However, there must be a core, an unvarying aspect of the disorder beneath the surface variations. Those who use standard definition of stuttering implicitly recognize that there is an unvarying core. The constraint of VOT on PTA irrespective age or duration of the problem is one such unvarying core beneath the surface variations. It is by isolating such unvarying aspects of the disorder, we accrue data fundamental to modelling PWRs and resolutions.

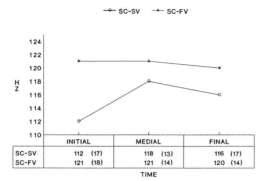

—◆— SC-SV   —✕— SC-FV

	INITIAL	MEDIAL	FINAL
SC-SV	112 (17)	118 (13)	116 (17)
SC-FV	121 (18)	121 (14)	120 (14)

TIME

Between status (initial) p = .001.

Figure 8. A graph of mean F0 at selected points for Short Vowels (SV) and Fluent Vowels (FV) in Speaking Context (SC). The table below the graph shows means and standard deviations (in parentheses).

As VOT shifts from long-lag end of the continuum towards "0" VOT (where release and voice onset are coincidental) there is a concurrent increase in percentage of Frg+Vs. If VOTs are on the other side of the continuum (prevoicing or lead VOT region) would this trend persist? When a voiced stop is produced with a lead VOT, voicing starts during closure, continues through release into the following vowel. Prevoicing depends upon maintenance of trans-glottal pressure difference which is rapidly enhanced when the stop is released. This is conducive for continuation of voicing and appearance of vowel. Hence, we hypothesize that when a stutterer repeats a word beginning with prevoiced stops he will produce Frg+Vs and thus conform with the trend established for lag end of the continuum. We are currently planning an investigation of this issue in Spanish stutterers. Unlike English, where, lead VOTs are not phonemically relevant and hence unpredictably used, Spanish uses lead VOTs phonemically and predictably. This fact ensures adequate samples of resolutions with prevoicing.

Linguistic stress and rate of production of words affect target VOT. Slowing down increases lag VOT; speeding up decreases it. Stress on the syllable with initial stop increases VOT and a shift of stress from initial syllable to a different syllable in the word decreases it. Thus, these factors indirectly constrain PTA through their effect on lag VOT. Do these factors have similar effect on lead VOTs? Are these factors (rate and stress) of any consequence when a stutterer terminates a prevoiced stop in view of the aerodynamic setting outlined in the previous paragraph?

The results of analysis of acoustic dynamics immediately before termination shows (1) Frg-V and Frg+SV differ from resolution in certain subsegmental phases, and (2) for most part there is no difference in samples from speaking and reading context

Frg-Vs have significantly longer gap phase than resolutions. These durational deviations are likely to be subperceptual. They signify inappropriate management of closure phase of stop+vowel sequence. As to why this phase deviates frequently for target words with voiceless stops is an interesting unanswered question. A clue for the frequency difference may lie in laryngeal and aerodynamic setting differences during gap phase for voiced and voiceless stops. Inappropriate management of closure phase seems to be the proximate cause for termination of Frg-V.

None of the spectral and temporal variables preceding the termination of Frg+LVs are significantly different from resolutions. In fact, the defining attribute of Frg+LV provided the only difference - fragment vowels, on an average, were longer than fluent vowel by 30 msec. Why an attempt which is unfolding as planned is terminated? The answer may lie in the realm of timing and anticipatory adjustments. The plan for production of a word includes specification of the duration of individual syllables (Keller, 1989). In implementing such a plan, a speaker makes appropriately timed articulatory adjustments to produce seamless sequence of component sounds. Articulatory adjustments may involve switching and/or combining of sources (laryngeal, upper articulatory) and anticipatory adjustment of filter (such as velar lowering). Hence, we hypothesize that stutterers terminate Frg+LV because of inept articulatory timing.

The results with Frg+SVs present a different picture. Short Vowels differed from fluent vowel spectra-temporally. We argued at great length (Viswanath & Neel, 1995) that the results with F1, F2 and F0, taken together, suggest a breakdown in synergistic organization of articulators (jaw, tongue and vocal folds) in achieving a common acoustic target, i.e., vowel. Hence, the proximate cause for termination of Frg+SV is this breakdown in articulatory synergy.

PWRs and resolutions drawn from speaking and reading context did not differ significantly. From a practical standpoint this is important information because samples for future studies can be drawn exclusively from more controllable reading context. However, since the sample size for this conclusion is not large (Viswanath & Neel, 1995) more data need to be collected from a larger sample of subjects before making a firm conclusion on this issue.

We summarized, discussed, raised questions and suggested fresh hypotheses regarding PWRs and resolutions with reference to the issues of where and why a stutterer terminates an aborted attempt. We are currently testing several of these hypotheses. The broad hypothetical conclusions stated in the paper may be revised in the light of new data, data grouped by subject, linguistic and production variables. The analysis of consecutive acoustic phases of stop+vowel sequence in terminated attempts and resolutions is time-intensive. Nevertheless, it is a important way of obtaining a dynamic picture of the most characteristic form of fluency failure in developmental stutterers.

Acknowledgments

This research is partly based on USPHS Grant RR-05425. We gratefully acknowledge the Benjamin-Jeremiah-Gideon-Abigail-Rebekah- Maida-Lowin Foundation and the M. R. Bauer Foundation for their generous support.

REFERENCES

Howell, P., & Williams, M. (1992). Acoustic analysis of perception of vowels in children's and teenager's stuttered speech. *Journal of the Acoustical Society of America, 84*, 80-89.

Joullian, A. (1995). An Acoustic Study of Young Stutterers' Part - Word Repetitions. Unpublished Master's thesis, University of Houston, Texas, USA.

Keller, E. (1989). Speech motor timing. In W.J. Hardcastle, & A. Marchal (Eds.), *Speech Production and Speech Modelling*, 403-439, Boston: Kluwer Academic.

Klatt, D. (1974). Voice Onset Time, Frication, and aspiration in Word - Initial Consonant Clusters. *Journal of Speech and Hearing Research, 18*, 686 - 706.

Lisker, L., & Abramson, A.S. (1964). A cross-language study of voicing in initial stops: Acoustical measurements. *Language and Speech, 10*, 1-28

Viswanath, N., & Neel, A. (1995). Part - Word Repetitions in persons who stutter: Fragment Types and Their Articulatory Processes. *Journal of Speech and Hearing Research, 38*, 740 -750.

Viswanath, N., & Joullian, A. (1995). Consequences of the relation between VOT and types of fragments in part-word repetitions. In C.W. Starkweather, & H.F.M. Peters (Eds.), *Stuttering: Proceedings of the First World Congress of Fluency Disorders*, Vol 1, University Press Nijmegen, The Netherlands.

Viswanath, N., & Rosenfield, D.B. (1991). Inter-gestural temporal co-ordination in stutterers. In H.F.M Peters, W. Hulstijn, & C.W. Starkweather (Eds.), *Speech Motor Control and Stuttering*, Pp 347 - 353, Elsevier Science Publishers, Amsterdam.

Wayland, Miller, & Voltis (1994). The influence of sentential rate on the internal structure of phonetic categories. *The Journal of the Acoustical Society of America, Vol 95, No. 5*, Pt.1, 2694-2701.

1997 Elsevier Science B.V.
Speech Production: Motor Control, Brain Research and Fluency Disorders
W. Hulstijn, H.F.M. Peters and P.H.H.M. Van Lieshout, editors

Chapter 38

THE ELECTROGLOTTOGRAPHIC SIGNAL AS A DEVICE FOR STUTTERING EVALUATION

Ulrich Natke, Karl Th. Kalveram and Lutz Jäncke

The electroglottographic (EGG) signal is related to temporal alterations of the vocal fold contact area. Combined with the acoustic speech signal it uncovers the working mechanisms of the phonatory apparatus. Today's computer equipment provides an easy to handle and low cost two-channel recording technique to pick up the EGG and acoustic speech signal in parallel. These records can be used to extract direct and derived parameters from both signals like voice onset time, open quotient, or degree of audio-phonatoric coupling. With regard to stuttering, this technique is useful as a training aid, with which ongoing speech production can be monitored. In addition, this equipment provides feedback of speech related parameters, for instance those indicating gentle onset, "pull-out", or vocal fry. These measurements are useful to evaluate progress during therapeutical interventions. We here give examples of speech- and EGG-recordings of stutterers and some hints concerning computerized analysis of these signals. It is concluded, that this noninvasive technique for investigation of laryngeal behavior is useful both for research and therapy.

INTRODUCTION

In the past many authors have related stuttering to laryngeal disturbances, either by measuring muscular activity in the larynx or by measuring vocal fold activity (Conture et al., 1977; Yoshioka & Löfqvist, 1981; Borden et al., 1985; Conture et al., 1986). These measures have been found to be atypical even during perceptual fluent utterances. However, until now it is unclear whether these laryngeal disturbances are the reason for stuttering or a consequence of it.

Nevertheless, during stuttering therapy, the modification of laryngeal activity is a main focus of intervention. For instance, voice initiation, voice shaping, gentle onset of voicing, vocal fry, blow up techniques, or Van Riper's pull-outs are typical examples for these interventions. Thus, it might be useful to monitor the EGG signal for examination of the phonatory apparatus during stuttering therapy. The measurement of vocal vibration by means of electroglottography is accomplished noninvasively by measuring changes in the electrical conductance of the larynx. For this purpose a pair of electrodes is attached above the thyroid cartilage. If the distance between the vocal folds decreases the electrical conductance between both electrodes increases. Applying proper equipment, there is a proportional relationship between the electrical conductance and the vocal fold contact area. Therefore, the EGG signal is a relative signal enabling absolute measures only in temporal direction.

EQUIPMENT AND DEFINITION OF EGG-WAVEFORM CHARACTERISTICS

We are using an electroglottograph (Laryngograph, Kay Electronics) together with a headset type microphone (Ramsa WM S10), which is mounted directly in front of the mouth. Both signals (EGG and speech) are supplied directly to the computer, which is equipped with a stereo soundcard (Soundblaster 16, Creative Labs). These signals are each allocated to a separate channel of the soundcard. This soundcard processes the signals without considerable attenuation of certain frequencies (Schwirzke & Hilgefort, 1995). The recording is controlled by standard software delivered with most of the soundcards (e.g. Creative WaveStudio, Creative Labs), which is also used for off-line processing. A sampling frequency of 20 kHz ensures a satisfying sound quality. For the EGG signal a frequency of 10 kHz is sufficient. The unfiltered EGG signal can show large baseline fluctuations caused by movements of the tongue, velum or extrinsic laryngeal musculature. These fluctuations usualy are removed with an analog 50 Hz high-pass filter. Dependent of the filter type the shape of the EGG signal can be distorted. This again can have great effects on the derived parameters. Rothenberg & Mashie (1988), therefore, recommend a linear phase filter, which equally delays all frequency portions of the signal. Another possibility is to determine the baseline for one period in a way that the areas above and below the baseline are equalized. If one likes to use the possibilities of digital filtering or to make observations at the unfiltered EGG signal (cf. below), the signal must be recorded unfiltered. With a sampling depth of 16 bit also small amplitudes of the EGG signal are sufficiently resolved. With the help of techniques such as ultrahighspeed cinematography the EGG waveform characteristics and their relationships to the vibratory modes of the vocal folds were confirmed (for an overview see Childers & Krishnamurty, 1984). These characteristics for period i can be operationally defined as seen in Table 1.

The *closing instant* is related to a sharp rise of the EGG signal indicating the abrupt closure caused by the Bernoulli effect. This can be detected by a sharp positive peak of the derivative dEGG/dt (Figure 1), which defines the instant of glottal closure $t_{c,i}$. As can be seen in Figure 1, the opening of the vocal folds by subglottal air pressure is a slower process. Therefore the instant of opening can not be detected as easily as the instant of closing. But the point of inflection of the decreasing EGG signal is close to the real instant of opening so it can be used for defining the *opening instant* $t_{o,i}$. It corresponds to a negative peak of the derivative.

With these instants *open phase*, *closed phase* and the related durations $T_{o,i}$ and $T_{c,i}$ can be defined. The *duration of glottal cycle* T_i can be defined as the interval between two successive closing instants. Therefore the *fundamental frequency* for period i can be calculated to $F_{0,i}=1/T_i$. The *open quotient* OQ_i is defined as the quotient between duration of open phase and

Table 1. Definition of EGG waveform characteristics for period *i*

closing instant	$t_{c,i}$	maximum of derivative $dEGG/dt$
opening instant	$t_{o,i}$	minimum of derivative $dEGG/dt$
duration of open phase	$T_{o,i}$	$= t_{c,i} - t_{o,i}$
duration of closed phase	$T_{c,i}$	$= t_{o,i+1} - t_{c,i}$
duration of glottal cycle	T_i	$= t_{c,i+1} - t_{c,i}$
fundamental frequency	$F_{0,i}$	$= 1/T_i$
open quotient	OQ_i	$= T_{o,i}/T_i$
contact closing to contact opening instant	$t_{co,i}$	maximum of *EGG*
contact index	CI_i	$= \left((t_{o,i+1} - t_{co,i}) - (t_{co,i} - t_{c,i}) \right) / T_{c,i}$

glottal period. A *closed quotient* can be defined analogous. The error which is combined with the opening instant is transmitted to the open quotient, which must be noticed. For definition of the *contact index*, the instant of contact closing to contact opening $t_{co,i}$ must be determined. It corresponds to the maximum of the EGG signal.

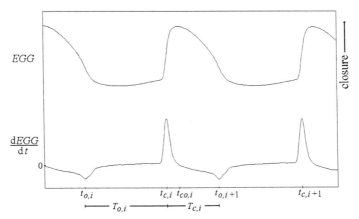

Figure 1. EGG-signal and via differential quotient approximated derivative $dEGG/dt$ over time t; i index of period, $t_{o,i}$ opening instant, $t_{c,i}$ closing instant, $t_{co,i}$ contact closing to contact opening instant, $T_{o,i}$ duration of open phase, $T_{c,i}$ duration of closed phase.

The contact index CI_i is now defined as the quotient between the durational difference of the contact closing and contact opening phases and the duration of the contact phase. An open index can be defined analogous. The meaning of these characteristics is explained below. The mean durations, mean frequency and mean open quotient are calculated by building the mean value for periods $i=1,...,n$.

Also the values can be plotted over time t to detect changes in the time course e.g. of the fundamental frequency $F_0=F_0$ (t) within a word.

USE IN RESEARCH

The *degree of stuttering severity* as measured in research as well as in well documented therapies can be determined e.g. with the 'stuttering-severity-instrument' of Riley (1972). With the equipment described above, the stuttering severity measurement can be completed by recording of EGG and the acoustic speech signal. The standard software allows selection of single passages for playing repeatedly and thus more exact investigation. During the assessment one can concentrate on secondary symptoms, e.g. head or limb movements.

The EGG signal can serve for detecting *'silent blocks'*, because unperceivable convulsions in the larynx are clearly observable in the EGG signal (Figure 2). During voiced periods sometimes unusual changes of the fundamental frequency can be discovered. The observation of this or other atypical laryngeal movements by applying the EGG signal enables the differentiation of fluent and unfluent utterances more exactly. This can have great influence on investigations which deal with fluent utterances of stuttering subjects (see last section of this chapter).

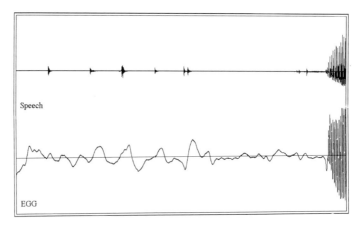

Figure 2. Recording of speech and unfiltered EGG signal during a 'silent block'. The irregular course of the EGG signal emphasizes unperceivable convulsion in the larynx.

The two channel recording technique enables an easy classification of *voice / unvoiced / silence*-periods. In addition, this classification can be accomplished automatically in real time. In order to do so, the EGG signal must first be high-pass filtered (analog or digital) and a threshold alignment to the subject is necessary. Applying this procedure an automatic *speech rate* estimation is possible.

For a first approximation voiced periods are taken as indicators of syllables. If further evaluation reveales that the speech rate measured with this procedure deviates from real speech rate a correction factor can be determined and included in the estimation. In order to investigate the coordination of phonation and articulation parameters such as *duration of phonation* or *voice onset time* (VOT) can be calculated with the help of the classification stated above. For single words the VOT can be measured directly with standard software by measuring the time from the beginning of articulation to the beginning of vocal fold vibrations. This measurement can easily be accomplished using a computer mouse with which the relevant events are marked resulting in an automatic time intervall measurement. For extensive investigation an automatic analysis can easily be implemented, for which the sound file is used as the data base. For example MATLAB (The Mathworks, Inc.), a common programming tool for matrix computations, can be used to read the sound file and process the data. These computer controlled analyses enables a very precise determination of the durations. Furthermore bigger data amounts can be processed almost automatically.

The *open quotient* (see above) derived from the EGG signal reflects the relation between subglottal air pressure and the vocal fold tone and in this way gives information about phonatory hypo- or hyperfunction. The open quotient depends on speech pitch and loudness, which must be considered in interindividual comparisons. In addition, vocal fold abduction and adduction measures can be derived from this open quotient (Rothenberg & Mahshie, 1988).

The *contact index* (see above) serves for measuring symmetry of the closed phase. It can take values between -1 and 1. A value of -1 indicates a vanishing contact closing phase, 0 indicates a symmetric closed phase and 1 a vanishing contact opening phase. The contact index is assumed to reflect vocal fold tonus and to be sensitive to mucosal dynamics within the vertical plane (Orlikoff, 1991).

In experiments with prematured and delayed auditory feedback with very short, unperceivable time displacements a reflex-like mechanism between the auditory feedback of the beginning of phonation and the duration of phonation was discovered. This mechanism was called audio-phonatoric coupling (APC). In non-stuttering people this coupling is found only in stressed syllables. In stuttering people the coupling seems to be stronger and it also works in unstressed syllables. Furthermore this depends on the stuttering severity (Kalveram & Jäncke, 89; Kalveram, 1991; Jäncke, 1991). With modified auditory feedback and measuring the duration of phonation the *degree of audio-phonatoric coupling* can be determined.

In many investigations the phonation is determined from the speech signal with the help of filter techniques. With the aid of the EGG signal the phonation is directly available resulting in a more precise measurement of phonatory events. Further applications of the EGG signal are proposed in spectral analysis, speech synthesis, and speech recognition (cf. Childers & Larar, 1984).

USE IN THERAPY

In this section we present some examples in which the EGG combined with the acoustic speech signal can be used in stuttering therapy for monitoring and visualization of the practiced behavior. The EGG signal clearly shows the *shape of onset of phonation*. Gentle onset of voicing is a main object in fluency shaping therapies. Figure 3 depicts a typical gentle onset of phonation while uttering the vowel /a/ in a stutterer, who has successfully passed a fluency shaping therapy. Additionally, an EGG signal is shown generated by a stutterer without such a therapy experience. It shows an abrupt rise of the EGG signal typically found for stutterers without gentle onset experience and for non-stuttering subjects. However, Peters & Boves (1988) observed abrupt onsets of voicing more often in stuttering people than in non-stuttering people suggesting a possible key disturbance for the initiation of phonation in stuttering subjects.

For measuring the gentle onset of voicing the EGG signal is more suitable than the acoustic speech signal. The latter often rises gradually, although the vibration of the vocal folds does not. On the other hand, smooth contacts during speech production can be controlled indirectly by controlling gradual rises of the speech signal. Computer programs can supervise the rise and decline of the phonation and other characteristics of speech such as loudness, velocity, or pauses. In order to monitor these events the signal must be rectified and low-pass filtered to get its envelope.

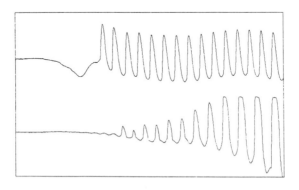

Figure 3. Unfiltered EGG signal while uttering the vocal /a/. Top: stutterer, who has not passed a fluency shaping therapy, bottom: stutterer, who has successfully passed a fluency shaping therapy

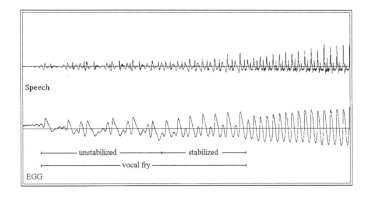

Figure 4. Speech and unfiltered EGG signal while uttering the vocal fry before /a/.

Real time programs can theoretically record over an unlimited time, which is an advantage over off-line working programs. Thus, everyday situations as conversation on the phone can be monitored and fed back by the computer which is important for daily training and adaptation of therapeutic techniques to everyday situations. The program can supervise gradual changes in the gentle onset from its extreme to a naturally sounding gentle onset. Thus, it can serve as a measuring device for therapy progress.

As in all feedback-therapies the client must be tought to achieve control over body functions independent of the computer feedback. Regarding gentle onset this can be done by 'sensing' the activity of the larynx. Therefore, the visual feedback must be switched off in the end phase of therapy. The analysis of the 'blind' spoken material is performed afterwards.

Often *continuous phonation* is applied in stuttering therapies. According to the remarks about classification a program for automatic supervising is easy to implement.

Even in so called stuttering modification therapies the use of EGG feedback can be useful. In these therapies the subject has to learn how to influence the speech production during or when anticipating a stuttering event. Van Riper's *pull-outs* (Van Riper, 1973) consist of slowing down the speech production in such a moment, thus automatically producing a kind of gentle onset. These onsets do not reach the degree of gentle onsets in fluency shaping therapies, but supervising it by EGG feedback can be useful, too.

The *vocal fry* can be an aid for stuttering people to break down a fixation of the vocal folds or to prevent such a fixation (Van Riper, 1973). The vocal fry can be visualized with the EGG signal. Figure 4 shows this kind of voice initiation before uttering the vocal /a/. Here the vocal fry is first indicated by irregular vibrations followed by a stable phase, in which periods with small and large amplitudes alternate. Such double vibratory patterns are typical for the vocal fry (Moorc, 1958).

FINAL REMARKS

The described technique to record the acoustic speech and EGG signal in parallel with a standard computer is an easy to use and low cost method with many applications in research as well as in therapy. Therefore, it is suitable as a standard method for evaluating the speech of stuttering subjects. The application in research and in therapy goes hand in hand. On one side the functioning of the phonatory apparatus combined with the articulators can be investigated. On the other side the procedure is helpful for direct use in stuttering therapy and seems to be superior to isolated feedback of the speech signal.[2] In addition, changes, e.g. in speech rate, degree of gentle onset, or degree of audio-phonatoric coupling can be measured during therapy in order to measure therapy progress as well as to uncover underlying processes. We suppose the core problem to lie in the inversion of the tool transformations necessary to coordinate phonation and articulation during speech acquisition, especially those enabling the realization of linguistic stress (cf. Kalveram & Natke, chapter 6). The described technique enables the investigation of these processes.

There are many investigations of "fluent" utterances of stuttering subjects. The different opinion or uncertainty what is meant by "fluent" can have considerable influence on the results (cf. Armson & Kalinowski, 1994). Conture et al. (1986) pointed out, that beneath perceptual criteria also physiological criteria have to be used in declaring an utterance as fluent. The EGG signal can be a useful aid for developing such criteria. But the problem arises whether the effects distinguishing "fluent" speech of stuttering from that of non-stuttering subjects can disappear because of this precise classification. This represents the entire problem of such investigations.

NOTES

[1]   This study was supported by the Deutsche Forschungsgemeinschaft (DFG).
[2]   No assessments of single therapy techniques were made, because obviously there is not only one therapy for all stutterers until now. Individual stutterers can profit very much from individual techniques, so the object seems to be to find out the right one.

REFERENCES

Armson, J., & Kalinowski, J. (1994). Interpreting results of the fluent speech paradigm in stuttering research: difficulties in separating cause from effect. *Journal of Speech and Hearing Research, 37,* 69-82.

Borden, G.J., Baer, T., & Kenney, M.K. (1985). Onset of voicing in stuttered and fluent utterances. *Journal of Speech and Hearing Research, 28,* 363-372.

Childers, D.G., & Krishnamurty, A.K. (1984). A critical review of electroglottography. *CRC Critical Reviews in Biomedical Engineering, 12,* 131-161.

Childers, D.G., & Larar, J.N. (1984). Electroglottography for laryngeal function assessment and speech analysis. *IEEE Transactions on Biomedical Engineering, 12,* 807-817.

Conture, E.G., McCall, G.N., & Brewer, D.W. (1977). Laryngeal behavior during stuttering. *Journal of Speech and Hearing Research, 20,* 661-668.

Conture, E.G., Rothenberg, M., & Molitor, R.D. (1986) Electroglottographic observations of young stutterers' fluency. *Journal of Speech and Hearing Research, 29,* 384-393.

Jäncke, L. (1991). The audio-phonatoric coupling in stuttering and non-stuttering adults: Experimental contributions. In H.F. Peters, W. Hulstijn, & C.W. Starkweather (Eds.), *Speech motor control and stuttering* (pp. 171-180). North Holland: Elsevier.

Kalveram, K.Th. (1991). How pathological audio-phonatoric coupling induces stuttering: A model of speech flow control. In H.F. Peters, W. Hulstijn, & C.W. Starkweather (Eds.), *Speech motor control and stuttering* (pp. 163-170). North Holland: Elsevier.

Kalveram, K.Th., & Jäncke, L. (1989). Vowel duration and voice onset time for stressed and nonstressed syllables in stutterers under delayed auditory feedback condition. *Folia Phoniatrica, 41,* 30-42.

Kalveram, K.Th., & Natke, U. (this volume) Stuttering and misguided learning of articulation, or why it is extremely difficult to estimate the physical parameters of limbs. In W. Hulstijn, H.F.M. Peters & P.H.H.M. Van Lieshout (Eds.), *Speech production: motor control, brain research and fluency disorders.* Amsterdam: Elsevier Science.

Moore, P., & Leden, H.v. (1958). Dynamic variation of the vibratory pattern in normal larynx. *Folia Phoniatrica, 10,* 205-238.

Orlikoff, R.F. (1991). Assessment of the dynamics of vocal fold contact from the electroglottogram: data from normal male subjects. *Journal of Speech and Hearing Research, 34,* 1066-1072.

Peters, H.F., & Boves, L (1988). Coordination of aerodynamic and phonatory processes in fluent speech utterances of stutterers. *Journal of Speech and Hearing Research, 31,* 352-361.

Riley, G.D. (1972). A stuttering severity instrument for children and adults. *Journal of Speech and Hearing Disorders, 37,* 314-322.

Rothenberg, M., & Mahshie, J.J. (1988). Monitoring vocal fold abduction through vocal fold contact area. *Journal of Speech and Hearing Research, 31,* 338-351.

Schwirzke, K., & Hilgefort, U. (1995). Klangwerk, 24 aktuelle PC-Soundkarten im Test. *c't 2,* 118-144.

Yoshioka, H., & Löfquist, A. (1981). Laryngeal involvement in stuttering. A glottographic observation using a reaction time paradigm. *Folia Phoniatrica, 33,* 348-357.

Van Riper, C. (1973). The Treatment of Stuttering. Englewood Cliffs, NJ: Prentice-Hall.

1997 Elsevier Science B.V.
Speech Production: Motor Control, Brain Research and Fluency Disorders
W. Hulstijn, H.F.M. Peters and P.H.H.M. Van Lieshout, editors

Chapter 39

SIMULTANEOUS ANALYSIS OF LIP, JAW AND TONGUE MOVEMENTS WITH AN INTEGRATED OPTICAL TRACKING AND EPG SYSTEM.

Emanuela Magno Caldognetto, Claudio Zmarich, Francesca Bettini, Giancarlo Ferrigno

The new system for the simultaneous recording and analysis of the lips, jaw and tongue movements consists of two integrated parts. ELITE makes it possible to analyse movement and velocity of speech articulators such as lips and jaw, as well as phonetically and phonologically relevant parameters, such as labial opening, width, and protrusion. The spatio-temporal evolution of the linguopalatal contacts is analyzed with a RION DP-20 electropalatograph (EPG), using flexible acrylic palates supporting 63 receptive electrodes. The two systems have been integrated via hardware and software and now the obtainable data permit to study the temporal and spatial features of the speech and nonspeech oral movements. The authors exemplify the method through the analysis of the alveolar voiceless plosive /t/ in the italian word /tata/ produced by one stutterer and one nonstutterer.

INTRODUCTION

A new system for simultaneous recording and analysis of lip, jaw and tongue movements has been developed by the authors. Lips and jaw articulatory movements are recorded with ELITE, a fully automatic, real-time movement analyzer for 3D kinematic data acquisition, while tongue-pseudopalate contacts are recorded with the electropalatograph RION DP-20 (Figure 1). The first component of the system, ELITE, ensures a high degree of accuracy and minimum discomfort to the subject. In fact, only small, non-obtrusive, passive markers of 2 mm in diameter, made of reflective paper, are attached onto the subjects' face. Subjects are placed at 1.5 metres in front of two CCD TV cameras which capture the lighting of the markers due to an infrared stroboscope. ELITE is characterized by a two-level architecture. The first level includes an interface to the environment and a fast processor for shape recognition (FPSR), which receives the output signal from the TV cameras at a frame rate of 100 Hz. The coordinates of the recognized markers are sent to the second level which consists of a general purpose PC. This level provides for 3D coordinate reconstruction, starting from 2D perspective projections. Simultaneously with the articulatory signals, ELITE also records the coproduced acoustic signal.

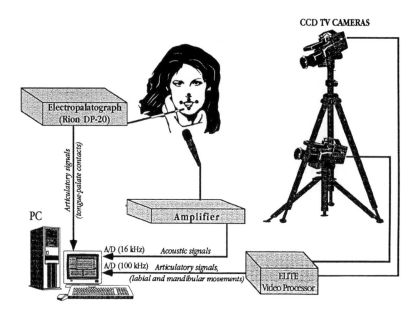

Figure 1. A schematic representation of the recording assembly with the ELITE and EPG integrated system.

The markers for phonetic research are placed on the central points of the vermilion border of the upper and lower lips, at the corners of the lips and at the center of the chin. Other markers, placed on the tip of the nose and on the lobes of the ears, serve as reference points to eliminate the effects of head movements. Thanks to a software reference model of the speech articulators implemented by the authors, these markers are recognized and subsequently processed for producing 3D articulatory trajectories. However, ELITE makes it easy to change the reference model in order to adapt the analysis to a new object. For each articulator, it is also possible to analyze the movement and velocity, as well as to calculate phonetically and phonologically relevant parameters, such as labial opening, width, and protrusion (Ferrigno & Pedotti, 1985; Magno Caldognetto et al., 1995; Zmarich et al., 1995). The spatio-temporal evolution of the linguopalatal contacts is analysed with a RION DP-20 electropalatograph (EPG), using flexible acrylic pseudopalates supporting 63 receptive electrodes (Figure 2). The linguopalatal contacts are sampled at 64 Hz. The pseudopalates are of six different sizes and can be easily fixed to the palatal arch of almost every subject. On our system, the EPG was integrated with ELITE, so that all the signals are simultaneously recorded on the same PC, where they can all be analyzed.

Through selection of appropriate options in the software developed by the authors, it is possible to analyze linguopalatal contacts, including the place of articulation (e.g. alveolar zone, palatal zone, external arch, etc.) and articulatory modes (e.g. presence of oral cavity occlusion, constriction, lateral aperture, etc.). While standard options are provided (see the five regions in Figure 3 below, following [4]), it is possible to define any new region

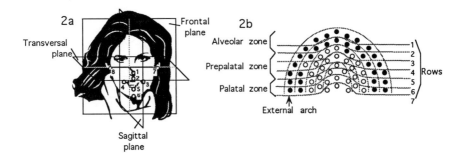

Figure 2. Placing of markers and disposition of the three virtual reference planes in ELITE (a), and the schematic representation of the RION pseudopalate (b). The filled circles represent the activated electrodes for the maximal occlusion relative to the second /t/ of /tata/. See text for explanation.

according to preference.

The spatio-temporal trajectories for some of the articulatory parameters recordable by this integrated system are shown in Figure 3, which refers to a normal production of the utterance "(dic)o 'tata chiaramente" (/ɗiko 'tata kjaraĥente/ = "say 'tata clearly"):

- *horizontal intercorner lip distance* corresponding to the distance between the markers placed at the corners of the lips and correlated with the *rounded / unrounded* feature;
- *anterior-posterior* movement of the *upper lip* and *lower lip*, calculated as the distance between the markers placed on the central points of either the upper or lower lip and the plane passing through the markers located on the lobes of the ears. This parameter correlates with the *protruded / retracted* feature;
- *horizontal movement* of the *left corner* and *right corner* of the lips, calculated as the distance between the marker on either the left or right corner and the sagittal plane;
- *vertical movement* of the *upper lip* and *lower lip*, calculated as the distance between the markers placed on the central point of either the upper lip or lower lip and the transversal plane passing through the tip of the nose and the markers on the ear lobes;
- *vertical jaw movement* , i.e. the distance between the markers situated at the centre of the chin and the transversal plane, primarily due to the jaw movement but also influenced by the movement of the skin on the chin. This parameter is correlated with the *high/low* feature;
- *interlabial vertical distance,* calculated as the distance between the markers placed on the central points of the upper and lower lips, and correlated with the feature *high/low;*
- *total linguopalatal contacts*, the percentage of activated electrodes on the total number;
- *external arch*, the percentage of activated electrodes on the border of the pseudopalate;
- *alveolar zone*, the percentage of activated electrodes on rows 1 & 2;
- *prepalatal zone*, the percentage of activated electrodes on rows 3, 4 & 5;
- *palatal zone*, the percentage of activated electrodes on rows 6 & 7.

The following example will provide a clear explanation of how the integrated

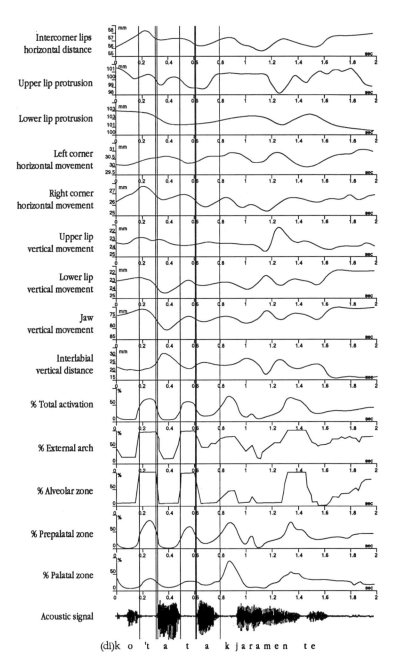

Figure 3. Schematic representation of the whole set of movement curves and acoustic signal for /(di)ko 'tata kjaraṁente/. See text for explanation.

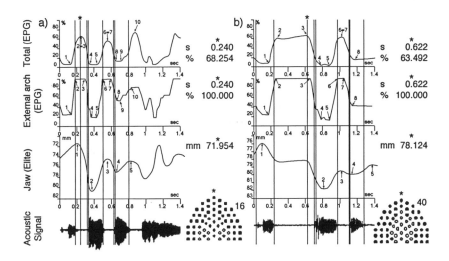

Figure 4. Representation of the temporal evolution of the % of total electrode activation (high), external arch electrodes activation (middle) and jaw movement (low), and the acoustic signal for a normal (a) and stuttered (b) performance of the sentence /ɖiko 'tata kjaraḿente/.

ELITE+EPG system describes (in a quantified manner) the kinematic anomalies in stutterers' speech. In Figure 4, two occurrences of the word /tata/ embedded in the carrier sentence *dico tàta chiaramente* are compared. Since tongue and jaw are the articulators most implicated in the production of the unvoiced alveolar plosives, the *external arch* and the *vertical jaw movement* are represented together with the acoustic signal. The contact profiles of the percentages of *external arch* and *total linguopalatal contacts* make it possible to identify the following:
- beginning (p.1) and end (2) of the closing movement for the first /t/;
- holding of the closure (2-3) for the first /t/;
- beginning (3) and end (4) of the opening movement for the first /t/;
- holding of the maximal open phase (4-5) for the first stressed /a/;
- beginning (5) and end (6) of the closing movement for the second /t/;
- holding of the closure (6-7) for the second /t/;
- beginning (p.7) and end (8) of the opening movement for the second /t/;
- holding of the open phase (8-9) for the final unstressed /a/;
- beginning (9) and end (10) of the closing movement for /kjaraḿente/.
    During normal production (4 a), the trajectory of the jaw movement does not provide evidence of any steady state and displays a continuous opening and closing movement from the maximal rising point (p.1) relative to the acoustic end of the /o/ to the slight final rising point for /k/(5), through the maximal lowering (2) within the stressed /a/, the relative rising point (3) for the second /t/ and the lowering (4) for the unstressed /a/. The stutterers' production of the same sequence (Figure 4 b) is perceived as a prolongation of the initial /t/

of the word /tata/. The external arch displays a minimal linguopalatal contact at the beginning of the closing movement (p.1), followed by the attainment and holding of the occlusion (2-3) for an abnormally long time (406 ms). The mandibular signal reaches the highest point when the acoustic waveform of the vowel /o/ begins (p.1), and successive lowering is interrupted midway by a "freezing" of the movement from 290 ms (2) to 600 ms (3), after which the jaw completes its downward movement at 830 ms (4).

It is worthwhile to note that the articulatory blockage begins and terminates firstly in the jaw with respect to the total activation profile, suggesting a probable causative role for this articulator and that, despite the obvious morphological diversity between normal and stutterers' gestures in the production of the first syllable /ta/, both subjects make the final downward movement point of the tongue (4) and jaw (2) coincide.

REFERENCES

Ferrigno, G., & Pedotti, A. (1985). ELITE: A digital dedicated hardware system for movement analysis via real-time TV signal processing. *IEEE Transactions of Biomedical Engineering, 32*, 943-50.

Farnetani, E., Vagges, K., & Magno Caldognetto, E. (1985). Coarticulation in Italian /VtV/ sequences: A palatographic study. *Phonetica, 42*, 78-99.

Magno Caldognetto, E., Vagges, K., & Zmarich, C. (1995). Visible articulatory characteristics of the italian stressed and unstressed vowels. *Proceedings XIIII International Congress of Phonetic Sciences,* Stockholm, vol. 1, 366-9.

Zmarich, C., Magno Caldognetto, E., & Vagges, K. (1995). Variability in the articulatory kinematics of lips and jaw in repeated /pa/ and /ba/ sequences in italian stutterers. *Proceedings XIIII International Congress of Phonetic Sciences,* Stockholm, vol.4, 536-9.

Chapter 40

VERBAL DELAYED REACTIONS. A STUDY OF PREFRONTAL FUNCTIONAL IMPAIRMENTS IN NEUROPSYCHIATRIC PATIENTS

Paolo Pinelli

The chronometric study of verbal reactions involves many phases, from programming and adjusting processes (Temporal Bridging) to the final neuromotor execution phase. Verbal Delayed Reactions allow us to investigate the processes of Temporal Bridging. These processes imply prefrontal functions (particularly area 46) and control not only the motor responses (as is the case in speech) but also the behavior at a high premotor level.

Verbal Delayed Reactions were studied in 3 stutterers, 4 patients with spastic dysphonia, a large number of dysarthric patients (with various pathologies including amyotrophic lateral sclerosis and cerebellar disease), 17 schizophrenics and 96 age-matched normal controls. Reaction times were measured, from the acoustic and EMG signals, in a reading task with single word stimuli. A so-called intermediate process ratio (IR) was defined as the ratio of the RT at a 1.5 sec foreperiod and the RT at trials without a foreperiod (immediate responses). A specific increase in IR, without any decrease in RT at immediate responses, was found in 12 of the 17 schizophrenics. In contrast, the IR was decreased in stutterers. The impairment of delayed reactions in schizophrenia could be attributed to a functional impairment of the prefrontal system, which is involved in the timing of sequential purposeful actions like speech. This process implies inhibitory processes which play a fundamental role in motor control. In stutterers, contrary to schizophrenics, inhibitory processes are diminished and successive actions are therefore impaired.

INTRODUCTION

Verbal reaction studies were planned to investigate, not only the final neuromotor executions, but also the brain processes that are held responsible for the programming and adjusting of the sequence of motor actions that generate the utterance of a word. To identify separately the programming and execution phases it is required that the subject performs two series of reactions. The first are *simple reactions*, which can yield useful cues on the activation of the neuromuscular executors and the contraction of the muscles that give rise to the expiring air flow and the modulation of the vocal tract. The second are *choice reactions* which include central programming processes. The visual neural processes and visuo-motor transport are common in both kinds of reactions (Pinelli, 1997).

Further series of investigations concerned *delayed reactions* (dR) that are known to involve prefrontal functions (particularly area 46). These investigations focused on two targets of assessment each with a different foreperiod (F). The foreperiod duration which discriminates between these two targets is 400 ms. This is the time required to develop the whole chain of programming - execution processes in the brain: visual perception, visuo-motor transformation, adjusting and integrating processes, and finally execution. First, delayed reactions with $F < 400$ ms involve parallel diffuse processes (PDP) of the earliest preprogramming. Second, delayed reactions with $F > 400$ ms are performed with reverberating internal circuits of programming during the foreperiod interval until the "go" signal appears. This kind of "working memory" has been called temporal bridging (T.B.).

In order to differentiate autonomous unconscious T.B. (or T.B. 1) from Short Term Memory (STM)-dependent T.B. (or T.B. 2), the word-stimulus in the series of dRs at $F = 0.5$ sec and $F = 1.5$ sec was continuously shown on the monitor up to the appearance of the "go" stimulus (to assess T.B.1) , whereas in a second series of dRs at $F = 4$ sec it disappeared after 1.5 sec.

METHODS

The word stimulus used in the simple reaction task was a disyllabic word, /mare/ , which was presented in a series of 24 trials. In choice reactions and delayed reactions three stimuli were presented in a random order. In addition to /mare/ , they included /ma/ and a sentence /mare è bello/, with 12 repetitions each. First a series of *immediate* ($F = 0$) reactions was performed. In two further series *delayed* reactions had to be given, in combinations of $F = 0.1$ sec and $F = 1.5$ sec, and of $F = 0.5$ sec and $F = 4$ sec respectively, each F occurring at random.

Equipment and recorded responses, stimulus presentation and measurements were the same as those reported in the papers by Colombo et al. (chapter 41) and by Spinatonda et al. (chapter 42). Two specific indices - the early process ratio (ER) and the intermediate process ratio (IR) - were calculated by taking ratio's of reaction times at specific foreperiods (see also Colombo et al., chapter 41; Spinatonda et al., chapter 42). The early process ratio (ER) was defined as the delayed RT with a 0.1 sec foreperiod divided by the immediate RT. The intermediate process ratio (IR) was defined as the delayed RT with a 1.5 sec foreperiod divided by the immediate RT. The evaluation of these indices in terms of related functional brain processes requires that some precise conditions are carefully fulfilled. For IR's this means that the acoustic RT at $F = 0$ should not be greatly reduced compared to mean normal values, as might occur after very intensive training and repetitions of the same reactions in a period of several months. Moreover, *acoustic and EMG reaction times* must not be larger than the foreperiod, to avoid a condition that would cause a "busy line" effect with upwards information to the programming and control systems through internal feedback.

Table 1. Acoustic reaction time (tACG) at three foreperiods (F), and intermediary process ratio's (IR) and early process ratio's (ER) for dysfluent subjects.

	N	Age	tACG F=0	tACG F=1.5s.	tACG F=0.1s	IR	ER
Normals	9	30	377	319	301	0.84	0.94
		s.d.12	s.d.47	s.d.62	s.d.60	s.d.0.07	s.d.0.11
Stutterers	3						
	S.C.	38	423	360	430	0.85	1.01
	M.D.	18	585	352	589	0.49	1.01
	B.G.	40	735	482	706	0.55	0.87
Spastic dysphonia 4		46	843	625	-	0.74	-
		57	795	658	-	0.82	-
		33	841	2194	-	2.6	-
		58	784	592	-	0.75	-
T.P.N.I.	1-V.A.	55	610	461	550	0.75	0.91
Laryngeal spasm	1-C.A.	44	425	279	364	0.63	0.85
Depressive syndrome	1-C.A.	58	592	436	407	0.73	0.68

MAIN FINDINGS

Normal controls

It has been found, in agreement with the lower threshold of the grammatical buffer (Pinelli, 1996), that the acoustic RT for /s/, in spite of the duration of the acoustic signal being more than double that of /b/, may be equal or shorter than the acoustic RT for /b/.

ER and IR have been calculated in a large normal population of 246 subjects, ranging from 4 to 81 years of age. To pre-school children choice picture naming tests were applied with schematic figures of a male and a female corresponding to the utterances /papà/ and /mamma/. From the age of 7 years onwards ER was found to be smaller than 0.9 and IR smaller than 0.85. Two groups of controls with different ages, culturally matched to the patient groups, were chosen for comparison (see Table 2).

Dysfluencies and neuro-psychiatric patients

The results obtained in stutterers, spastic dysphonia and laryngeal spasms are given in Table 1.

Table 2. Intermediary process ratio's (IR) and early process ratio's (ER) for 8 groups of neurological patients (see text) and 2 control groups.

	N	IR,F=1.5s.(s.d.)	ER (s.d.)
Normals 16 to 45	41	0.82 (0.12)	0.89 (0.11)
Normals 46 to 81	55	0.76 (0.16)	0.99 (0.17)
AP	7	0.68 (0.09)	0.97 (0.12)
HMSN	14	0.69 (0.11)	0.91 (0.12)
ALS	52	0.73 (0.08)	0.94 (0.10)
MFCV	16	0.80 (0.12)	1.08 (0.13)
TNPI	9	0.88 (0.13)	1.22 (0.14)
FD	13	0.76 (0.14)	0.97 (0.12)
PD	14	0.87 (0.13)	1.32 (0.26)
AD	18	0.92 (0.14)	1.51 (0.35)

Stutterers with an acoustic RT and EMG-RT longer than the foreperiod of the particular dRs were omitted owing to the "busy line" effect that causes pseudo-increases in IR. One case of spastic dysphonia with an acoustic RT longer than the foreperiod (F) is included in the table.

The results obtained in neurological patients are given in Table 2. They include acquired polyneuropathies (AP), hereditary degenerative neuropathies (HMSN), amyotrophic lateral sclerosis (ALS), multifocal cerebral vasculopathies (MFCV), traumatic neural chronic impairments (TNPI), focal dystonia's (FD), Primary Parkinson disease (P.D.), and Alzheimer Disease (AD). The results of chronic schizophrenic patients with positive symptoms (C.P.) and recent paranoid patients (RPS) are reported in Figure 1.

DISCUSSION

In normal subjects the Index IR is always smaller than one. In dysarthric patients of very different pathology the mean values of IR were also always smaller than one (see the IR's of the patient-groups listed in Table 2). However, single patients can show values of IR up to 1.2, but, in contrast to schizophrenics, these patients were characterized by relatively high values of acoustic RT at F=0 sec, as well as by a high ER and by rather typical abnormalities in the EMG patterns.

In stutterers, reported in Table 1, a peculiar finding is represented by a "lateral facilitation" effect revealed by a very low IR (case MD) or ER (case BG). Additional results obtained in spastic dysphonia, before and after botulinum local treatment, show that the improvement in the executive processes produced a statistically significant decrease in "central times", at least in cases lasting no longer than 17 years (and then without upwards neuroplastic changes).

A statistically significant increase in IR, without a decrease in acoustic RT at F=0

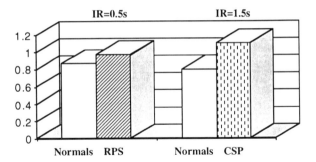

Figure 1. Intermediary process ratio's (IR) for two groups of schizophrenic patients, i.e. recent paranoid patients (RPS) and chronic schizophrenic patients (CSP), and their respective control subjects.

sec, was observed in schizophrenic patients, at F= 0.5 sec in recent paranoidal syndromes, and at F=1.5 and F=4 sec in positive syndromes.

CONCLUDING REMARKS

The delayed verbal-reaction methodology developed in the Veruno laboratory allows an analysis of the phases of brain processes involved in speech production. The internal programming circuits and feedbacks, developing in the cortico-basal ganglia-cerebellar systems, are reflected in the ratio between the acoustic RT at F=0 in choice reactions and the acoustic RT in simple reactions. The "temporal bridging", occurring in the inter- mediary processes between early programming and adjusted execution, is measured with delayed reactions.

Speaking is equivalent to a series of sequential complex purposeful actions. The sequence of brain processes, mentioned above, is operating in all psychomotor activities. *Specific convertors (Formulators) and afferent and efferent channels* characterize different kinds of actions. Speech is only one of these actions, although it is unique in man.

Temporal bridging, occurring in delayed reactions with F>400 ms, is necessary in maintaining the thread of the speech, as well as in thinking and decisional voluntary actions, even although in the last cases the responses take place at a higher premotor level.

REFERENCES

Ceriani, F., et al. (1992). Speech reaction times: an EMG and ACG study in healthy subjects. *Functional neurology, Suppl. 4, vol 7*, 77-90.
Colombo, R., Spinatonda, G., Conti, R., Pasetti, C., Pinelli, P., & Minuco, G. (this volume). Functionality indices for the evaluation of speech production. A study in normal subjects. In W. Hulstijn, H.F.M. Peters, & P.H.H.M. Van Lieshout (Eds.), *Speech production: motor control, brain research and fluency disorders*. Amsterdam: Elsevier Science.

Pinelli, P. (1992). Neurophysioloogy in the science of speech.- Current Opinion in Neurology and *Neurosurgery, 5,* 744-755.

Pinelli, P. (1997). Brain Control of Behaviour. An analysis of verbal delayed reactions and their impairment in Mental Disorders. Basel, Switzerland: Karger.

Pinelli, P., & Ceriani, F. (1992). Rappresentazioni e processi del parlare. Milano, Italy: Ambrosiana.

Spinatonda, Capodaglio, E., Colombo, R., Conti, R., Imbriani, M., Pinelli P., Pasetti, C., & Minuco, G. (this volume). Chronometry of the brain processes during speech production. A quantitative test to monitor exposition to neurotoxic solvents. In W. Hulstijn, H.F.M. Peters, & P.H.H.M. Van Lieshout (Eds.), *Speech production: motor control, brain research and fluency disorders.* Amsterdam: Elsevier Science.

Speech Production: Motor Control, Brain Research and Fluency Disorders
W. Hulstijn, H.F.M. Peters and P.H.H.M. Van Lieshout, editors

Chapter 41

FUNCTIONALITY INDEXES FOR THE EVALUATION OF SPEECH PRODUCTION: A STUDY IN NORMAL SUBJECTS

Roberto Colombo, Gianluca Spinatonda, Roberto Conti, Carlo Pasetti, Paolo Pinelli, Giuseppe Minuco

The measurement of reaction times (RT) in response to suitable stimuli may provide insight into the separate functional blocks corresponding to diverse speech production mechanisms. The quantitative evaluation of speech motor performance provides useful information for the early detection and long-term monitoring of many neurological diseases.

Speech motor performance and the effect of age were investigated by measuring vocal reaction times (VRT) and speech durations, in a group of thirty normal subjects divided into three age groups (18-44, 45-59, 60-80). VRTs were measured by using an immediate and delayed reaction stimulation paradigm. Analysis of the acoustic and electromyographic signals indicated that reaction times increased with age in both the immediate and delayed tasks; also the acoustic signal durations increased with age. The analysis of variance showed that the difference between the young and elderly groups was statistically significant.

In an attempt to classify the performace obtained in the execution of the reading tasks, and detect interference phenomena, some functionality indexes were computed.

INTRODUCTION

Reaction Time (RT) has been widely used in clinical fields such as neuropsychology, psychology, neurology and physical medicine to assess the performance of the diverse cerebral processes involved in the execution of a given task or in the production of a response generated by external stimuli. In recent years, the RT paradigm has also been used in the investigation of lack of vocal fluency and stuttering, suggesting that stutterers may have difficulty in the motor programming of speech (Watson, 1987; Peters, 1989).

Since speech disorders affect a very large proportion of patients with neurological diseases, the quantitative evaluation of speech motor performance can provide useful information for the early detection and long-term monitoring of many neurological diseases. In fact, other studies have focused their attention on speech impairment occurring in degenerative neural processes such as Parkinson's Disease (Streifler, 1984), or Amyotrophic Lateral Sclerosis (Kent, 1992). Consequently we decided to investigate vocal reaction times (VRT) as a possible parameter in quantifying chronic and degenerative neural processes.

The aim of this paper is to investigate speech motor performance and the effect of age on VRTs in a group of normal subjects. Some functionality indexes are introduced in the attempt to discriminate pathological from normal subjects and to quantitatively evaluate their performance.

METHOD

In order to outline the functions responsible for VRTs, we will consider a modified version of the "speaker as information processor" proposed by Levelt (Levelt, 1989), as this seems the most appropriate for describing our experiments. It consists of the following main blocks:

The *Visual Process* is the first block we will consider because the tasks in our experiments consist in reading a word presented on the screen of a stimulus unit (visual stimuli). The *Formulator* is the process that translates a conceptual structure into a linguistic structure. This is a two-step process involving: a) the grammatical encoding of the message and b) the phonological encoding that selects the appropriate phonetic or articulatory plan for each lemma and for the required utterance. In simple terms, the formulator receives fragments of messages as input and produces a phonetic plan as output. Our experiments include the phonological but not the grammatical encoding step.

The *Articulator* converts the phonetic plan into overt speech by means of the musculature of the respiratory, laryngeal, supra-laryngeal and oromandibular systems. Synchronizing articulation with the selected speech rate may necessitate temporary storage of the phonetic plan. This storage is known as the *Articulatory Buffer*.

The closed loop control of speech production is performed by the *Auditory Process* involving both the audition and, in some cases, the speech comprehension components. The *Conceptualizer* refers to the sum of mental activities exerted during intentional speech. In our experiments this process is secondary to the visual process involved in the reading of words.

Stimulation Procedure

Two stimulation paradigms were used : an immediate reading task and a delayed reading task. The immediate reading task is the analogue of a typical choice reaction time task. The subject is requested to utter a word immediately after it is presented on a computer screen. It is worth stressing that in this task the subject is unable to program the motor commands in advance. The processes involved are visual perception, formulation and articulation of speech.

In the delayed reading task the subject has to wait for a response signal before starting to speak. In this case the word is presented in advance on the screen prior to the response signal, and at the onset of voicing the visual perception and formulation processes have already been executed as well as the phonetic plan of the word stored in the Articulatory Buffer; the subject needs only to retrieve it. Only the articulation time is required to complete the task. The delay between the presentation of the word and the presentation of the response signal is called the foreperiod.

The difference between the RT obtained in the immediate reading task and the RT obtained in the delayed reading task should depend solely on the performances of the Visual Perception and Formulation processes. We will refer to this time as the Central Processing Time (CPT) because it takes into consideration the processes of pattern recognition and programming of the movement, but not its execution.

The experimental set-up consisted of two computerised units: the Words-Images Presenter (WIP) and the Signal Acquisition System (SAS). The WIP presented sequences of words or images as visual stimuli to the subject under examination, implementing both immediate and delayed presentation tasks. The SAS consisted of a personal computer with a 12 bit A/D interface (Microstar Laboratories - DAP 2400) able to manage acquisition, processing and data storage of the acoustic, electroglottographic, electromyographic and lip and jaw kinematic signals (Colombo, 1995).

The study population consisted of 30 normal subjects (15 males, 15 females) divided into three age groups defined as: YOUNG(18-44, n=9), MIDDLE-AGED (45-59, n=10) and OLD (60-80, n=11). An experimental session involved three tasks, an immediate reading task and two delayed reading tasks, in which the foreperiod was randomly varied on the basis of two alternatives (0.1, 1.5 s for one task, and 0.5, 4 s for the other task). Twenty-four visual stimuli were used in each task. The words were presented for 3 s in random sequence, and a 3 - 6 s interval elapsed between stimuli. In all three tasks the two-syllable words /MARE/ (sea) and /MURO/ (wall) were used. These were selected because they are well-matched in terms of frequency, initial sound and utterance complexity. Each word was presented 12 times in the immediate reading task and 6 times for each foreperiod in the delayed reading tasks. In order to avoid learning effects the words and foreperiods were randomly distributed in each sequence.

RESULTS AND DISCUSSION

In the present paper, we report the results of the speech reaction time analyses based on the acoustic and EMG signals, and those of the duration of the acoustic signal. We considered each subject's mean VRTs in the three tasks. A preliminary statistical analysis did not show significant differences as a function of the stimulus word (paired Student's t test), so we analysed the data by grouping the results of the two words. The analysis of variance was applied to test differences between tasks within age groups and to compare results among the three groups.

Figure 1a shows the means and standard deviations (S.D.) of the RTs as measured by the acoustic and electromyographic signals for each task in the three age groups. It clearly shows that for the acoustic signal both RTs and S.D.s increased with age. The greatest S.D. increase was observed in the OLD group. In all groups the longest RTs were recorded in the immediate reading task and in the 0.1, 0.5 foreperiod reading tasks. The best RT performance corresponded to the 1.5 s foreperiod reading task.

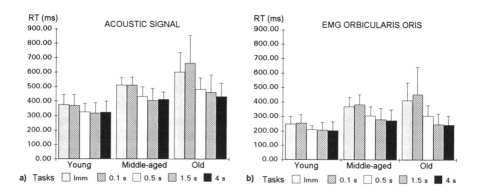

Figure 1. Reaction times based on the (a) Acoustic and (b) EMG Orbicularis Oris signals of a group of 30 normal subjects. The two panels report the measurements obtained in both the immediate (Imm) and delayed (foreperiods = 0.1, 0.5, 1.5, 4 s) reading tasks

Elderly subjects attained their lowest RT values on the 4 s foreperiod reading task. Furthermore, in this group RTs were longer, but not significantly, during the 0.1 s foreperiod reading task as compared to the immediate reading task, this probably being due to an interference phenomenon between visual and formulation processes. An interpretation of this fact may be given considering the visual and formulation as concurrent processes. So, the slowing of performance in the elderly may imply a conversion from concurrent to sequential execution of these processes; however this remain only a speculative hypothesis.

Between-group comparisons showed a significant difference between the performances of the YOUNG vs. MIDDLE-AGED subjects and of the YOUNG vs. OLD subjects on each task. Within-group analysis showed that in all groups RTs significantly decreased during the 1.5 and 4 s foreperiod reading tasks as compared to the immediate reading task.

Figure 1b shows mean and S.D. of the RTs based on the EMG signal of the orbicularis oris muscle. The increase in the mean values as a function of age was very similar to that obtained for the acoustic signal . The S.D. of the OLD group was higher than that of the other groups, but in the case of the orbicular oris muscle only for the immediate and 0.1 s foreperiod tasks. Between-group comparisons revealed that only the YOUNG group differed significantly from the other groups. The measurements for the digastric muscle showed very similar results. The within-group analysis showed results quite similar to those obtained for the acoustic signal.

The comparison between normal and pathological conditions may be a very difficult task because of the many factors influencing the RT values. The effect of age on VRTs has been described, but other factors such as fatigue, stress, and diverse language or dialect may influence the RT measurement. So a comparison between diverse conditions would require a large number of subjects and/or very well-matched groups. Therefore in an attempt to evaluate and classify the individual performance obtained during the execution of the reading tasks some functionality indexes were computed:

1) the difference between the RTs obtained in the immediate reading tasks and those obtained in the delayed reading task with foreperiods of 1.5 s and 4 s. These values should correspond to the central processing times (CPT) relative to the formulation and visual perception processes;
2) the early process ratio defined as ER=RTf0.1/RT immediate (i.e. the delayed RT with foreperiod 0.1 s divided by the immediate RT). This index should be > 1 when the interference phenomenon is present and < or = 1 in the other case.
3) the intermediate process ratio IR=RTf1.5/RT immediate (i.e. the delayed RT with foreperiod 1.5 s divided by the immediate RT).

Figure 2 shows the CPTs based on the acoustic and electromyographic signals for the two foreperiods considered. Mean and S.D. values clearly increased, consistent with the theory that the aging phenomenon is accompanied by a slowing of the motor planning processes.

Figure 3 reports the values of the IR and ER indexes obtained in the three age groups plus, in addition, in a group of schizophrenic patients. The IR index shows a slight decrease with age in the normal subjects with a mean value ranging from .85 to .75. It seems that even if the VRTs increase with age, the performance of the so-called intermediate processes (the IR index) remains about the same under the delayed reading task condition. However, this performance index is significantly different when measured in a group of schizophrenic patients. This result obviously needs a more detailed analysis.

On the contrary the ER mean values showed an age dependent increase (0.98-1.1 range), which could be explained by an age dependent sensitivity to the above described interference phenomenon. Also the schizophrenic group showed increased ER values that were significantly different from an age-matched group of normal subjects.

The data relative to schizophrenic patients are not the focus of this paper, but have been reported simply to clarify the application of the above-mentioned performance indexes.

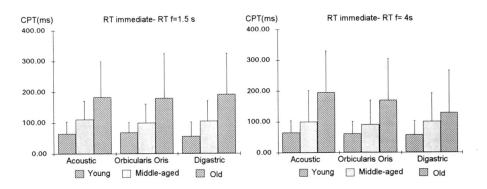

Figure 2. Central Processing Times based on the Acoustic, EMG Orbicularis Oris and EMG Digastric signals.

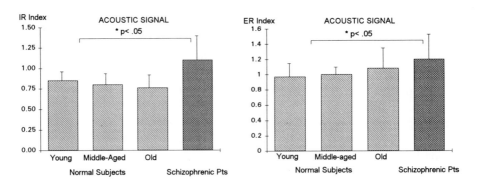

Figure 3. Intermediate Processes Index (IR) and Early Process Index (ER) computed in a group of 30 normal subjects and in a group of 20 schizophrenic patients.

CONCLUSIONS

The results of this study show that by using the VRT measurement technique it is possible to obtain qualitative and quantitative information about the processes involved in speech production. Evidence of an age-dependent slowing in the motor planning processes was obtained in a group of normal subjects.

Some performance indexes have been introduced in order to evaluate and classify the individual performance of the subjects examined. The preliminary results seem to indicate an alteration of performance, such as happened in the group of schizophrenic patients considered.

The Acoustic and EMG signals seem to provide similar information in this sample of normal subjects, but the application of this method to the study of patients with neurological diseases, in whom preinnervation, coinnervation and hyperinnervation phenomena are generally evident, should highlight the neural and the mechanical components of the VRTs.

REFERENCES

Colombo, R., Parenzan, R., Minuco, G., et al. (1995). Multiparametric quantitative evaluation of the speech production system: a study in normal subjects. *Functional Neurology, Vol. X, 1*, 3-16

Kent, F.J., Kent, R.D., Rosenbek, J.C., et al. (1992). Quantitative description of the dysartria in women with amyotrophic lateral sclerosis. *Journal of Speech and Hearing Research, 35*, 723-733.

Levelt, W.J.M. (1989). The speaker as information processor. In: Joshi A. (ed) *Speaking from intention to articulation* (p. 1-28). London, MIT Press.

Peters, H.F.M., Hulstijn, W., & Starkweather, C.W. (1989). Acoustic and Physiological reaction times of stutterers and nonstutterers. *Journal of Speech and Hearing Research, 32*, 668-680.

Streifler, M., & Hofman, S. (1984). Disorders of verbal expression in parkinsonism. *Advances in Neurology, 40*, 385-393.

Watson, B.C., & Alfonso, P.J. (1987). Physiological bases of acoustic LRT in nonstutterers, mild stutterers and severe stutterers. *Journal of Speech and Hearing Research, 30*, 434-447.

Speech Production: Motor Control, Brain Research and Fluency Disorders
W. Hulstijn, H.F.M. Peters and P.H.H.M. Van Lieshout, editors

Chapter 42

CHRONOMETRY OF THE BRAIN PROCESSES DURING SPEECH PRODUCTION: A QUANTITATIVE TEST TO MONITOR EXPOSITION TO NEUROTOXIC SOLVENTS

Gianluca Spinatonda, Edda M. Capodaglio, Roberto Colombo, Roberto Conti, Marcello Imbriani, Paolo Pinelli, Carlo Pasetti, Giuseppe Minuco

The aim of this study was to evaluate the effects of exposition to neurotoxic solvents in a group of laundry operators by means of Vocal Reaction Times (VRTs) measurements. A group of normal subjects, matched for age and educational level, constituted the controls.
Vocal Reaction Times were measured by a device that presented to each subject a sequence of words on a computer screen, acquired the acoustic signal and measured VRTs and durations. During the test a random sequence of words was presented to the subjects; the protocol consisted of an immediate reading task and two delayed reading tasks. The test was performed using the concrete words /MARE/(sea) and /MURO/(wall) and the meaningless words /ABAVEK/ and /UBAVEK/.
Statistical analysis of the acoustic signals showed that reaction times were longer for the exposed group than for the controls. The differences between durations were significant for the delayed reading tasks using concrete words and for all tasks using meaningless words. These findings suggest that the two sorts of words used may provide different information: VRTs with /MARE/ and /MURO/ seem to be more specific for evaluating motor planning processes, while duration data for /ABAVEK/ and /UBAVEK/ seem to be better for testing the muscle command preparation and execution stages.

INTRODUCTION

The damages to the Central Nervous System (CNS) caused by a prolonged exposition to organic solvents such as perchloroethylene have been well known for several years, but their long term effects are still not clear. They mainly consist of an increase in the activation threshold of cognitive functions, such as memory, concentration, attention and rapid responses, activated during complex motor functions such as manual dexterity and visuo-motory coordination. Besides, it is likely that progressive alterations due to chronic exposition to neurotoxic agents may be initially compensated by the redundancy of resources typical of the CNS, so that in an early stage of involvement only the activation of complex functions may manifest a dysfunction or a reduced performance in execution.

The most frequently used methods for assessing the nature of these dysfunctions are standard assessment tests evaluating attention, such as the Stroop test and the digit cancellation test. More recently, the measurement of Reaction Times (RTs) has been introduced in order to obtain a quantitative and qualitative evaluation (Anshelm Olson et al., 1981; Camerino et al., 1993). In particular, the study of the brain processes underlying speech production has been found to be a sensitive method, able to provide information related to the early detection of sub-clinical alterations of the CNS and the long-term monitoring of neurological diseases (Kent et al., 1992; Pinelli et al., 1993).

In this paper we describe a method based on the measurement of Vocal Reaction Times (VRT) and speech durations for the quantitative evaluation of CNS dysfunctions due to chronic exposition to organic solvents. A group of laundry workers has been considered for this purpose.

METHOD

The measurement of vocal reaction times, after suitable stimuli, may provide information on the separate functional stages corresponding to cognitive, articulatory, and biomechanical components of speech production. In particular, by an appropriate stimulation paradigm, it is possible to highlight the motor plan assembly and the muscle command preparation and execution stages of the speech (Levelt, 1989; Van Lieshout et al., 1996). The former corresponds to the phonological and phonetic encoding of the message. It consists of the procedures that select the appropriate articulatory or phonetic plan. The latter constitute the articulatory process that converts the phonetic plan into overt speech by means of setting and executing the commands for the musculature of the respiratory, laryngeal and oromandibular systems.

The architecture employed consisted of a personal computer presenting sequences of words as visual stimuli to the subject under examination and acquiring vocal responses to measure the related VRTs and speech durations. To be able to use this test outside the laboratory a notebook PC combined with a small external audio amplifier, microphone and A/D converter were selected. Further details about the method are reported in another paper by Colombo et al. (chapter 41).

Experimental protocol

To evaluate the effects of exposition to neurotoxic organic solvents a group of 35 laundry workers (36 ± 11 years old), who were exposed to perchloroethylene (PCE), was selected. To quantitatively infer the degree of exposure, the environmental conditions of the workplace were measured and reported as PCE concentration (mg/m^3). A group of 39 normal subjects (36 ± 10 years old), matched for age and for educational level, was used as controls.

The stimulation paradigm included two types of tasks: an immediate reading task followed by a delayed reading task. In the former the subject was requested to pronounce a word appearing on the PC screen immediately after its presentation; in the latter the subject had to wait for a response signal (two lines of asterisks above and below the presented word) before starting to speak. It is worth underlining that in the immediate reading task the subject under test was unable to assemble in advance the specific motor plan. In contrast, in the delayed reading task subjects had time to create a phonetic motor plan before the onset of the response signal. In this case time delays in completing the task can be attributed to muscle command preparation and execution processes only. The delay between the presentation of the word and the presentation of the response signal is called foreperiod (F).

An experimental session consisted of two sequences of an immediate reading task followed by a delayed reading task, with foreperiods 0.1 s and 1.5 s. The concrete two-syllabic words /MARE/(sea) and /MURO/(wall) were used in the first sequence (i.e. first and second tasks) and the meaningless three-syllabic words /ABAVEK/ and /UBAVEK/ were used in the second sequence (i.e. third and fourth tasks). The meaningless words were introduced to explore more complex formulation processes and to increase the sensitivity of the test for the speech duration measurement.

Each experimental session consisted of 96 presentations of the selected words in the four tasks outlined above where the stimuli were randomly sequenced. The laundry workers were tested directly in the work place, while the control group was examined in our laboratory.

RESULTS AND DISCUSSION

In order to test for group differences, the t-test for independent samples was performed on the diverse tasks and types of words (concrete and meaningless). The results are shown in Table 1.

Table 1. VRTs, durations and between-group differences for the immediate and delayed tasks and for concrete and meaningless words (* $p < 0.05$, ** $p < 0.005$, *** $p < 0.0005$).

		Vocal Reaction Times (ms)			Durations (ms)		
		Controls	Exposed	D%	Controls	Exposed	D%
	Imm.	427 ± 68	495 ± 112	16% **	303 ± 75	332 ± 77	10%
/MARE/ - /MURO/	0.1 s	435 ± 94	556 ± 169	28% ***	279 ± 66	328 ± 82	18% *
	1.5 s	345 ± 88	425 ± 140	23% **	292 ± 67	340 ± 86	16% *
	Imm.	553 ± 134	568 ± 132	3%	361 ± 82	413 ± 67	14% **
/ABAVEK/ - /UBAVEK/	0.1 s	540 ± 121	595 ± 161	10%	341 ± 93	400 ± 71	17% **
	1.5 s	394 ± 90	453 ± 150	15% *	361 ± 84	417 ± 75	16% *

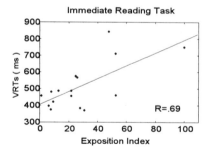
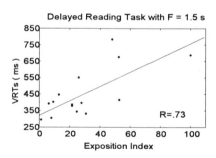

Figure 1: Correlation analysis between VRTs in the immediate and delayed (F=1.5 s) reading tasks and Exposition Index (logarithm of PCE concentration multiplied by Years of Work) for a sub-group of 16 subjects that, due to the particular duty assigned, were more exposed to organic solvents vapour inhalation. (p < .005)

The reaction times obtained in the group of subjects exposed to PCE were significantly longer than those obtained in the control group when concrete words were used. The increase in VRTs was evident both in the immediate and in the delayed reading tasks. The 0.1 s foreperiod task showed the largest difference between groups and seemed to produce an interference phenomenon similar to what is described in aging (Colombo et al., 1995). The VRTs obtained with meaningless words showed a slight but not significant increase in the exposed subjects. The major difference was obtained in the delayed reading task with 1.5 s foreperiod. Therefore we can conclude that subjects exposed to PCE are characterised by a general slowing down of the brain processes underlying speech production. Furthermore, the 1.5 s foreperiod task did not show the same performance facilitation for the subject group as for the control group.

The analysis of speech durations showed that the exposed subjects had higher values than controls with both types of words. The differences were larger for the meaningless words, probably because they involve more complex processes. For both groups speech duration seemed unrelated to the type of task.

In order to model the relationship between exposition to PCE and VRTs we selected a sub-group of 16 subjects that, due to the particular duty assigned, we presumed to be more exposed to organic solvents vapour inhalation. Figure 1 reports the regression analysis, with the concrete word set, between VRTs and an Exposition Index (EI) in the immediate reading task and in the delayed reading task with a foreperiod duration of 1.5 s.

Because of the non-normal nature of PCE concentration distribution, the exposition index was computed by multiplying the natural logarithm of the PCE concentration by the years of work. Regression analysis showed a correlation coefficient $r=0.69$ (p<.005) in the immediate reading task and $r=0.73$ (p<.005) in the delayed reading task (with 1.5 s foreperiod). These correlations confirm the direct dependence of VRT increase on the dose in subjects chronically exposed to organic solvents.

CONCLUSIONS

These results show that the laundry workers examined in this study are characterised by a slowing down phenomenon of the speech production mechanisms both in the motor plan assembly and in the muscle command preparation and execution stages. A consistent correlation was found between VRTs and exposition to organic solvents, confirming the hypothesis that the VRT measurement technique may be considered a useful tool for the assessment of the preclinical alterations of CNS in the monitoring of individuals chronically exposed in the workplace to neurotoxic agents.

REFERENCES

Anshelm Olson B., Gamberale F., & Grönqvist B. (1981). Reaction time changes among steel workers exposed to solvent vapor. A longitudinal study. *International Archives of Occupational and Environmental Health, 48*, 211-218.

Camerino D., Cassitto M.G., & Gilioli R. (1993). Prevalence of abnormal neurobehavioural scores in populations exposed to different industrial chemicals. *Enviromental Research, 61(2)*, 251-7.

Colombo R., Parenzan R., Minuco G., Conti R., Miscio G., Pisano F., & Pinelli P. (1993). Multipara metric quantitative evaluation of the speech motor system. Technology and Health Care. *Proceedings 2nd European Conference on Engineering and Medicine*, 403-404.

Colombo R., Parenzan R., Minuco G., Conti R., Miscio G., Pisano F., & Pinelli P. (1995). Multipara metric quantitative evaluation of the speech production system: a study in normal subjects. *Functional Neurology, 1*, 3-16.

Kent J.F., Kent R.D., & Rosenbek J.C., et al. (1992). Quantitative description of the dysartria in women with amyotrophic lateral sclerosis. *Journal of Speech and Hearing Research, 35*, 723-733.

Levelt, W.J.M. (1989). *The speaker as information processor.* In A. Joshi (Ed.), Speaking from intention to articulation. London: MIT Press (pp. 1-28).

Peters H.F.M., Hulstijn W., & Starkweather C.W. (1989). Acoustic and Physiological reaction times of stutterers and nonstutterers. *Journal of Speech and Hearing Research, 32*, 668-680.

Pinelli P., Pisano F., & Miscio G., et al. (1993). Fluctuations in speech reaction times: The effect of aging and non-dominant hemisphere motor area lesions. Technology and Health Care. *Proceedings 2nd European Conference on Engineering and Medicine* (pp. 68-69).

Scott S., Caird F.I., & Williams B.O. (1984). Evidence for an apparent sensory speech disorder in Parkinson's disease. *Journal of Neurology, Neurosurgery, & Psychiatry, 47*, 840-843.

Streifler M., & Hofman S. (1984). Disorders of verbal expression in parkinsonism. *Advances in Neurology, 40*, 385-393.

Van Lieshout P.H.H.M., Hulstijn W., & Peters HFM (1996). Speech production in people who stutter: Testing the motor plan assembly hypotesis. *Journal of Speech and Hearing Research, 39*, 76-92.

Speech Production: Motor Control, Brain Research and Fluency Disorders
W. Hulstijn, H.F.M. Peters and P.H.H.M. Van Lieshout, editors

Chapter 43

EN ROUTE TO A SPEECH MOTOR TEST: A FIRST HALT

Pascal H.H.M. van Lieshout, Herman F.M. Peters, Annette J. Bakker

In clinical practice the assessment of speech motor behavior is in most cases restricted to perceptual descriptions of speech characteristics, from which general conclusions are drawn about underlying problems of speech motor behavior. However, these subjective indices of motor performance need to be substantiated with objective measurements in the acoustic, physiological, and kinematic domain to unlock the dynamic principles underlying normal and nonfluent speech motor production. In this study, using a choice and simple reaction time paradigm we tried to access the influence of syllable onset or coda complexity, stress location, syllable frequency, and word size on acoustic reaction time and word duration. The data collected from two small groups of stuttering and matched nonstuttering subjects showed that in spite of sometimes even clear main effects for a certain type of manipulation, stuttering individuals as such did not show major differences with the data from the control subjects. In contrast, measures extracted from glottographic, myographic and respiratory signals, may offer better possibilities to find clear differences between verbal motor skills of stuttering and nonstuttering subjects. To illustrate this point, some preliminary motor data will be presented and discussed with respect to the further development of a speech motor test.

INTRODUCTION

Fluency disorders are characterized by a variety of speech motor symptoms which to some extent have a highly idiosyncratic nature. These symptoms can be related to the speech production stages of motor plan assembly, muscle command parametrization, and, muscle command execution (Van Lieshout et al., 1996a; 1996b). In order to achieve an objective and quantitative assessment of these symptoms it is necessary to develop a standardized approach in which measures of speech motor activity as related to speech respiration, phonation, and articulation are collected simultaneously with the acoustic signal under various linguistic and motor demands (Peters et al., 1995). These demands include the manipulation of the amount of preparation time preceding the verbalization of a test word by using a simple (delayed) and choice (immediate) verbal reaction time paradigm. Since changes in muscle command preparation (including motor initiation) and execution time can be studied more or less in isolation in a simple reaction time-task (cf. Peters et al., 1989), the use of two different reaction time paradigms with the same stimuli allows for a distinction between effects that arise at an earlier stage (motor plan assembly or planning) and those that arise at later stages (muscle command parametrization and execution). Furthermore, by manipulating specific aspects of the verbal stimuli, the demands on the processing time for specific stages can be varied. In this paper we present the first results on acoustic reaction time and word duration of an experiment in which two small groups of stuttering and nonstuttering subjects were asked to name a number of verbal stimuli that were manipulated in terms of syllable onset or coda complexity, stress location, syllable frequency, and word size. Furthermore, some preliminary data will be presented on specific motor aspects of fluent and nonfluent speech production.

METHODS

Subjects

For this study the data of six people who stutter (age range 18 - 26 years) and five people who do not stutter (age range 23 - 34 years), matched for highest level of education were used. From the six people who stutter two had less then a minimum amount of perceptually fluent utterances (25%), leaving the data of four stuttering subjects for further analysis on verbal reaction times and word durations. None of the subjects reported problems in hearing acuity, language development, voice quality or motor development. Stuttering severity was determined by an experienced speech pathologist based on a standard protocol used at the Department of Voice and Speech Pathology at the ENT clinic of the University Hospital Nijmegen and ranged from slightly moderate to severe.

Procedure

In this study four different stimulus manipulations were used in a simple (SRT) and choice reaction time (CRT) paradigm. To exclude influences of higher order linguistic stages that precede the motor plan assembly stage, only pronounceable nonwords were selected. If not indicated otherwise, all syllable frequencies were low. The four manipulations were as follows, with the more complex stimuli underlined:

1. *Cluster* (CL): monosyllabic nonwords with a single (1C) or a multiple (2C) consonant onset or in case with a vowel onset (see below), a single or a multiple consonant coda (e.g., /bir/ vs. /bri/ or /oos/ vs. /oks/).

2. *Stress location* (SL): disyllabic nonwords with the primary stress on either the first (1st syl) or second (2nd syl) syllable, to the subjects indicated by capital letters on the screen (e.g., /MOTlik/ vs. /motLIK/);

3. *Syllable frequency* (SF): disyllabic nonwords with either a high (high) or low (*low*) second syllable frequency (e.g., /bamzon/ vs. /bamnit/);

4. *Word size* (WS): monosyllabic (1 syl) vs. disyllabic (2 *syl*) nonwords (e.g., /praamt/ vs. /pemnal/) matched for number of graphemes;

These manipulations were selected because they are known for their influence on stuttering frequency and/or for their processing demand on at least one of the speech motor production stages mentioned above (cf. Van Lieshout, 1995). For each of the two levels of a stimulus manipulation there were twelve different nonwords, half of them starting with a consonant, the other half starting with a vowel. Furthermore, half of the consonant-initial nonwords and vowel-initial nonwords involved lip activity for the purpose of electromyographic registrations. So, in total each manipulation included 24 different words. For all four manipulations together the total number of trials in one block added up to 96 for each task (simple or choice reaction time). The presentation of this block of 96 randomized trials was halfway interrupted by a short break. The same stimuli were used for the simple and choice reaction time task, only the order of trials was different across tasks.

Measurements

For each subject the following measures, the selection of which was based on earlier research (Van Lieshout et al., 1996a, 1996b), were taken:

a. Using Respitrace recordings of thoracic and abdominal movements:
    - The onset of thoracic and abdominal inspiration and expiration
b. Using Fourcin Laryngograph recordings of Electroglottographic activity (EGG):
    - The onset and offset of voice related activity, as well as (if present) the onset of the first glottal pulse
c. Using Integrated surface Electromyographic (IEMG) recordings of M. Orbicularis Oris superior and inferior:
    - The onset and offset, as well as peak amplitude location of IEMG for lip consonants and vowels
d. Using Acoustic recordings:
    - The onset and offset of the speech acoustic signal

Data were collected and analyzed with custom-made software that was developed using Viewdac data acquisition and analysis tools (Asyst, V. 2.1, Keithley Instruments Inc.). Automatic algorithms were used to detect onsets and offsets in signals, based on thresholds (= mean noise level + three standard deviations) in the signal, except for the respitrace signals, where velocity zero crossings were used to detect onsets and offsets of relevant events.

Analysis

A first analysis showed no systematic main effects for sound category (consonant vs. vowel). Therefore, for each subject the selected measure for central tendency (median) was based on a maximum of twelve trials per stimulus manipulation level, regardless the type of initial sound. Medians instead of means were taken to counteract a bias of outliers in the data set. In this paper individual data will be presented on the average difference between the median values of the complex level and the less complex level of each manipulation for verbal reaction time and word duration, separated for the simple and the choice reaction time task. We expect that the more complex stimuli have longer reaction times and word durations than their less complex counterparts. More in particular, we expect for cluster to find a main positive effect on word duration, for stress location a main positive effect on choice reaction time   and possibly word duration   (based on longer final vowel duration for second syllable stress location), for syllable frequency a main effect for choice reaction time   and word duration   (cf. Levelt & Wheeldon, 1994), and finally, for word size, we expect main effects on choice and simple reaction time   as well as on word duration   (cf. Van Lieshout, 1996b). These main effects are expected to be stronger for the stuttering subjects, if they encounter problems in processing the stimuli in (at least) one of the speech motor production stages mentioned above.

RESULTS AND DISCUSSION

In Figure 1 data are presented for each stimulus manipulation on the average difference in verbal reaction time (RTd) and word duration (WDd) for individual subjects who stutter (ST) and who do not stutter (NS) for the simple (SRT) and choice (CRT) reaction-time task. As can be seen from this figure there are notable between-subject differences in both groups. Regarding the main effect of each stimulus manipulation it was found that in line with our expectations:

- For cluster, 83 % of all cases show positive word duration differences, indicating longer word durations for nonwords with more than one consonant in initial or coda position compared to nonwords with a singleton consonant onset or coda. However, contrary to our expectations these more complex nonwords also show (with only one exception) shorter verbal reaction times in the simple reaction time task (for the choice reaction time task the effect is less consistent). To date, we have no obvious explanation for the latter effect.
- For stress location, choice reaction time differences were all positive, indicating that nonwords with stressed second syllable have longer choice reaction times than nonwords with stressed first syllable[1]. In 75% of the cases (both tasks) word duration differences were positive, thus indicating that nonwords with stress on the second syllable also show longer word durations.
- For syllable frequency, there was a small majority of cases (67%) showing positive choice reaction time differences, indicating that nonwords with low frequency second syllable have longer choice reaction times than nonwords with high frequency second syllable. A clear unexpected group difference is seen for the simple reaction time task, where reaction time differences indicate that four out of five nonstutterers show longer reaction times for the nonwords with high frequency second syllable, whereas the stutterers in three out of four cases show longer reaction times for the nonwords

with low frequency second syllable. The latter might suggest that for stutterers even in the later stages of motor processing, words with lower frequency second syllable are more difficult to handle.

Also, there is a rather consistent (89% of all cases in both tasks) unexpected effect for word duration differences, indicating longer word durations for nonwords with a high frequency second syllable. This is most evident for the stuttering subjects in the simple reaction time task. Why subjects take more time to verbalize nonwords with a relatively high second syllable frequency is unknown. It might relate to the fact that these high frequency second syllables often had to be syllables with a meaning when spoken in isolation, which might induce a different (more precise and thus slower) mode of articulation.

- For word size, positive choice and simple reaction time differences were found in most cases (83%), indicating longer reaction times for bisyllabic nonwords compared to monosyllabic nonwords. Similarly, positive word duration differences were found in all cases, indicating longer word durations for bisyllabic words.

Despite these clear main effects for each stimulus manipulation, there are only a few examples of conspicuous differences between stuttering and nonstuttering subjects, except of course for the already mentioned but unexpected group difference in the simple reaction time task for the syllable frequency manipulation. One example concerns ST1, who shows a relatively long delay in choice reaction time for the nonwords with stress on the second syllable. Likewise, he is also slower than any of the other subjects in verbalizing these nonwords, as shown in his average word duration difference for the same task. Another example is ST2, who shows a clear effect of word size in his choice reaction time. However, in general, clear individual outliers in the data of the stuttering subjects are not readily apparent. In particular this is true, because the nonstuttering subjects are almost as different from each other as they are from stuttering individuals. This might suggest that a speech motor test based on this set-up lacks sufficient sensitivity to detect differences between stuttering and nonstuttering individuals as related to motor plan assembly, muscle command parametrization and execution. Or, as an alternative explanation, that the chosen manipulations are of less relevance to characterize such differences. In either case the set-up of the test will have to change to make it a useful tool to discriminate between the motor performance of a person who stutters and a normal speaker.

Of course, just looking at verbal reaction times and word durations limits the scope of our investigation. For this reason, we included the physiological measures on respiration, phonation, and articulation as described above. There is not enough space to discuss the merits of using these measures to characterize individual differences between stuttering and nonstuttering subjects, but an example might illustrate the point.

Figure 2 shows three typical examples of perceptually fluent utterances (in all cases the nonword ['m k.s t]), spoken by a control speaker (left part), and two stuttering

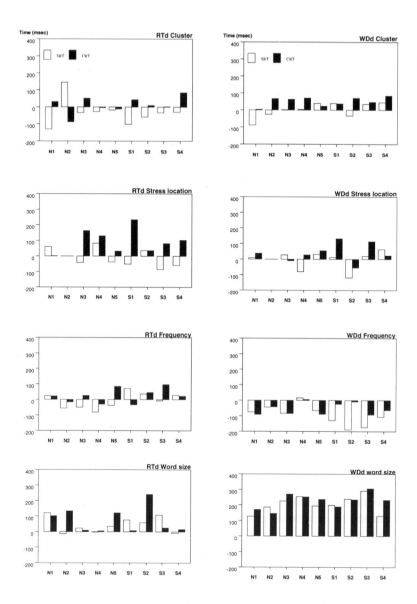

Figure 1. Between stimulus manipulation-levels differences in verbal reaction time (RTd) and word duration (Wdd) for individual subjects who stutter (S#) and who do not stutter (N#) for the simple reaction time task (SRT) and the choice reaction time task (CRT) regarding Cluster (2C minus 1C), Stress location (2nd Syl minus 1st Syl), Frequency (low minus high), and Word size (2 syl minus 1 syl).

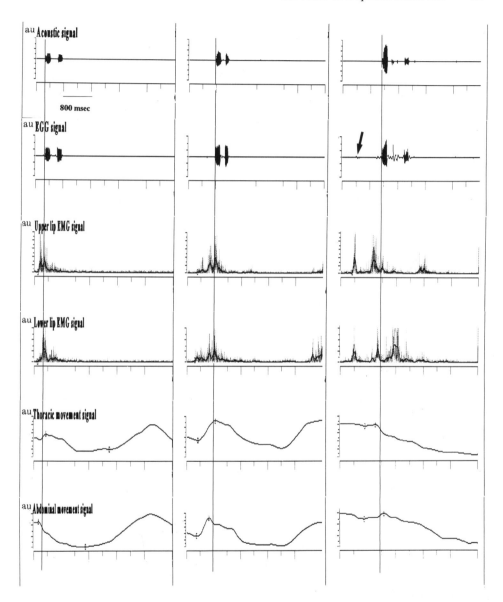

Figure 2. Examples of a perceptually fluent token of the nonword ['m k.s t] for a normal speaker (left part of the figure), and two persons who stutter (middle and right part of the figure). From top to bottom are displayed: acoustic signal, EGG signal, upper lip EMG (including integrated EMG signal shown in dark line overlaying grey colored rectified raw EMG), lower lip EMG (see upper lip), thoracic movement signal, and abdominal movement signal. Vertical lines indicate line-up point of onset speech. The arrow in the EGG signal of the right part of the figure shows the onset of a laryngeal block (See text for more details).

subjects (middle and right part) in a simple reaction time-task. The fluent speaker shows adequate motor control in the synchronization of upper lip and lower lip IEMG and the asynchronous onset of expiratory movements as seen in the thoracic and abdominal wall displacement signals. The asynchronous timing of these onsets for expiration displays the same event as described earlier by Baken et al. (1979), which was attributed to a control mechanism for regulating ventilatory pressures prior and during phonation. For the person who stutters in the middle part of Figure 2, it can be seen that his speech onset is delayed, compared to the control speaker. This delay most likely is related to a similar delay in the onset and duration of his inspiration movements, as well as in the onset and peak EMG latency of upper and lower lip muscle activity. The sequence of events is normal. This pattern is also described by Van Lieshout et al. (1996a), and attributed to the use of a particular type of motor control strategy, in which a stronger emphasis than normally is placed on incoming sensory information to update input to the verbal motor effector system.

A different pattern is seen for the second person who stutters (right part of Figure 2). Although like the other two subjects his speech output was classified perceptually as fluent, there are clear instances of non-adequate motor behavior. In the IEMG signals there are early activations, paralleled by an unsuccessful attempt to start phonation (laryngeal block, see arrow in EGG signal) and delays in the onset of expiration, including a reversed sequence (as compared to normal speaker and other stutterer) of abdominal and thoracic onset. Similar inadequacies in terms of motor control can also be found in his dysfluent speech, suggesting that there is some kind of (individual) threshold that determines whether or not inadequacies in motor behavior will generate a perceptually nonfluent speech output (cf. Peters & Boves, 1988; Peters et al., 1995). Of course, much more data are needed to test this and other assumptions and to validate the observations on the few subjects used thus far. But, to us it is obvious that these kind of data will help to improve our diagnostic tools with respect to the source(s) of stuttering behavior and the type of therapy that could or should be used.

NOTE

[1]   The data for NS2 were discarded, since he made too many errors in assigning stress to the indicated syllable.

REFERENCES

Baken, R.J., Cavallo, S.A., & Weissman, K.L. (1979). Chest wall movements prior to phonation. *Journal of Speech and Hearing Research, 22,* 862-872.
Levelt, W.J.M. (1989). *Speaking: From intention to articulation.* Cambridge, MA: MIT Press.
Levelt, W.J.M., & Wheeldon, L. (1994). Do speakers have access to a mental syllabary? *Cognition, 50,* 239-269.
Peters, H.F.M., & Boves, L. (1988). Coordination of aerodynamic and phonatory processes in fluent

speech utterances of stutterers. *Journal of Speech and Hearing Research, 31*, 352-361.

Peters, H.F.M., Hulstijn, W., & Starkweather, C.W. (1989). Acoustic and physiological reaction times of stutterers and nonstutterers. *Journal of Speech and Hearing Research, 32*, 668-680.

Peters, H.F.M., Hietkamp, R.K., & Boves, L. (1995). Aerodynamic and phonatory processes in dysfluent speech utterances of stutterers. In C.W. Starkweather and H.F.M. Peters (Eds.), *Proceedings First World Congress on Fluency Disorders* (Volume I), International Fluency Association Publication. Nijmegen, The Netherlands: University Press.

Peters, H.F.M., Hulstijn, W., & Van Lieshout, P.H.H.M. (1995). Toward a Nijmegen Speech Motor Test. In C.W. Starkweather, & H.F.M. Peters (Eds.), *Stuttering: Proceedings of the first world congress on fluency disorders* (pp. 15-18). The International Fluency Association: Nijmegen University Press.

Van Lieshout, P.H.H.M. (1995). *Motor planning and articulation in fluent speech of stutterers and nonstutterers.* Unpublished Doctoral dissertation (NICI Technical Report 95-07), University of Nijmegen, The Netherlands.

Van Lieshout, P.H.H.M., Hulstijn, W., & Peters, H.F.M. (1996a). Speech production in people who stutter: Testing the motor plan assembly hypothesis. *Journal of Speech and Hearing Research, 39*, 76-92.

Van Lieshout, P.H.H.M., Hulstijn, W., & Peters, H.F.M. (1996b). From planning to articulation in speech production: What differentiates a person who stutters from a person who does not stutter? *Journal of Speech and Hearing Research, 39*, 546-564.

Speech Production: Motor Control, Brain Research and Fluency Disorders
W. Hulstijn, H.F.M. Peters and P.H.H.M. Van Lieshout, editors

Chapter 44

LINGUISTIC STRESS AND THE RHYTHM EFFECT IN STUTTERING

Ann Packman, Mark Onslow, Janis van Doorn

The authors have developed a proximal model of stuttering that links stuttering to the variability of linguistic stress. One prediction of the model is that stuttering is suppressed in speaking conditions that reduce the variability of syllabic stress. Ten stuttering adults and ten matched controls spoke under control conditions, a slow rate condition, and a rhythmic speech condition. Variability of syllabic stress, as measured by the standard deviation of vowel duration, decreased during rhythmic speech as did stuttering. This reduction in variability was independent of reduction in speech rate. The findings support the model.

INTRODUCTION

For centuries, people have recognised the beneficial effects on stuttering of speaking in rhythm (for reviews see Ingham, 1984; Wingate, 1976). Rhythmic speech is one of the most effective of the ameliorative speaking conditions and the rhythm effect has been so widely and consistently verified that Wingate (1976) referred to it as universal. However, despite considerable theoretical and empirical investigation, the rhythm effect has never been explained.

A new model of stuttering (Packman et al., 1996) provides a possible explanation for the beneficial effects of rhythmic speech on stuttering. Zimmermann (1980) suggested that the speech motor systems of people who stutter are unstable and are therefore more easily perturbed by variability. The variability model (Vmodel) proposed by Packman et al. (1996) suggests that speaking in rhythm suppresses stuttering by reducing the perturbing effects on the speech motor system of variable syllabic stress. Reduction in the variability of syllabic stress has already been identified as a feature of prolonged-speech, another novel speech pattern that suppresses stuttering (see Onslow et al., 1992; Packman et al., 1994). In those studies, vowel duration (VD) was measured during perceptually stutter-free speech and was found to be less variable during prolonged-speech; that is, the standard deviation of VD was reduced during prolonged-speech. Vowel duration is one acoustic correlate of linguistic stress (Crystal & House, 1988a) and thus, it was argued, prolonged-speech involves a reduction in stress contrasts.

A number of writers have suggested that reduced stress contrasts are a feature of rhythmic speech (Andrews & Harris, 1964; Starkweather, 1987; Wingate, 1976; 1981); however, there is no empirical support for the idea. Accordingly, the aims of the present study were to provide such empirical evidence and, at the same time, test a prediction of the Vmodel. The main hypothesis of the study is that rhythmic speech reduces the variability of syllabic stress. Ingham and Andrews (1971) found that stutterers were unable to use syllable-timed speech at normal speech rates. Thus the present study includes a reduced rate condition as well as a rhythmic speech condition so that differential effects on variability of the two conditions can be determined. The study did not set out to compare a stuttering group with a group of matched controls but rather to (a) demonstrate with a group of individuals who stutter that the rhythm effect is accompanied by reduction in variability of VD, and (b) demonstrate in a group of normally fluent speakers, without the confound of stuttering, the effects of slowing down and rhythmic speech on variability of VD.

METHOD

Subjects

Subjects were 10 adults who stutter and 10 controls matched for age, sex and educational level. The mean age of the stuttering subjects was 25 years (range 18-42 years) and of the nonstuttering subjects was 25 years (range 18 -39 years). There were two women and eight men in each group. Twenty four subjects originally participated in the study. However, the investigator judged that two stuttering subjects and two nonstuttering subjects did not use rhythmic speech correctly and so they were excluded from the investigation.

Instrumentation

Subjects sat alone in a sound-treated booth for all speaking conditions. Speech was recorded with a Beyer Dynamic microphone M88N(C), at a microphone-to-mouth distance of 15 cm, on to one track of a Sony DAT recorder (TCD D10 PRO). In the rhythmic speech condition, customised software on an IBM 386 PC provided a rhythmic stimulus of 190 beats per minute which was delivered to the subject through an earpiece. The investigator listened to the subject's speech through headphones and conversed with the subject through an intercom system.

Speaking conditions

Each subject spoke under two control conditions (CONTROL 1, CONTROL 2), a reduced speech rate condition (SLOW) and a rhythmic speech condition (RHYTHM). The order of conditions was CONTROL 1, SLOW, CONTROL 2 and RHYTHM and was the same for all subjects. The RHYTHM condition was placed last because of the possibility of carry-over of the rhythm effect to other speaking conditions (see Andrews et al., 1982). To counteract a possible order effect there was a break of approximately one week between SLOW and CONTROL 2. Each condition was a 5-min session during which each subject spoke in continuous monologue. At 30-s intervals during SLOW the investigator said "remember to slow down" over the intercom. The timer for the session was deactivated during this instruction. Prior to RHYTHM, the investigator modelled syllable-timed (ST) speech and the subject practised it for 10 min. The subject was instructed to say each syllable in time to the computer beat and to pause normally, for example to take a breath. An independent judge later confirmed from the audiotape recordings that the subjects used ST speech satisfactorily during RHYTHM.

Speech rate and stuttering measures

From the audiotape recordings, the investigator measured speech rate in syllables per minute (SPM) and stuttering in percent syllables stuttered (%SS) using a two-button electronic counter-timer device (see Packman et al., 1994, for details). The SPM measures included pauses. Intrarater and interrater reliability of %SS and SPM measures was calculated on 10% of the data. Differences in the rate-rerate %SS scores were all less than one percentage point and differences in the investigator and independent %SS scores were all less than three percentage points. None of the differences in SPM scores were more than 10%. Correlation coefficients for the pairs of SPM scores were 1.0 (rate-re-rate) and .95 (investigator and independent scores).

Acoustic measures

The investigator measured VD from the audiotape recordings of SLOW, CONTROL 2 and RHYTHM for the 10 nonstuttering subjects, and of CONTROL 2 and RHYTHM for the 10 stuttering subjects. Measures were made from only one CONTROL condition because there were no significant differences in either SPM or %SS scores for these two conditions (see *Results*). Vowel duration was not measured in SLOW for the stuttering group because there was no significant difference in SPM across conditions in this group (see *Results*). The investigator made the VD measures from the speech waveforms displayed on a Kay DSP Sona-Graph 5500 using the procedure described in Onslow et al. (1992) and Packman et al. (1994). All measurable vowels that were perceptually stutter-free were measured. The reliability of the investigator's judgment that vowels were perceptually stutter-free was assessed by having an independent clinician mark perceived stutterings on an orthographic transcript of the middle minute of each CONTROL 2 session for each stuttering subject. Of the 232 vowels that had been measured in these minutes by the investigator, only 5 (2.2%) were judged to be stuttered by the independent clinician.

RESULTS

Speech rate and stuttering measures

All subjects spoke in almost continuous monologue. A repeated measures ANOVA for the *stuttering group* showed no significant difference in SPM across conditions, $F(2,18) = 3.21$. However, it is difficult to interpret this result because it is confounded by stuttering. Friedman's analysis of variance by ranks was used to analyse %SS because many of the scores were zero. This analysis showed significant differences in %SS scores across speaking conditions, $Xr^2 (2) = 21.09$, $p < .01$. The mean ranks for the conditions were 3.45, 2.20,

3.25, and 1.10 respectively. Clearly, there was little difference between the ranking of %SS scores for the two CONTROL conditions, the %SS scores for SLOW were clearly ranked lower than those for the CONTROL conditions, and the %SS scores for RHYTHM were clearly ranked lower than those for SLOW. The means for SPM and %SS measures for CONTROL2, SLOW and RHYTHM are presented in Table 1.

The SPM measures for the *nonstuttering group* are not confounded by stuttering and so indicate how the experimental conditions influenced overall speech rate. A repeated measures ANOVA showed a significant effect across conditions, $F(2,18) = 34.54, p < .01$. A Scheffe test showed that the means of SPM for the two experimental conditions were significantly lower than for the CONTROL2 condition, $p < .01$, and that there was no significant difference between the two experimental conditions. In other words, as a group the subjects slowed down significantly, and to the same extent, in both SLOW and RHYTHM. The means for SPM measures for CONTROL2, SLOW and RHYTHM are presented in Table 1.

Acoustic measures

The means, SD, and number (and ranges) of measures for VD for the *stuttering group* across the speaking conditions are presented in Table 1. The mean of VD for RHYTHM was significantly greater than the mean of VD for CONTROL 2, $t = 7.23, p < .01$, df = 9 and the mean SD of VD for RHYTHM was significantly less than the mean SD for CONTROL 2, $t = 4.75, p < .01$, df = 9.

The means, SD, and number (and ranges) of measures for VD for the *nonstuttering group* across the speaking conditions are presented in Table 1. A repeated measures ANOVA showed a significant effect in VD across conditions, $F(2,18) = 20.79, p < .01$. A Sheffe test showed that VDs were significantly longer in SLOW and RHYTHM than in CONTROL 2, $p < .01$, but that there was no significant difference in VD between the two experimental conditions. For SD, there was a significant effect across conditions, $F(2,18) = 35.1, p < .01$. Mean of SDs in RHYTHM was significantly smaller than in both CONTROL 2, $p < .01$, and SLOW, $p < .01$, and mean SD in SLOW was significantly greater than in CONTROL 2, $p < .05$.

Table 1.   Means for speech rate, stuttering, and VD measures for the two groups across three conditions.

| | Stuttering group | | | Stuttering group | | |
	Control	Slow	Rhythm	Control	Slow	Rhythm
SPM	116	95	117	224	154	140
%SS	10.8	9.5	1.2	-	-	-
VD (ms)	102.3	-	135.4	81.3	98.1	111.4
SD of VD (ms)	64.7	-	41.2	55.9	67.0	36.9
No.(and range)	161	-	191	281	238	245
of VD Measures	(26-298)	-	(98-236)	(181-441)	(164-395)	(139-355)

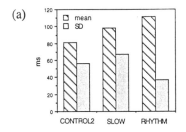 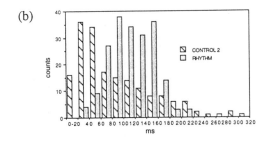

Figure 1. Mean VD and SD of VD for the nonstuttering group in CONTROL2,SLOW and RHYTHM (a), and the distribution of VD for a nonstuttering subject in CONTROL2 and RHYTHM (b)

The effects of slowing down and speaking in rhythm, without the confound of stuttering, are shown in Figure 1. Figure 1(a) summarises the effect of SLOW and RHYTHM on VD for the nonstuttering group. The findings of Crystal and House (1988b) suggest that SD should increase as VD increases and this indeed occurred in SLOW. However, it is clear that RHYTHM had the opposite effect on SD. In other words, although subjects slowed down and increased VD in RHYTHM, variability decreased rather than increased, as would have been expected. The effect of RHYTHM on the distribution of VD for a typical control subject, N5, is shown in Figure 1b. The positively skewed (1.35) distribution of VD in CONTROL resembles that of other normal speakers reported by Crystal and House (1988a) while in RHYTHM, the distribution of VD is smaller and less skewed (.07).

CONCLUSIONS

A prediction of the Vmodel — that variability of syllabic stress reduces during rhythmic speech — was confirmed by the findings of the present study. The use of a control group in the present study meant that the effects on linguistic stress of rhythmic speech could be studied free from the effects of changes in stuttering. The reduction in variability during rhythmic speech was independent of a reduction in speech rate because variability should have increased rather than decreased with the decrease in speech rate. The findings also provide empirical support for previous suggestions that reduced stress contrasts are a feature of rhythmic speech.

NOTES

This research was conducted when Ann Packman and Mark Onslow were affiliated with the School of Communication Disorders, The University of Sydney.

REFERENCES

Andrews, G., & Harris, M. (1964). *The syndrome of stuttering*. London: Heinemann.

Andrews G., Howie, P. M., Dosza, M., & Guitar, B. (1982). Stuttering: Speech pattern characteristics under fluency-inducing conditions. *Journal of Speech and Hearing Research, 25,* 208-216.

Crystal, T.H., & House, A.S. (1988a). Segmental durations in connected-speech signals: Syllabic stress. *Journal of the Acoustical Society of America, 83,* 1574-1585.

Crystal, T.H., & House, A.S. (1988b). A note on the variability of timing control. *Journal of Speech and Hearing Research, 31,* 497-502.

Ingham, R.J. (1984). *Stuttering and behavior therapy: Current status and experimental foundations*. San Diego: College-Hill.

Ingham, R.J. & Andrews, G. (1971). Stuttering: The quality of fluency after treatment. *Journal of Communication Disorders, 4,* 277-288.

Onslow, M., van Doorn, J., & Newman, D. (1992). Variability of acoustic segment durations after prolonged-speech treatment for stuttering. *Journal of Speech and Hearing Research, 35,* 529-536.

Packman, A., Onslow, M., Richard, F., & van Doorn, J. (1996). Syllabic stress and variability: A model of stuttering. *Journal of Clinical Linguistics and Phonetics.* (in press).

Packman, A., Onslow, M., & van Doorn, J. (1994). Prolonged-speech and modification of stuttering: Perceptual, acoustic and electroglottographic data. *Journal of Speech and Hearing Research, 37,* 724-734.

Starkweather, C.W. (1987). *Fluency and stuttering*. Englewood Cliffs, NJ: Prentice-Hall.

Wingate, M.E. (1976). *Stuttering: Theory and treatment*. New York: Irvington Publishers Inc.

Wingate, M.E. (1981). Sound and pattern in artificial fluency: Spectrographic evidence. *Journal of Fluency Disorders, 6,* 95-118.

Zimmermann, G.N. (1980). Stuttering: A disorder of movement. *Journal of Speech and Hearing Research, 23,* 122-136.

Speech Production: Motor Control, Brain Research and Fluency Disorders
W. Hulstijn, H.F.M. Peters and P.H.H.M. Van Lieshout, editors

Chapter 45

PROSODIC DISTURBANCES IN STUTTERING ADULTS

Lutz Jäncke, Anne Bauer, Karl-Theodor Kalveram

Two experiments were conducted in order to investigate whether stutterers exhibit difficulties to produce changing prosodic patterns flexibly. In experiment 1, 15 adult stutterers had to utter the testword /tatatas/ repeatedly with stress on the second syllable (block1). In the following blocks 2 and 3, subjects were required to shift stress from the second to the first syllable. This demand to utter the testword with a different metric structure evoked an increase in stuttering frequency (from 2% of dysfluent words in block 1 to 20% in block 2). In experiment 2, 10 adult stutterers and 10 adult nonstutterers had to utter the testword /papapas/ repeatedly with stress on the second syllable. In one experimental condition, subjects were unexpectedly required to shift stress from the second to the first syllable, while in another experimental condition, they were unexpectedly required to shift stress from the second to the third syllable. In contrast to nonstutterers, stutterers were generally unable or deficient in switching stress immediately from one syllable to another with respect to the suprasegmental aspects of prosody (duration, intensity, and F_0). These results are interpreted as supporting the view of stuttering as a prosodic disturbance.

INTRODUCTION

Wingate (1979, 1984) developed an influential view of stuttering as a 'prosodic defect' manifested as an intermittent disorder of actualizing stress increase. Thus, stuttering is viewed as a defect in the transition to stressed syllables. Although this view is broadly discussed in many textbooks on stuttering there is a considerable lack of empirical work on this topic. Among the few studies investigating possible deficiencies in speech prosody in stutterers are those of Bergmann (1986) and ours (Jäncke, 1991; Kalveram & Jäncke, 1989). Bergmann demonstrated that stuttering frequency decreased while stutterers were reading poems comprising a metric structure. Our own research demonstrated an extraordinary strong 'audiophonatoric coupling' (APC) in stutterers. This atypical strong APC was thought to be the result of the deficiency in switching the APC according to the stress pattern.

The present study was designed to further investigate possible prosodic defects in stutterers. First, we evaluated whether the unexpected demand to change intra-word stress might increase stuttering frequency (experiment 1). Second, we examined whether the stutterers were able to adapt their pattern of suprasegmental measures (duration, intensity, and fundamental frequency) to an unexpectedly changing stress pattern (experiment 2). We hypothesized that nonstutterers would be able to change the suprasegmental measures according to the required stress pattern while stutterers would not accomplish the necessary suprasegmental shifts as precisely as the nonstutterers even in fluent utterances.

EXPERIMENT 1

Subjects

Fifteen adult native German speaking stutterers (mean age/SD in years: 35/7, 9 female and 6 male) participated in this study. According to the 'Stuttering Severity Instrument' (SSI) of Riley (1972), 6 stutterers were judged as mild, 5 as moderate and 4 as severe. All stutterers had previously participated in various speech-related therapies. However, none of these therapies were conducted in the last two years before the experiment. All stutterers had no known neurological or hearing disorder and were paid for their participation.

Speech task

Subjects had to utter the meaningless testword /tatatas/ in two different speech rates (fast, slow) and two different stress patterns. These two stress patterns were: 1.) baseline stress condition (first and third syllable unstressed and second syllable stressed) and 2.) experimental condition (first syllable stressed and second and third syllable unstressed). Before each utterance, the prosodic pattern was prescribed by a sequence of three sine tones, each tone representing the duration of one syllable. The duration of tones indicating unstressed syllables was 150 ms (fast speech rate) and 200 ms (slow speech rate). The duration of tones indicating stressed syllables was 300 ms (fast) and 400 ms (slow). These tone durations were applied since previous experiments have demonstrated that they were appropriate to evoke the required speech rates and stress patterns (Jäncke, 1994; Kalveram & Jäncke, 1989). Subjects were instructed to listen to the tones which were presented via loudspeaker and then to utter the testword in the prescribed speech rate and stress pattern. Prior to the experiment, the subjects were required to utter the testword in the three stress conditions. The experimenter immediately gave feedback whether the subjects placed stress correctly on one of the three syllables. We chose the stress pattern with stress on the second syllable as baseline stress condition because we have the impression that this pattern is more convenient for German speakers than the other patterns. The experimental section was divided into three blocks. In block 1 the testword was uttered under baseline stress condition while in blocks 2 and 3 the testword had to be uttered under the experimental stress condition. All three blocks were realized once with fast or normal speech rate. The order of speech rate was randomized across subjects. Each block comprised 50 trials resulting in a total of 300 trials (150 trials for each speech rate).

Data acquisition and analysis

During the experiment, subjects were seated in a sound-isolated chamber. They had to speak into a microphone that was placed 15 cm in front of their head. Experimental control was managed by a laboratory computer (VME-bus computer ELTEC Eurocom 7). The acoustic speech output was recorded on a high-quality audio tape recorder and off-line evaluated for speech dysfluencies by a trained phonetician (L.J.). The frequency of stuttering events was measured and subjected to statistical evaluation.

RESULTS

Stuttering frequency was calculated for each block and summed across both speech rates because prior data inspection revealed no substantial influence of this factor on stuttering frequency. Thus, a total of 100 speech trials was the basis for calculating stuttering frequency in the each of the three blocks. We found that stuttering frequency significantly increased from baseline (block 1) to block 2 (Wilcoxon matched pairs sign rank test, $p < .001$). In block 3 we also found an increased stuttering frequency compared to block 1 ($p < .05$) but this increase was smaller than for block 2 ($p < .05$) (Table 1).

EXPERIMENT 2

Subjects

Ten adult stutterers (mean age/SD in years: 34/7, 6 female and 4 male) participated in this study. According to the SSI, 4 stutterers were judged as mild, 5 as moderate and 1 as severe. All stutterers had previously participated in various speech-related therapies. However, none of these therapies were conducted in the last two years before the experiment. The control group consisted of 10 normal speaking adults, (34/6, 6 female and 4 male). All subjects were native German speakers and none of them had a known neurological or hearing disorder. All subjects were paid for their participation.

Speech task

Subjects had to utter the meaningless testword /papapas/ in two different speech rates (fast, slow) and three different stress patterns. These three stress patterns were: 1.) baseline stress condition (first and third syllable unstressed and second syllable stressed), 2.) stress condition A (first syllable stressed and second and third syllable unstressed), and 3.) stress condition B (third syllable stressed, first and second syllable unstressed). As in experiment 1 the prosodic pattern was prescribed by a sequence of three sine tones, each tone representing the duration of one syllable. The duration of tones indicating unstressed syllables was 150 ms (fast speech rate) and 200 ms (slow speech rate). The duration of tones indicating

Table 1. Median and range of stuttering frequency for the three blocks. Stuttering frequency was pooled across speech rates (fast and normal).

	Median	Range
block 1 (baseline)	2%	0-10%
block 2 (1. block requiring the changed stressed pattern)	20%	5%-38%
block 3 (2. block requiring the changed stressed pattern)	7%	5%-15%

stressed syllables was 300 ms (fast) and 400 ms (slow). Experimental procedure and instructions to the subjects were similar as in experiment 1.

The experimental section was divided into blocks. Each block comprised the initial repeated utterance of the testword under baseline stress condition followed by uttering the testword under one of the stress conditions A or B. Speech rate was held constant within each block but randomized across blocks. Each block was repeated 5 times with randomized order for each subject. The frequency of utterances under baseline stress condition ranged randomly from 2 to 8. Hereafter, the prescribing tone sequence changed (without announcement) and then was presented five times, requiring the subjects to speak repeatedly in a new stress pattern (stress condition A or B). This procedure was introduced in order to make the point in time when changing in stress was required more unforseeable.

Data acquisition and analysis

During the experiment, subjects were seated in a sound-isolated chamber. They had to speak into a microphone that was placed 15 cm in front of their head. Experimental control, the delivering of the tones and the storage of data was managed by a laboratory computer. The acoustic speech signal was off-line lowpass-filtered (400 Hz, 24 dB/octave), rectified and again lowpass-filtered (40 Hz, 24 dB/octave) resulting in the phonation signal. The filtered and rectified data were digitized at a rate of 1000 Hz (12 bit resolution), stored in computer memory, and afterwards automatically analyzed by a computer algorithm. In addition, fundamental frequency (F_0) was calculated off-line from the stored acoustic speech signal applying the auto-correlation algorithm proposed by Rabiner and Shafer (1978). For each trial, the mean duration and amplitude of phonation as well as the mean F_0 for each syllable were calculated. Furthermore, the computer was instructed to reject all speech responses with fewer than three phonations and speech responses which do not fit into a prescribed time frame of duration of phonation. After this automatic preselection, the remaining responses were rated as to whether they showed any further perceptual dysfluencies. None were detected. Then the respective means and standard deviations for baseline and experimental conditions were computed separately for stutterers and nonstutterers.

RESULTS

Initial tests (by means of nonparametrical analysis) revealed no strong differences between stutterers and nonstutterers with respect to the suprasegmental measures (duration, intensity, and F_0). The only exception was that stressed phonations were produced with shorter duration in stutterers than in nonstutterers while they were speaking slowly ($p < .01$). In addition, we confirmed that the suprasegmental measures varied according to speech rate and stress pattern. Stressed phonations were produced with longer durations, higher F_0, and larger intensity (all p-values $< .01$). Fast speech rate was mainly realized by decreasing durations of phonation. F_0 and intensity of phonation was mainly unaffected by speech rate.

The main question of the present experiment was whether stutterers replace an intra-word stress pattern by another pattern with similar precision as nonstutterers? In order to answer this question we calculated for each syllable separately the difference between the duration of phonation under baseline condition (stress on the second syllable) and the duration of phonation under the stress conditions A or B. These difference scores are depicted in Figures 1 to 3. As can be seen on these Figures, when stress A is required, nonstutterers change the suprasegmental measures according to the required stress pattern (all p-values <0.01). The second syllable is getting shorter, generated with reduced intensity and F_0 while the first syllable is getting longer, generated with increased intensity and F_0. Analogues, when stress pattern B is required, nonstutterers change the suprasegmental measures with changing stress pattern (all p-values <0.01). The second syllable is getting shorter, generated with reduced intensity and F_0 while the third syllable is getting longer, generated with increased intensity and F_0. Stutterers, on the other hand, changed the suprasegmental measures either to a lesser extent than nonstutterers (*duration*: stress A fast and slow speech rate; *intensity*: stress A slow speech rate; F_0: stress A: fast and slow speech rate) or they were unable to install the new stress pattern (*duration*: stress B fast and slow speech rate; *intensity*: stress B slow speech rate; F_0: stress B: fast and slow speech rate). These results were confirmed by nonparametrical analysis (Mann-Whitney U-tests).

Furthermore, we were able to demonstrate that stutterers do generally not speak monotonously in a pattern of reduced variability in suprasegmental measures.

In order to evaluate whether stuttering severity affects the present results, we inspected the individual data and found that the severe stutterer revealed a pattern of speech measures

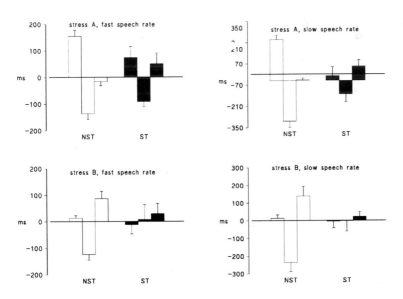

Figure 1. Mean *change of duration of phonation* (in msec) from baseline to the two stress conditions (A and B). A positive value indicates an increase and a negative value a decrease in duration. □: indicates nonstutterers, ■: indicates stutterers. The first bar of each subfigure represents the 1.syllable, the 2. bar the 2. syllable, and the 3. bar the 3. syllable. Vertical lines indicate standard deviations.

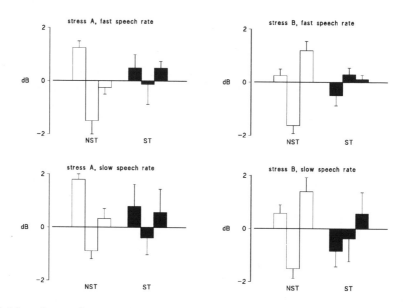

Figure 2. Mean *change of intensity of phonation* (in dB) from baseline to the two stress conditions (A and B). A positive value indicates an increase and a negative value a decrease in intensity. □: indicates nonstutterers, ■: indicates stutterers. The first bar of each subfigure represents the 1.syllable, the 2. bar the 2. syllable, and the 3. bar the 3. syllable. Vertical lines indicate standard deviations.

similar as it was found for the entire stutterer group, thus, mitigating the possibility that the observed effects are a function of stuttering severity.

DISCUSSION

While nonstutterers were able to change quickly their stress pattern in terms of the suprasegmental measures, stutterers showed some problems in performing this stress adaptation. First, the unexpected demand to change intra-word stress increased stuttering frequency. Second, when speaking fluent the stress adaptation was accompanied only by small, inappropriate or no shifts in the suprasegmental measures. There was no strong difference between stutterers and nonstutterers with regard to suprasegmental measures for the baseline stress condition. Strong differences only emerged when a change in intra-word stress was required.

These results support the hypothesis of stuttering as a prosodic disturbance (Bergmann, 1986; Wingate, 1984; Wingate, 1979). These authors demonstrated that stuttering episodes were located mainly on stressed syllables. In addition, unexpected changes in prosodic structure increased stuttering frequency whereas a foreseeable prosodic structure as in poems with regular meter reduced stuttering frequency (Bergmann, 1986). In the light of these results, stuttering can be described as a 'prosodic defect' manifested as an intermittent disorder of actualizing stress increase and stress change.

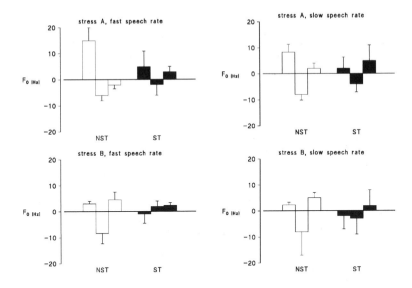

Figure 3. Mean *change of fundamental frequency* (in Hz) from baseline to the two stress conditions (A and B). A positive value indicates an increase and a negative value a decrease in fundamental frequency. □: indicates nonstutterers, ■: indicates stutterers. The first bar of each subfigure represents the 1.syllable, the 2. bar the 2. syllable, and the 3. bar the 3. syllable. Vertical lines indicate standard deviations.

When emphasizing prosody as one of the major factors in stuttering one has to consider that stressed syllables are important features for many aspects associated with speech production: First, stressed speech elements are central for the timing structure of utterances (Kalveram, 1991a; Kalveram, 1991b; Fowler, 1986; Dauer, 1983; Martin et al., 1975). On the basis of current knowledge of speech motor timing it is most likely to assume that the succession of stressed syllables determine some kind of time or rhythm frame in which the unstressed syllables are embedded. Even for two or three-syllabic words with only one stressed syllable the position of the stressed syllable within the word affects the surrounding unstressed syllables (Kalveram, 1991a; Kalveram, 1991b; Faure et al., 1980). Second, there is considerable evidence that emotional expression in speech is mainly executed with stressed syllables (Ladd et al., 1985). Furthermore, certain aspects of the stress structure are essential for the linguistic functions of intonation as well as for the pragmatic and emotional functions of intonation. Because of the relative importance of stress structures for communication, these elements of speech require adequate control on the part of the speaker. If we assume a close link between emotional and motoric disturbances while speaking it is reasonable to expect disfluencies to occur at these central points of stress. Thus, one can speculate about an interaction between emotional states and the motoric execution of stressed syllables mediated by person-dependent and communication-related psychological factors.

Because of the tight link between intra-word stress and stuttering frequency and the fact that stress is mainly realized by variation in duration, intensity and pitch of phonation, the physiological mechanisms for the production of the phonation are becoming more important in elucidating stuttering causes. Thus, it should be more valuable in future studies to examine phonatory processes, i.e. subglottal airpressure build-up (Peters & Boves, 1988), and coordination of phonation with articulation (Perkins et al., 1976) than to look for specific articulatory disturbances in stutterers.

REFERENCES

Bergmann, G. (1986). Studies in stuttering as a prosodic disturbance. *Journal of Speech and Hearing Research*, *29*, 290-300.

Dauer, R.M. (1983). Stress-timing and syllable-timing reanalyzed. *Journal of Phonetics*, *11*, 51-63.

Faure, G., Hirst, D.J., & Chafcouloff, M. (1980). Rhythm in English: Isochronism, pitch, and percieved stress. In L.R. Waugh & C.H. Schooneveld (Eds.), *The melody of language*. (pp. 71-79). Baltimore: University Park Press.

Fowler, C. (1986). An event approach to the study of speech perception from a direct-realist perspective. *Journal of Phonetics*, *14*, 3-28.

Jäncke, L. (1991). The "audio-phonatoric coupling" in stuttering and nonstuttering adults: Experimental contributions. In H.F.M. Peters, A. Hulstijn, & C.W. Starkweather (Eds.), *Speech Motor Control and Stuttering*. (pp. 171-180). Amsterdam: Elsevier Scientific Publishers.

Jäncke, L. (1994). Variability and duration of voice onset time and phonation in stuttering and nonstuttering adults. *Journal of Fluency Disorders*, *19*, 21-37.

Kalveram, K.T. (1991a). Sensumotorik des Sprechens oder Wie man "ta-ta-tas" spricht und gegebenenfalls dabei stottert The perceptual motor processes of speech, or how one utters "ta-ta-tas" and sometimes stutters when doing it. *Psychologische Beitraege*, *33*, 94-121 Note: Erscheint.

Kalveram, K.T. (1991b). How pathological audio-phonatoric coupling induces stuttering: A model of speech flow control. In H.F.M. Peters, W.H. Hulstijn, & C.W. Starkweather (Eds.), *Speech motor control and stuttering*. (pp. 117-122). Amsterdam: Elsevier Science Publishers.

Kalveram, K.T., & Jäncke, L. (1989). Vowel duration and voice onset time for stressed and nonstressed syllables in stutterers under delayed auditory feedback condition. *Folia Phoniatrica et Logopaedica*, *41*, 30-42.

Ladd, D.R., Silverman, K.E.A., Tolkmitt, F., Bergmann, G., & Scheerer, K.R. (1985). Evidence for the independent function of intonation contour type, voice quality, and F_0 range in signalling speaker affect. *Journal of the Acoustical Society of America*, *78*, 435-444.

Martin, R., St Louis, K., Haroldson, S., & Hasbrouck, J. (1975). Punishment and negative reinforcement of stuttering using electric shock. *Journal of Speech and Hearing Research*, *18*, 478-490.

Perkins, W., Rudas, J., Johnson, L., & Bell, J. (1976). Stuttering: Discoordination of phonation with articulation and respiration. *Journal of Speech and Hearing Research*, *19*, 509-522.

Peters, H.F., & Boves, L. (1988). Coordination of aerodynamic and phonatory processes in fluent speech utterances of stutterers. *Journal of Speech and Hearing Research*, *31*, 352-361.

Rabiner, L., & Shafer, R. (1978). *Digital processing of speech signals*. Englewood Cliffs: Prentice-Hall.

Riley, G.D. (1972). A stuttering severity instrument for children and adults. *Journal of Speech and Hearing Research*, *37*, 314-322.

Wingate, M.E. (1979). The first three words. *Journal of Speech and Hearing Research*, *22*, 604-612.

Wingate, M.E. (1984). Stuttering as a prosodic disorder. In R. Curlee & W. Perkins (Eds.), *Nature and treatment of stuttering*. (pp. 215-235). San Diego: College-Hill.

Speech Production: Motor Control, Brain Research and Fluency Disorders
W. Hulstijn, H.F.M. Peters and P.H.H.M. Van Lieshout, editors

Chapter 46

INSTRUCTING STUTTERERS TO SING: EFFECT ON STUTTERING FREQUENCY AT TWO SPEAKING RATES

Helen Glover, Joseph Kalinowski, Andrew Stuart, Michael Rastatter

Singing as a fluency-enhancing mechanism is well established. The fluency derived by singing has been attributed to a reduced speech rate, memorized material, semantically reduced content, and/or an imposed rhythm. In this study, an attempt was made to control each of these conditions. Twelve participants who stutter were instructed to read or sing each of four different passages of prose under the following conditions: reading at a normal rate, reading at a fast rate, singing at a normal rate, and singing at a fast rate. Participants exhibited a statistically significant decrease in stuttering frequency (75% overall) while singing as compared to reading. There was no difference in stuttering frequency with rate conditions. Current findings suggest that stutterers are capable of internally generating fluent speech production by imposing some derivation of melody when asked simply to sing. There is no claim that these participants were singing, as skills and capabilities varied tremendously, only that participants achieved dramatic fluency enhancement after they were instructed to sing. Since fluency was maintained in both the normal and fast rates of production, alternatives to the traditional explanations cited above must be held accountable for these findings.

INTRODUCTION AND REVIEW OF THE LITERATURE

The fluency-enhancing effects of singing for stutterers is well documented (e.g., Fletcher, 1928; Bloodstein, 1950; Johnson & Rosen, 1937; Reid, 1946; Wingate, 1969; Healey et al., 1976; Colcord & Adams, 1979; Andrews et al., 1982; Starkweather, 1982; Andrews et al., 1983). Throughout the literature, however, there has not been universal agreement as to the underlying mechanisms that are responsible for fluency during singing. Wingate's (1969) proposal of a parsimonious explanation for conditions known to enhance fluency was "altered vocalization". He discounted the notion that fluent singing was due primarily to the effect of rhythm on the words. That is, "in singing, a person intentionally emphasizes vocalization to express a pattern of stresses centering on the syllable nuclei" (p. 680). Others have suggested that the rhythmic nature of singing is the main factor which induces fluency under this condition (e.g., Starkweather, 1982). In general, the fluency-enhancement associated with singing has been attributed to reduced speech rate, memorized material, semantically reduced content, and/or an imposed rhythm. The present study was designed to account and control for each of these alternative explanations for fluency during productions following instructions to sing.

To account for reduced speech rate, participants were instructed to sing at their normal rate and at a fast rate. If stutterers could sing fluently during the increased rate, this finding would contradict the notion that a reduced rate is responsible for the fluency. To the best of our knowledge, no one has asked stutterers to sing at both a normal and fast rate. We have recently reported that stutterers can produce fluent speech under conditions of delayed auditory feedback and frequency-altered feedback at both normal and fast rates of speech (Kalinowski et al., 1993; Hargrave et al., 1994; MacLeod et al., 1995; Kalinowski et al., 1996; Stuart et al., 1996). These studies provided evidence that a reduced speech rate is not required for enhancement of fluency under such conditions.

To control for memorized material (i.e., familiar words and/or melody of a song), passages of prose which were novel to the participants were utilized. Instructions were given to sing the passage, not by using a well-known melody, but instead by generating idiosyncratic sequences of pitches. Other studies of singing and stuttering have incorporated well-known songs. Typically a new set of lyrics made to fit the melody of a song such as "Home on the Range" were read and sung by the participants (although the researchers failed to validate that singing occurred). To control for any possible fluency-enhancing effects of a well-known melody or memorized words, it seemed intuitive that novel passages of prose be used rather than familiar songs.

Semantically, songs are often very simple and/or redundant. To control and account for the notion that a song's semantically-reduced content contributes significantly to any fluency enhancement during singing, this study employed prose rather than lyrical material. Further, no text was repeated within the passages.

Finally, to control for the influence of external rhythms on any fluency enhancement during singing, no instrumental accompaniment was present during the experiment. Further, any rhythmic beat which would be inherent in a well-known tune was also absent . Thus, any rhythms produced by the participants during the singing conditions were entirely internally generated.

METHODS

Twelve stutterers who were classified as moderate to severe (aged 18 to 47) served as participants. Each test session was video recorded. Participants were given instructions both via a demonstration videotape played at the beginning of each test session and the same instructions repeated aloud prior to each test condition. Participants read or sang aloud from different junior-high level passages of prose containing historical information at a normal and fast rate of production. (G. Sims, 1987, *Explorers*, Creative Teaching Press, Inc., and C. Taylor, 1985, *Inventions*, Creative Teaching Press, Inc.) Passages were randomized among participants while test conditions were counter-balanced. During the fast rates, subjects were instructed to go as fast as they could while remaining intelligible.

Following each condition, a five-point Likert scale was presented to the participants asking them to judge their singing performances. While this rating scale does not provide perceptual or acoustical measures of the singing performances, it does allow for some experiential verification from the participants that they were singing. All participants indicated that they felt they were in a singing mode during most, if not all of the singing tasks. That is, following instructions to sing the passages of prose, they subjectively reported experiencing singing. To the best of our knowledge, previous studies investigating stuttering and singing have not validated that participants were, in fact, singing on any level, perceptual, acoustic, or experiential.

Two trained graduate students determined stuttering frequency for the first 300 syllables of each passage from the recorded videotaped samples of all participants. Interjudge syllable-by-syllable agreement was determined to be .85, as indexed by Cohen's *kappa*. (Cohen's *kappa* values greater than .75 represent excellent agreement beyond chance.)

Speech rate was calculated from the audio track of each videotaped sample. Perceptually fluent portions containing 50 contiguous syllables were transferred onto the hard drive of a personal computer (Apple Model Power Macintosh 7100/80) via a videocassette deck (Samsung Model VR8705) interfaced with an analog to digital input/output board (Digidesign Model Audiomedia II NuBus). Sampling frequency was 10,000 Hz. Waveforms of the samples were generated by a commercially available speech and sound signal analysis application (InfoSignal Inc. Model Signalyze 3.0). The criterion of 50 contiguous fluent syllables was set to allow participants to "get up to speed" following a stuttering moment. In three and five normal and fast reading conditions, respectively, participants did not produce the required number of contiguous fluent syllables. In these cases, a minimum of 43 syllables was accepted. Duration of these samples was determined from the acoustic onset of the first syllable to the offset of the last syllable. Pauses greater than 100 ms within the samples were extracted. These pauses were usually audible inspirations at the ends of phrases and sentences. Speech rate, in syllables per second, was then determined by dividing the syllable count by the sample duration. (See Kalinowski et al., 1993, for a detailed explanation of the speech rate calculation procedure.)

RESULTS

Mean stuttering frequency as a function of speech mode (reading vs. singing) and speech rate condition (normal vs. fast) are presented in Figure 1. As the stuttering frequency data were positively skewed with unequal variances, a square root transformation was applied to the data prior to conducting inferential statistical analysis. A two-factor analysis of variance with repeated measures was then performed to investigate the effect of speech mode and speech rate condition on stuttering frequency. Only a significant main effect of speech mode was found ($p < .0001$). That is, participants exhibited a statistically significant 75% reduction in stuttering frequency for the singing conditions. No significant main effect of speech rate was found ($p > .05$), nor was there a significant speech mode by speech rate interaction ($p > .05$).

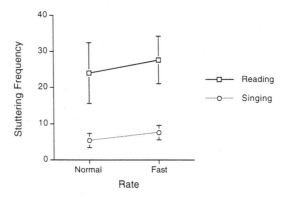

Figure 1. Mean stuttering frequencies (i.e., number of stuttering episodes/300 syllables) as a function of speech mode and speech rate conditions (*N* = 12). Error bars represent plus/minus one standard error.

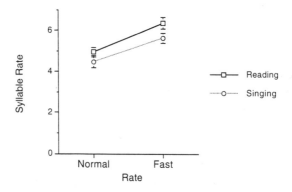

Figure 2. Mean speech rates (syllables/s) as a function of speech mode and speech rate conditions. Error bars represent plus/minus one standard error. *Note:* Means were calculated from 9, 7, 12, and 12 values for the normal reading, fast reading, normal singing, and fast singing conditions, respectively.

Mean speech rates (syllables/s) as a function of speech mode and speech rate condition are presented in Figure 2. A two-factor analysis of variance with repeated measures was also performed to investigate the effect of speech mode and speech rate condition on speech rate. Significant main effects of speech mode (p=.011) and speech rate condition (p<.0001) were found. The interaction of speech mode by speech rate condition was not significant (p>.05).

DISCUSSION

The most important finding of this study is that significant fluency enhancement occurred when participants followed instructions to sing at both fast and normal rates. The overall reduction in stuttering disfluencies observed here, however, is not as robust as that reported in other studies investigating the singing of common melodies. One may speculate the reason for such an occurrence was the inability of stutterers to remain in the "singing" mode during the current experiment.

It may also be noted that participants in the present experiment displayed faster rates of speech under the nonsinging conditions relative to the singing conditions under both the normal and fast rate conditions. This result may appear to support the notion that fluency enhancement during singing can be attributed, at least in part, to a reduction in speech rate. However, for two reasons, it seems unlikely that the reductions in rate shown in the singing conditions can be responsible for the enhancement of fluency which occurred in these conditions. First, even though the average syllable rate obtained under the fast singing conditions, (i.e., 5.6 syllables/s), was slower than that for the fast reading conditions, (i.e., 6.3 syllables/s), the average fast singing rate clearly exceeded values for normal conversational rates of between 4 to 5 syllables/sec. (e.g., Netsell, 1981; Pickett, 1980; Walker & Black, 1950). Second, the fast singing condition yielded fluency enhancement similar in magnitude to the normal singing condition, despite the significant increase in rate. Thus, our participants were able to sing at a fast rate and still show a substantial decrease in stuttering. This finding diminishes the notion that increases in vowel durations are responsible for increased fluency. Simply put, the current results showed significant improvement in fluency under the normal and the fast singing conditions, but not for the reading tasks.

While such findings are consistent, in part, with past studies showing the effects of singing on the frequency of stuttering, the current data also shadow the findings of investigations on exogenous fluency-enhancing conditions. Although there has been little general agreement as to the mechanisms that facilitate fluency in altered auditory feedback conditions (e.g., delayed auditory feedback and frequency-altered feedback) it is well documented that these stimulus-input conditions enhance fluency, regardless of speaking rate (Hargrave et al., 1994; MacLeod et al., 1995; Kalinowski et al., 1993).

Singing constitutes a self-generated enhancer of fluency that enables a stutterer to maintain a fluent speaking pattern without the implementation of a specific motoric strategy or altered auditory feedback. The current experimental paradigm required the subjects to self-generate the temporal and rhythmic sequences underlying their singing output, which differed across the subject pool. Singing sequences were idiosyncratic to each participant, allowing variation in the strategies used in the generation of melody. External, experimental influences on the encoding events underlying singing were eliminated. Also, the passages did not contain semantically reduced content or an imposed rhythm and were not memorized or sung with continuous phonation (variables held in the past to account for improved fluency of stutterers during singing).

Within the constraints of this experimental design, stutterers were capable of improving their fluency simply by imposing an idiosyncratic melodic structure on their speech. Consequently, one may speculate that some neuro-processing mechanism(s) may have been actuated, or on the other hand inhibited, to facilitate fluency. Alternatively, one may hypothesize that production of "singing-like speech has less timing and precision demands relative to reading. The appeal of the latter hypothesis is weak, however. Recall that participants were able to sing the prose at accelerated rates while maintaining intelligibility. This being the case, it is conceivable that timing and precision demands were increased, rather than reduced, during the fast singing conditions. Beyond speculation, attempts to identify the exact underlying mechanisms/processes of singing that induce fluency, based on these data alone, would be conjecture.

Finally, neuro-imaging techniques such as positron emission tomography (PET-scans), magnetic resonance imaging (MRI), and electroencephalography (EEG) are currently being applied in stuttering research. We are currently using topographic EEG mapping technology to investigate the neurophysiology of exogenous fluency-enhancing conditions (altered auditory feedback) in stuttering. Data from these experiments may help elucidate the mechanism(s) or process(es) underlying the events generating enhanced fluency during altered auditory feedback. Similar experimentation to test the neurophysiology of endogenous fluency-enhancing conditions (singing) may be of benefit in further understanding the aspect of singing or song-like speech which is responsible for enhancing the fluency of stutterers.

REFERENCES

Andrews, G., Craig, A., Feyer, A., Hoddinott, P., & Neilson, M. (1983). Stuttering: A review of research findings and theories circa 1982. *Journal of Speech and Hearing Disorders, 45,* 287-307.

Andrews, G., Howie, P.M., Dozsa, M., & Guitar, B.E. (1982). Stuttering: Speech pattern characteristics under fluency-inducing conditions. *Journal of Speech and Hearing Research, 25,* 208-216.

Bloodstein, O. (1950). A rating scale study of conditions under which stuttering is reduced or absent. *Journal of Speech and Hearing Disorders, 15,* 29-36.

Cohen, J. (1960). A coefficient of agreement for nominal scales. *Educational and Psychological Measurement, 20,* 37-46.

Colcord, R.D., & Adams, M.R. (1979). Voicing duration and vocal SPL changes associated with stuttering reduction during singing. *Journal of Speech and Hearing Research, 22,* 468-479.

Fletcher, J.M. (1928). *The problem of stuttering.* New York: Longmans, Green.

Hargrave, S., Kalinowski, J., Stuart, A. Armson, J., & Jones, K. (1994). Stuttering reduction under frequency-altered feedback at two speech rates. *Journal of Speech and Hearing Research, 36,* 1313-1316.

Healey, E.C., Mallard, A.R., & Adams, M.R. (1976). Factors contributing to the reduction of stuttering during singing. *Journal of Speech and Hearing Research, 19,* 475-480.

Johnson, W., & Rosen, P. (1937). Studies in the psychology of stuttering: VII. Effect of certain changes in speech pattern upon stuttering frequency. *Journal of Speech Disorders, 2,* 105-109.

Kalinowski, J., Armson, J., Roland-Mieszkowski, M., Stuart, A., & Gracco, V.L. (1993). Effects of alterations in auditory feedback and speech rate on stuttering frequency. *Language and Speech, 36,* 1-16.

Kalinowski, J., Stuart, A., Sark, S., & Armson, J. (1996). Stuttering amelioration at various auditory feedback delays and speech rates. *European Journal of Disorders of Communication 31, 259-268.*

MacLeod, J., Kalinowski, J., Stuart, A., & Armson, J., (1995). Effect of single and combined altered auditory feedback on stuttering frequency at two speech rates. *Journal of Communication Disorders, 28,* 217-228.

Netsell, R. (1981). The acquisition of speech motor control: A perspective with directions for research. In R. Stark (Ed.), *Language behavior in infancy and early childhood*. Amsterdam: Elsevier-North Holland. pp. 127-153.

Pickett, J.M. (1980). *The Sounds of Speech Communication: A Primer of Acoustic Phonetics and Speech Perception*. Baltimore: University Park Press.

Reid, L.D. (1946). Some facts about stuttering. *Journal of Speech Disorders, 11,* 3-12.

Starkweather, C.W. (1982). Stuttering and laryngeal behavior: a review. (*ASHA Monographs 21*) Rockville, MD: American Speech-Language-Hearing Association.

Stuart, A., Kalinowski, J., Armson, J., Stenstrom, R., & Jones, K. (1996). Fluency effect of frequency alterations of plus-minus one-half and one-quarter octave shifts in stutterers' auditory feedback. *Journal of Speech and Hearing Research, 399,* 396-401.

Walker, C., & Black, J. (1950). *The Intrinsic Intensity of Oral Phrases* (Joint Project Report No. 2). Pensacola, FL: Naval Air Station, United States Naval School of Aviation Medicine.

Wingate, M.E. (1969). Sound and pattern in "artificial" fluency. *Journal of Speech and Hearing Research, 12,* 677-686.

Speech Production: Motor Control, Brain Research and Fluency Disorders
W. Hulstijn, H.F.M. Peters and P.H.H.M. Van Lieshout, editors

Chapter 47

ON THE MECHANISMS OF SPEECH MONITORING

Albert Postma

It has recently been proposed that disfluencies and stuttering may derive from self-repairing of speech programming flaws (Postma & Kolk, 1993). Following this proposal, the present paper elaborates upon the mechanism of speech monitoring: the process by which speakers verify the correctness of the speech flow and install repairs if necessary. A crucial distinction concerns the question whether speech monitoring is perception based or production based. The former view holds that speakers inspect their own speech by the same system they use for analyzing other-produced speech: the speech comprehension system. Monitoring as such is a centrally (consciously) controlled activity. In contrast, the production based view assumes the existence of multiple, distributed monitors, each connected to a distinct processing component in the speech production sequence. These monitors may function autonomously. The major differences between the two approaches will be discussed. The distinction in types of speech monitoring is extended to stuttering.

ON THE MECHANISMS OF SPEECH MONITORING

In 1993 a new view on disfluency and stuttering was put forward by Herman Kolk and myself, termed "the Covert Repair Hypothesis" (CRH) (Postma & Kolk, 1993). Basically, we contended that disfluencies and stutterings are side-results of repair activities of some covert, i.e. not yet externalized, flaw in the speech production sequence. As the central source of flaws in stutterers, a defect in phonological encoding was hypothesized. As such we could potentially account for certain deviancies in speech motor control, as the phonological encoding stage forms the interface between central linguistic planning and subsequent speech motor execution. Moreover, it allowed us to deal with findings on linguistic factors in stuttering, for example the concomitance of stuttering with various phonological disorders in children (see LaSalle & Conture, 1995; Yaruss & Conture, 1996)

It is evident that speakers closely attend their utterances. More than half of their errors are followed by an immediate or shortly delayed self-correction. Repair activities in speech production are the function of the speech monitor. In this paper I will review the mechanisms of speech monitoring. In addition, I will try to extend the CRH by further applying certain monitoring principles to stuttering.

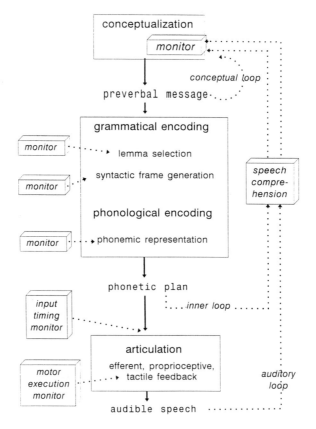

Figure 1. Production stages and (hypothetical) monitoring components in the speech production system. Monitors to the left can be regarded as being production based, while those to the right reflect the perception based view.

Stages in speech production

Speech output is achieved by a series of processing stages. At each stage potentially errors can occur. The middle part of figure 1 presents the general scheme of production components proposed by Levelt (1989) and others. Speaking starts with conceptualization (planning an utterance's meaning and purpose). Next, there is grammatical encoding (syntactic planning and lexical selection). Phonological encoding (building a morpho-phonological representation) may be subdivided in the assemblage of an abstract phonemic representation, and the subsequent construction of a context-dependent, phonetic representation (or articulatory plan) (see Levelt & Wheeldon, 1994 for more details). Finally, there is articulation: translating the phonetic codes into speech motor movements.

Perception based monitoring

Where in this model does monitoring take place? Levelt adheres a so called *percepti-*

on based monitoring approach. Speech monitoring is essentially achieved by the same system which analyzes speech of others: the speech comprehension system. This approach has two important characteristics. First, the number of channels to be monitored is limited. A conceptual loop allows the verification of the preverbal message; an inner loop entails inspection of the phonetic plan prior to its execution; and the auditory loop comprises the hearing of one's own speech. The inclusion of particularly these channels follows from the fact that they are accessible by the speech comprehension system. Moreover, monitoring as such does not apply to all types of intermediate processing results, but only to certain "end products". A second, important characteristic is that perception based monitoring is a central, consciously controlled mechanism.

Production based monitoring

Alternatively, there is the *production based monitoring approach.* Monitoring may involve each step in the sequence from thought to articulation. As in the model proposed by Laver (1980), each processing component is equipped with its own specialized comparator. Several of such comparators have been proposed: one for lemma selection, one for timing asynchronies between phonological encoding and articulatory unpacking of the phonetic plan, and monitors for efferent, proprioceptive and tactile feedback (see also Postma & Kolk, 1993).

Critics of production monitors

According to Levelt (1989) production monitors suffer several weaknesses. First, an important criticism of production based monitors concerns 'reduplication of knowledge'. In order to monitor a given processing stage, they would have to access the same information as used by that process. Moreover in doing so, it might mean a duplication of the capabilities of perception at large. The strength of this criticism may be doubted, however. It all depends upon what exactly the monitor is doing. For example, Blackmer and Mitton (1991) propose a sort of restart or repair device at the articulator which checks whether there is input (not what the input is). Second, production based monitors would essentially be hold up monitors. That is, they delay further processing of information while inspecting it. Indeed, such could seriously hinder progress of speech processing. However, production monitors may as well be of the flow-through type: further processing is allowed during monitoring (cf. Blackmer & Mitton, 1991). Third, while perception monitors inspect only 'end products', production monitors scrutinize intermediate results as well. When one assumes that monitoring takes place at a central level this may become a problem. The inner workings of processing modules can typically not be assessed consciously, only their final results. This point of concern, however, is less critical, when monitors are placed at a local level, and work rather autonomously.

Characteristics of Production and Perception Monitors

The idea that speech is somehow controlled by perceptual monitor mechanisms is without dispute. We all attend to, hear, and become aware of our errors. However, in contrast with the foregoing critics, one can not a priori rule out the possibility of production monitoring. Perhaps not all of the production monitors shown in figure 1 are realistic, but some of them could be. There is more empirical evidence needed here. Let me summarize the major distinctive characteristics between the two approaches, completing the remarks made earlier.

First, there is the issue of speed. In perception based monitors detection and interruption can take place very quickly by the conceptual loop. But for linguistic form errors the mechanisms seem slower. Indeed, firstly all the processing stages have to be completed, and secondly time consuming analyses by the speech comprehension system have to be performed. However, very fast error detection-and-reaction events are known to occur, as indicated by interrupt-to-repair times of 0 msec (Blackmer & Mitton, 1991). One attempt to deal with this problem has been to insert an articulatory buffer between the phonological encoding stage and the articulator. Parts of the speech plan may thus be buffered sometime prior to their articulation. The whole problem is less serious for production based monitors which can take action almost immediately after the conception of an error. So, to simplify things, we may take perception monitors to be relatively slower than production monitors, or to be more sensitive to speech output rate[1].

Second, an important point is the level at which the monitor resides. Perception based monitors are central and consciously managed, and potentially resource limited. Hence, you can not divide attention over too many channels at one time. Production based monitors are more or less autonomously, and may function automatically and greatly subconsciously (cf. Berg, 1992). In a study by Postma and Noordanus (in press), we had subjects report their own speech errors. We observed that in several cases subjects made self-repairs, but did not explicitly report the error. This may suggest that self-repair can be virtually automatic.

Third, perception monitors can be more flexible with regard to the specific criteria

Table 1. Differences between perception and production based speech monitors.

	Perception Based Monitoring	Production Based Monitoring
Speed	slow	fast
Location	central	distributed
Awareness	conscious	automatic, reflexological
Capacity	limited by attentional resources	autonomous resources
Aspects of Speech Flow Scrutinized	flexible	fixed
Repair Proper	elaborated revision, coordinated with original utterance in order to aid the listener	simple retrace and restart / postpone; repair "on the fly"
Speech Comprehension	related to comprehension skills	no relation

against which the speech flow is checked. For example, in reading aloud lists of words you would be more focused upon lexical status than you would be when dealing with lists interspersed with nonwords (cf. Baars et al., 1975). In addition, it may be the case that under special conditions perception monitoring may be directed to completely new types of information (or monitoring loops) than the regular ones. For example, as is common in stuttering therapies, speakers may deliberately chose to monitor proprioceptive feedback. Production monitors as such appear more rigid. That is, they can only work at those points which they are prewired to control, either genetically or by abundant practice[2,3].

Fourth, the step following error detection is executing the repair proper. There is evidence that speakers not always simply interject the correct elements, but sometimes construct their revisions more elaborately in order to serve their audience. Speculating, one may expect the two types of monitors to differ in this respect. That is, perception monitors would be more involved in the just mentioned manner of repair, while production monitors underlie a restricted repair mode.

Finally, in the perception based approach self-repair behaviour and comprehension skills should be correlated whereas this is not the case for production monitors. Schlenck et al. (1987) observed that the frequencies of certain classes of self-repairs - i.e. prepairs or covert repairs - were unaffected in aphasic patients with severe comprehension problems.

Stuttering and Production Monitoring

How does this all apply to stuttering and disfluencies? Though a repair explanations appears to be generally accepted for disfluencies in normal speakers, there is considerable disagreement about its potential for stuttering (cf. Van Lieshout, 1995). A crucial question seems to be whether or not qualitative differences between normal and disordered disfluency exist. Focusing upon part word repetitions, it has often been claimed that these incidents are faster, include shorter interfragment intervals, and are less controllable (which eventually may result in a sense of loss of control) than normal sound repetitions. It would be of interest to see how well the distinction between perception and production based monitors accounts for this hypothesized difference. More precisely, I want to speculate here upon the possibility that perception based monitoring is mainly responsible for normal disfluencies, and production based monitoring applies primarily to stuttering.

Two notions in the literature attest that there may be some truth in this speculation. Blackmer and Mitton (1991) ascribe multiple, fast sound repetitions in normal speakers to a monitor device which signals discrepancies between the arrival of new material from the phonological encoding stage and the articulator waiting for a new piece of speech plan to execute. If new input is too late, the articulator simply starts anew with the old plan. A similar mechanism might explain stuttered repetitions. Moreover, Throneburg and Yairi (1994) have suggested that stuttering children exhibiting faster repetitions than controls indicates a heavier reflexological role in the disfluencies of the former. To quote them: "In normal speakers the system allows sufficient time to make necessary adjustments between one attempt and the next. For the most part, such adjustments are satisfactory. In stutterers, however, corrective responses may be reflexively rigid, allowing only brief intervals for readjusting. Thus the chance is greater for an unsatisfactory outcome that requires additional repetitive corrective attempts" (Throneburg & Yairi, 1994; p. 1074).

This description very aptly resembles what a production monitor might do. To conclude, future research in stuttering might further elaborate upon the distinction between perception and production based monitoring as an account of normal and disordered disfluency[4].

NOTES

[1]   Speeding up speaking rate would virtually annihilate the 'look ahead range' of the articulatory buffer. Hence, under the perception based approach the delay between error onsets and self-repair onsets would increase drastically when speech becomes faster. For production monitors one might expect a more moderate increase in error-to-repair times since the working of these monitors may be presumed to accelerate in proportion to the rate of the associated processing component.

[2]   Mackay (1992) presents a model with distributed, partly autonomous monitors, which react specifically to 'novelty' in utterances. Though it allows for flexibility in production monitors, novelty here applies mostly to the level of the individual error and not to the overall criteria used for monitoring.

[3]   Being rigid does not mean that production monitors are totally detached from internal or external influences. For example, if speakers strive for high accuracy of their utterances, this may indirectly increase the scrutiny of production monitors.

[4]   Depending upon which types of production monitors will be shown likely, it may broaden the range of potential speech errors or motor control deviances which are 'repaired' in a stuttering event.

REFERENCES

Baars, B.J., Motley, M.T., & MacKay, D.G. (1975). Output editing for lexical status in artificially elicited slips of the tongue. *Journal of Verbal Learning and Verbal Behaviour, 14*, 382-391.

Berg, T. (1992). Productive and perceptual constraints of speech error correction. *Psychological research, 48*, 133-144.

Blackmer, E.R., & Mitton, J.L. (1991). Theories of monitoring and the timing of repairs in spontaneous speech. *Cognition, 39*, 173-194.

LaSalle, L.R., & Conture, E.G. (1995). Clustering of between- and witin-word disfluencies in the speech of children who do and do not stutter. *Journal of Speech and Hearing Research, 38*, 965-999.

Laver, J.D.M. (1980). Monitoring systems in the neurolinguistic control of speech production. In V.A. Fromkin (Ed.), *Errors in linguistic performance: slips of the tongue, ear, pen, and hand.* New York: Academic Press.

Levelt, W.J.M. (1989). *Speaking: from Intention to Articulation.* Cambridge, MA: M.I.T. Press.

Levelt, W.J.M., & Wheeldon, L.R. (1994). Do speakers have access to a mental syllabary? *Cognition,*

50, 239-269.

MacKay, D.G. (1992). Awareness and error detection: New theories and research paradigms. *Consciousness and Cognition, 1*, 199-225.

Postma, A., & Kolk, H.H.J. (1993). The covert repair hypothesis: prearticulatory repair processes in normal and stuttered disfluencies. *Journal of Speech and Hearing Research, 36*, 472-487.

Postma, A., & Noordanus, C. (in press). Production and detection of speech errors in inner, mouthed, noise masked, and normal auditory feedback speech. *Language and Speech.*

Schlenk, K., Huber, W., & Wilmes, K. (1987). "Prepairs" and repairs: different monitoring functions in aphasic language production. *Brain and Language, 30*, 226-244.

Throneburg, R.N., & Yairi, E. (1994). Temporal dynamics of repetitions during the early stage of childhood stuttering: an acoustic study. *Journal of Speech and Hearing Research, 37*, 1067-1075.

Van Lieshout, P.H.H.M. (1995). Motor planning and articulation in fluent speech of stutterers and nonstutterers. Doctoral dissertation, Nijmegen University.

Wheeldon, L.R., & Levelt, W.J.M. (1995). Monitoring the time course of phonological encoding. *Journal of Memory and Language, 34*, 311-334.

Yaruss, J.S., & Conture, E.G. (1996). Stuttering and phonological disorders in children: Examination of the covert repair hypothesis. *Journal of Speech and Hearing Research, 39*, 349-364.

Speech Production: Motor Control, Brain Research and Fluency Disorders
W. Hulstijn, H.F.M. Peters and P.H.H.M. Van Lieshout, editors

Chapter 48

MENTAL EFFORT AND SPEECH FLUENCY

Hans-Georg Bosshardt

The aim of the present investigation was to test the assumption that speech disfluencies can be the result of interference between the execution of speech movements and concurrent cognitive processes. During speech production information related to subsequent speech is retrieved from short-term memory and translated into a phonetic code while previously planned portions of speech are being produced. Presumably persons differ in the extent to which they are able to perform speech movements unimpeded by simultaneous cognitive processes. It was assumed that speech disfluencies can be experimentally induced with a dual-task paradigm. In each trial a sequence of three unrelated nouns had to be repeated ten times (speech production task). Under dual-task conditions a mental addition task had to be performed concurrently with the speech production task. The result of the mental addition had to be kept in mind until after the word repetition task was completed. In each experimental session participants were required to perform the mental addition, the speech production, and the dual task in three successive blocks of ten trials each. The total experiment consisted of three sessions on three separate days. Four adult persons who stutter and four persons who do not stutter were asked to perform the two tasks both separately and concurrently. The effects of dual-task conditions on stuttering rate were statistically evaluated in a single-subject design. Data on speech fluency revealed that individuals differ in the extent to which mental calculation interferes with overt speech production and that they used different speech maneuvers to cope with the requirements of the dual-task situation. The implications of these results for a theory of speech production and stuttering are discussed.

INTRODUCTION

In the present paper it is proposed that speech disfluencies can be the result of an interference between the execution of speech movements and concurrently performed cognitive processes. Although speaking is often assumed to be as automatic and effortless, it actually involves a highly complex coordination of processing and storage (Danemann & Green, 1986). During speech production subsequent portions of the utterance are planned or retrieved from short-term memory while earlier portions are being produced (Ferreira, 1991, 1993). Therefore it is assumed that the processing load continuously fluctuates during speech production (see also Power, 1985; Ford & Holmes, 1978) and that these fluctuations are correlated with variations in the frequency of stuttering.

Empirical support for this thesis can be found in studies with persons who stutter. From these studies it can be concluded that stuttering and disfluencies tend to occur with higher frequencies at clause boundaries (Wall et al., 1981), in longer and more complex sentences (Bernstein Ratner & Sih, 1987; Bloodstein & Gantwerk, 1967; Bloodstein & Grossman, 1981; Gordon et al., 1986; Jayaram, 1984; Howell & Au-Yeung, 1995; Kadi-Hannifi & Howell, 1992; Martin et al., 1990; Peters et al., 1989; Rommel et al., 1992; Rommel, 1993; Ryan, 1992; Tornick & Bloodstein, 1976; Wells, 1979), and on words bearing a higher information load (Soderberg, 1966, 1967). Bernstein Ratner (1995) and St.Louis (1979) provide more detailed reviews of the empirical work which relates stuttering to linguistic variables. Peters and Starkweather (1990; Starkweather, 1991; see also Starkweather, 1995) concluded from these facts that speech planning and motor execution of speech might interfere with each other.

It seems to be a well-established fact that stuttering rate is related to some aspects of linguistic complexity. But there are two reasons why this relationship cannot be taken as conclusive evidence for the interference assumption. One reason is that variations in linguistic complexity can be correlated with prosodic changes, which could be the actual determinant of stuttering rate (Wingate, 1988, p.175 f.). Another reason why the relationship between linguistic complexity and stuttering cannot be regarded as conclusive evidence for the interference assumption is related to the fact that processing load during speech production is only partially dependent on variations in linguistic complexity. In a sentence reproduction experiment Bosshardt (1995) obtained some evidence suggesting that at least adult participants are able to reduce the processing load imposed by highly complex sentences by breaking them into smaller units. Linguistic material can be processed in a flexible way (Folkins, 1991) and therefore processing load during sentence production can only be partially controlled by variations in linguistic complexity.

For these reasons and against the background of the empirical results of Caruso et al. (1994; Caruso et al., chapter 18) it seemed more promising to experimentally manipulate the processing load during speech production. In the present experiment a dual-task paradigm was used to investigate whether higher-level cognitive processing can induce speech disfluencies and in which way the speech processes of persons who stutter differ from persons who do not stutter. Under dual-task conditions an automatic word repetition task had to be performed concurrently with mental addition as a secondary task. In the oral word-repetition task, participants were required to continuously repeat a sequence of three words until the experimenter stopped them after the tenth repetition. From Baddeley's empirical (Baddeley et al., 1981) and theoretical work (1990; Gathercole & Baddeley 1993) it can be inferred that this task can be almost automatically performed in the phonological loop system, i.e., with minimal demand on attention and central processing capacity.

A mental addition task in which three summands had to be added was used as a secondary task. Under dual-task conditions the participants were instructed to continuously articulate three words while mental calculations had to be performed concurrently. The result of the mental calculations had to be kept in mind until after they finished the word repetition task.

Presumably, overt articulation can be seen essentially as a product of the phonological loop and of the articulatory systems, whereas the mental addition task is largely based on central executive processes (Hitch, 1978). The central executive is a limited capacity system which is responsible for the control of mental processes and short-term retention with one strategy for the latter being use of the phonological loop. In contrast to finger-tapping, which was used in earlier dual-task experiments with persons who stutter (Brutten & Trotter, 1985, 1986; Sussmann, 1982), the mental addition task of the present experiment demands more attention and is a purely mental task which does not require any overt reaction concurrently to word repetition.

From a motor control perspective of stuttering as developed by Van Lieshout et al. (1995; Van Lieshout et al., 1996a,b; Van Lieshout et al., chapter 11) it has been proposed ".. that persons who stutter may use different motor control strategies to compensate for a reduced verbal motor skill .." (Van Lieshout et al., 1996a, p. 76). In a similar vein it is proposed here that persons who stutter are able to resort to a "supervised form of speaking" which is based on processes within the central executive system and which result in a reduction of stuttering rate. If the speech of persons who stutter is based to a greater extent on control processes in the central executive system, then their speech is more liable to interference from concurrent mental calculations than that of persons who do not stutter.

The opposite prediction can be derived from the covert repair hypothesis (Postma & Kolk, 1993). In contrast to the motor control perspective, Postman and Kolk assume that stuttering *is the audible result* of covert repair processes by which the persons who stutter try to compensate for inaccurate phonological coding. It follows from this assumption that the speech of persons who stutter is based to a greater extent on central executive functions and that their speech should become more fluent under concurrent mental load because under these conditions the probability of speech monitoring and of covert repairs is reduced. Against this theoretical background it is further expected that the speech of persons who do not stutter depends to a smaller extent on processes in the central executive system and that therefore their fluency is comparably less affected by concurrent mental calculations.

The aim of the present study was to investigate how speech fluency is affected by processes in the central executive system. More specifically, the following research questions were addressed: 1) How is the fluency of the word repetitions influenced when mental calculation has to be concurrently performed? Theoretically such an interference is taken as an indication that the word repetition and mental addition tasks impose overlapping demands on the speech production system. 2) How do persons differ in the way with which mental calculation changes the fluency of word repetitions? Instead of providing information about global between-group differences the results of individual participants were statistically evaluated. 3) The final research question to be addressed by the present experiment was whether the effects of dual task on stuttering are moderated by pause rate and breathing. It is conceivable that the amount of temporal overlap between mental arithmetic and word repetition can be reduced by increasing the frequency of pausing and breathing.

METHOD

Subjects

The results of four adult persons who stutter (age range: 23 to 52 years) and of four persons who do not stutter (age range: 20 to 29 years) will be reported. The persons who stutter were recruited from self-help groups and were paid for their participation (30,00 DM). They differed in their socio-economic background (a registered hospital nurse, two craftsmen and a student). As determined in oral reading of a newspaper text of 200 words these persons stuttered (silent prolongations, prolongations and repetitions of sounds, syllables, and one syllable words) on 2.5% (S14), 11.5% (S15), 1.5% (S17), and 2.0% (S19) of the words. In a subsequent free report of this text the stuttering rates were 12.7% (S14), 20.6% (S15), 7.5% (S17), and 10.6% (S19). In no case was the duration of the three longest blocks longer than a second. The participants who do not stutter were undergraduate psychology students who participated in the experiment to fulfill their course requirements.

Material

The words for the repetition task were drawn from a pool of ten three-syllabic compound nouns: Bohnentopf, Blattspinat, Buttermilch, Reissalat, Suppenkraut, Knoblauchbrot, Kokosnuss, Sauerkraut, Traubensaft, Weizengrieß [pot of beans, leafy spinach, buttermilk, rice salad, pot-herb, bread with garlic, coconut, pickled cabbage, grape-juice, semolina]. These nouns are all common words from the semantic field foodstuff, have three syllables, are pronounced with primary stress on the first syllable, and begin or end with plosives or fricatives. From this pool, 30 sequences of three words were constructed in a pseudo-random way with the restriction that at every position each word appeared at least in one and maximally in six sequences. Ten sequences were used at each of the three sessions.

A total number of 30 addition tasks was constructed. For these tasks the first addends were between 21 and 44, the second between 11 and 18, and the third between 2 and 9. The sum of the first two addends required no carrying but addition of the third always did. Ten addition tasks were used on each of three days of the experiment.

Procedure

The experiment was run in three sessions on three days. The single and dual task in every session consisted of ten trials. A particular trial began as soon as the participants had pushed a button. Operation of the push button by the participants caused a computer program to present three words on the monitor (Screen 1). Screen 2, consisting of the same three words plus three numbers, was exposed for the duration of three seconds as soon as the experimenter operated one of his buttons. After three seconds Screen 2 was automatically replaced by Screen 1. The same words were presented on both screens but the numbers for the mental calculation were only presented on Screen 2.

The same material was presented visually in all single- and dual-task conditions. In the mental addition part of the investigation, participants were instructed to disregard the words, to calculate the sum and to produce the result as fast as possible. In the word repetition part, the same material was presented again with the instruction to repeat the three words continuously as fast as possible and to disregard the numbers. After ten vocal repetitions of the words the experimenter indicated the end of the trial and cleared the computer screen. In the dual-task part of the investigation, participants were instructed to mentally calculate while concurrently repeating the word list. The persons were again instructed to repeat the words continuously as fast as possible. The experimenter exposed the numbers (Screen 2) at the end of the third repetition of the words when the stressed syllable of the third word was being pronounced. The participants were instructed to continuously repeat the words until the experimenter announced the end of the trial. Thus, under dual-task conditions participants performed the first three word repetitions with the expectation that they will be required to mentally add the summands as soon as Screen 2 had been exposed. Consequently, only the word repetitions after the third one had to be produced concurrently with the secondary mental addition task. After the tenth repetition the end of the trial was announced and the subjects produced the result of their mental addition.

Dependent Variables

Stuttering rate. All repetitions, exchanges of sounds, syllables, or words together with lengthening of vowels and consonants and all indications of tension (intensity and duration) were counted as stuttering. The number of syllables stuttered was added over blocks of three repetitions of three words (repetitions one to three, four to six, and seven to nine). Thus, for every trial three stuttering rates were obtained, one for each block. The factor block (one through three) was an additional repeated measurement factor.

Inhalation. All audible signs of inhalation were registered and summed over blocks of three repetitions of three words. The factor block (one through three) was an additional repeated measurement factor.

Pauses. Filled and silent pauses were perceptually identified and summed over blocks of three repetitions. Silent pauses were only scored when no audible signs of inhalation and no indications of tension were present. Pauses between words were only scored when they had a minimum duration of 250 ms, and pauses within words a minimum of 150 ms. Filled pauses were only scored in those cases where no audible signs of inhalation or tension could be detected and which were not a sound or syllable exchange. These scores were also summed over blocks of three repetitions. The factor block (one through three) was added as a repeated measurement factor to the design.

Reliability. The criteria for scoring were defined by two raters using the verbal repetitions of one participant (N04). Then these raters independently scored the verbal repetitions of all persons. Interrater agreement was determined for a total of 16128 syllables (from two persons who stutter and one person who does not stutter). The raw percentages of syllables that were scored identically by both raters were 99.3% for stuttering, 99.6% for pauses and 99.7% for inhalation. After correcting for chance (Scott, 1955) the agreement between the raters was 79.8% for stuttering, 59.5% for pauses, and 95.2% for inhalation.

While the reliability of the stuttering and inhalation rates were considered to be adequate a further effort was made to define pauses more precisely. To increase the objectivity of the definition of silent pauses in between-word positions they were scored only if their duration (c.f. Goldman-Eisler, 1968) was 250 ms or longer and in within-word positions only if their duration was 150 ms or longer. All scores used in this analysis were checked by both raters and discrepant scores were corrected by mutual decision.

Design

The effects of the factors block and task (single or dual task) on stuttering rate, inhalation and pauses were evaluated with separate analyses of variance for every participant. In a multivariate mixed design, stuttering rate, inhalation and pauses were treated as separate dependent variables with day as a between-groups factor and with block and task as repeated measurement factors. To protect the statistical decisions against inflation of α-error, univariate results for each dependent variable were only interpreted when the averaged F-values corresponding to multivariate tests for all variables were significant. The criterion of statistical significance was set at $\alpha = 0.05$ throughout this study.

RESULTS

Stuttering rate

The stuttering rate of only one participant who does not stutter (N05) was significantly influenced by the interaction task by block ($F (2,54)=5.73$, $p<.01$). The stuttering rates of the other participants who do not stutter were not significantly influenced by task, block or by the interaction. It can be seen from the top of Figure 1 that person N05 had a lower stuttering rate under dual- than under single-task conditions in Block 1. Under dual-task condition participants performed the word repetitions in Block 1 with the expectation that in the Blocks 2 and 3 they will be required to mentally calculate and to keep the result in mind. Thus, the significant reduction of the stuttering rate of person N05 in Block 1 is actually an effect of the person's expectation about what she will have to do during the following repetitions (i.e. in Blocks 2 and 3). The results of person N05 suggest that she reduced her stuttering rate by speaking in a controlled or supervised form in the first block. This form of speaking cannot be maintained when the mental calculations have to be performed concurrently with speech and consequently in Blocks 2 and 3 the stuttering rates increase to a level that is comparable to that of single-task conditions (see top part of Figure 1).

Under dual conditions the stuttering rates of two persons who stutter (S17 and S19) were significantly influenced by the factor task (S17: $F(1,27)=22.39$, $p<.001$; S19: $F(1,27)=4.59$, $p<.05$) but the interaction of task by block was significant only for one person (S17: $F(1,27)=12.13$, $p<.001$; S19: $F(1,27)=0.08$, n.s.). For participant S17 the difference between the stuttering rates for speaking under dual and under single-task conditions was significantly more pronounced in Block 2 than in the other blocks (cf. bottom part of Figure 1). In contrast, the stuttering rate of participant S19 was significantly influenced only by the main effect task, indicating that her stuttering rate in all blocks was generally higher under dual- in comparison to single-task conditions. Thus, the results for person S19 indicate that even before the mental addition actually had to be performed, her stuttering rate was increased. The stuttering rates of two other persons who stutter were not significantly influenced by task and its interaction with block.

Pause rate

The pause rate of one person who does not stutter (N04: $F(2,54)=5.44, p<.01$) and of one person who stutters (S19) was significantly influenced by the interaction between task and block ($F(2,54)=4.18, p<.05$). Both persons increased their pause rates under dual-task as compared to single-task speaking. This increase was significantly more pronounced in Block 2 than in the other blocks. One interpretation of these results could be that in the dual-task situation, pauses reduce the amount of temporal overlap between the two tasks. This could be one of the maneuvers speakers use to overcome the constraints of the dual-task situation. In this case pause and stuttering rate should negatively correlate with one another. On the other hand it could equally be maintained that pausing is another form of disfluency caused by the processing load of the dual-task condition. In this case it is to be expected that pause and stuttering rates are positively correlated. An analysis of intercorrelations among the variables will be postponed until after the presentation of the results of the inhalation rate.

Inhalation rate

One person who does not stutter (N05) showed a significant main effect of task ($F(1,27)$ $=4.17, p<.05$), and the interaction of task by block was significant for two other persons who do not stutter (N04: $F(2,54)=15.76, p<.001$; N06: $F(2,54)=13.73, p<.001$) and for two persons who stutter (S15: $F(2,54)=5.11, p<.01$; S19: $F(2,54)=15.29, p<.001$). Under dual-task conditions, the inhalation rate of person N05 was generally increased in all blocks whereas the inhalation rate of the other persons were increased in Blocks 1 and 2, and reduced in Block 3. As with pauses the position at which participants inhale could be another maneuver which relieves speakers from concurrently performing mental calculations and speaking and thereby reduces stuttering. Therefore the intercorrelations between stuttering, pauses, and inhalation will be analyzed in the following section.

Intercorrelations among the dependent measures

Multiple regression technique was used to analyse how stuttering was related to pause and inhalation rate. Separate regression analyses were calculated for every participant and for the single- and dual-task conditions. Only two of these eight regressions were significant (N06: R=.79, F(2,27) = 22.33, p<.000; S19: R=.50, F(2,27) = 4.40, p<.02). In both cases pause rate was a significant predictor of stuttering rate. But in both cases pause rate was *positively* related to stuttering rate.

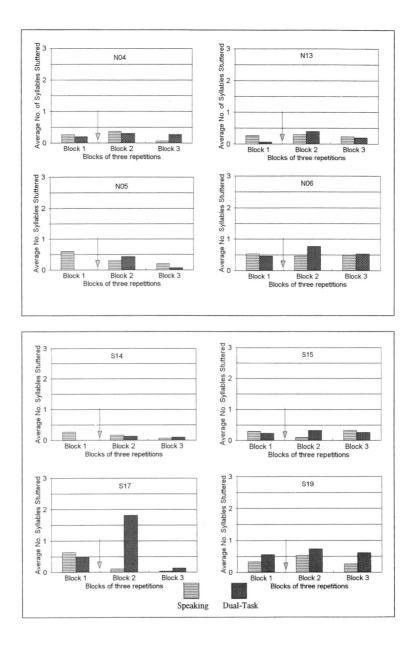

Figure 1. Average number of syllables stuttered per block for four participants who do not stutter (top part) and for four participants who stutter (bottom part). The arrows indicate the point in time at which the numbers were presented.

From these results it can be concluded that we obtained no indication for a negative relationship between the frequency of stuttering and either pause or inhalation rate, which suggests that pausing and inhalation cannot be interpreted as maneuvers for the prevention of stuttering. Rather, all these measures can be seen as some sort of disfluency the frequency of which increased under dual-task conditions.

Conclusions

The present results can be most economically interpreted with the assumption that some persons - irrespective of whether they stutter or not - can produce speech in some "supervised" form which requires processing space within the central executive system and which reduces the stuttering rate relative to an "unsupervised" form of speaking. This form of speaking may be based to a greater extent on auditory feedback than unsupervised forms (see Van Lieshout et al., 1996a) but most importantly our results suggest that its efficiency is reduced by a secondary task which draws on the capacity of the central executive system. The data of the present study, generally did not support the expectations derived from the covert repair hypothesis (Postma & Kolk, 1993). In those cases in which task significantly affected the stuttering rate at all, we obtained no indication that the stuttering rate was reduced under dual-task conditions.

The results of two persons who stutter and of one person who does not stutter can be adequately interpreted by reference to the assumption of supervised speech. It is assumed that two persons who stutter were able to maintain a low stuttering rate under single-task conditions because they closely supervised their speech. Under dual-task conditions their stuttering rate increased significantly because they were not able to maintain this supervised mode of speaking. The results suggest that at least for some persons who stutter the expectation to be required to speak under dual-task conditions is sufficient to stop the supervised form of speaking and increase the stuttering rate. One of the persons who do not stutter supervised her speech carefully in the first block of repetitions thereby reducing her stuttering rate in this block even below the level of single-task conditions. This observation cannot be taken as evidence for Postma and Kolk's (1993) covert repair hypothesis because when the secondary task had actually been presented this form of speaking could not be maintained any further and consequently the stuttering increased to the level characteristic of unsupervised speech.

The theoretical framework developed so far adequately accounts for the results of those participants who were significantly influenced by the task conditions. But it remains to be determined why other persons who stutter and who do not stutter were not significantly affected by the dual-task conditions of the present experiment. From a therapeutic perspective it could be very important to learn more about the conditions under which a person's speech becomes less susceptible to interference from concurrent cognitive processing. One can speculate that apart from supervised speech, which requires attention in a limited capacity system, there are probably other modes of speech control which are based on different subsystems of the speech production apparatus. Another task for future research is to describe supervised forms of speech in terms of other characteristics (for example timing) which are observable independently of their hypothesized effects on speech fluency.

ACKNOWLEDGMENTS

[1] The author gratefully acknowledges that his work is influenced by stimulating discussions with Hans Fransen, Brigitte Gäßler, and Waltraud Ballmer-Omar. Heiko Hübner realized the technical basis of this experiment and Serena L'hoest and Thorsten Zirkwitz helped to run the experiment and to analyze the results. Donald Goodwin helped to improve the English style of the present text. This work was supported by grant no. 827/3-2 from the Deutsche Forschungsgemeinschaft (DFG), Germany.

REFERENCES

Baddeley, A., Eldridge, M., & Lewis, V. (1981). The role of subvocalisation in reading. *Quarterly Journal of Experimental Psychology, 33A*, 439-454.

Baddeley, A. (1990). *Human memory*. Boston: Allyn and Bacon.

Bernstein Ratner, N.E., & Sih, C.C. (1987). Effects of gradual increases in sentence length and complexity of children's dysfluency. *Journal of Speech and Hearing Disorders, 52*, 278-287.

Bernstein Ratner, N. (1995). Stuttering. A psycholinguistic perspective. In R. Curlee & G. Siegel (Eds.), *Nature and treatment of stuttering: New directions*. Boston: Allyn & Bacon.

Bloodstein, O., & Gantwerk, B.F. (1967). Grammatical function in relation to stuttering in young children. *Journal of Speech and Hearing Research, 10*, 786-789.

Bloodstein, O. & Grossman, M. (1981). Early stutterings: Some aspects of their form and distribution. *Journal of Speech and Hearing Research, 24*, 298-302.

Bosshardt, H.G. (1995). *Syntactic complexity, short-term memory and stuttering* (Paper read at the 1995 ASHA Convention in Orlando, USA). Bochum: Ruhr-Universität Bochum, Fakultät für Psychologie.

Brutten, G.J., & Trotter, A.C. (1985). Hemispheric interference: A dual-task investigation of youngsters who stutter. *Journal of Fluency Disorders, 10*, 77-85.

Brutten, G.J., & Trotter, A.C. (1986). A dual-task investigation of young stutterers and nonstutterers. *Journal of Fluency Disorders, 11*, 275-284.

Caruso, A.J., Chodzko-Zajka, W.J., Bidinger, D.A., & Sommers, R.K. (1994). Adults who stutter: Responses to cognitive stress. *Journal of Speech and Hearing Research, 37*, 746-754.

Caruso, A.J., & Max, L. (this volume). Application of motor learning theory to stuttering research. In W. Hulstijn, H.F.M. Peters, & P.H.H.M. Van Lieshout (Eds.), *Speech production: motor control, brain research and fluency disorders*. Amsterdam: Elsevier Science.

Cohen, J., & Cohen, P. (1975). *Applied multiple regression/correlation analysis for the behavioral sciences*. Hillsdale, N.J.: L. Erlbaum.

Danemann, M., & Green, I. (1986). Individual differences in comprehending and producing words in context. *Journal of Memory and Language, 25*, 1-18.

Ferreira, F. (1991). Effects of length and syntactic complexity on initiation times for prepared utterances. *Journal of Memory and Language, 30*, 210-233.

Ferreira, F. (1993). Creation of prosody during sentence production. *Psychological Review, 100*, 233-253.

Folkins, J.W. (1991). Stuttering from a speech motor control perspective. In H. F. M. Peters, W. Hulstijn, & C. W. Starkweather (Eds.), *Speech motor control and stuttering* (pp. 561-570). Amsterdam: Excerpta Medica.

Ford, M., & Holmes, V.M. (1978). Planning units and syntax in sentence production. *Cognition*, *6*, 35-53.

Goldman-Eisler, F. (1968). *Psycholinguistics: Experiments in spontaneous speech*. NewYork: Academic Press.

Gathercole, S.E., & Baddeley, A.D. (1993). *Working memory and language*. Hillsdale: Lawrence Erlbaum.

Gordon, P.A., Luper, H.L., & Peterson, H.A. (1986). The effects of syntactic complexity on the occurrence of disfluencies in 5 year old stutterers. *Journal of Fluency Disorders*, *11*, 151-164.

Hitch, G.J. (1978). The role of short-term working memory in mental arithmetic. *Cognitive Psychology*, *10*, 302-323.

Howell, P. & Au-Yeung, J. (1995). Syntactic determinants of stuttering in the spontaneous speech of normally fluent and stuttering children. *Journal of Fluency Disorders*, *20*, 317-330.

Jayaram, M. (1984). Distribution of stuttering in sentences. Relationship to sentence length and clause position. *Journal of Speech and Hearing Research*, *27*, 338-341.

Kadi-Hanifi, K., & Howell, P. (1992). Syntactic analysis of the spontaneous speech of normally fluent and stuttering children. *Journal of Fluency Disorders*, *17*, 151-170.

Martin, R., Felsenfeld Parlour, S., & Haroldsen, S. (1990). Stuttering and level of linguistic demand. *Journal of Fluency Disorders*, *15*, 93-106.

Peters, H.F.M., Hulstijn, W., & Starkweather, C.W. (1989). Acoustic and physiological reaction times of stutterers and nonstutterers. *Journal of Speech and Hearing Research*, *32*, 668-680.

Peters, H.F.M. & Starkweather, C.W. (1990). The interaction between speech motor coordination and language processes in the development of stuttering. *Journal of Fluency Disorders*, *15*, 115-125.

Postma, A., & Kolk, H. (1993). The covert repair hypothesis: Prearticulatory repair processes in normal and stuttered disfluencies. *Journal of Speech and Hearing Research*, *36*, 472-487.

Power, M.J. (1985). Sentence production and working memory. *The Quarterly Journal of Experimental Psychology*, *37A*, 367-385.

Rommel, D. (1993). Psycholinguistische Aspekte des Stotterns. In H.S. Johannsen (DGPP) & L. Springer (DBL) , *Stottern, Tagungsbericht Münster* (pp. 59-73). Ulm: Phoniatrische Ambulanz.

Rommel, D., Moldaschel, S., Müller, M., Schulze, H., Johannsen, H.S., & Sieron, J. (1992). *Psycholinguistische Merkmale des Sprechverhaltens stotternder Kinder unterschiedlicher Altersstufen in verschiedenen Sprechsituationen* (Paper read at the XXIInd World Congress of the International Association of Logopedics and Phoniatrics). Hannover, Germany.

Ryan, B. (1992). Articulation, language, rate and fluency characteristics of stuttering and nonstuttering preschool children. *Journal of Speech and Hearing Research*, *35*, 333-342.

Scott, W.A. (1955). Reliability of content analysis: the case of nominal scale coding. *Public Opinion Quarterly*, *19*, 321-325.

Soderberg, G.A. (1966). The relations of stuttering to word length and word frequency. *Journal of Speech and Hearing Disorders*, *9*, 584-589.

Soderberg, G.A. (1967). Linguistic factors in stuttering. *Journal of Speech and Hearing Research*, *10*, 801-810.

St. Louis, K. (1979). Linguistic and motor aspects of stuttering. In N. J. Lass (Ed.), *Speech and Language*. Vol. 1 (pp. 89-210). New York: Academic Press.

Starkweather, C.W. . (1991). The language-motor interface in stuttering children. In H.F. M. Peters, W.

Hulstijn, & C.W. Starkweather (Eds.), *Speech motor control and stuttering* (pp. 385-391). Amsterdam: Excerpta Medica.

Starkweather, C.W. (1995). A simple theory of stuttering. *Journal of Fluency Disorders, 20,* 91-116.

Sussman, H.M. (1982). Contractive patterns of intrahemispheric interference to verbal and spatial concurrent tasks in right-handed, left-handed and stuttering populations. *Neuropsychologia, 20,* 675-684.

Tornick, G., & Bloodstein, O. (1976). Stuttering and sentence length. *Journal of Speech and Hearing Research, 19,* 651-654.

Van Lieshout, P.H.H.M. (1995). *Motor planning and articulation in fluent speech of stutterers and nonstutterers.* Nijmegen: University Press Nijmegen.

Van Lieshout, P.H.H.M., Hulstijn, W., Alfonso, P.J., & Peters, H.F.M. (this volume). Higher and lower order influences on the stability of the dynamic coupling between articulators. In W. Hulstijn, H.F.M. Peters, & P.H.H.M. Van Lieshout (Eds.), *Speech production: motor control, brain research and fluency disorders.* Amsterdam: Elsevier Science.

Van Lieshout, P.H.H.M., Hulstijn, W., Peters, F.M. (1996a). Speech production in people who stutter: testing the motor plan assembly hypothesis. *Journal of Speech and Hearing Research, 39,* 76-92.

Van Lieshout, P.H.H.M., Hulstijn, W., Peters, F.M. (1996b). From planning to articulation in speech production: What differentiates a person who stutters from a person who does not stutter?. *Journal of Speech and Hearing Research, 39,* 546-564.

Wall, M.J., Starkweather, C.W., & Cairns, H.S. (1981). Syntactic influences on stuttering in young child stutterers. *Journal of Fluency Disorders, 6,* 345-352.

Wells, G. B. (1979). Effect of sentence structure on stuttering. *Journal of Fluency Disorders, 8,* 123-129.

Wingate, M. (1988). *The structure of stuttering.* New York: Springer Verlag.

Speech Production: Motor Control, Brain Research and Fluency Disorders
W. Hulstijn, H.F.M. Peters and P.H.H.M. Van Lieshout, editors

Chapter 49

THE EFFECTS OF FORMAL AND CASUAL INTERVIEW STYLES ON STUTTERING INCIDENCE

Peter Howell, Anuparma Kapoor, Lena Rustin

It is necessary that a variety of speech recordings are made in order to ensure that an accurate reflection of a child-stutterer's problem is obtained. One type of speech deemed important is dialogue interaction with a fluent speaker. The involvement of the second speaker potentially introduces extra variables which might affect the child's speech. One of these variables is the style of speech that the interviewer adopts. In this study, the role of interviewer's style is investigated. Although analysis of the interviewer's speech shows that the speakers adopted the required style, this had no effect on the proportion of dysfluencies emitted by the child-stutterers.

INTRODUCTION

Assessing a child's speech is an important way of diagnosing stuttering and ascertaining whether the treatment the child is being given is successful. It has been considered that assessments of various forms of speech should be made: A typical set of recordings might include a read text, a piece of monologue and when the child is involved in dialogue with a speech therapist. The dialogue differs from the other forms of speech insofar as it involves a second speaker and the intention is to establish how the child is able to respond in dialogue interaction. It is assumed that, since experienced pathologists do the interviewing, any difference in speech behaviour which is observed during dialogue are due to how the child handles communicative interaction. However, since different interviewers are used with different children it is legitimate to ask whether the pathologist's style of speech influences the behaviour of the child who stutters.

One variable that may be important in this regard is the difference between formal and casual style of speech (Picheny et al., 1985). Picheny et al. (1985) reported that speakers can volitionally change their speech from formal to casual and that hearing impaired listeners recognize 10% more words when listening to formal speech. To date, there have been no studies which have investigated whether the style of speech an interviewer adopts affects the speech that the interviewee produces. It seems possible that it might: Children who stutter may produce more dysfluencies in their speech when the interviewer has a formal style.

This hypothesis is tested in the experiment reported in this chapter. Each child is interviewed twice, once by an interviewer who is required to adopt a formal interview style and once when an interviewer adopts a casual style. The interviews are analyzed in two ways: First, each interviewer's speech is analyzed to check that their speech has differences that are known to occur between formal and casual styles. Second, the dysfluencies that the child produced are assessed. The hypothesis predicts that the children will produce more dysfluencies when being interviewed by the interviewer who speaks in a formal style. Since familiarity with the interview situation may affect a child's response, three groups of children are tested: A group of stuttering children who had attended a speech pathology clinic regularly, a group of stuttering children who were attending for the first time and a control group of fluent children. It is expected that the children who had attended the clinic regularly would have most experience of the interviewing situation and might show less reaction to a change in interviewing style.

The available literature indicates what speech changes should occur when an interviewer is adopting a formal style. Picheny et al. (1985) found that in clear speech speaking rate is decreased both by inserting pauses and by lengthening the duration of individual speech sounds. Clark et al. (1988) have also shown that formal speech involves adjustments for rate and level as well as pitch of the voice. Fairbanks and Miron (1957) made measurements of /s-vowel-s/ syllables which differed in "conversational effort". The maximum value of intensity on each of the three phonemes was measured. There was found to be little difference between the intensity of the consonant (initial or final) and the vowel for casual speech. In formal speech, however, the intensity of the vowel was appreciably higher than the consonant.

Chen et al. (1983) have reported differences in voice onset times (VOT) of syllable-initial voiced and voiceless plosive stop consonants. Voiced and voiceless plosives differ in when voicing starts relative to the release gesture (VOT); the VOT distributions for voiced plosives showed considerable overlap with the voiceless distribution for speech samples drawn from conversation, but there was no overlap for either speaker in the clear speech. Thus, the task of separating out these two classes of syllable-initial plosive stop consonants would be easier for listeners who heard clear speech.

A set of measures was selected based on the studies reviewed to check whether the interviewer was varying her speech between formal and casual. The measures taken were vowel intensity, duration of selected vowels and stop closure VOT in plosives. In the formal style it is expected that vowel intensity will be higher, vowel duration and VOT stop closure will be longer than in the casual speech of these same speakers.

METHOD

Recordings

Two types of subjects were involved in the experiment referred to as interviewers and interviewees. Two interviewers were selected for the study based on a preliminary experiment conducted with fluent speakers to establish whether they could vary their speech style (established from the occurrence of significant differences between the formal and casual speech metrics mentioned above and described more fully below). All interviewers who participated in this experiment had significant differences on all measures. The two speakers were chosen as they are both female and in their early twenties, both of which might affect a child's interaction (neither of these was a speech pathologist).

All interviewers were instructed during the course of this preliminary experiment on what topics to cover and approximately how time should be shared between the speakers (roughly 50% each as the interviewee's speech is as important as the interviewer's). The topics of conversation were chosen from home/parents, school, social interaction, television, leisure activities food and holidays. Interviews were three minutes long and a varying number of the topics (between one and three) would be covered depending on what interested the child. Topics employed in the formal interview were not employed in the casual interview. Further guidance about what topics to cover were not given to stop the interviews being over-contrived.

Twelve children were interviewed aged between 9 and 12. Four of these had been attending a speech pathology clinic for over a year. Four were recorded on their first visit. Four control children from the same area of the city and with similar socio-economic and educational backgrounds to the stuttering children were recruited and recorded in the same manner.

In the interviews themselves the interviewer and the child sat facing one another making sure each other's face could be clearly seen. The child and interviewer was positioned so that distance and direction of the recording microphone did not vary between interviews. Recordings were made in the same quiet room throughout on a Sony TCD-D3 DAT recorder. Calibrations were checked frequently to ensure that intensity did not drift over time. A Sennheiser K6 microphone was used to transduce the sound. The DAT tape recordings were then transferred to a Sun. Each child was interviewed by one of the interviewers formally and casually by the other (the orders of which speaker this was and which style the child received first was counterbalanced over children within each sub-group of four speakers).

ASSESSMENT OF DYSFLUENCIES IN THE CHILD'S SPEECH

The assessment procedure employed is parallel in most regards to those described in Howell et al. (chapter 34). First word boundaries have to be added to the speech and a classification of the word as fluent (F), prolongation (P), repetition (R) or other type of dysfluency (O) made. The words in the child speech were marked by an experienced judge who is known from reliability assessments that have been made to show close agreement with a second highly-trained judge. The position where each word ended was located with the aid of two travelling cursors which were superimposed on the speech waveform display. Each cursor position was independently adjusted with a mouse. The first cursor was initially placed at the start of the speech. The second cursor was positioned slightly before where the end of the first word was thought to be located. The section of speech between the first and second cursors was then played and listened to over an RS 250-924 headset, to check whether the end of the word had been correctly located. The second cursor was then adjusted further forward and played. Once the judge had adjusted past the end of the word, the judge adjusted the cursor back in time into the file. The judge continued crossing backwards and forwards across the boundary at the end of word until he was satisfied that he had located it accurately. This marker was stored and the subject proceeded to locate the boundary between the next words in the sequence in the same way (this procedure is similar to that used by Osberger and Levitt, 1979).

Assessment procedures for dysfluencies

After the word-endpoint boundaries had been obtained, two experienced judges made fluency assessments about the child's words. Words were defined as the interval from the end of one word to the end of the next. Each word in the speech of the child was judged once each.

For each of the three complete set of judgments, the procedure was identical: First, a random sequence specifying presentation order of all words from all speakers was computed. The words were randomized so that the global context in which all judgments are made is as constant as possible. The first randomly-selected word was then heard in isolation. After a short pause the test word was heard along with the word that had preceded it (the two words had the same timing and were in the same order as in the original recording). Consequently, pauses were apparent when they occurred between the context and test word. The test word alone and this same word with the word that preceded it could be heard as many times as the judge required by hitting the return key on the computer keyboard. Thus, presentation of the test and context words were initiated by the judge and the current trial terminated and the next trial commenced after the judge entered his responses (detailed in the following paragraphs). The full context was not available at the beginning of the recording (in these cases, the word to be judged was still played in isolation beforehand). It was stressed to the judges that judgments were being made about the first word that was played.

The two judgments obtained about each word, were a rating about how comfortably the word "flowed" and a categorisation of the word as fluent (F), or as a dysfluent prolongation (P), repetition (R) or other (O) dysfluency. It was stressed that the rating scale was *not* a finer-grained indication of whether a word is fluent or dysfluent: A word low in "flow" might nevertheless be categorised as F or vice versa (as does happen in the data). The 5-point scale indicated the extent to which the judge agreed with the statement that "the speech is flowing smoothly" (1 = agree, 5 = disagree with intermediate values indicating intermediate levels of agreement).

Judges were self-paced in that they terminated the judgment session when they began to feel fatigued. On recommencing, they started at the point in the random sequence they had left off. Typically judges would judge about 200 words before taking a rest.

Assessment procedure for interviewer's style

Forty vowels and forty plosive stop consonants (twenty voiced and twenty voiceless) spoken by the interviewer were selected at random from each interview for analysis (24 interviews in all). The vowels and plosives were delimited from oscillograms using the Osberger and Levitt (1979) procedure. Peak intensity and duration of the vowel were obtained directly from the oscillograms. VOT was measured for each plosive as the gap between sound onset and visible onset of voicing. The average vowel duration and intensity were obtained for each interview. The difference between average voiceless and voiced VOTs was obtained for each plosive again for each interview.

RESULTS AND DISCUSSION

The vowel duration and speech intensity as well as the difference between voiceless and voiced VOTs of the interviewers was analyzed to check that they had made the appropriate adjustments to their speech style, whether this varied between interviewer and whether this differed across the three child sub-groups. For each measure an ANOVA was performed with interviewer (the two speakers) and interview style (formal and casual) as factors. Interview style was the only factor that was significant in either analysis ($p < 0.001$ in each case). In the formal style the intensity was 2.7 times greater than in the casual style, vowel durations were on average 19.8 ms longer and the difference between voiceless and voiced plosives was 15 ms greater than for the casual style. For each of these measures, then, it appears that the speakers followed the interview-style instructions.

Did this have any effect on the dysfluencies that the stutterers produced? This question was addressed by an ANOVA which had the factors speaker groups and interview style. The measures analyzed were various all attempting to characterize difficulties the child speaker might have. The main ones investigated were percentage of dysfluent words out of all words spoken and average flow rating over all words spoken. In each case, there was a main effect of speaker group with the child stutterers exhibiting more dysfluencies than the controls. However, no differences were found in any of these measures between formal and casual styles. Thus, it appears from these data that interview style does not affect the dysfluencies emitted. This particular variable, then, would not appear crucial when obtaining speech samples.

ACKNOWLEDGEMENT

This research was supported by a grant from the Wellcome Trust.

REFERENCES

Chen, F.R., Zue, V.W., Picheny, M.A., Durlach N.I., & Braida, L.D. (1983). Speaking clearly: Acoustic characteristics and intelligibility of stop consonants. *Speech Communication Group, MIT: Working Papers*, 2, 1-8.

Clark, J., Lubker, J., & Hunnicutt, S. (1988). Some preliminary evidence for phonetic adjustment strategies in communication difficulty. In R. Steele, R., & T. Threadgold (Eds.), *Language Topics:*

Essays in Honour of Michael Halliday (pp. 161-180). John Benjamins, Amsterdam.

Fairbanks, G., & Miron, M.S (1957). Effects of vocal effort upon the consonant-vowel ratio within the syllable. *Journal of the Acoustical Society of America, 29,* 621-626.

Howell, P., Sackin, S., Glenn K., & Au-Yeung, J. (this volume). Automatic stuttering frequency counts. In W. Hulstijn, H.F.M. Peters, & P.H.H.M. Van Lieshout (Eds.), *Speech production: motor control, brain research and fluency disorders.* Amsterdam: Elsevier Science.

Osberger, M.J., & Levitt, H. (1979). The effect of timing errors on the intelligibility of deaf children's speech. *Journal of the Acoustical Society of America, 66,* 1316-1324.

Picheny, M.A, Durlach, N.I., & Braida, L.D. (1985). Speaking clearly for the hard of hearing II: Acoustic characteristics of clear conversational speech. *Journal of Speech and Hearing Research, 29,* 434-446.

Speech Production: Motor Control, Brain Research and Fluency Disorders
W. Hulstijn, H.F.M. Peters and P.H.H.M. Van Lieshout, editors

Chapter 50

EVALUATING SPEECH QUALITY BEFORE AND AFTER STUTTERING THERAPY

Marie-Christine Franken, Renée van Bezooijen, Louis Boves

The purpose of the present study was to develop an instrument to evaluate the changes in the speech quality as a result of stuttering therapy. Listeners judged the suitability of speech of people who stutter (N = 10) at three stages of therapy (before, after, and six months after) and that of people who do not stutter (N = 10), using an anchored 10-point scale, for 10 speaking situations which supposedly make different demands. Listeners consisted of three groups: unsophisticated listeners (N = 17), clinicians specializing in the treatment of stuttering (N = 17), and stuttering listeners (N = 17). Results indicate that the rating instrument can be scored reliably, that listeners can discriminate the speech of the people who stutter from the speech of the reference speakers, and that unsophisticated listeners were less tolerant in their judgments than clinicians and stuttering listeners.

INTRODUCTION

Which measures adequately describe the speech of a person who stutters? Traditionally, stuttering severity (percentage syllables stuttered), and speech rate (number of syllables per second) were measured to describe the speech fluency. Clinical experience and research (Franken et al., 1992) has learned that *speech quality* is a very important issue for investigating improvement. Percentage syllables stuttered and number of syllables per second are not sufficient to describe the overall post-treatment speech quality.

To describe speech quality of people who stutter during and after treatment a naturalness scale has been advocated: a 7- or 9-point equal-appearing interval scale with one extreme defined as 'highly natural' and the other extreme defined as 'highly unnatural' (Martin, Haroldson & Triden, 1984; Onslow & Ingham, 1987).

What are the most relevant criteria for the evaluation of post-(stuttering) treatment speech quality? In our opinion, the following two are particular important:

(1) the *speaker* judges that he/she feels *sufficiently comfortable* in the speaking situation concerned.

(2) the *listener* judges the speech quality of the speaker to be *sufficiently suitable* for the speaking situation concerned;

In this paper, we will restrict ourselves to the development of tools regarding the second criterion. The naturalness scale described by Martin et al. (1984) shows several psychometric problems to suffice as a measurement tool for this criterion. First, ratings on equal-appearing interval scales do not allow one to determine whether the speech is *sufficiently* natural, not to be distinguishable from that of average speakers. Second, the naturalness judgments are given without relating it to specific speech situations, while research indicates that norms applied to speech are stricter as the speaking situation becomes more formal: the type of speech that may be acceptable in the privacy of one's home differs from what is allowed or expected in the public domain with listeners unknown to the speaker. Thus, judgments on speech quality should be related to the speaking situation.

In attempts to minimize the psychometric limitations of the naturalness scale when evaluating speech quality, we propose the concept of communicative suitability (i.e., the speaking situation-dependent adequacy of speech as judged by listeners).

The purpose of the present study was to develop and evaluate a global instrument for assessing the communicative suitability of speech. The aim was to develop a measurement tool that could be used to make absolute judgments and link the judgments to the speaking situation.

METHOD

10 stutterers were recorded in the clinic pre-treatment, post-treatment, and six months follow-up treatment, each time commenting on a different topic. Also, 10 non-stuttering reference speakers were recorded. Stimuli for the judgment experiment were selected from a semi-spontaneous speech task in which speakers summarized and commented upon a newspaper article for about five minutes. The reference speakers were recorded on two topics during a single session. Stimulus material selected consisted of fragments of about 45 seconds, semi-spontaneous speech. The total number of stimuli judged was 50 (10 stutterers X 3 recordings + 10 reference speakers X 2 recordings).

The listeners rated the suitability of the speech, using a 10-point scale, for 10 speaking situations which supposedly make different demands. Table 1 shows the rating scale and gives an overview of the 10 speaking situations.

Listeners consisted of three groups: adults who stutter ($N=17$), adults who do not stutter ($N=17$), and clinicians specializing in the treatment of stuttering ($N=17$). The listeners rated the suitability of the speech, using a 10-point scale, for use in each of 10 speaking situations which supposedly make different demands. The reason for choosing these 10 situations is explained elsewhere (Franken et al., in press). Listeners judged the suitability on the 10-point suitability scale, keeping in mind the grading scale that is commonly used in the Dutch educational system (1: very bad <-> 10: excellent). Therefore, the scale can be considered an anchored 10-point scale, allowing interpretation of the judgments of communicative suitability in absolute terms. Order of presentation of the 10 situations to be rated was random and changed every 10 stimuli.

Table 1. 10-point suitability scale and the 10 speaking situations for which communicative suitability was rated.

*How **suitable** do you judge the speech of this speaker for:*
1. talking about everyday events with a friend

| 1 | 2 | 3 | 4 | 5 | 6 | 7 | 8 | 9 | 10 |

(1: very bad   6: just sufficient;
2: bad;   7: amply sufficient;
3: moderate;   8: good;
4: insufficient;   9: very good;
5: just insufficient; 10: excellent).

2. telling a housemate about one's new job
3. chatting with housemates during a party game
4. giving a speech at a family celebration
5. making conversation with a friend in the train
6. ordering bread from the baker around the corner
7. getting into contact with a stranger on the bus
8. asking a bypasser for directions
9. instructing a group at a dancing school
10. giving a lecture to a newly founded professional association

Table 2. Mean communicative suitability ratings ($N=51$) for 10 reference speakers for 10 speaking situations (10-point scales), ordered from lowest to highest suitability.

Speaking situation	Mean	SD
9. instructing a group at a dancing school	5.7	2.2
10. giving a lecture to a newly founded professional association	5.8	2.2
4. giving a speech at a family celebration	6.7	2.0
7. getting into contact with a stranger on the bus	7.3	1.6
8. asking a bypasser for directions	7.5	1.5
6. ordering bread from the baker around the corner	7.7	1.4
3. chatting with housemates during a party game	7.7	1.4
5. making conversation with a friend in the train	7.7	1.3
2. telling a housemate about one's new job	7.7	1.4
1. talking about everyday events with a friend	8.0	1.3

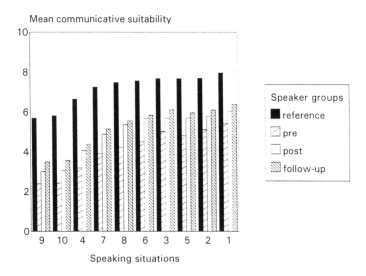

Figure 1: Mean suitability ratings (N=51) for the 10 speaking situations separately for the three moments of measurement of the stuttering speakers, and for the reference speakers. The 10 situations are ordered from low to highly demanding cf. the means for the reference speakers in Table 1. For the meaning of the speaking situations, see Table 1.

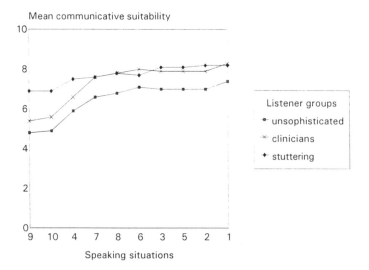

Figure 2. Interaction between speaking situation and listener group (unsophisticated listeners, clinicians, and stuttering listeners) for the speech of the reference speakers. Suitability ratings (10-point scales) for the 10 speaking situations. The 10 situations are ordered from low to highly demanding cf. the means for the reference speakers in Table 2. For the meaning of the speaking situations, see Table 1.

RESULTS

Results indicate that the rating instrument can be scored reliably (all Cronbach's alpha exceeded .93).

Analysis of variance for the mean ratings (51 listeners) of the reference speakers showed that the factor speaking situation had a significant effect ($p < .001$) on the suitability ratings, with more demanding situations receiving lower suitability scores than the less demanding ones.

Table 2 shows the mean communicative suitability ratings for the reference speakers for each of the 10 selected speaking situations ($N = 51$).

Analyses of variance showed that the speech of the people who stutter (pre-treatment, post-treatment, and six months follow-up) was judged significantly less suitable ($p \leq 0.001$) than the speech of the reference speakers. This result is illustrated in Figure 1.
Furthermore, analyses of variance showed that nonstuttering, unsophisticated adults were less tolerant in their judgments than clinicians and persons who stutter. Figure 2 illustrates that unsophisticated listeners were less tolerant ($p < 0.001$) in their judgments than clinicians and stuttering listeners, regarding the speech of the reference speakers.

CONCLUSIONS

1. The relevance of the concept of "communicative suitability" was confirmed. The data showed that speech qualities which are just good enough for low demanding situations are judged unsuitable for highly demanding situations. Speech from people who stutter could be discriminated from speech from reference speakers.
2. Distinguishing between non-formal, slightly formal, formal and very formal speaking situations seems relevant when judging communicative suitability.
3. Our data suggest that "the man in the street" is less tolerant in his judgments than clinicians specializing in stuttering and listeners who stutter.

REFERENCES

Franken, M.C., Boves, L., Peters, H.F.M., & Webster. R.L. (1992). Perceptual evaluation of the speech before and after fluency shaping stuttering therapy. *Journal of Fluency Disorders, 17*, 223-241.

Franken, M.C., van Bezooijen, R., & Boves, L. Stuttering and communicative suitability of speech. *Journal of Speech and Hearing Research*, in press.

Martin, R., Haroldson, S., & Triden, K. (1984). Stuttering and speech naturalness. *Journal of Speech and Hearing Disorders, 49*, 53-58.

Onslow, M., & Ingham, R.J. (1987). Speech quality measurement and the management of stuttering. *Journal of Speech and Hearing Disorders, 52*, 2-17.

PART E

Developmental aspects of speech production and fluency disorders

© 1997 Elsevier Science B.V. All rights reserved.
Speech Production: Motor Control, Brain Research and Fluency Disorders
W. Hulstijn, H.F.M. Peters and P.H.H.M. Van Lieshout, editors

Chapter 51

NEURONAL GROUP SELECTION AND EMERGENT OROFACIAL MOTOR CONTROL: TOWARDS A UNIFYING THEORY OF SPEECH DEVELOPMENT

Steven M. Barlow, Don Finan, Rich Andreatta

The wealth of multimodal mapping available to the brain for speech motor control represents an excellent example of a complex behavior that may be heavily determined by neuronal selectionist mechanisms and multisensory registration in space and time. In sharp contrast to instructionist notions, selectionist models (Edelman, 1978, 1987, 1992) embrace variation as centrally important to an organism in achieving good adaptive performance. The variability in the intergestural dynamics of speech is consistent with this principle of selectionism. Significant relations exist between selectionist mechanisms and neuroplasticity in developing and mature organisms. Recent experimental evidence and hypotheses are reviewed concerning some of the mechanisms of plasticity available to the nervous system. It is hypothesized that the sensory consequences of speech movement are continually encoded and serve as the catalyst for change (plasticity). The potency of mechanosensory input is demonstrated by recent orofacial entrainment experiments in human neonates.

INTRODUCTION

Applying Selectionist Principles to a Neurobiological Model of Speech Development and Production.

The wealth of multimodal mapping available to the brain for speech production represents a complex motor behavior that lends itself well to the potent shaping influences favored by neuronal selectionist mechanisms. Although competing theories in biological systems have traditionally been either instructionist or selectionist (Sporns, 1994), there is mounting experimental evidence for selectionist principles operating at different levels of the nervous system for the acquisition and maintenance of motor skills (Edelman, 1978, 1987, 1992). This theoretical stance embraces variation as centrally important to an organism in achieving good adaptive performance. Sporns (1994) stated that eventhough variability may be structural or dynamic, structural differences between functional elements can give rise to additional variability in the ensuing dynamics. The variability in the intergestural orofacial dynamics of sucking, babbling, and speech is consistent with this principle of selectionism.

The topographical maps of our brains basically provide an experiential indication of what we have done, and suggest what we can do. The sensory consequences of movement are continually encoded and mapped in the brain. Motor action produces multiple and simultaneous sensory maps, so that movement and its visual, proprioceptive, auditory and tactile consequences continually converge and are temporally correlated in multiple sites in the CNS. Neural network principles demonstrate that such multiple reentrant maps can lead to the selection of categories of actions that are both stable and flexible (Edelman, 1987; Thelen & Smith, 1994). According to Thelen and Smith (1994), these ideas turn the usual development stories backward; multimodal correspondences are the *cause* of development rather than a *product* of development. Therefore, to understand orofacial control we feel it is imperative to look at its assembly during development. *The hypothesis is that while the status of the neuromotor system determines the behavioral output, the behavior itself changes the neuromotor system.* Our entrainment studies in neonates and infants are designed to test this notion.

Establishing perceptual categories is an important element of selection for the developing talker. To the neonate who lacks the experience or pre-wiring, the world is an "unlabeled place" (Edelman, 1987) The partitioning of this stimulus world into meaningful categories depends on individual experience and the adaptive value that this partitioning has for the neonate. Similar problems exist in the formulation of movement patterns and synergies during development. Motor and sensorimotor coordination develop gradually and most oral movements are not "given" or hard-wired but depend in their realization on actual performance and experience. The ongoing growth and morphological change of the orofacial sensorimotor apparatus demand that the neural structures controlling the orofacial apparatus be capable of following changes adaptively by forming and dissolving motor categories when needed. This seems logical given the transition from primitive total body reflex actions, to sucking, eating, babbling, gesture and speech. It seems highly unlikely that a programmed system (instructionist) would be able to anticipate fully the demands made on an organism by its environment in the course of a lifetime, a key argument for the operation of somatic selection mechanisms (Sporns, 1994).

We have learned that babies and young children differ significantly in their movement patterns for sucking, smiling, eating, and speech. The progression from a set of simple 'synergies' to well-adapted movements can be viewed as a process of selection of movements from a repertoire (Sporns & Edelman, 1993). During ongoing experience and interaction with the environment, appropriate movements are selected and others are eliminated, in response to global value signals related to the salience of these movements. Developmental and experience-dependent processes are of central importance in a selectionist theoretical framework and seem especially important in the emergence of speech production.

Correlation and Reentry

In order to assure that comparison and association of neuronal responses registered in separate cortical maps take place, the theory advocates that neuronal responses must become *correlated* with each other. Correlation is attained through *reentry* (functional reciprocity between neuronal groups), the ongoing and reciprocal exchange of signals between neural maps. There is strong empirical evidence for the existence of multisensory maps in the mammalian nervous system which are driven by spatial and temporal correlation. Barry Stein and his colleagues (see Stein et al., 1995 for review) have conducted an elegant series of experiments outlining the multisensory properties of the tectum and cerebral cortex in cat and have generated a series of integrative rules which bear special relevance to a selectionist theory of motor development.

Spatial Rule:

The overall spatial registry among the different sensory maps (superior colliculus) extends to the different sensory receptive fields of an individual multisensory neuron. Thus, a visual and somatosensory stimulus originating from the same location in space will fall within the excitatory receptive fields of a visual-somatosensory multisensory neuron. The physiological result of this stimulus pairing to a single event is an enhancement of the neurons' response. Many more impulses are evoked by the stimulus combination than by either stimulus alone. Instead of a simple additive effect, the increase in neural activity is multiplicative. Enhancement and depression are dynamic properties that depend on the relative spatial relations of stimuli and the receptive fields of the neuron.

Temporal Rule:

Multisensory interactions are very common in the superior colliculus and cerebral cortex despite the substantial latency differences among the inputs from the different modalities. Responses to auditory stimuli range from 6-25 ms, somatosensory stimuli 12-30 ms, and visual stimuli 40-120 ms. The large differences in conduction time would appear to preclude any possibility for neural interaction. Fortunately, most stimuli initiate excitatory or inhibitory events that last far longer than these intersensory latency differences. This provides a long processing window, thereby enabling the inputs to interact despite their significant differences in arrival time (Meredith et al., 1987). Overlapping the periods of peak activity of the unimodal discharge train seems to optimize multisensory interaction.

Magnitude or Inverse Effectiveness Rule:

The magnitude of a multisensory interaction is defined as $[CM - SM_{max}/SM_{max} \times 100]$, where CM is the combined modality response and the SM_{max} is the best single modality response (Stein et al., 1995). In general, the more effective the unimodal stimuli, the lower the magnitude of the enhancement they generate in combination, a phenomenon referred to as *inverse effectiveness*. As previously noted, multisensory enhancements appear multiplicative. For example, a response to a combined stimulus might be 10 or more impulses, whereas response to an individual stimulus might be 2 impulses or fewer. In fact, some individual stimuli evoke no activity. It is only when the stimuli are combined that a vigorous response occurs (Meredith & Stein, 1986). For behavior, this makes good sense. Potent unimodal stimuli need no enhancement to be effective. The combinations of relatively weak unimodal stimuli may be an efficient mechanism for establishing new correlations in the formation of novel sensory and motor maps. The utility of multisensory enhancement becomes obvious when considering the dynamic environment of the neonate who is very busy associating new faces with voices, correlating oromotor performance with tactile, kinesthetic, and acoustic features, in the pursuit of speech and language acquisition.

Receptive Field Preservation Rule:

The unimodal receptive field properties of multisensory superior colliculus [SC] neurons (receptive field borders, direction sensitivity, velocity sensitivity) remain unaltered in the presence of a stimulus from another modality (Stein et al., 1993).

Cortical neurons integrate multisensory information in the same way as do superior colliculus neurons. Multisensory neurons in cortex display spatial overlap of receptive fields, regardless of location in the brain or the species in which they are found (Stein et al., 1993). Consistent with the spatial rule, multisensory neurons in cortex display responses to each unimodal stimulus when presented individually, and manifest an enhanced response when the stimuli were presented simultaneously and in spatial register. According to the *temporal rule*, the magnitude of the response was greatest when the peak periods of the unimodal responses was overlapped. Combinations of two weak unimodal stimuli resulted in the largest interaction, known as *inverse effectiveness*.

These integrative principles appear to be universal properties of multisensory neurons, regardless of location or species (rat cortex, cat, primate cortex, and human EP studies). Integrative information systems in the brain act to enhance responses to stimuli that originate from the same event and to inhibit responses to unrelated stimuli. This is a dynamic process that may be central to the formation of new perceptual and motor categories.

Neuronal Groups

According to Edelman and Sporns, *neuronal groups* (NGŝ) offer several advantages. It reduces the need for point-to-point wiring in map formation. NGŝ permit units with fixed anatomy (i.e., somatosensory cortex) to undergo functional reorganization as required by changing needs and growth of the organism. They also permit essential reciprocal mappings between distant cortical areas to be maintained during such reorganization. NGŝ permit signals reflecting sensory context to have consistent effects on units with related function by placing those units in close spatial proximity. NGŝ permit selective changes in synaptic efficacy to be coordinated among collections of neurons with related functions and facilitate long-term stability of connections receiving common patterns of correlated input.

The Relation Between Selectionist Mechanisms and Neuroplasticity.

The topographically ordered mapping between the body surface and the surface of the somatosensory cortex is not fixed and anatomically hardwired, even in the adult animal, but is capable of dynamically readjusting to changes in the input (Merzenich et al., 1984; Calford & Tweedale, 1990). These changes in input may result from different activities engaging the organism, or alterations in the input due to injury or deprivation. There appear to be a variety of mechanisms, some reflecting short-term adaptive processes (almost immediate) likely due to changes in synaptic efficacy, and other long-term changes affecting the structure of interconnections. The plasticity of the brain has been the subject of intense study in recent years and a number of paradigms have opened up the neurobiological possibilities for a variety of selectionist mechanisms. The capacity of the nervous system to change its wiring in response to changes in behavioral patterns or sensory environment has been described for the visual system (Miller, 1992; Tamura et al., 1992; Pettet & Gilbert, 1992; Shatz, 1994), auditory system (Edeline & Weinberger, 1991; Sanes & Takacs, 1993), spinal motor systems (Kalb & Hockfield, 1992; Lo & Poo, 1991), and somatosensory systems (Billy & Walters, 1989; Fox, 1994; Meftah & Rispal-Padel, 1994; Recanzone et al., 1990). A major finding common to these studies is that the development and stability of synaptic connections in the nervous system are clearly influenced by the pattern of electrical activity and competitive interaction between adjacent nerve terminals (Garraghty et al., 1994). In essence, *'neurons wire together, if they fire together'* (Sporns, 1994).

Shaping Neuronal Connections and Group Formation.

There are important lessons to be learned from the exciting neurobiological literature on synaptic competition and activity-dependent change that bear directly on our thinking about orofacial development and motor control. It is generally thought that the formation of precise neural connections involves two distinct mechanisms: those that are *activity-independent* and those that require *neuronal activity* (Goodman & Shatz, 1993; Shatz, 1994). The *activity-independent* mechanisms occur early in fetal life and involve "molecular sensing' for axon outgrowth, pathfinding, and target selection. In contrast, the refinement of initially diffuse connections within targets almost always requires neuronal activity. For the human orofacial system, this process of refinement seems to span a protracted period of development that begins *in utero* and extends well into infancy and childhood. In her award winning paper, Shatz (1994) suggested that neuronal activity affords the post-natal organism with a mechanism for adaptation, i.e, the maturing nervous system can be modified by experience itself (adaptability). As previously described, adaptability is a hallmark feature of the orofacial system given the expanding repertoire of motor behaviors played out through this anatomy (sucking, smiling, gesture, drinking and eating, hand-mouth manipulation, cooing, babbling, and speech). Neuronal activity is a genetically conservative means of achieving a high degree of specificity and precision in neuronal wiring. Applied to the trigemino-thalamic projection, specification of each neural connection between primary trigeminal afferents and the VP_m thalamus using specific molecular markers would require an extraordinary number of genes, given the thousands of connections formed. The alternative, to specify precise pathways and targets using the rules of activity-dependent sorting and multimodal mapping to achieve ultimate precision in connectivity, is far more economical. We strongly believe this form of activity-dependent neuronal plasticity is an essential mechanism of normal development *and could be applied as a powerful habilitative tool in human neonates at-risk for orosensory and oromotor disorders.*

Model of Area 3b Organization

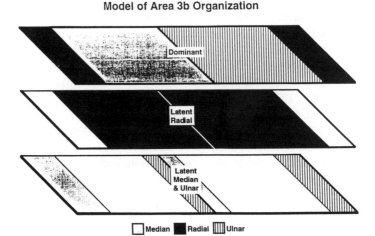

Figure 1. Schematic representation of the hypothetical 'dominant' and 'latent' domains of the three peripheral nerves to the hand in area 3b of cortex. [With permission from Garraghty, Hanes, Florence & Kaas, 1994].

Injury-Dependent Change.

   One way to explore neural selection mechanisms is to experimentally deprive the brain of its input(s). This general approach has been effective in revealing patterns of dominant and latent inputs conveyed over the median, ulnar, and radial nerves to primary somatosensory cortex. Garraghty et al. (1994) have developed a model of Area 3b organization (see Figure 1) based on 5 different experimental manipulations involving :
(1) transection of the median nerve where reorganization is complete and accomplished largely by expansion of radial nerve representation (Merzenich et al., 1983a, b); (2) transection of the median and ulnar nerves where reorganization is complete and accomplished solely by expansion of radial nerve representation (Garraghty & Kaas, 1991); (3) transection of the median and radial nerves where reorganization is incomplete (Garraghty et al., 1994); (4) transection of the ulnar and radial nerves where reorganization is incomplete (Garraghty et al., 1994); and (5) multiple-digit amputation where reorganization is incomplete (Merzenich et al., 1984). When analyzed collectively, these studies suggest that the median and ulnar nerves have large zones of dominance in somatosensory cortex, with limited representation by latent inputs. In contrast, the radial nerve normally has a small cortical territory which is dominant, but the extent of its latent inputs overlap completely with the zones of median and ulnar nerve dominance (Garraghty et al., 1994).

   Two hypotheses have been proposed to account for the reorganization that occurs in cortical and subcortical structures following an interruption of somatosensory inputs (Garraghty et al., 1994). These hypotheses are summarized schematically in figure 2. The left half of this figure shows the proposed outcome of eliminating inputs where parts of projecting axonal arbors are not equally effective in activating postsynaptic neurons under normal

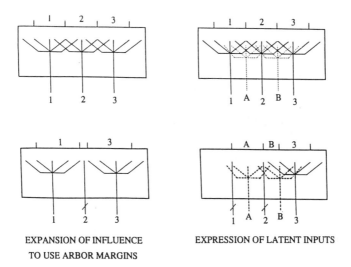

EXPANSION OF INFLUENCE   EXPRESSION OF LATENT INPUTS
TO USE ARBOR MARGINS

Figure 2. A set of schematic diagrams illustrating two potential mechanisms for cortical and subcortical map reorganizations after an interruption of their inputs. On the left is the predicted outcome of eliminating inputs where parts of projecting axonal arbors are not equally effective in activating postsynaptic neurons under normal circumstances. In the top left, the axonal arbors providing inputs '1', '2', and '3' are broader than the areas of the map which are dominated by their inputs. As shown in bottom left panel, elimination of input '2' causes the lateral-most arbors of neurons '1' and '3' to become effective, and the regions of cortex where these inputs dominate appear to expand. On the right, a normally latent set of inputs, labeled 'A' and 'B,' are added to the model. As shown on the top, their inputs are normally not expressed, however if inputs '1' and '2' are eliminated, neurons 'A' and 'B' are permitted to express themselves [With permission from Garraghty, Kaas & Florence, 1994].

circumstances. In the top left, the axonal arbors providing inputs '1', '2', and '3' are broader than the areas of the map which are dominated by their inputs. If input '2' is removed, the adjacent lateral-most portions of arbors '1' and '3' become effective , and the regions of cortex where these inputs dominate thus appear to expand. The initial conditions are repeated on the right side of figure 2 with the addition of a normally latent set of inputs designated 'A' and 'B.' As illustrated at the top, their inputs are normally not expressed. If inputs '1' and '2' are eliminated, then 'A' and 'B' are permitted to express themselves.

These concepts support the notion that neural plasticity in the mature brain is partially due to a change in the effectiveness of existing connections. Deprivation studies also provide evidence suggesting that neural plasticity is actually the result of multiple processes, varying greatly in the time of expression. It is well known in somatosensory cortex that some neurons deprived of their normal inputs by nerve transection immediately express new receptive fields (Garraghty et al., 1994). The rapid change in receptive field properties implies the pre-existence of relevant circuitry in the form of latent architecture which become 'unmasked' following peripheral nerve transection. This is quite different from the mechanisms associated with neural sprouting which occur over a protracted period of time.

It was hypothesized that NMDA receptors (glutamatergic) are necessary for the reorganization that follows within four weeks (Garraghty & Muja, 1996). In three monkeys in which NMDA receptors were concurrently blocked, most the deprived cortex remained unresponsive. It was concluded that much of the cortical recovery that typically follows peripheral nerve injury in adult monkeys is apparently dependent on NMDA receptors and may well be due to Hebbian-like changes in synaptic strength.

According to Garraghty and Muja (1996), there appear to be two phases of reorganization following deafferentation. Initially, some deprived neurons immediately express new receptive fields (Merzenich et al., 1983b; Cusick et al., 1990; Calford & Tweedale, 1991). This initial phase of recovery is likely due to changes in synaptic efficacy arising from reductions in afferent-driven inhibition (Alloway & Burton, 1991). This is known as the '*unmasking*' of latent inputs (Merrill & Wall, 1972).

In the second phase, the remaining majority regain responsiveness over a period of weeks or months (Merzenich et al., 1983a, b; Garraghty & Kaas, 1991). This phase may be due to the increased efficacy of previously existing synapses (Garraghty & Sur, 1990). Converging evidence suggests that ACh is involved in the 2nd phase of reorganization. ACh depletion acts to prevent the activation of N-methyl-d-aspartate (NMDA) glutamatergic receptors, and that the activation of these receptors was necessary for the emergence of new receptive fields in injury-deprived cortex. It was further argued that elimination of the normally dominant inputs to median nerve cortex permits the gradual strengthening of correlations between the activity of the formally impotent presynaptic and deprived postsynaptic elements. These enhanced correlations may also have been made possible by reductions in intracortical inhibition as a necessary not sufficient condition. Experiments such as this currently assume that mechanisms involved in developmental synaptic plasticity persist into adulthood, and account for environmentally induced changes in the mature brain (Rauschecker, 1991).

The grain of primary cortical maps is finer than that of the thalamocortical afferents. The spread of thalamocortical axonal arbors is typically much larger than the zone in the cortex where the receptive fields of the incoming afferents are normally represented. This anatomical feature of cortex makes it possible to express a 'subset' of degenerate inputs. Electrophysiological mapping of cortical topography reflects modifications in this selection process. According to Garraghty and Muja (1996), when **GABA** *ergic* activity is disrupted with antagonists, the receptive fields of many cortical neurons are found to enlarge dramatically suggesting that the expressed subset of degenerate inputs involves selection via inhibitory elimination. The existence of immediate changes in somatosensory, motor, visual, and auditory cortex following injury suggests that a permissive anatomical infrastructure is normally present and that the map normally expressed in cortex represents a dominant fraction of all available inputs.

Activity-Dependent Change.

A growing body of evidence from experiments on CNS plasticity leads us to believe that sensorimotor control is established through use. Many experiments have controlled the sensory experience or induced motor cortex in order to quantitatively assess the plastic nature of central neural representations. In a recent study by Xerri, Stern and Merzenich (1994), alterations of the cortical representation of the rat ventrum were induced by rat pup nursing behavior. The primary sensory cortex representation of the ventral trunk skin of lactating rats was nearly two times larger than in matched postpartum non-lactating controls. The expansion of SI cortical areas for ventral trunk was greatest for nipple bearing skin between the forelimbs and hindlimbs, and was associated with receptive fields about one-third the sizes of those recorded in matched nonlactating or virgin controls. It is likely that these representational differences for nipple-bearing and non-nipple-bearing ventrum skin are exaggerated due to the behavioral significance of the activity. Experiments such as these point to the importance of experience and activity-dependent mechanisms in shaping neural structure and function. According to Xerri et al. (1994), once sucking is begun, the heavy schedule of novel afferent inputs that is generated produces changes in brain representation that are presumed to modify the sensory experience associated with sucking. These experience-driven neurological changes become an intrinsic part of the behavior. The robustness of activity-dependent plasticity is underscored by Merzenich's observation that experienced-induced changes have been documented and mapped in every sensory and motor area studied thus far (Merzenich et al., 1990). It seems quite probable that human sucking, oromotor play, prevocalization, and babbling en route to speech, results in substantial representational remodeling in most if not all somatosensory areas, as well as in a number of motor and premotor regions.

Application of Activity-Dependent Mechanisms for Orofacial Motor Control

Compared with newborns of other species, the human neonate is relatively helpless in motor capabilities and relatively precocious in sensory capabilities. There is evidence that specialization of the perioral sensorimotor apparatus begins very early in life. Bosma (1970) stated that "suckling, maintaining the airway, and responding to tactual stimuli are 'mature' neonatal oral functions" that are highly adaptive to local sensory experience and integrated with the whole of the organism (p.550). This is consistent with the time course and pattern of neurogenesis in the orofacial region.

Humans, like other mammals, are born with the ability to produce sucking movements and other cyclic movements. But like all other rhythmic movements, sucking is not just endogenous, but emergent from rhythm-generating circuits and subject to modification by external inputs. For example, rapid adjustment of sucking to the presence of fluid in the mouth and the entrainment of swallowing, respiration when nutritive sucking. Some recent experimental findings suggest that the organization of centrally patterned orofacial movements can be modified by applying controlled mechanical inputs to this region during non-nutritive sucking (Finan & Barlow, 1996).

Entrainment of Rhythmic Motor Outputs.

Entrainment is defined as the synchronization of an endogenous oscillator to external periodic events (Pavlidis, 1973; Glass & Mackey, 1988: Kriellaars et al., 1994). For a given stimulus with fixed amplitude and period, a stable phase relationship between the stimulus and oscillator must exist to satisfy the conditions for entrainment. One such endogenous oscillator in the neonate is the non-nutritive suck rhythm generator represented by its motor output, and the external periodic event is the pulsating surface of the baglet (nipple) of the motor driven ACTIFIER. The ability of an oscillator to synchronize to an external periodic signal provides adaptive and predictive control that allows fast and reliable responses to external changes (Pavlidis, 1973). This type of control would aid in adapting the suck rate set by higher brain centers to variations in pacifier compliance and physical characteristics. The ability of a peripheral signal to entrain suck demonstrates the potential for on-line integration of mechanosensory events into the suck rhythm generating circuitry. Entrainment stimulation techniques have been shown in a variety of animal preparations to be an effective means of regulating and modifying the rhythm of central pattern generators (CPGs) involved in the control of cyclic motor behaviors such as stepping and locomotion (Conway et al., 1987; Pearson et al., 1992), and mastication (Rossignol et al., 1988).

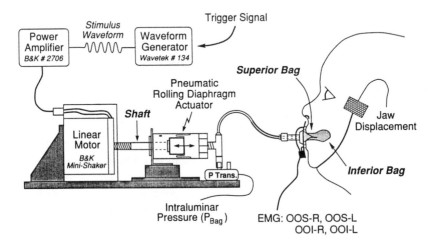

Figure 3. A schematic diagram of the actifier system developed for neurophysiological studies of oromotor entrainment, electromyography, and perioral reflex modulation in neonates and infants. The system consists of a modified pacifier, an array of 4 miniature linear motors for mechanical stimulation of perioral tissue, and a large linear motor/rolling diaphragm assembly designed to regulate conformational dynamics of the latex nipple [baglet]. The Bruel & Kjaer minishaker linear motor is coupled to a pneumatic rolling diaphragm actuator in order to regulate intraluminal pressure of the latex baglet. Movement of the rolling diaphragm to the left produces a negative pressure within the cylinder of the diaphragm which causes the baglet to collapse whereas displacement of the diaphragm to the right produces a positive pressure and a subsequent expansion of the baglet.

The use of mechanical entrainment effectively strengthens the temporal and spatial correlation between sensory experience and the ongoing motor pattern.

Neonate Oromotor Entrainment

Recently, entrainment techniques have been applied to the study of oromotor control and non-nutritive suck in human neonates. As shown in figures 3 and 4, a new instrument has been designed and built that permits investigation of oromotor entrainment and sensorimotor integration during non-nutritive sucking in neonates and infants. It is referred to as an actifier (see details in Finan & Barlow, 1996). The design consists of 4 linear motors integrated into the housing of a pacifier equipped with 8 miniature Ag/AgCl EMG electrodes (allows sampling of 4 EMG channels around the oral opening). The 4 linear motors are strategically located for independent stimulation of the upper and lower lip margin to permit detailed investigations of perioral reflex modulation.

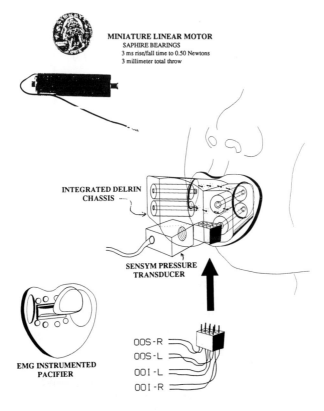

Figure 4. An expanded schematic of the electrode arrays and linear motor arrangement integral to the actifier. These linear motors translate carbon shafts on sapphire bearings and can produce a +/- 1.5 mm displacement with a 3 ms rise/fall time at 0.5 Newtons.

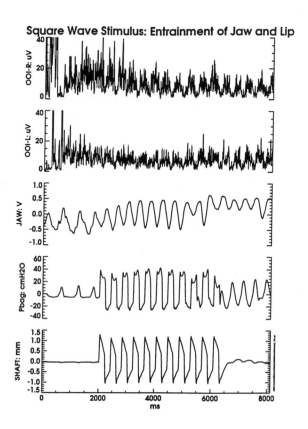

Figure 5. Entrainment of jaw and lips with a 2.5 Hz square wave stimulus. Data were sampled from a female infant at 3 weeks of age. The top two channels show the electromyograms [rectified and integrated] for the orbicularis oris inferior recording sites, followed by jaw displacement, intraluminal pressure of the latex baglet, and linear motor shaft displacement. [Finan & Barlow, 1996].

A fifth, more powerful linear motor which is pneumatically coupled to the baglet (nipple), allows the shape and intraluminal pressure of the baglet to be dynamically controlled by a digital computer. Based on our experience with non-nutritive suck dynamics in healthy term infants, we have been able to digitally synthesize control (input) signals to drive the baglet and produce a spectrally rich mechanical stimulus that produces 1:1 oromotor entrainment during non-nutritive suck. This feature of the device transforms the pacifier-cutaneous stimulator array into an active instrument which explains why we like the term 'actifier.'

Thus far, the actifier has been used to investigate the responsiveness of the suck CPG to cyclic mechanical stimulation of the intraoral and perioral mechanoreceptors in 8 human neonates. An example of 1:1 entrainment, sampled from a 3-week old baby girl, is shown in figure 5. The sequence of signals includes EMGs from the left and right divisions of the orbicularis oris inferior, jaw strain gage, intraluminal pressure of the baglet (nipple), and

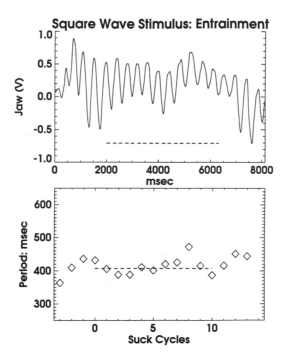

Figure 6. Additional detail on the oromotor entrainment from the previous figure. Jaw motion [inferior-superior] are shown in the top panel. The bottom panel represents the suck cycle period as measured on the jaw waveform. The dashed line indicates the frequency and duration of the square wave stimulus waveform. This infant begins the non-nutritive suck burst at a relatively slow rate [suck periods ~ 530 - 580 ms] but resets suck cycle period [1:1 *entrainment*] upon stimulus onset.

linear motor shaft displacement. Phasic bursts in the rectified and integrated EMG waveforms correspond to the individual suck cycles generated by this neonate. The onset of the entrainment stimulus is indicated in the shaft displacement signal (bottom trace). The degree of mechanically induced entrainment is shown in figure 6. Jaw movements and lip EMGs became phasically synchronized to the entraining input signal throughout the duration of the stimulus burst. The neonate modified her suck cycle period from 500-600 ms to the 400 ms period of the entraining input for the duration of the stimulus. A second example of entrainment shown in figures 7 and 8 illustrates a higher rate suck (350 ms period) that was modified to match the 400 millisecond period of the entraining stimulus within two cycles of stimulus onset. These findings provide strong evidence that the temporal characteristics of the suck CPG can be rapidly modified by afferent feedback.

The richness of the somatic sensory experience offered by the dynamic baglet of the actifier affords some exciting possibilities for the habilitation of an aberrant suck pattern generator. The actifier can be configured to provide a true multimodal experience for the baby. Mechanically activated bells or whistles, pleasing to the infants, can be coupled in

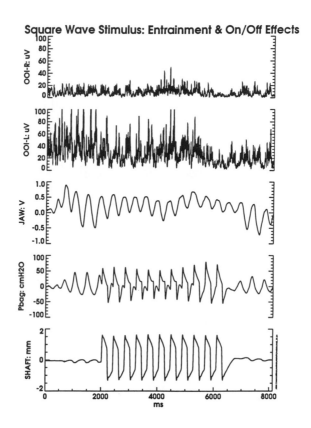

Figure 7. Another example of oromotor entrainment using a 2.5 Hz square wave stimulus. Data were sampled from a female infant at 3 weeks of age. The top two channels show the electromyograms [rectified and integrated] for the orbicularis oris inferior recording sites, followed by jaw displacement, intraluminal pressure of the latex baglet, and linear motor shaft displacement. [Finan & Barlow, 1996].

parallel to the throw of the linear motor that is used to drive the baglet. With this configuration, we can produce acoustic cues that are temporally correlated with the entrainment stimulus of the pulsating baglet. Consistent with the entrainment and neuronal plasticity literature (Thelen & Smith, 1994), we expect the multimodal experience will provide the nervous system with more highly correlated spatial and temporal information, effectively enhancing multisensory information processing. This stimulus condition is expected to influence entrainment patterns.

The use of 'natural' forms of stimulation is preferred to preserve the physiologic nature of recruitment pattern in the hopes of synthesizing a sensory experience that can be reinforced through motor activity. Use of a mechanical entrainment stimulus also has the distinct advantage of being safe and comfortable for the neonate. It is hypothesized that a highly controlled regimen of entrainment stimulation using a motorized pacifier baglet will lead to

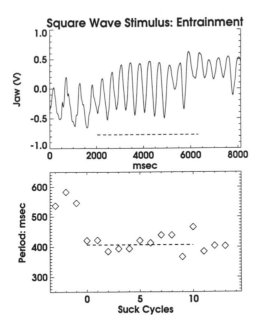

Figure 8. Additional detail on the oromotor entrainment from the previous figure. Jaw motion [inferior-superior] are shown in the top panel. The bottom panel represents the suck cycle period as measured on the jaw waveform. The dashed line indicates the frequency and duration of the square wave stimulus waveform. In this example, the infant initiates the non-nutritive suck burst at a relatively high rate [suck period ~ 370 ms] progressing to a slower rate of suck by the third cycle [~ 440 ms]. Upon stimulus onset, the infant reset the oromotor pattern generating output to approximate the period of the entrainment stimulus [~ 400 ms].

changes in the spatiotemporal organization of the non-nutritive suck, and ultimately lead to a change in the central neural representation for somatic sensation and corresponding motor maps in neonates manifesting oromotor dysfunction. We expect to find concomitant changes in the modulation and specificity of mechanically evoked perioral reflexes as the non-nutritive suck becomes more organized. The exact time course of this predicted change is unknown for the orofacial system, however, the principles of activity-dependent change and neuronal group selection should play a dominant role in the motor reorganization.

REFERENCES

Alloway, K., & Burton, H. (1991). Differential effects of GABA and bicuculline on rapidly- and slowly-adapting neurons in primary somatosensory cortex of primates. *Experimental Brain Research, 85,* 598-610.

Billy, A.J., & Walters, E.T. (1989). Long-term expansion and sensitization of mechanosensory receptive field in aplysia support an activity-dependent model of whole-cell sensory plasticity. *The Journal of*

Neuroscience, 9, 1254-1262.

Bosma, J.F. (1970). Summarizing and perspective comments: Part V. Form and function in the infant's mouth and pharynx. In J.F. Bosma (Ed.), Second Symposium on Oral Sensation and Perception. Charles C. Thomas Publisher, Springfield, Illinois, pp. 550-555.

Calford, M.B., & Tweedale, R. (1990). Interhemispheric transfer of plasticity in the cerebral cortex. *Science, 249,* 805-807.

Conway, B.A., Hultborn, H., & Kiehn, O. (1987). Proprioceptive input resets central locomotor rhythm in the spinal cat. *Experimental Brain Research, 68,* 643-656.

Cusick, C.G., Wall, J.T., Whiting, J.H., & Wiley, R.G. (1990). Temporal progression of cortical reorganization following nerve injury. *Brain Research, 537,* 355-358.

Edeline, J-M. & Weinberger, N.M. (1991). Thalamic short-term plasticity in the auditory system: Associative retuning of receptive fields in the ventral medial geniculate body. *Behavioral Neuroscience, 105,* 618-639.

Edelman, G.M. (1978). Group selection and phasic re-entrant signalling: A theory of higher brain function. In *The Mindful Brain* (G.M. Edelman, & V.B. Mountcastle, Eds.), pp. 51-100. MIT Press, Cambridge, MA.

Edelman, G.M. (1987). *Neural Darwinism: The theory of neuronal group selection.* Basic Books, New York.

Edelman, G.M. (1992). *Bright air, brilliant fire: on the Matter of the Mind.* Basic Books, New York.

Finan, D.S., & Barlow, S.M. (1996). The actifier: A device for neurophysiologic studies of orofacial control in human infants. *Journal of Speech and Hearing Research, 39,* 833-838.

Fox, K. (1994). The cortical component of experience-dependent synaptic plasticity in the rat barrel cortex. *The Journal of Neuroscience, 14,* 7665-7679.

Garraghty, P.E., Hanes, D.P., Florence, S.L., & Kaas, J.H. (1994). Pattern of peripheral deafferentation predicts reorganizational limits in adult primate somatosensory cortex. *Somatosensory and Motor Research, 11,* 109-117.

Garraghty, P.E., & Kaas, J.H. (1991). Large-scale functional reorganization in adult monkey cortex after peripheral nerve injury. *Proceedings of the National Academy of Science* USA 88, 6976-6980.

Garraghty, P.E., & Kaas, J.H. (1992). Dynamic features of sensory and motor maps. *Current Opinion in Neurobiology, 2,* 522-527.

Garraghty, P.E., Kaas, J.H., & Florence, S.L. (1994). Plasticity of sensory and motor maps in adult and developing mammals. In V.A. Casagrande, & P.G. Shinkman (Eds.), *Advances in Neural and Behavioral Development,* Vol. 4, Ablex, Norwood, NJ,pp. 1-36.

Garraghty, P.E., & Muja, N. (1996). NMDA receptors and plasticity in adult primate somatosensory cortex. *The Journal of Comparative Neurology, 367,* 319-326.

Garraghty, P.E., & Sur, M. (1990). Morphology of single intracellularly stained axons terminating in area 3b of macaque monkeys. *Journal of Comparative Neurology, 294,* 583-593.

Glass, L., & Mackey, M.C. (1988). *From Clocks to Chaos: The rhythms of Life.* Princeton, NJ: Princeton University Press.

Goodman, C.S., & Shatz, C.J. (1993) Developmental mechanisms that generate precise patterns of neuronal connectivity. *Neuron, 10,* 1-20.

Kalb, R.G., & Hockfield, S. (1992). Activity-dependent development of spinal cord motor neurons. *Brain Research Reviews, 17,* 283-289.

Kriellaars, D.J., Brownstone, R.M., Noga, B.R., & Jordan, L.M. (1994). Mechanical entrainment of fictive locomotion in the decerebrate cat. *Journal of Neurophysiology, 71(6),* 2074-2086.

Lo, Y-J., & Poo, M-M. (1991). Activity-dependent synaptic competition in vitro: Heterosynaptic suppression of developing synapses. *Science, 254,* 1019-1022.

Meftah, E.M., & Rispal-Padel, L. (1994). Synaptic plasticity in the thalamo-cortical pathway as one of the neurobiological correlates of forelimb flexion conditioning: Electrophysiological investigation in the cat. *Journal of Neurophysiology, 72,* 2631-2647.

Meredith, M.A., Nemitz, J.W., & Stein, B.E. (1987). Determinants of multisensory integration in superior colliculus neurons: I. Temporal factors. *Journal of Neuroscience, 10,* 3215-3229.

Meredith, M.A., & Stein, B.E. (1986). Visual, auditory, and somatosensory convergence on cells in superior colliculus results in multisensory integration. *Journal of Neurophysiology, 56,* 640-662.

Merrill, E.G., & Wall, P.D. (1972). Factors forming the edge of a receptive field: The presence of relatively ineffective afferent terminals. *Journal of Physiology* (London), *226,* 825-846.

Merzenich, M.M., Kaas, J.H., Wall, J., Nelson, R.J., Sur, M., & Felleman, D. (1983a). Topographic reorganization of somatosensory cortical areas 3b and 1 in adult monkeys following restricted deafferentation. *Neuroscience, 8,* 33-55.

Merzenich, M.M., Kaas, J.H., Wall, J., Sur, M., Nelson, R.J., & Felleman, D. (1983b). Progression of change following median nerve section in the cortical representation of the hand in areas 3b and 1 in adult owl and squirrel monkeys. *Neuroscience, 10,* 639-665.

Merzenich, M.M., Nelson, R.J., Stryker, M.P., Cynader, M., Schoppman, A., & Zook, J.M. (1984). Somatosensory cortical map changes following digit amputation in adult monkeys. *Journal of Comparative Neurology, 224,* 591-605.

Merzenich, M.M., Recanzone, G.H., Jenkins, W.M., & Nudo, R.J. (1990). How the brain functionally rewires itself. In *Natural and Artificial Parallel Computations* M. Arbib, & J. Robinson (Eds.), 177-210. Cambridge, MA: MIT Press.

Miller, K.D. (1992). Models of activity-dependent neural development. *Seminars in the Neurosciences, Vol 4, No. 1,* 61-73.

Pavlidis, T. (1973). Entrainment of oscillators by external inputs, In *Biological Oscillators: Their mathematical analysis.* London: Academic, 71-98.

Pearson, K.G., Ramirez, J.M., & Jiang, W. (1992). Entrainment of the locomotor rhythm by group Ib afferents from ankle extensor muscles in spinal cats. *Experimental Brain Research, 90,* 557-566.

Pettet, M.W., & Gilbert, C.D. (1992). Dynamic changes in receptive-field size in cat primary visual cortex. *Proceedings of the National Academy of Science, 89,* 8366-8370.

Recanzone, G.H., Allard, T.T., Jenkins, W.M. & Merzenich, M.M. (1990). Receptive-field changes induced by peripheral nerve stimulation in SI of adult cats. *Journal of Neurophysiology, 63,* 1213-1225.

Rauschecker, J.P. (1991) Mechanisms of visual plasticity: Hebb synapses, NMDA receptors, and beyond. *Physiological Review, 71,* 587-615.

Rossignol, S., Lund, J.P., & Drew, T. (1988). The role of sensory inputs in regulating patterns of rhythmical in higher vertebrates. In Cohen, A., Rossignol, S., & Grillner, S. (Eds.), *Neural Control of Rhythmic Movements in Vertebrates.* John Wiley and Sons, New York, 201-283.

Sanes, D.H., & Takacs, C. (1993). Activity-dependent refinement of inhibitory connections. *European Journal of Neuroscience, 5,* 570-574.

Shatz, C.J. (1994). Role for spontaneous neural activity in the patterning of connections between retina and LGN during visual system development. *International Journal of Developmental Neuroscience, 12,* 531-546.

Sporns, O. (1994). Selectionist and instructionist ideas in neuroscience. In *Selectionism and the Brain.* O. Sporns, & G. Tononi (Eds.), Academic Press, New York.

Sporns, O., & Edelman, G.M. (1993). Solving Bernstein's problem: A proposal for the development of coordinated movement by selection. *Child Development, 64,* 960-981.

Stein, B.E., Meredith, M.A., & Wallace, M.T. (1993). Nonvisual responses of visually responsive neurons. *Progress in Brain Research, 95,* 79-90.

Stein, B.E., Wallace, M.T., & Meredith, M.A. (1995) . Neural mechanisms mediating attention and orientation to multisensory cues. In *The Cognitive Neurosciences.* S. Michael, & S. Gazzaniga (Eds.), A Bradford Book, MIT Press. 683-702.

Tamura, H., Tsumoto, T., & Hata, Y. (1992). Activity-dependent potentiation and depression of visual cortical responses to optic nerve stimulation in kittens. *Journal of Neurophysiology, Vol 68, No. 5,* 1603-1612.

Thelen, E., & Smith, L.B. (1994). Dynamic systems approach to the development of cognition and action. MIT Press/Bradford Books Series in Cognitive Psychology.

Wallace, M.T., Meredith, M.A., & Stein, B.E. (1992). Integration of multiple sensory modalities in cat cortex. *Experimental Brain Research, 91,* 484-488.

Xerri, C., Stern, J.M., & Merzenich, M.M. (1994). Alterations of the cortical representation of the rat ventrum induced by nursing behavior. *The Journal of Neuroscience, 14,* 1710-1721.

1997 Elsevier Science B.V.
Speech Production: Motor Control, Brain Research and Fluency Disorders
W. Hulstijn, H.F.M. Peters and P.H.H.M. Van Lieshout, editors

Chapter 52

SPEAKING RATE AND SPEECH MOTOR CONTROL: THEORETICAL CONSIDERATIONS AND EMPIRICAL DATA

Kelly D. Hall, Ehud Yairi

Certain aspects of overall speaking rate as well as segment duration are believed to reflect, in part, the level of maturity of the speech motor control mechanism. Numerous investigations have been designed to explore speaking rate in normally-speaking children as well as the effect of aging on speaking rates. Recent years have seen a growing interest in the speaking rate of children who stutter. Theoretically, inasmuch as stuttering is viewed as a disorder of motor speech control, one may speculate that young stuttering children would differ from nonstuttering children with regard to speaking rate performance both near the onset of the disorder as well as when the disorder progresses. Speaking rate has also become an important factor in clinical approaches to stuttering. Available research on speech rate both for normally speaking children and for children who stutter is insufficient and often conflicting. Noticeably, there have been no longitudinal studies related to this variable. The present paper presents a review of models of speech rate control, relating them to motor aspects of stuttering, evaluates current information on speaking rate in children who stutter, and presents initial findings of a longitudinal study of speech rate of young preschool children who developed persistent stuttering in comparison with a control group of nonstuttering children.

A BRIEF REVIEW OF THE LITERATURE

Because speaking rate reflects motor control, it has been an ideal parameter for the investigation of sensorimotor control of the speech production system (Gracco, 1991). Understanding speech timing in normal speakers is important both for establishing developmental norms as well as furthering treatment strategies for disordered speech. From this perspective, better understanding of the parameter of speaking rate within the complex of speech motor control, particularly in children, appears to be very relevant to research pertaining to the nature and treatment of stuttering.

Several theories and models have been advanced to explain the strategies that a speaker uses to monitor and control speaking rate. The linear model suggests that changes in rate of speech are accomplished by speech motor commands controlling a mechanism that simply compresses or contracts the durations of articulatory movements in consonant and vowel segments sequentially by a constant factor (Allen, 1973; Lindblom, 1968). In contrast to the traditional view of speech rate control, the nonlinear model suggests that a reorganization of the timing of successive speech movements occurs (Gay, 1981; Hughes & Abbs, 1976). Gay

(1981) provides evidence to show that increasing rate can cause changes in segmental duration that are nonproportional across consonant and vowel categories. Vowel durations were compressed proportionally greater than consonant closure duration. Gay inferred that because a speaker alters the degree of overlap of consonants and vowel segments, the timing of the movement comprising the entire articulatory gesture must be reorganized when rate is changed. This suggests a nonlinear reduction in the duration of speech segments that indicates restructuring of the temporal pattern of speech rather than a linear change in the timing of motor commands to the articulators. Tuller et al. (1982) found that instead of an absolute temporal change applied to each segment sequentially, relative intersegmental timing of consonants and vowels remains constant across various speaking rates. Thus, there are nonlinear changes in adjacent segments when rate is altered.

As models are explored and challenged, it has become apparent that no single mechanism is solely responsible for control of speaking rate. One possibility is that different motor speech programs are responsible for controlling different temporal speech events, for example, words, syllables and/or vowel duration vs. duration of overall speaking rate. In fact, the traditional view of speech motor control speculates that individual strategies are controlled independently from one another (Van Lieshout, 1995). There has been evidence, however, to negate such independent systems for control of rate across temporal speech events (Kelso et al., 1983; Linville & Folkins, 1982). According to the Task Dynamic model, the coordination of such a variety of possible strategies during speech is achieved by neuromotor control of functionally related speech movements in which individual articulatory movements are linked together in a highly coordinated articulatory "gesture" (Gracco, 1994; Saltzman, 1991; Van Lieshout, 1995). Thus, while speaking rate varies, the underlying principles that control the coordination of the strategies remain stable (Gracco, 1994).

Regardless of the specific model, variability in such temporal speech events as overall speaking rate and segment duration (i.e., words, syllables and/or vowel duration) is believed to reflect, in part, the level of maturity of the speech motor control mechanism. That is, decreased variability in the temporal characteristics of speech production may reflect increased speech motor control (Kent & Forner, 1980).

To date, there have been numerous investigations designed to explore normal development of motor speech timing control in children (Kubaska & Keating, 1981; Tingley & Allen, 1975; Walker et al., 1992). In addition to interest in the relationship between speaking rate and stuttering (Kelly & Conture, 1992; Myers & Freeman, 1985; Pindzola et al., 1989) there are numerous investigations of the relationship between rate and speech-related neurological impairments (Darley et al., 1975; Kent, 1984).

By far, the most consistent finding in the literature is that there appears to be considerable individual variability in speech rate measures (Miller et al., 1984; Shewan & Henderson, 1988). Of special relevance to the present discussion however, are findings showing that duration of speech segments is greater and more variable in young children as compared to older children and adults (DiSimoni, 1974a, 1974b; Gilbert & Purves, 1977; Tingley & Allen, 1975). It should be pointed out, however, that the developmental decrease in segment duration is not necessarily linear (Kubaska & Keating, 1981; Nittrouer, 1993; Robb & Saxman, 1990).

Although the theory of neurologic maturation can explain some of the variance in temporal characteristics of children's speech, it does not account for temporal variability in adult speech. Specifically, adult speakers have been shown to vary considerably in their speaking rate during conversational speech (Miller et al., 1984). Several investigators (Kent & Forner, 1980; Smith et al., 1983) have argued that variability is a statistical artifact of longer segment durations, not neuromuscular control. Others, however, attempted to identify the actual dynamics that affect segment duration and control of speaking rate (Robb & Saxman, 1990; Schwartz, 1995). Speaking rate alterations, such as from slow to fast or vice versa, both within and across speakers, appear to be accomplished by either changing pause time, increasing/decreasing the occurrence of pauses, and/or changing articulation rate which, in turn, affects segment duration variability (Goldman-Eisler, 1956; Grosjean, 1980; Miller et al., 1984). A wide range of other variables also assert influence. Among those are linguistic factors such as length of the utterance (Malecot et al., 1972; Starkweather, 1985), phonetic features (Umeda, 1977), speaking context (Duchin & Mysak, 1987; Goldman-Eisler, 1956; Kowal et al., 1973; Walker et al., 1992), cross-linguistic differences (Griffiths, 1990; O'Connell & Kowal, 1971), linguistic proficiency (Ryan, 1992), and syntactic complexity (Cook et al., 1974; Hawkins, 1971). A different class of variables explored includes IQ (Dawson, 1929), gender (Kowal et al., 1975; Walker et al., 1992), motivation (Smith et al., 1983), and speaker identification (Meyers & Freeman, 1985).

In general, the findings of the studies listed above have been inconclusive and typically require replication, modification, and expansion. However, several consistent trends, emerge. For example, speech rate in adults is slower in shorter utterances and faster in longer utterances (Malecot et al., 1972; Starkweather, 1985). This trend is not as clear in children and appears to be age-dependent (Walker et al., 1992). In children, speech rate tends to increase with age (Kowal et al., 1975; Tingley & Allen, 1975; Walker et al., 1992) although there is conflicting evidence (Pindzola et al., 1989). To date, there have been no longitudinal investigations of speech rate development in children.

Thus, it would appear that speaking rate, although typically influenced by neurological maturation, is a complex phenomenon that is highly affected and controlled by diverse variables both internal (e.g., neurologic maturation, linguistic complexity, etc.) and external (e.g., speaking task, speaker identification, motivation). Therefore, comparison of speech rate studies which focus on different factors is difficult. This is further complicated by the vast differences in methodologies employed in analysis of speech rate timing.

Within a theoretical framework of stuttering as a disorder of timing and motor discoordination (Kent, 1984; Van Lieshout, 1995; Van Lieshout et al., 1996; Van Riper, 1982; Webster, 1974; Webster, 1990), the role of speaking rate may be quite intriguing. Inasmuch as variability in temporal speech parameters, including overall speaking rate and segment duration, reflects the level of maturity of the speech motor control mechanism (less variability is indicative of greater speech motor control), and inasmuch as stuttering is viewed as a disorder of motor speech control, one may speculate that the perceptually fluent utterances of young stuttering children near the onset of the disorder would differ from that of their peers with regards to speech motor control as reflected in their speaking rate (Van Riper, 1982). Furthermore, such differences would become more pronounced over time as the disorder persists and becomes chronic. Additionally, differences in speaking rate would also be expected between children who persist in stuttering and those who recover.

A review of the theoretical and research literature in stuttering reveals that, for the most part, rate has been implicated in the disorder in secondary or indirect ways. First, with regards to the rate of the movement of the articulators, Webster (1974) hypothesized that stuttering persists in individuals whose coarticulatory movements are too rapid. Support for this assumption comes from the studies showing young stutterers produce faster articulatory movements in either fluent (Kowalczyk & Yairi, 1995; Pindzola, 1987) or disfluent speech (Throneburg & Yairi, 1994; Zebrowski, 1994). Other investigators have provided data indicating that stutterers' speech movements are slower than normal (Adams, 1987; Zimmermann, 1980), and still others reported little differences (Healey & Ramig, 1986; Zebrowski et al., 1985).

Second, the relationship between overall speaking rate and stuttering is likely to be much more complex than a problem of peripheral motor execution as it may also involve higher, premotor levels. On the one hand, theorists have proposed that stuttering may occur when longer linguistic processing or longer phonological processing is needed prior to motor execution (cf Peters et al., 1989; Postma & Kolk, 1993; Nudleman et al., 1989). According to these hypotheses, people who stutter would be disfluent when additional preparation time is required for processing speech, that is, assembling the motor plan prior to its translation into a muscle movement program. Thus, we would expect stutterers' overall speaking rate during both fluent and disfluent speech to be slower than that of nonstutterers. Postma, Kolk and Povel's (1990) findings that speaking rates of stutterers were slower than that of nonstutterers support this assumption. On the other hand, Conture et al. (1993) theorized that children who stutter speak *faster* than their ability to achieve correct phonological encoding and subsequently make inappropriate phonological selections that necessitate correction, in this case, disfluencies. This hypothesis would be difficult to test experimentally. Yaruss and Conture (1996) were unable to corroborate this tenet with their data for children ages 4 to 6.

The hypothesis that stutterers who did not receive clinical treatment are inherently faster speakers has been particularly influential in treatment strategies for stuttering. Reducing speech rate has been shown to increase fluency (Evesham & Huddleston, 1983; Franck, 1980; Spencer, 1976). Indeed, Andrews et al.(1982) found that when adult stutterers spoke under the fluency enhancing conditions of delayed auditory feedback or speaking with a metronome, they slowed their rate of speech. In contrast, Stephenson-Opsal and Bernstein Ratner (1988) and Zebrowski (1991) found that speech fluency was associated with an *increased* rate of speaking in stuttering children.

The few studies that have compared rate of speaking in children who do and those who do not stutter have yielded conflicting results. For example, Meyers and Freeman (1985) found that the fluent conversational speech of children who stutter (ages 4.1 to 5.11; M = 58 months) was significantly slower by one-half syl/sec than their nonstuttering peers and this difference was due primarily to the contribution of the severe stutterers. Ryan (1992), on the other hand, found no differences in speaking rate of children (age range 2.10 to 5.9, M = 52 months) who do and do not stutter. Kelly and Conture (1992) also found no differences in speaking rate in stuttering and nonstuttering children (ages 3.3 to 4.8; M = 48 months). Negative findings were also reported by Yaruss and Conture (1995) for children ranging from 4 to nearly 7 years old. Thus, the relationship between speaking rate and stuttering, particularly in children, remains unclear. Furthermore, comparisons among studies are difficult to make because of methodological differences and the many factors reviewed earlier that influence rate. It should be noted, for example, that Ryan (1992) used all utterances, fluent and disfluent, in the calculation of syllables per minute.

As stated earlier, overall speaking rate is believed to reflect in part the level of maturity of speech motor control. If true, then one may speculate that young stuttering children who have not yet received therapy would differ from their nonstuttering peers with regards to their time-related speaking rate development. Past research has been inconclusive as to whether children who stutter speak perceptually fluent utterances with a different (Meyers & Freeman, 1985; Richardson, 1985) or similar rate (Kelly & Conture, 1992; Ryan, 1992) when compared to their nonstuttering peers. Furthermore, in the absence of longitudinal studies of either stuttering or rate, the relation between the development of the disorder and the development of this indicator of motor speech control is not known. The purpose of this preliminary study was to compare the development of speaking rates of young stuttering children near the onset of stuttering with the rates of matched nonstuttering children in a longitudinal study.

THE STUDY

Method
A total of 12 subjects, six (four males and two females) in each group, ranging in age from 37 to 49 months, participated. At the initial data acquisition point, close to stuttering onset, the mean age of the stuttering group was 43.8 months. Our longitudinal records indicate that all six children eventually persisted in stuttering for a period longer than three years and were still stuttering as this report was prepared. (See Yairi et al., 1996). The control group's mean age was 41.3 months.

Articulatory rate in terms of syllable per second was calculated from spontaneous speech recorded during conversation with adults at three sessions, 12 months apart. From each subject's speech sample, 45 to 50 fluent utterances were selected for analysis. Articulatory rate was determined for each of the digitized utterances of a subject. An utterance was defined according with criteria described by Gollinkoff and Ames (1979). No utterance contained disfluency, non-speech sounds, or a pause longer than 250 msec (Miller et al., 1984). Using CSpeech version 4.0 (Milenkovic, 1987), a time waveform and corresponding

FFT-based spectrographic display of each utterance were verified through playback of the auditory signal. Durational measures in msec were made by placing the left cursor at the enhanced onset and offset of each utterance (see Throneburg & Yairi, 1994, Yairi & Hall, 1993). Each subject's mean for the duration of his/her utterances was determined.

Findings

Group means of syllables per second were calculated based on each individual's mean duration. For the persistent stuttering group, the means for the three testing visits (with 12-month intervals between visits) were 3.94, 3.92, and 4.30. The respective means for the control group were 3,67, 3.79, and 3.93. A two-way analysis of variance with repeated measures indicated no significant differences across visits (p = 0.109). Thus, the trend indicated in our longitudinal data is not strong enough to fall in line with previous reports of cross-sectional studies showing an increase across time in speaking rate of children (Amster & Starkweather, 1987; Kent & Forner, 1980; Kowal et al., 1975; Tingley & Allen, 1975; Walker et al., 1992). Of greater interest are the findings showing no significant differences (p = .30) in the articulatory rate of normally fluent children and young children who stutter at the early stage of stuttering as well at subsequent recording sessions as they persisted in stuttering.

Our findings are the first longitudinally gathered articulatory rate data for preschool age children, whether stuttering or nonstuttering. Considering the longitudinal nature of the study, large speech samples, the strict procedures and criteria used in selecting utterances, and the computer-based measuring technique, the results reported herein appear to be among the more valid data currently available on the speaking rate development of young children. Although the number of subjects is not large, an equivalent cross-sectional study would have involved 36 children but yield less valid developmental data. It is also important to note that the present results are within the range of data found in current literature. For example, Walker et al. (1992) reported 3.69 syl/sec for normally-fluent 3-year olds. For normally fluent and stuttering children ages 3 to 4 years Kelly and Conture (1992) reported a rate of 3.01 and 3.34 syl/sec respectively while for children ages 4 to 6 Yaruss and Conture (1996) reported a rate from 3.62 to 3.88 syl/sec, depending on the subgroup and speech samples.

For our normally-fluent subjects, although some increase in rate was expected across time, there is evidence from past research indicating the possibility of nonlinearity in speech rate development in children (Pindzola et al., 1989). Perhaps a faster rate of speech appears at a somewhat older age after the child's linguistic skills grow. The main motivation of this study, however, was to compare the speech rate of children who stutter at the beginning of the problem with normally fluent children as they grow older. Bearing in mind the limitations of this study, at present the negative findings do not support the notion that deficits in timing of speech movement, specifically, differences in either faster or slower than normal articulatory rate (Postma & Kolk, 1993; Kolk et al., 1991; Conture et al., 1993), is a major factor in the incipient stage of stuttering or as the disorder persists in early childhood. Boutsen et al. (chapter 53) also found no differences between children who stutter and nonstuttering children. Perhaps rate becomes a more prominent factor at later stages of the disorder. It is also possible that articulatory rate, as conventionally defined, is too gross a measure to examine speech motor control differences in children who and do not stutter. Finally, it may be that children who stutter use different motor strategies, such as more restricted movements, to control their articulatory rate that are not tapped by our measures.

SUMMARY

The review of the literature presented several theoretical models of speaking rate control and many variables that could influence this parameter of verbal behavior. It also emphasized the lack of longitudinal data in the body of research on the development of speaking rate. The possible implications of rate to the disorder of stuttering and the present conflicting data on this topic were discussed. Our preliminary study presents an important initiative toward a systematic, more valid approach to age-related speaking rate development in both stuttering and nonstuttering children. As this project expands to include more subjects, as well as a subgroup of children who have recovered from stuttering, our analyses will include other factors that were found relevant to rate. For example, additional analyses of linguistic influences, as well as additional metrics, such as phone rate, are being incorporated. Results will be presented in future reports.

ACKNOWLEDGMENTS

This research was supported by grant #R01-DC00459 from the National Institute On Deafness and Other Communication Disorders, National Institutes Of Health. Principal Investigator: Ehud Yairi.

REFERENCES

Adams, M.R. (1987). Voice onsets and segment durations of normal speakers and beginning stutterers. *Journal of Fluency Disorders, 12*, 133-139.

Allen, G.D. (1973). Segmental timing control in speech production. *Journal of Phonology, 1*, 207-225.

Amster, B.J. & Starkweather, C.W. (1987). Articulatory rate, stuttering and speech motor control. In H.F.M. Peters, & W. Hulstijn (Eds.) *Speech motor dynamics and stuttering* (pp. 317-328). New York: Springer-Verlag.

Andrews, G. Howie, P.M., Dozsa, M., & Guitar, B.E. (1982). Stuttering: Speech pattern characteristics under fluency inducing conditions. *Journal of Speech and Hearing Research, 25*, 208-216.

Boutsen, F., & Hood, S. (this volume). Determinants of speech rate and fluency in fast and slow speaking normally fluent children. In W. Hulstijn, H.F.M. Peters, & P.H.H.M. Van Lieshout (Eds.), *Speech production: motor control, brain research and fluency disorders*. Amsterdam: Elsevier Science.

Conture, E.G., Louko, L.J., & Edwards, M.L. (1993) Simultaneously treating stuttering and disordered phonology in children: Experimental therapy, preliminary findings. *American Journal of Speech-Language Pathology: A Journal of Clinical Practice, 2*, 72-81.

Cook, M., Smith, J., & Lalljee, M.G. (1974). Filled pauses and syntactic complexity. *Language and*

Speech, 17, 11-17.

Darley, F., Aronson, A.E., & Brown, J.R. (1975). *Motor speech disorders.* Philadelphia: W.B. Saunders Company.

Dawson, L. (1929). A study of the development of the rate of articulation. *Elementary School Journal, 29,* 610-615.

DiSimoni, F. (1974a). Influence of vowel environment on the duration of consonants in the speech of three-, six-, and nine-year old children. *Journal of the Acoustical Society of America, 55,* 360-361.

DiSimoni, F. (1974b). Influence of consonant environment on the duration of vowels in the speech of three-, six-, and nine-year old children. *Journal of the Acoustical Society of America, 55,* 362-363.

Duchin, S.W., & Mysak, E.D. (1987). Dysfluency and rate characteristics of young adult, middle-aged and older males. *Journal of Communication Disorders, 20,* 245-257.

Evesham, M., & Huddleston, A. (1983). Teaching stutterers the skill of fluent speech as a preliminary to the study of relapse. *British Journal of Disordered Communication, 18,* 31-38.

Franck, R. (1980). Integration of an intensive program for stutterers within the normal activities of a major acute hospital. *Australian Journal of Human Communication Disorders, 8,* 4-15.

Gay, T. (1981). Mechanisms in the control of speech rate. *Phonetica, 38,* 148-158.

Gilbert, J., & Purves, B. (1977). Temporal constraints on consonant clusters in child speech production. *Journal of Child Language, 4,* 417-432.

Gollinkoff, R., & Ames, C. (1979). A comparison of fathers' and mothers' speech with their very young children. *Child Development, 50,* 28-32.

Goldman-Eisler, F. (1956). The determinants of the rate of speech output and their mutual relations. *Journal of Psychosomatic Research, 1,* 137-143.

Gracco, V.L., (1991). Sensorimotor mechanisms in speech motor control. In H. Peters, W. Hulstijn, & C.W. Starkweather (Eds.), *Speech motor control and stuttering (pp. 53-78).* North Holland: Elsevier.

Gracco, V.L., (1994). Some organizational characteristics of speech movement control. *Journal of Speech and Hearing Research, 37,* 4-27.

Griffiths, R. (1990). Speech rate and comprehension: A preliminary study in time-benefit analysis. *Language Learning, 40,(3),* 311-336.

Grosjean, F. (1980). Temporal variables within and between languages. In Dechert, Taupach, Towards (Eds.). *A cross-linguistic assessment of speech production language,* Frankfurt am Main.

Hawkins, P.R. (1971). The syntactic location of hesitation pauses. *Language and Speech, 14,* 277-288.

Healey, E.C., & Ramig, P.R. (1986). Acoustic measures of stutterers' and nonstutterers' fluency in two speaking contexts. *Journal of Speech and Hearing Research, 29,* 325-331.

Hughes, O.M., & Abbs, J.H. (1976). Labial-mandibular coordination in the productions of speech: Implications for the operation of motor equivalence. *Phonetica, 33,* 199-221.

Kelly, E.M., & Conture, E.G. (1992). Speaking rates, response time latencies, and interrupting behaviors of young stutterers, nonstutterers, and their mothers. *Journal of Speech and Hearing Research, 35,* 1256-1267.

Kelso, S., Tuller, B., & Harris, K.S. (1983). A dynamic pattern perspective on the control and coordination of movement. In P.F. MacNeilage (Ed.), *The production of speech.* Springer, New York.

Kent, R.D., & Forner, L.L. (1980). Speech segment durations in sentence recitations by children and adults. *Journal of Phonetics, 8,* 157-168.

Kent, R.D. (1984). Anatomical and neuromuscular maturation of the speech mechanism: Evidence from acoustic studies. *Journal of Speech and Hearing Research, 19,* 421-447.

Kolk, H., Conture, E., Postma, & Louko, L. (1991). *The covert-repair hypothesis and childhood stuttering.* Paper presented at the annual convention of the American-Speech-Language-Hearing

Association, Atlanta, GA.

Kowal, S., O'Connell, D.C., O'Brien, E.A., & Bryant, E.T. (1973). Temporal aspects of reading aloud and speaking: Three experiments. *Journal of Psychology, 88*, 549-569.

Kowal, S., O'Connel, D.C., & Sabin, E.F. (1975). Development of temporal patterning and vocal hesitations in spontaneous narratives. *Journal of Psycholinguistic Research, 4*, 195-207.

Kowalczyk, P., & Yairi, E. (1995). *Features of F-2 transitions in fluent speech of children who stutter.* A paper presented at the national convention of the American Speech-Language-Hearing Association, Orlando.

Kubaska, C., & Keating, P. (1981). Word duration in early child speech. *Journal of Speech and Hearing Research, 24*, 615-621.

Lindblom, B.E.F. (1968). *Temporal organization of syllable production.* (Quarterly Progress and Status Report 2-3). Stockholm: Royal Institute of Technology.

Malecot, A., Johnston, R., & Kizziar, P.A. (1972). Syllabic rate and utterance length in French. *Phonetica, 29*, 235-251.

Meyers, S.C., & Freeman, F.J. (1985). Mother and child speech rates as a variable in stuttering and disfluency. *Journal of Speech and Hearing Research, 28*, 436-444.

Miller, J., Grosjean, F., & Lomanto, C. (1984). Articulation rate and its variability in spontaneous speech: An analysis and some implications. *Phonetica, 41*, 215-225.

Nittrouer, S. (1993). The emergence of mature gestural patterns is not uniform: Evidence from an acoustic study. *Journal of Speech and Hearing Research, 36*, 959-972.

Nudleman, H.B., Herbrich, K.E., Hoyt, B.D., & Rosenfield, D.B. (1989). A neuroscience model of stuttering. *Journal of Fluency Disorders, 14*, 399-427.

O'Connell, D.C., & Kowal, S. (1971). Cross-linguistic pause and rate phenomena in adults and adolescents. *Journal of Psycholinguistic Research, 1*, 155-163.

Peters, H.F.M., Hulstijn, W., & Starkweather, C.W. (1989). Acoustic and physiological reaction times of stutterers and nonstutterers. *Journal of Speech and Hearing Research, 32*, 668-680.

Pindzola, R.H. (1987). Durational characteristics of the fluent speech of stutterers and nonstutterers. *Folia Phoniatrica, 39*, 90-97.

Pindzola, R.H., Jenkins, M.M., & Lokken, K.J. (1989). Speaking rates of young children. *Language, Speech, and Hearing Services in the Schools, 20*, 133-138.

Postma, A., & Kolk, H. (1993). The covert repair hypothesis: Prearticulatory repair processes in normal and stuttered disfluencies. *Journal of Speech and Hearing Research, 36*, 472-487.

Postma, A., Kolk, H., & Povel, D-J (1990). Speech planning and execution in stutterers. *Journal of Fluency Disorders, 15*, 49-59.

Richardson, D. (1985). Speaking, stuttering, and disfluency rates of preshcool stutterers and their mothers. Unpublished masters thesis. California State University, Long Beach.

Robb, M., & Saxman, J. (1990). Syllable durations of preword and early word vocalizations. *Journal of Speech and Hearing Research, 33*, 583-593.

Ryan, B. (1992). Articulation, language, rate, and fluency characteristics of stuttering and nonstuttering preschool children. *Journal of Speech and Hearing Research, 35*, 333-342.

Saltzman, E. (1991). The task dynamic model in speech production. In H.F.M. Peters, W. Hulstijn, & C.W. Starkweather (Eds.), *Speech motor control and stuttering* (pp 37-53). Amsterdam: Elsevier Science Publishers

Schwartz, R.G. (1995). Effect of familiarity on word duration in children's speech: A preliminary investigation. *Journal of Speech and Hearing Research, 38*, 76-84.

Shewan, C.M., & Henderson, V.L. (1988). Analysis of spontaneous language in the older normal population. *Journal of Communication Disorders, 21*, 139-154.

Smith, B.L., Sugarman, M.D., & Long, S.H. (1983). Experimental manipulation of speaking rate for studying temporal variability in children's speech. *Journal of the Acoustical Society of America, 74*, 744-749.

Spencer, G. (1976). The status of environmental and group cohesiveness in the treatment of stuttering. *Australian Journal of Human Communication Disorders, 4*, 140-145.

Starkweather, W. (1985). The development of fluency in normal children. In H. Gregory (Ed.), *Stuttering therapy: Prevention and intervention with children, (pp. 9-42)*. Memphis, TN: Speech Foundation of America.

Stephenson-Opsal, D., & Ratner, N. (1988). Maternal speech rate modification and childhood stuttering. *Journal of Fluency Disorders, 13*, 49-56.

Throneburg, R.N., & Yairi, E. (1994). Temporal dynamics of repetitions during the early stage of childhood stuttering: An acoustic study. *Journal of Speech and Hearing Research, 37*, 1067-1075.

Tingley, B.M., & Allen, G.D. (1975). Development of speech timing control in children. *Child Development, 46*, 186-194.

Tuller, B., Harris, K.S., & Kelso, J.A.S. (1982). Stress and rate: Differential transformations of articulation. *Journal of the Acoustical Society of America, 71*, 1534-1543.

Umeda, N. (1977). Consonant duration in American English. *Journal of the Acoustical Society of America, 61*, 846-858.

Van Lieshout, P.H.H.M. (1995). *Motor planning and articulation in fluent speech of stutterers and nonstutterers*. University Press Nijmegen, The Netherlands.

Van Lieshout, P.H.H.M., Hulstijn, W., & Peters, H.F.M. (1996). Speech production in people who stutter: Testing the motor plan assembly hypothesis. *Journal of Speech and Hearing Research, 39*, 76-92.

Van Riper, C. (1982). *The nature of stuttering (2nd ed.)*. Englewood Cliffs, NJ: Prentice Hall.

Walker, J.F., Archibald, L.M.D., Cherniak, S.R., & Fish, V.G. (1992). Articulation rate in 3- and 5-year old children. *Journal of Speech and Hearing Research, 35*, 4-13.

Webster, G.W. (1974). Behavior analysis of stuttering: treatment and theory. *Innovative Treatment Methods in Psychopathology*. New York: Wiley & Sons.

Webster, G.W. (1990). Motor performance of stutterers: A search for mechanisms. *Journal of Motor Behavior, 22*, 553-571.

Yairi, E., & Hall, K. (1993). Temporal relations within repetitions of preschool children near the onset of stuttering: A preliminary report. *Journal Of Communication Disoders, 26*, 231-244.

Yairi, E., Ambrose, N., Paden, E., & Throneburge, R. (1996). Predictive factors of persistence and recovery: Pathways of childhood stuttering. *Journal of Communication Disorders, 29*, 51-77.

Yaruss, S., & Conture, E. (1995). Mother and child speaking rates and utterance lengths in adjacent fluent utterances: Preliminary observations. *Journal of Fluency Disorders, 20*, 257-278.

Yaruss, S., & Conture, E. (1996). Stuttering and phonological disorders in children: Examination of the Covert Repair Hypothesis. *Journal of Speech and Hearing Research, 39*, 349-364.

Zebrowski, P.M. (1991). Duration of the speech disfluencies of beginning stutterers. *Journal of Speech and Hearing Research, 34*, 254-263.

Zebrowski, P.M. (1994). Duration of sound prolongations and sound/syllable repetition in children who stutter: Preliminary observations. *Journal of Speech and Hearing Research, 37*, 254-263.

Zebrowski, P.M., Conture, E.G., & Cudahy, E.A. (1985). Acoustic analysis of young stutterers' fluency: Preliminary observations. *Journal of Fluency Disorders, 10*, 173-192.

Zimmerman, G. (1980). Articulatory dynamics of fluent utterances of stutterers and nonstutterers. *Journal of Speech and Hearing Research, 23*, 95-107.11

Speech Production: Motor Control, Brain Research and Fluency Disorders
W. Hulstijn, H.F.M. Peters and P.H.H.M. Van Lieshout, editors

Chapter 53

DETERMINANTS OF SPEECH RATE AND FLUENCY IN FAST AND SLOW SPEAKING NORMALLY FLUENT CHILDREN

Frank R. Boutsen, Stephen B. Hood

Research suggests that speech rate and fluency develop as children mature. Moreover, there are indications that development in either domain is related. That is, with increased age children tend to not only speak faster and produce longer sentences, their speech also contains more normal disfluencies. Though normally speaking youngsters are typically considered a homogenous population it is to be expected that some of its members are more or less fluent and speak with faster or slower habitual speech rates. In this paper preliminary data from fast and slow speaking normally fluent youngsters between the ages of 6-12 are presented with regard to predictors of speech rate and fluency. Speech rate, articulation rate, MLU and fluency were determined during conversational speech and picture description. These variables together with two motor speech measures (i.e., counting, and DDK) were included in a comparative and correlational analysis. Implications of the data with regard to fluency and stuttering will be discussed.

INTRODUCTION

As children mature, their speech timing approximates that of an adult. This is reflected in their speech rate as well as in their fluency. Starkweather (1987) has pointed out that the development of speech rate and fluency results from better control of the vocal tract, improved speech rhythm control and increased language skills. In addition, he has cited data from studies by Kowal et al. (1975) which suggest that speech rate and fluency develop in a similar pattern. That is, spurts and delays in speech rate and fluency development have been shown to occur at similar age intervals. Though these data suggest that speech rate and fluency are predictive of one another at least in development, the nature of their relation is not clear. This is because the effect of age was not partialled out in previous studies. In addition, whether or not variations in fluency or speech rate are caused by the same or different variables has not received much research attention in studies with children.

Most of the data pertaining to sources of variability in speech rate and fluency have come from studies with adults. Duchin and Mysak (1987) investigated the disfluency and rate patterns in adult males during oral reading, conversation and picture description. Results revealed that the speech tasks contributed significantly to differences in speech rate. Speech rates were faster during oral reading than during conversation. Picture description was associated with the slowest speech rate. In addition, normal disfluencies were more prevalent in conversation than in picture description and oral reading with no significant differences between the latter two conditions. Results further showed that among normal disfluencies phrase repetitions were positively correlated with rate. The influence of sentence length on speech rate and fluency has been investigated in a number of studies (Goldman-Eisler, 1954; Malecot et al., 1972). In general, the data show that longer sentences are associated with faster speech rates and increased disfluency.

Some of the findings in adult studies of speech and disfluency have been confirmed in children. For instance, Amster (1984) showed that in preschool children, longer sentences are associated with increased speech rates. In addition, there are several indications in the literature that as the length of the utterance is increased, the frequency of disfluency does also (Haynes & Hood, 1977; Pearl & Bernthal, 1980). In the aforementioned studies the speech context was not systematically varied, however. Therefore, it is not known to what extent the predictive relationships observed in these investigations was influenced by the speech context. In addition, it is not known whether similar results would be obtained in slow versus fast speaking normally fluent children.

This void led to the present investigation. Its purpose was to examine predictors of fluency and speech rate in slow and fast normally fluent children during conversational speech and picture description. Specifically, it was to investigate to what extent conversational speech rate and fluency in both groups can be predicted by speech rate during picture description and measures of articulation rate and mean length of utterance during both conversation and picture description. Additionally, it was to investigate whether maximum performance measures including DDK and rapid counting contribute to the prediction of these parameters as well. Maximum performance tasks were included in the set of predictor variables because research suggests that rapid repetition tasks are positively correlated to speech rate (Tiffany, 1980). Yet, their relation to normal disfluencies has thus far not been explored. Secondly, unlike the other measures, maximum performance indices are obtained in a nonpropositional speech task and, thus, are less contaminated by language factors.

Investigation of the predictors of speech rate and fluency in slow and fast speaking children is expected to provide further insight in the processes of speech rate and fluency. In addition, knowledge of what determines these processes in subsets of the normal population can aid to our understanding of populations whose rate or fluency is disordered.

METHODS

Subjects

Subjects were 80 children, 20 at each of 4 age groups (4:6-6:0; 6:6-8:0; 8:6-10:0; 10:6-12:0). They had been judged by their teachers and parents as having no physical, psychological or behavioral disorders. Half the number of children were identified by the parent or teacher as a "slow" talker while the other half included children identified as a "fast" talker. All subjects scored within normal limits on an age-appropriate speech and language screening test. The screening instruments included the Fluharty Preschool Speech and Language Screening Test (Buono-Fluharty, 1978) and the Clinical Evaluation of Language Functions -Elementary Screening Test (Messing-Semel & Wiig, 1980). In addition, all subjects passed a hearing screening test for frequencies of 1000, 2000 and 4000 Hz at 20 dB HL.

Speech tasks and analysis

The speech tasks included conversational speech, picture description, rapid repetition of the syllables /pʌ/, /tʌ/ and /kʌ/ and rapid counting form 1-10. Conversational speech was elicited in response to open-ended questions from the examiner about favorite toys, games, family and friends. In picture description, the subjects were asked to describe sequenced picture cards (Perkins, 1968). During rapid repetition tasks subjects were instructed to rapidly produce the numbers 1-10 and repeat /pʌtʌkʌ/ for a period of 5 seconds as fast as possible. Each of the repetition tasks was conducted three times.

The speech samples were tape recorded using a Uher professional tape recorder. The microphone was placed directly in front of the subject. Speech samples during conversational speech and picture description were transcribed verbatim for the purpose of word and syllable counts. For both speech conditions, speaking rate, articulation rate, mean length of utterance (MLU) and fluency were determined as follows. Speaking rate and articulation rate were based on speech samples from which the first ten utterances were omitted. Speaking rate was expressed in words per minute. Articulation rate was expressed as the average number of syllables per second across six fluent utterances. Both measures were determined with the stopwatch method. Disfluent segments were identified in the conversation and picture description samples using Johnson's (1961) classification system of disfluencies. Specifically, the transcripts were coded for part-word repetitions, interjections, prolongations, and revisions/incomplete phrases. The total percent disfluent in either speech context was calculated by dividing the sum of all disfluencies by the total number of words spoken. In addition, MLU was determined for both conditions by dividing the total number of morphemes by the total number of words spoken. As for the repetition tasks, only the second trial was used for analysis. The measures of time lapsed during counting from one to 10 and number of repetitions of /pʌtʌkʌ/ over 5 seconds were derived with the stopwatch method.

Reliability.

Inter-judge and intra-judge reliability measures were obtained six weeks following the initial calculations of the speaking rates and articulation rates. Reliability data were based on the remeasurement of the speech samples of 4 subjects who were randomly selected out of each age group. Both the inter and intra-judge reliability measures for disfluency type ranged from 93 % to 100% agreement, with an average of 98.4 %. Reliability coefficients for rate measures exceeded $r = .90$.

RESULTS AND DISCUSSION

The descriptive statistics (mean and standard deviation) for each of the variables are summarized in table 1. There, it can be seen that children identified as fast talkers had faster speech, articulation and DDK rates than those who were identified as slow talkers.

In addition, the means of MLU, fluency and articulation rate differed slightly during conversational speech and picture description. Standard deviations were similar in each group.

In order to investigate the group (fast vs. slow) and speech task (conversation vs. picture description) effect on speech rate, articulation rate, MLU and fluency two-way analyses of variance were conducted. In addition, T-tests were computed to see if the groups differed on the maximum repetition tasks. The results of these analyses are summarized in table 2. As can be seen in the table, between-group differences were significant for the rate variables during conversational speech and picture description and for DDK. The means were similar for measures of MLU, fluency and counting from 1-10. A significant effect for speech context (conversation vs. picture description) was observed for articulation rate and for fluency.

Inspection of the means, however, suggests that high statistical power rather than meaningful differences between task produced the statistically significant effects.

In order to examine linear relations between the variables in each group Pearson correlations were computed for the groups separately.

Table 1. Descriptive statistics (mean & standard deviation) for speech rate, articulation rate, MLU, fluency, counting, and DDK in slow and fast talkers.

Variable	Context	Slow Talkers		Fast Talkers	
		Mean	SD	Mean	SD
Speech Rate	conversation	121.3	26.08	167.9	25.39
(words/min)	picture description	131.5	31.25	161.1	33.81
Arctic. Rate	conversational	4.26	0.70	5.48	1.12
(syllables/sec)	pict. description	4.10	0.96	5.04	0.80
MLU	conversational	9.05	3.38	10.33	3.19
	pict. description	9.57	3.14	10.19	3.20
Disfluency	conversational	6.2	2.9	6.1	3.0
(% total)	pict. description	4.6	2.7	5.6	3.1
Counting (secs.)	counting	4.63	1.85	4.16	1.81
DDK (reps / 5 secs.)	DDK	6.90	1.63	7.95	1.86

Table 2. ANOVA and t -test results for the analyses of conversational speech, picture description and maximum repetition tasks (counting and diadochokinetic rate {DDK}) in slow and fast talkers.

ANOVA

Dependent Variables	Effect	F-value	P
Speech Rate	Group (Fast vs. Slow)	67.320	0.0001
	Task (Conversational vs. Picture)	0.13	0.7160
	Group vs. Task	3.38	0.0679
Articulation Rate	Group (Fast vs. Slow)	55.72	0.0001
	Task (Conversational vs. Picture)	4.38	0.0381
	Group vs. Task	0.99	0.3212
MLU	Group (Fast vs. Slow)	3.47	0.0643
	Task (Conversational vs. Picture)	0.14	0.7105
	Group vs. Task	0.42	0.5185
Fluency	Group (Fast vs. Slow)	0.85	0.3591
	Task (Conversational vs. Picture)	5.02	0.0265
	Group vs. Task	1.33	0.2509
t-Test		**t-value**	**P**
Counting	Group (Fast vs. Slow)	1.53	.13
DDK	Group (Fast vs. Slow)	2.5	.01

The correlations of interest to this study are summarized in table 3. There, it can be seen that in the fast speaking group conversational speech rate correlated significantly and positively to the other three rate measures obtained during conversation and picture description, MLU and DDK.

Fluency, on the other hand, was significantly negatively correlated to speech rate. Thus, slower speech rates in the fast speaking group are associated with increased disfluency, as can be expected. As for fluency during conversation, it was positively correlated with fluency during picture description and negatively with both measures of MLU and conversational speech rate. The table further makes apparent that the pattern of correlations between these variables was different in the slow speaking group. That is, although conversational speech rate revealed positive correlations with the other three rate measures, MLU and DDK the correlations with the measures of fluency were nonsignificant. Moreover, fluency during conversational speech was unrelated to any of the variables except for fluency during picture description to which it was positively related.

Separate stepwise regression analyses were conducted for each group to determine the extent to which conversational speech rate and fluency can be predicted in each group. The alpha level for a variable to be entered in the analysis was set at .05.

Table 3. Predictors of conversational speech rate and fluency in slow and fast talkers.

	Slow Talkers		Fast Talkers	
	Conv. Speech Rate	Conv. Fluency	Conv. Speech Rate	Conv. Fluency
Conv. Speech Rate	1.00	-0.01	1.00	-0.43*
Pict. Speech Rate	0.61*	0.13	0.66*	-0.26
Conv. Articulation Rate	0.64*	0.06	0.66*	-0.30
Pict. Articulation Rate	0.63*	0.15	0.37*	-0.09
Conv. MLU	0.71*	0.15	0.62*	-0.41*
Pict. MLU	0.68*	0.07	0.67*	-0.37*
Conv. Fluency	-0.01	1.00	-0.43*	1.00
Pict. Fluency	0.05	0.47*	-0.39*	0.34*
Counting	-0.17	0.08	0.09	-0.25
DDK	0.80*	0.10	0.44*	-0.03

$* = p < .05$

Results of these analyses are summarized in table 4.

This table makes apparent that predictors of speech rate and fluency were different in the slow and fast talkers as well as in the conversational versus speech conditions. Specifically, among the fast talkers MLU and speech rate during picture description explained 55% of the variance in conversational speech rate. On the other hand, 60% of the variance in speech rate during picture description was accounted for by DDK and conversational speech rate. Speech context also affected the prediction of fluency. That is, fluency during conversational speech was predicted by conversational speech rate, which accounted for 19% of the variance. However, fluency during picture description was predicted by MLU during picture description. The predictors of speech rate and fluency in the slow speaking group revealed a different pattern than that observed in the fast speaking group. That is, different variables accounted for the variance explained in conversational speech rate (69%) and speech rate during picture description (57%). Specifically, DDK and articulation rate during picture description predicted conversational speech rate whereas articulation rate during picture description and MLU were predictive of speech rate during picture production. Finally, fluency during conversational speech was unaccounted for by any of the variables in the slow speaking group.

Overall, the results of this investigation suggest that speech rate and fluency are differently determined in fast and slow speaking children. This result cannot be explained in terms of a differential effect of speech task conditions on speech rate or fluency in either

Table 4. Summary of stepwise regression analyses for speech rate and fluency during conversation and picture description in slow vs. fast talkers.

	Slow Talkers		Fast Talkers		
Conversational Speech Rate	R**2	F	Conversational Speech Rate	R**2	F
DDK	0.64	68.49	Picture MLU	0.44	30.18
Picture Arctic. Rate	0.69	5.24	Picture Speech Rate	0.55	8.83
Picture Speech Rate			Picture Speech Rate		
Picture Arctic. Rate	0.49	36.88	DDK	0.45	31.13
Conv. MLU	0.57	6.20	Conv. Speech Rate	0.60	5.14
No Variable Retained			Conversational Fluency		
			Conv. Speech Rate	0.19	8.74
			Picture Fluency		
			Picture MLU	0.26	3.41

group. Thus, speech rate and fluency, may not be unitary constructs in the normally fluent population. It is noteworthy that although language related measures were important predictors of speech rate and fluency among the fast talkers, the amount of disfluencies was not related to any of the variables in the slow talkers. This raises the possibility that normal disfluency among slow talkers, like the disfluencies of stutterers, are not easily predicted. In this regard, more research is needed to determine whether the normal disfluencies of stutterers are similar to those of the slow talkers and dissimilar to those of fast talkers.

REFERENCES

Amster, B. (1984). The development of speech rate in normal preschool children. Ph.D. Dissertation, Temple University Philadelphia.

Buono-Fluharty, N. (1978). Fluharty Preschool Speech and Language Screening Test. Hingham, M.A., Teaching Resources Corporation.

Duchin, S., & Mysak, E. (1987). Disfluency and rate characteristics of young adult, middle-aged and older males. *Journal of Communication Disorders*, 20, 245-257.

Goldman-Eisler, F. (1954). On the variability of the speed of talking and on its relation to the length of utterance in conversation. *British Journal of Psychology*, 45, 94-107.

Haynes, W., & Hood, S. (1977). Language disfluency variables in normal speaking children from discrete chronological age groups. *Journal of Fluency Disorders*, 2, 57-74.

Johnson, W. (1961). Measurement of oral reading and speaking rate and disfluency of adult male and female stutterers and nonstutterers. *Journal of Speech and Hearing Disorders:* Monograph Supplement Number, *7*, 1-20.

Kowal, S., O'Connell, D., & Sabin, E. (1975). Development of temporal patterning and vocal hesitations in conversational narrative. *Journal of Pyscholinguistic Research*, *4*, 195-207.

Malecot, A., Johnston, R., & Kizziar, P. (1972). Syllabic rate and utterance length in French. *Phonetica, 26,* 231-251.

Messing-Semel, E., & Wiig, E. (1980). *Clinical Evaluation of Language Functions*. Columbus, OH: Charles E. Merril Publishing Co.

Pearl, S.Z., & Bernthal, J.E. (1980). The effects of grammatical complexity upon the disfluency behavior in nonstuttering children. *Journal of Fluency Disorders*, *5*, 55-68.

Perkins, S. (1968). Sequence Picture Cards. Tulsa, Oklahoma: Speech and Language Materials, Inc.

Starkweather, C. (1987). *Fluency and Stuttering*. Englewood Cliffs: Prentice-Hall, Inc.

Tiffany, W. (1980). The effects of syllable structure on diadochokinetic and reading rates. *Journal of Speech and Hearing Research*, *23*, 894-908.

Speech Production: Motor Control, Brain Research and Fluency Disorders
W. Hulstijn, H.F.M. Peters and P.H.H.M. Van Lieshout, editors

Chapter 54

IMPROVING ASSESSMENT OF CHILDREN'S ORAL MOTOR DEVELOPMENT IN CLINICAL SETTINGS

J. Scott Yaruss

Speech-language pathologists (SLPs) often measure oral diadochokinetic (DDK) rates as a possible indicator of a child's oral motor development. Unfortunately, the diagnostic implications of fast or slow DDK rates are far from clear. This is particularly true for young children between the ages of 3 and 7, when many disorders of speech and language are most likely to be diagnosed. This paper proposes two alternative ways to use the DDK task in a clinical setting in order to better assess young children's oral motor development. The first technique measures aspects of the DDK task other than rate, such as the accuracy and fluency of DDK productions. The second technique utilizes alternate speech and non-speech target strings that may be easier for young children to produce. Preliminary results with normally developing children as well as children who stutter indicate that these techniques may improve the utility of DDK tasks for assessing children's oral motor development in clinical settings.

INTRODUCTION

Children's oral motor abilities are frequently assumed to play at least some role in the onset, development, or maintenance of stuttering in young children (e.g., Perkins et al., 1975; Riley & Riley, 1979, 1986; see reviews in Bloodstein, 1995; Conture, 1991). For this reason, speech-language pathologists (SLPs) are often encouraged to obtain measures of children's oral diadochokinetic (DDK) rates as one indication of their oral motor development (Conture, 1990; Conture & Caruso, 1987; Curlee, 1993; Riley & Riley, 1985). Typically, the DDK task involves having a child produce a string of nonsense syllables as quickly as possible (e.g., Canning & Rose, 1974; Fletcher, 1972; Kent et al., 1987; Riley & Riley, 1985; Robbins & Klee, 1987). Examples of commonly used target strings include repeated monosyllables (e.g., "puh puh puh ..." or "tuh tuh tuh..."), bisyllables (e.g., "puh-tuh puh-tuh..." or "tuh-kuh tuh-kuh..."), and trisyllables (e.g, "puh-tuh-kuh puh-tuh-kuh..."). As will be discussed in more detail below, real words, such as "buttercup" or "pattycake" have also been used with young children (Canning & Rose, 1972; Robbins & Klee, 1987). Different articulators can be independently assessed based upon the stimuli chosen for production (e.g., "puh" assesses labial abilities); however, it appears that young children's rates for various monosyllables and bisyllables are strongly correlated with their rate for trisyllabic tokens (Wolk et al., 1993). Thus, in a clinical setting, the trisyllabic tokens "puh-tuh-kuh" or "pattycake" may be among the more useful measures to obtain.

CLINICAL MEASUREMENT OF CHILDREN'S DDK RATES

Benefits of DDK measures.

There are several potential benefits to using DDKs to assess children's oral motor skills. First, the measure is relatively easy to obtain. To calculate DDK rates, the SLP can either determine the length of time required for the child to produce a given number of iterations ("time-by-count" measurement, after Fletcher, 1972) or count the total number of iterations a child is able to produce during a set amount of time ("count-by-time" measurement, e.g., Robbins & Klee, 1987). In general, the "time-by-count" measurement technique is considered easier since the SLP is only required to count the number of iterations produced while production time is recorded via a stopwatch (Kent et al., 1987). Second, since the DDK task uses repeated syllables, it approximates conversational speech but is presumed to be "free from the imponderable phonological complications" (Tiffany, 1980) that plague other speech tasks. Finally, compared to other measures of maximum performance, DDK productions are believed to be relatively stable indicators of oral ability (Kent et al., 1987).

Complicating factors.

Unfortunately, the diagnostic implications of fast or slow DDK rates for young children are far from clear (Kent et al., 1987; McDonald, 1964; Tiffany, 1980; Winitz, 1969). This is particularly true for children between the ages of 3 and 7, when stuttering and other developmental speech and language disorders are most likely to be diagnosed. There are several explanations for this difficulty. First, obtaining reliable DDK productions from very young children can be quite problematic – the task requires that children follow relatively complex instructions, and young children can fatigue during repetitive tasks (Canning & Rose, 1974). Also, producing nonsense syllables may be too abstract or unnatural for young children (Canning & Rose, 1974; Wit et. al., 1993). For this reason, Canning and Rose utilized the real word "buttercup" rather than "puh-tuh-kuh" for subjects younger than 5½ years of age. Canning & Rose also reported that younger subjects made a number of articulation errors during their DDK productions, though no specific analysis of the errors was provided.

Because of the difficulty of obtaining DDK productions from young children, there have been relatively few normative studies of young children's DDK rates (Canning & Rose, 1974; Robbins & Klee, 1987), and those studies that have been conducted have utilized differing methodologies. For example, as noted above, Canning and Rose (1974) used "buttercup" to test their younger subjects using a count-by-time method, while Robbins and Klee (1987) used "pattycake" and /pʌrəkək/ with a time-by-count method. Although it is true that time-by-count and count-by-time measurements are simply the reciprocal of one another, Robbins and Klee (1987) required children to produce the target string for 3 seconds, while Canning and Rose (1974) required children produce the target string for a longer period of time in order to reach 10 iterations. Some children were unable to do this in one breath, however, so "any inhalations were included in the overall time recorded in for the task" (p. 48), a procedure which may have lowered overall rates. Thus, there may be differences in these two sets of normative data that are due to methodological differences rather than to true differences in children's oral motor skills. Regardless of the exact causes of these differences, however, the result of these methodological differences is that it is somewhat difficult to interpret young children's DDK rates based upon available norms.

LINGUISTIC AND MOTOR INFLUENCES ON DDK PRODUCTION.

There is one additional factor that complicates the interpretation of children's (and adults') DDK productions. Recent studies of speech production in adults have revealed that the linguistic nature of the speaking material in a repetitive speech task can affect the accuracy and rate of production. For example, when adults repeat syllables with the same or similar initial consonants or CV sequences, there is an increased likelihood of articulation errors (e.g., Dell, 1984). It seems reasonable to assume that this "repeated phoneme effect" may also affect DDK tasks, since these, too, involve rapid repetitions of the same syllables. In addition, although there is some facilitative effect of rapidly repeating the same words, recent studies have also found that the repetition of syllables involving the same consonants or CV sequences can reduce production rate in a repetitive task (Sevald & Dell, 1994). (These findings have been explained in a connectionist model in terms of competition between phonemes to occupy a slot in a word frame.) Thus, it appears that rapidly repeating the same or similar segments, as in the DDK task, can actually *inhibit* rapid and accurate production of target strings for reasons that have more to do with the linguistic nature of the stimuli than with the oral motor skills of the speaker. It is not currently known to what extent these phenomena affect younger children's performance on DDK tasks. Still, it would appear that the DDK task may not be as free from linguistic influences as has traditionally been assumed.

DDK Rates of Children Who Stutter

When examining DDK rates of children with speech and language disorders such as stuttering, additional problems may be encountered. For example, the few empirical studies that have compared the DDK rates of children who stutter to children who do not stutter have failed to reveal significant deficits in stuttering children's DDK rates (Yaruss et al., 1995; Wolk et al., 1993). Similarly, numerous studies have failed to show consistent differences in DDK rates between *adults* who do and do not stutter (see reviews in Bloodstein, 1995; Starkweather, 1987). Thus, it is not entirely clear how slow DDK rates may be implicated in childhood stuttering. Recently, however, a review of the clinical diagnostic records of young children who stutter revealed that approximately 40% of children exhibited below-normal DDK rates (Yaruss et al., 1996). Also, Riley and Riley (1979, 1985, 1986) have reported that as many as 69% of children who stutter also exhibit problems with oral motor coordination on DDK tasks. Therefore, it appears that further investigation of the DDK task

– particularly relating to improving its clinical utility – may be warranted.

IMPROVING DDK MEASURES

Supplemental measures.

Aside from collecting additional normative data on very young children, one means for improving the clinical utility of the DDK task may be to supplement basic measures of rate with measures of other aspects of children's DDK productions. For example, Riley and Riley (1985) measure "smoothness of coarticulation" and "precision of articulation" as indicators of oral motor discoordination in young children. Similarly, Conture (1990) suggested that stuttering during DDKs may have prognostic implications. In order to maximize the clinical utility of any additional measures of DDK production, it would seem important for such measures to be based upon concepts and techniques that are already familiar to practicing SLPs, so little, if any, additional training would be required. The present author and colleagues have been investigating one technique for improving assessment of young children's oral motor abilities based on measurements of the *accuracy* (i.e., number of articulation errors) and *fluency* (i.e., number of speech disfluencies) of children's DDK productions (Yaruss et al., 1996). Preliminary results using this technique with 15 children aged 3 ½ to 5 ½ indicate that normally developing children produce frequent articulation errors, but relatively few speech disfluencies, when repeating the standard trisyllable "puh-tuh-kuh." In addition, normally developing children were quite variable when producing the nonsense trisyllables such as "puh-tuh-kuh," but more consistent when producing real words such as "pattycake." Preliminary results for 10 young children who stutter (Yaruss et al., 1995) have revealed a greater tendency toward the production of speech disfluencies during DDK productions, even though the repetitive nature of the DDK task might be assumed to enhance children's fluency. Although considerably more data, including normative data on the occurrence of articulation errors and speech disfluencies, are needed, preliminary results suggest that supplementing measures of DDK rate with additional measures of accuracy and fluency may hold promise for improving the clinical assessment of children's oral motor development. However, results also demonstrate the complexity and difficulty of the traditional DDK task for young children.

New target strings.

As noted above, children appear to have less difficulty during DDK tasks if they are asked to repeat real words rather than strings of nonsense syllables. The reason for this difference is not entirely clear, though the difference may be related to children's familiarity with target strings such as "pattycake." (If so, then production of "puh-tuh-kuh" might improve after sufficient exposure to this stimulus.) In addition, as noted above, repeating the same consonants in tasks similar to the DDK task may actually inhibit the rapid and accurate production of target strings. Thus, it seems that the *linguistic* nature of the syllables in this nonspeech motor task affects motoric performance, and may thereby affect the assessment of oral motor development. In order to sort out the relative contribution of linguistic and motor effects on children's repeated production of syllables in a DDK task, it may be helpful to examine children's DDK abilities using a different set of target strings than the ones that have traditionally been used. One such set of alternate target strings is presented in Table 1. Using these stimuli, it is possible to contrast children's production or real words (e.g., "puppy," "doggy") with phonetically similar nonsense words ("puh-puh," "duh-guh"). It is also possible to compare the rapid production of similar consonants ("daddy" or "duh-duh") with production of varied consonants ("doggy" or "duh-guh") for both real and nonsense stimuli.

In a preliminary study, six normally developing children, age 3 ½ to 5 ½, were asked to repeat real words and nonsense tokens, presented in random order, as rapidly as possible in a DDK task (each production required 10 repetitions of the target string following an examiner's model). Results supported prior findings that children are more accurate when producing real words. Specifically, children produced no articulation errors on bisyllabic real words such as "puppy" or "doggy," and they produced errors on only 5% of iterations for real trisyllables such as "pattycake," compared to 20% of iterations for nonsense syllables such as "puh-tuh-kuh." For both real and nonsense words, children produced very few speech disfluencies, and the few disfluencies they did produce occurred on the trisyllabic stimuli. Perhaps the most interesting findings from this preliminary analysis, however, were related to children's rate, and potential interactions between rate and accuracy. Specifically, one-half of the subjects exhibited faster rates for nonsense stimuli, while the other half exhibited faster rates for real words. A closer inspection of children's actual productions, however, revealed that those children who exhibited faster rates on nonsense stimuli actually did this at the expense of articulatory accuracy. When only accurate iterations were examined, all children were faster on real words than on nonsense syllables. These findings again highlight the difficulty of using the traditional DDK task with very young children and suggest that it may be appropriate to select different target strings in order to improve our ability to interpret young children's DDK productions as indications of oral motor development.

Table 1. Examples of alternate target strings for young children's DDK productions.

Repeated Consonants		Varied Consonants	
Real Words	Nonsense Words	Real Words	Nonsense words
puppy	puh-puh	patty	puh-duh
daddy	duh-duh	doggie	duh-guh
cookie	kuh-kuh	kitty	kuh-duh

CONCLUSIONS

In conclusion, the DDK task appears to hold promise as an indication of children's oral motor development because it is easy to administer in clinical settings. However, there are a number of potential problems with this technique that complicate the interpretation of young children's DDK productions. This paper has presented two potential solutions to these problems: first, measurement of aspects of DDK productions other than rate, including the occurrence of articulation errors and speech disfluencies; and second, use of target strings other than the traditional nonsense syllables to better identify the relative effects of linguistic and motor influences on children's DDK rates. It is believed that combining these techniques with additional normative data for very young children will ultimately improve the clinical utility of the DDK task as a meaningful indicator of children's oral motor development.

REFERENCES

Ackermann, H., Kertrich, I., & Hehr, T. (1995). Oral diadochokinesis in neurological dysarthrias. *Folia Phoniatrica et Logopedica, 47,* 15-23.

Bloodstein, O. (1995). *A Handbook on Stuttering.* San Diego: Singular Publishing.

Canning, B., & Rose, M. (1974). Clinical measurements of the speech tongue and lip movements in British children with normal speech. *British Journal of Disorders of Communication, 9,* 45-50.

Conture, E.G. (1990). *Stuttering* (2nd ed.). Englewood Cliffs, NJ: Prentice-Hall.

Conture, E.G., & Caruso, A.J. (1987). Assessment and diagnosis of childhood disfluency. In L. Rustin, D. Rowley, & H. Purser (Eds.), *Progress and Treatment of Fluency Disorders* (pp. 57-82). London: Taylor and Francis.

Curlee, R.F. (1993). Identification and management of beginning stuttering. In R.F. Curlee (Ed.), *Stuttering and Related Disorders of Fluency* (pp. 1-22). New York: Thieme Medical Publishers.

Dell, G. (1984). Representation of serial order in speech: Evidence from the repeated phoneme effect in speech errors. *Journal of Experimental Psychology: Learning, Memory, and Cognition, 22,* 22-233.

Fletcher, S.G. (1972). Time-by-count measurement of diadochokinetic syllable rate. *Journal of Speech and Hearing Research, 15,* 763-770.

Kent, R.D., Kent, J.F., & Rosenbek, J.C. (1987). Maximum performance tests of speech production. *Journal of Speech and Hearing Disorders, 52,* 367-387.

McDonald, E.T. (1964). *Articulation Testing and Treatment: A Sensory Motor Approach.* Pittsburgh, PA: Stanwix House.

Perkins, W.H., Rudas, J., Johnson, L., & Bell, J. (1976). Stuttering: Discoordination of phonation with articulation and respiration. *Journal of Speech and Hearing Research, 198,* 509-522.

Riley, G., & Riley, J. (1979). A component model for diagnosing and treating children who stutter. *Journal of Fluency Disorders, 4,* 279-293.

Riley, G., & Riley, J. (1985). *Oral motor assessment and treatment: Improving syllable production.* Austin, TX: Pro-Ed.

Riley, G., & Riley, J. (1986). Oral motor discoordination among children who stutter. *Journal of Fluency Disorders, 11,* 335-334.

Robbins, J., & Klee, T. (1987). Clinical assessment of oropharyngeal motor development in young children. *Journal of Speech and Hearing Disorders, 52,* 271-277.

Sevald, C. & Dell, G. (1994). The sequential cuing effect in speech production. *Cognition, 53,* 91-127.

Starkweather, W. (1987). *Fluency and stuttering.* Englewood Cliffs, NJ: Prentice-Hall, Inc.

Tiffany, W. (1980). The effects of syllable structure on diadochokinetic and reading rates. *Journal of Speech and Hearing Disorders, 23,* 894-908.

Winitz, H. (1969). *Articulatory Acquisition and Behavior.* Englewood Cliffs, NJ: Prentice Hall.

Wit, J., Maassen, B., Gabreëls, F.J.M., & Thoonen, G. (1993). Maximum performance tests in children with developmental spastic dysarthria. *Journal of Speech and Hearing Research, 36,* 452-459.

Yaruss, J.S., LaSalle, LR., & Conture, E.G. (1996). *Evaluating Stuttering in Young Children: Diagnostic Data.* Manuscript submitted for publication.

Yaruss, J.S., Logan, K.J., & Conture, E.G. (1995). Speaking rate and diadochokinetic abilities of children who stutter. In C.W. Starkweather & H.F.M. Peters (Eds.), *Stuttering: Proceedings of the First World Congress of Fluency Disorders* (pp. 283-286). Nijmegen, The Netherlands: University Press Nijmegen.

Yaruss, J.S., Logan, K.J., & Conture, E.G. (1996). *Assessing rate, accuracy, and fluency of young children's diadochokinetic productions: A preliminary study.* Manuscript submitted for publication.

© 1997 Elsevier Science B.V. All rights reserved.
Speech Production: Motor Control, Brain Research and Fluency Disorders
W. Hulstijn, H.F.M. Peters and P.H.H.M. Van Lieshout, editors

Chapter 55

CLOCK AND MOTOR VARIANCES IN LIP-TRACKING: A COMPARISON BETWEEN CHILDREN WHO STUTTER AND THOSE WHO DO NOT

Peter Howell, James Au-Yeung, Lena Rustin

Previous research shows that there was a deficit in a lip tracking task in stuttering children when compared to nonstuttering children. The current study tried to determine if the timing mechanism or the motor control of the speech articulator were at fault which led to the deficit. This paper presents the result from a pilot study which decomposed the lip tracking variances into clock and motor components. Both components were thought to be at fault in stuttering subjects although previous studies did not support a timing deficit hypothesis in stuttering subjects in general motor control. The preliminary results from our study showed that there is a deficit in the motor control of the speech articulator in stuttering subjects. Our results, however, did not support a timing deficit in stuttering subjects.

INTRODUCTION

Howell et al. (1995) have reported accuracy of tracking performance for the lower lip in response to a sinusoidally-moving visual target for stuttering and fluent children. It was found that children who stutter are less accurate than children who do not stutter in tracking the sinusoid. This finding is particularly important as in other studies in which articulator movements during speech performance have been measured in stuttering children, no deficits in articulation have been found relative to fluent controls (e.g., Conture et al., 1988).

Hulstijn et al. (1992) tested the timing of stuttering and nonstuttering subjects in a finger tapping and speech task and found that there was no difference between the two groups. They had only tested the subjects at a timing interval of 400ms. Zelaznik et al., (1994) further tested stuttering and control subjects with a simple timing task at various timing intervals and reported similar findings to those of Hulstijn and colleagues. Their experiments tested the general motor skills of stuttering subjects. Their basic assumption was that the same timing mechanism is utilised in general motor control and speech motor control. In this study, we are looking at the timing mechanism again but at a level near to speech production itself. Lip-tracking tests specifically the motor control of the articulator in a non-speech task. In order to track a sinusoidal target accurately, subjects must make movements that are precise in extent (termed motor variance by Wing & Kristofferson, 1973) and these movements must be co-ordinated over time (what Wing & Kristofferson call clock variance). Wing and

Kristofferson's analysis procedure is applied to decompose performance into motor and clock (timekeeper) variance components and were employed in the studies carried by Hulstijn et al. and Zelaznik et al.

Motor variance is expected to be higher in stuttering children due to the difficulty that they are reported to have in producing particular phonemes. Greater clock variance is suggested by the effectiveness of treating stuttering by techniques designed to control their speech rate (Andrews et al., 1982). Deficiency of the timekeeper in stutterers is also revealed in the fact that less stuttering is found in singing or choral reading where stutterers make use of an external timekeeper rather than that of their own (Shaffer, 1982).

METHOD

Subjects

Nine stuttering children (8 males and 1 female) age 9-10 who are attending therapy at the Michael Palin Centre for Stammering Children and five controls (4 males and 1 female) from a local school in London participated in the experiment.

Procedure

The procedure was similar to the Howell et al. (1995) study. Strain gauges were attached to the upper lip, the lower lip and the jaw of a subject. The subject was then asked to track a sinusoidally-moving cross displayed on a computer screen. The frequency of the moving cross varied between sessions at 1.2Hz (833ms period), 1.1Hz (909ms period), 1.0Hz (1000ms period), 0.9Hz (1111ms period), 0.8Hz (1250ms period) and 0.75Hz (1333ms period). The frequencies chosen were lower than those employed in Hulstijn et al. (1992) and Zelaznik et al. (1994) because the lip-tracking task employed was more difficult than their timing task with finger movements. Moreover, tracking at lower frequencies increased the timing variability (Michon, 1967). Our expectation was that under such tougher conditions we should be able to differentiate the performance of stuttering and nonstuttering subjects.

Each session of the experiment was divided into two phases, paced and unpaced. In the paced section, the 'synchronization phase', the moving cross appeared on the screen for 24 periods. During this phase, the subjects were asked to use their lower lip to control a hollow square displayed on the screen to trap the moving cross. The dimension of the square was the same as the cross's. The 'continuation phase' followed the 'synchronization phase' during which the cross was not displayed on the screen and the subjects were instructed to continue their lip movement to control the square on the computer screen, as best as they could, in the same speed as in the synchronization phase. The continuation phase lasted about 31 periods followed by an on screen visual message signalling the termination of the session. The frequencies were randomised across subjects and each subject was asked to perform the test twice for each frequency.

Analyses

Both stuttering and control subjects took a few cycles to track the target correctly in the synchronization phase and in the continuation phase some subjects lost their concentration or even started talking after the cross disappeared for a short while. So, for the analysis the 26th-35th periods (the beginning of the continuation phase excluding the first one) were used.

The procedure for analysis was adopted from Wing and Kristofferson (1973) where a stochastic clock was assumed, meaning thath the clock interval is rondom. For the *k*th response, the motor delay interval D_k was also assumed to be random. The inter-response interval (IRI) between two responses was given by I_j where $I_j = C_j + D_j - D_{j-1}$ and C_j was the timekeeper (clock) interval. Thus, the variance of the inter-response interval was the sum of the variance of the clock and twice the variance of the motor delay. Furthermore, the motor delay variance was found to be the negative value of the autocovariance at lag 1. The lag 1 autocorrelation was also found to be between the value of 0 and -0.5. Data lying outside this range was discarded in the analysis. Data from only five stutterers (4 males and 1 female) and four controls (4 males) were usable. For each frequency, at most one data set from each subject was used. In order to match the number of data points from each subject group, a total of 20 data sets from the controls and 20 data sets from the stuttering subjects satisfied the criteria that were used for analysis: 3 from 833ms, 4 from 909ms, 2 from 1000ms, 4 from 1111ms, 4 from 1250ms and 3 from 1333ms.

Results

The mean values of the Inter-Response Interval (IRI) and the mean values of the square root of Total Variance (TV, s_t^2), Clock Variance (CV, s_c^2) and Motor Delay Variance (MDV, s_D^2) were plotted against the period of the tracking target in Fig.1. No significant difference was found in the IRI between stuttering subjects and controls in an analysis of variance, $F(1,38) = 0.35$, $p < 1$.

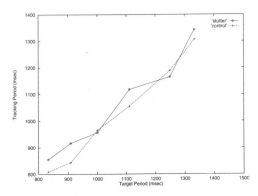

Figure 1a. The Inter-Response Interval (IRI) of stutterers and controls under each tracking period.

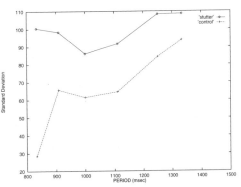

Figure 1b. The standard deviations of the Total Variance (TV) of stutterers and controls under each tracking period.

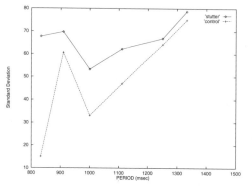

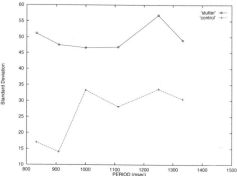

Figure 1c. The standard deviations of the Clock Variance (CV) of stutterers and controls under each tracking period.

Figure 1d. The standard deviations of the Motor Delay Variance (MDV) of stutterers and controls under each tracking period.

Table 1. The mean values of the Inter-Response Interval (IRI) in msec and the standard deviations of Total Variance (TV), Clock Variance (CV) and Motor Delay Variance (MDV) are given under each tracking period (in msec) for stuttering and control subjects. n is the number of data point employed in the analysis for each tracking period.

Tracking Period	n	Stuttering Subject				Control Subject		
		IRI	TV	CV	MDV	IRI	TV	CV	MDV
833	3	855	100.5	67.7	51.2	809	28.5	15.0	17.0
909	4	917	98.3	69.7	47.5	844	65.7	60.6	14.1
1000	2	957	86.2	53.2	46.6	966	61.5	33.1	33.4
1111	4	1119	91.7	62.2	46.9	1055	64.6	47.0	28.1
1250	4	1165	108.3	66.9	56.9	1189	84.3	64.2	33.7
1333	3	1344	108.6	78.8	48.9	1306	93.9	75.0	30.5

This showed that stuttering subjects could perform the tracking task in the continuation phase and produced periods of tracking similar to those of the nonstuttering controls. Analysis of variance, however, showed that stuttering subjects had significantly higher variances for tracking in general, for the total variance, TV, $F(1,38)=9.06$, $p<0.01$. For the clock variance, CV, no significant difference was found between stuttering and nonstuttering subjects $F(1,38)=2.53$, $p<0.5$. Finally, for the motor delay variance, MDV, $F(1,38)=16.55$, $p<0.001$, which showed that stuttering subjects had significantly higher motor variance in the control of their articulators than nonstuttering subjects. The mean values of the IRI and the standard deviations of Total Variance, Clock Variance and Motor Delay Variance are shown under each tracking period in Table 1.

CONCLUSION

The experiment reported in this paper tested the non-speech motor control of the stutterers. Our result supports the findings of Hulstijn et al. (1992) and Zelaznik et al. (1994) that there is no deficit in the timing mechanism of children who stutter when compared with those who do not stutter. However, a consistent trend is noted where the clock variance is higher for stuttering subjects than control subjects. This may need to be explored further with a larger subject group as Hulstijn et al. and Zelaznik et al. did not find such differences in general motor tasks which were much simpler tasks than the one employed by us and their tasks involved timing with higher clock frequencies which might be able to differentiate the clock performance of stuttering and nonstuttering subjects. On the other hand, a motor deficit is shown in the control of the lower lip of stuttering subjects which is consistent with Howell et al. (1995) where they found stuttering subjects to be less accurate in the lip-tracking task. Our result pinpoints the deficit of the accuracy in the motor control of the articulator. Our finding on a limited number of subjects makes the result preliminary in nature. Our ongoing research with larger subject groups should be able to verify our predictions and findings in this study. Further researches are planned to retest the stuttering subjects after their fluency enhancing therapy which includes the slowing down of speech rate. That would enable us to test if the therapies change the clock or the motor control of the articulators.

ACKNOWLEDGEMENT

This research was supported by a grant from the Wellcome Trust. We thank the staff, children and parents of the Michael Palin Centre for Stammering Children for making this study possible.

REFERENCES

Andrews, G., Graig, A., Feyer, A.M., Hoddinott, S., Howie, P., & Neilson, M. (1983). Stuttering: A review of research findings and theories circa 1982. *Journal of Speech and Hearing Disorders, 48,* 226-246.

Conture, E.G., Colton, R.H., & Gleason, J.R. (1988). Selected temporal aspects of coordination during fluent speech of young stutterers. *Journal of Speech and Hearing Research, 31,* 640-653.

Howell, P., Sackin, S., & Rustin, L. (1995). Comparison of speech motor development in stutterers and fluent speakers between 7 and 12 years old. *Journal of Fluency Disorders, 20,* 243-255.

Hulstijn, W., Summers, J.J., van Lieshout, P.H.M., & Peters, H.F.M. (1992). Timing in finger tapping and speech: A comparison between stutterers and fluent speakers. *Human Movement Science, 11,* 113-124.

Michon, J.A. (1967). *Timing in temporal tracking.* Soesterberg, The Netherlands: Institute for Perception-TNO.

Shaffer, L.H. (1982). Rhythm and timing in skill. *Psychology Review, 89,* 109-122.

Wing, A.M., & Kristofferson, A.B. (1973). Response delays and the timing of discrete motor responses. *Perception and Psychophysics, 14,* 5-12.

Zelaznik, H.N., Smith, A., & Franz, E.A. (1994). Motor performance of stutterers and nonstutterers on timing and force control tasks. *Journal of Motor Behavior, 26,* 340-347.

© 1997 Elsevier Science B.V. All rights reserved.
Speech Production: Motor Control, Brain Research and Fluency Disorders
W. Hulstijn, H.F.M. Peters and P.H.H.M. Van Lieshout, editors

Chapter 56

VISUOMOTOR TRACKING IN CHILDREN WHO STUTTER: A PRELIMINARY VIEW

Patricia M. Zebrowski, Jerald B. Moon, Donald A. Robin

The purpose of this study was to use a nonspeech task to explore the role of the speech motor system in the speech production of individuals who stutter. Four boys who stutter (mean age = 12 years; 11 months) and four age-matched nonstuttering boys served as subjects for the investigation. A target signal representing one of four different tracking conditions was displayed on an oscilloscope screen as a vertically moving horizontal bar. Movement signals from the lower lip and jaw were transduced via a standard strain gauge cantilever system, and were represented as a small dot on the oscilloscope screen. Each subject was required to track the presented target signal with either the jaw or the lip alone.
Cross-correlation analysis revealed that the stuttering children performed significantly poorer than their nonstuttering peers in using the lower lip to track predictable signals; however, there was no between-group difference observed for the jaw. Further, both groups showed decreased lip tracking accuracy with increased frequency of the predictable signal. Of interest is that the children who stutter showed better performance than the nonstuttering children in tracking the unpredictable target with both the lip and jaw. In general, findings support prior work in tracking with nonspeech structures (e.g., Noble et al., 1955; Flowers, 1978). Results suggest that some children who stutter may have difficulty either developing or accessing an internal model with which to predict articulator movement.

INTRODUCTION

A recurring question in the drive to understand both the etiology and development of stuttering has been: To what extent are stuttered disruptions related to a more pervasive deficit in motor control? One way to address this issue is to examine motoric control of the speech mechanism separate from the phonologic, semantic, syntactic and pragmatic demands placed on the system during ongoing speech. To that end, we have used a visuomotor tracking paradigm (e.g., McClean et al., 1987) to assess individual articulator function during a nonspeech task designed to mimic the lip and jaw opening and closing gestures used for speech (Moon et al., 1993; Hageman et al., 1994). Our long range goal is to use this paradigm to help us to grasp the role of the speech motor system across a variety of speech disorders, including stuttering, as well as in normal and "exceptional" speech.

METHOD

Subjects

Subjects for this study were four boys, with a mean age of 12:11 (years:months), who were enrolled in a six-week intensive residential stuttering therapy program. All children had a history of stuttering therapy, although in varying amounts. Results from administration of the *Stuttering Severity Instrument (SSI; Riley, 1980)* prior to treatment indicated that two of the four boys exhibited "moderate-severe" stuttering, while the remaining two displayed "moderate" and "severe" stuttering, respectively. A control group consisting of four age-matched nonstuttering boys was also included, and the data collected from these subjects will be displayed for comparison purposes. None of the subjects displayed additional speech, language, learning or hearing problems, with the exception of stuttering for the boys who stuttered.

Procedures

The procedures used in this preliminary study were identical to those described in detail by Moon et al. (1993). Briefly, a sinusoidal "target" signal representing one of three different tracking conditions (i.e., "predictable" sinusoids of 0.3, 0.6, and 0.9 Hz), and a complex, or "unpredictable" signal consisting of a range of frequencies from 0.1 to 1.0 Hz, was displayed on an oscilloscope screen as a vertically moving horizontal bar. Movement signals from the lower lip and jaw were transduced via a standard strain gauge cantilever system, and were represented as a small dot on the oscilloscope screen. For lower lip tracking, custom-made bite blocks which provided an 8-mm incisal gap, were used to fix the jaw.

For each condition, subjects were instructed to use either their lower lip or jaw to track the presented target bar throughout the extent of its excursion. As such, they were directed to "keep the dot on the bar." Presentation order for the three predictable (sinusoid) signals was counterbalanced, as was order of articulator (i.e., lower lip vs jaw). For each subject, tracking the unpredictable signal always followed sinusoid tracking.

Data Analysis

Target and transducer signals were digitized at 50 Hz. Within each tracking condition, six 10-second tracking runs for both the lower lip and jaw were submitted to a custom computer program that compared the transducer signals (i.e., lip and jaw) to the target signals vis a vis a number of variables, including: cross-correlation at 0-degree phase shift, best cross-correlation (i.e., regardless of phase), target-articulator gain ratio, target-articulator phase shift, and mean target-articulator amplitude difference. A detailed description of all measures is provided elsewhere (i.e., Moon et al., 1993); however, a brief summary follows:

Cross-correlation (0-degree phase shift) - derived by obtaining the inverse Fourier transform of the cross spectrum of the articulator movement and target signals, throughout a range of possible phase differences.

Best cross-correlation - the highest correlation coefficient obtained regardless of phase relationships between the target and articulator (i.e., phase shifted).

Target-articulator gain ratio and phase shift - gain ratio represents the frequency-specific target-articulator amplitude differences; phase shift indicates frequency-specific target-articulator timing differences(a negative phase shift reflects an articulator phase lead, while a positive shift indicates an articulator phase lag).

Target-articulator amplitude difference - Provides an overall indication of amplitude synchrony over time, regardless of target frequency.

Separate randomized block analyses of variance measures were conducted for each of the five variables measured. For purposes of this analysis, all correlations were transformed using the Fisher's Z transformation procedure. Model main effects were articulator (lip or jaw), and target frequency (0.3, 0.6 or 0.9 Hz). Further, analysis of target-articulator amplitude difference and the two correlation measures involved the addition of the unpredictable target signal (0.1-1.0 Hz).

RESULTS

Figures 1-5 provide mean and standard deviation values calculated for each measurement variable within each target-articulator condition. As indicated in Figures 1 and 2, correlational analyses revealed that in general, the stuttering children performed significantly poorer than their nonstuttering peers in using the lower lip to track predictable signals ($F(1, 331)=67.9$; $p \leq .0001$); however, there was no significant between-group difference observed for jaw tracking performance. Further, both groups showed significantly decreased lip tracking accuracy with increased frequency of the predictable signal ($F(3, 331)=61.9$; $p \leq .0001$), an observation consistent with earlier work describing the tracking abilities of normal talkers (Moon et al., 1993; Hageman et al., 1994).

Between-group comparison of tracking performance on the unpredictable target yielded interesting results. As Figures 1 and 2 indicate, the nonstuttering children's performance on this task was poorer than on any of the predictable signals, a similar observation to that made by Moon et al. and Hageman et al. for their normal subjects. The stuttering children, however, performed as well or better when tracking the unpredictable signal with the lower lip than they did while tracking the fastest predictable signal (0.9 Hz). Hageman et al. observed a similar pattern of performance for apraxic speakers. Further, the stuttering children in the present study performed significantly better than their nonstuttering counterparts in tracking the unpredictable target.

Figure 3 reveals that the nonstuttering children showed a greater gain ratio overall than the stuttering children; however, this between-group difference was nonsignificant. There was a significant difference between articulators for both groups, with a greater gain ratio observed for the jaw as opposed to the lower lip ($F(1, 248)=14.09$; $p \leq .0002$).

As suggested by Figure 4, while the nonstuttering children showed minimal changes in phase difference across the predictable signals, the children who stutter showed a declining target-articulator phase difference for lip tracking, associated with increased target frequency

Cross-Correlation (O-degree phase shift)

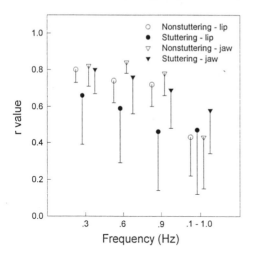

Figure 1. Mean and standard deviation correlation coefficients measured at 0-degree phase shift for each articulator by target frequency condition.

Best Cross-Correlation

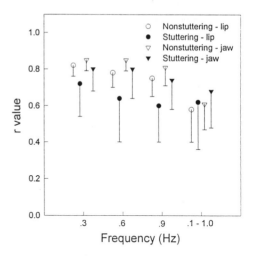

Figure 2. Mean and standard deviation correlation coefficients measured after phase shift for each articulator by target frequency condition.

Target - Articulator Gain Ratio

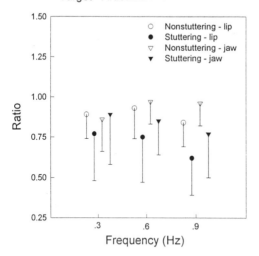

Figure 3. Mean and standard deviation target-articulator gain ratios for each articulator by target frequency condition.

Target - Articulator Phase Shift

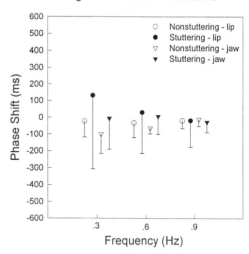

Figure 4. Mean and standard deviation phase shift values (in msec) for each articulator by target frequency condition. Negative values reflect articulator phase advancement relative to the target.

Target - Articulator Amplitude Difference

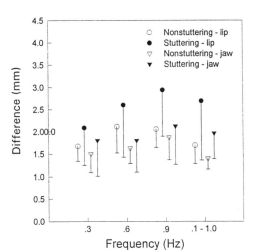

Figure 5. Mean and standard deviation target-articulator amplitude difference values (in mm) for each articulator by target frequency condition.

(i.e., changed from primarily phase "lag" while tracking 0.3 Hz target, to no or minimal phase difference for 0.6 and 0.9 signals).

Figure 5 shows the mean and standard deviation target-articulator amplitude difference values for the lower lip and jaw within each target condition. Overall, there was a significant difference between articulators, with the average difference greater for the lower lip than the jaw (F $(1, 331)$ = 80.75; $p \leq .0001$). Further, this difference was greater for the stuttering than the nonstuttering boys. For both groups, there was a tendency for the target-articulator amplitude difference to increase with target frequency from 0.3 to 0.9 Hz, with a decrease seen in the unpredictable target condition.

DISCUSSION

Present findings offer further support to earlier work with both normal and speech-disordered subjects in which the same or a similar tracking paradigm was used. That is, in general jaw tracking appears to be easier than lower lip tracking, as evidenced by higher cross correlations, smaller phase shifts, smaller target-tracker amplitude differences, and lower variability over most of the measures used.

Further, the poorer tracking performance exhibited by the stuttering children corroborates the results of prior investigations of the tracking behaviors of adults with apraxia of speech (Hageman et al., 1994) and children who stutter (Howell et al., 1995).

In a study of visuomotor tracking in a nonspeech system, Flowers (1978) suggested that individuals operate in a "predictive mode" while tracking a known signal. That is, they are able to maintain smooth, continuous tracking by developing an internal, higher-level model of a particular motion. This model allows for the accurate, spontaneous replication of the target movement with a minimum of attention paid to the target signal (with the exception of intermittent sampling). Flowers further suggested that people may change to a "responsive mode" when tracking an unknown, or unpredictable signal. In this responsive mode, the development of an internal model is not feasible, so continuous attention to the time-varying position of the target is necessary to accurately track the signal. For that reason, tracking unpredictable targets is thought to be more difficult, resulting in poorer performance overall when compared to tracking predictable signals.

In this preliminary study, the children who stutter performed more poorly than the nonstuttering children in tracking predictable signals. Further, unlike their normally fluent peers, the stuttering children improved their performance while tracking the unpredictable target. These findings suggest that individuals who stutter may have difficulty in either developing or accessing an internal model or plan of articulatory movements required for speech production. As a result, we speculate that people who stutter may function better in a more responsive mode, where they are required to make use of various feedback modes (e.g., visual or kinesthetic) to produce smooth and continuous articulator movement.

FUTURE RESEARCH

Presently, we are in the process of acquiring additional tracking data from a larger number of stuttering children and a group of age- and gender-matched nonstuttering peers. We intend to examine the possible relationship between nonspeech motor control (vis a vis visuomotor tracking) and speech by correlating tracking performance with perceptual judgments of speech (dis)fluency, as well as with measures of interarticulator coordination obtained from both fluent and disfluent speech samples.

REFERENCES

Flowers, K. (1978). Some frequency response characteristics of parkinsonism on pursuit tracking. *Brain, 101,* 19-34.

Hageman, C.F., Robin, D.A., Moon, J.B., & Folkins, J.W. (1994). Oral motor tracking in normal and apraxic speakers. *Clinical Aphasiology, 22,* 219-229.

Howell, P., Sackin, S., & Rustin, L. (1995). Comparison of speech motor development in stutterers and fluent speakers between 7 and 12 years old. *Journal of Fluency Disorders, 20*(3), 243-255.

McClean, M., Beukelman, D., & Yorkston, K. (1987). Speech-muscle visuomotor tracking in dysarthric and nonimpaired speakers. *Journal of Speech and Hearing Research, 30,* 276-282.

Moon, J.B., Zebrowski, P., Robin, D.A., & Folkins, J.W. (1993). Visuomotor tracking ability of young adult speakers. *Journal of Speech and Hearing Research, 36,* 672-682.

Noble, M., Fitts, P., & Warren, C. (1955). The frequency response of skilled subjects in a pursuit tracking task. *Journal of Experimental Psychology, 4,* 249-256.

Riley, G. (1980). *Stuttering Severity Instrument for Children and Adults.* Pro-Ed.

Speech Production: Motor Control, Brain Research and Fluency Disorders
W. Hulstijn, H.F.M. Peters and P.H.H.M. Van Lieshout, editors

Chapter 57

LINGUISTIC BEHAVIORS AT THE ONSET OF STUTTERING

Nan Bernstein Ratner

This pilot investigation sought to operationally define linguistic demands on children's fluency. A cohort of children near stuttering onset (N=8; ages 2;5-3:4) completed a battery of standardized and spontaneous language and fluency measures. Additionally, self-monitoring of speech output was tested by exposure to Delayed Auditory Feedback (DAF). Results suggest the possibility that stuttering children have discrepancies between their expressive and receptive lexical skills, and that stuttered utterances are likely to have high type-token ratios (higher lexical demand) and lower levels of grammaticality than fluent utterances. Additionally, stuttering children appear to be atypically sensitive to the effects of DAF, suggestive of developmental hyperfunction of self-monitoring abilities.

INTRODUCTION

Stuttering is a unique developmental communication disorder. With the possible exception of some autistic syndromes, no other speech/language disorder of childhood has a developmental profile of ostensibly normal communicative development and function, followed by onset of atypical behaviors (Van Riper, 1982; Yairi, 1983). This staging process highlights the need for a greater understanding of the child's functioning close to the onset of stuttering symptoms, to isolate possible precipitators of the condition.

One long-standing hypothetical answer to the question of why stuttering has an onset is that the demands of some aspect of the child's developing linguistic system stress or overwhelm the capacities of his speech motor system (the "Demands and Capacities Model" (c.f., Adams, 1982; Starkweather, 1987). This is an attractive notion if it can in fact be qualified and quantified. However, few models of this sort appear to posit specific and generalizable definitions of either capacity or demand, or propose what specific limitations exist within the speech production system to lead to the specific type of fluency failure we call stuttering. Clinical application of some Demands and Capacities models to individual children appear to resemble the opposite of the Procrustean bed described in other chapters in this volume. Rather, the Demands and Capacities bed appears to fit all who lie in it merely because its borders are so poorly defined. If one looks far enough, one can discover relative limitations on function for any speaker. I believe that the challenge of validating or falsifying a Capacities and Demands model goes somewhat further than this. It needs to explain why stuttering has its onset when it does, rather than existing at the onset of speech and language development. It would seem apparent that even one year old conversationalists experience communicative stress, but such demand does not appear to map to stutter behaviors; this phenomenon appears later in communicative development. The C&D model needs to define, for individual children, and for the population as a whole, what apparent limitation leads to speech production breakdown, and to explain why the breakdown resembles stuttering, rather than normal disfluency. Finally, the model needs to delineate whether some capacity limitation in the child is of a transient or more permanent nature, and why, if it is the former, the stuttering may persist after mismatches between capacity and demand no longer exist.

Clearly, understanding children's speech motor development is an important factor in addressing these concerns, as other authors, such as Kent (this volume), have indicated. In this paper, I will confine my observations to aspects of the child's *linguistic* development. I describe some pilot work we are currently doing at Maryland to isolate relationships between linguistic behaviors and stutters close to the onset of stuttering in children. Our goal is to determine whether and how language factors are involved in a demands/capacities model.

Past research has suggested that changes in syntactic demand adversely affect fluency patterns in young children between the ages of four and eight who stutter (see Bernstein Ratner, 1997 for summary); newer research suggests that the influence of syntactic demand on stuttering wanes over the course of development into adolescence (Silverman & Bernstein Ratner, in press). However, because such research has typically involved children well past the onset of symptoms, it is as yet unclear what types of linguistic demand might exert either a causal or exacerbating influence on fluency in 30-38 month old children, the age at which stuttering onset is typically reported.

There are a number of candidates for linguistic stressors in child development in the age range between 30-38 months (Bernstein Ratner, 1997). Among them are the transition from an asyntactic system of utterance generation to one which is syntactically governed and driven (e.g., Locke, 1993); specific acquisition of grammatical representations/forms which signal quantum changes in the nature of the child's grammar (Radford, 1994), and concurrent "bursting" in cross-domain talents, such as morphology and the lexicon (Bates et al., 1995).

We have begun to collect data from children within three months of onset of stuttering symptoms (range 1-3 months) to examine profiles of linguistic functioning at the time that stuttering begins. In this paper, I will report preliminary data from eight children selected from a larger cohort being followed longitudinally.

In this work, we have made an assumption about the ways in which we think the Demands and Capacities Model of stuttering is best tested. In order for such a theory not to be vacuous because of its lack of specification, we presume that *individuals* have capacities and demands placed upon them, whereas *groups* do not. This implies that within-subject behavior is an important focus for the evaluation of this model. In doing so, we fully recognize the fine line between a theory of behavior that twists itself to the nuances of individual behavior in the absence of an overarching account of the behaviors of larger groups. In particular, I have no desire to create a smorgasbord of 100 varieties of developmental stuttering, each apparently dependent upon the vagaries of presenting symptoms. Rather, we hope that by exploring within-subject behaviors across a group of young stuttering children, we may eventually capture some regularities which *do* apply to stuttering children as a group, or to a significant sub-group, in much the same way as major subgroups of individuals with diabetes have been identified.

METHOD

In brief, the current study tracks children longitudinally starting within a three month period following identification of the onset of stuttering symptoms. To refine the accuracy of this timing, we canvass parents of children within SIX months of stuttering onset, and follow only those children with closer onset times. In addition, ALL intake information is gathered independently from both father and mother, to assure agreement about the timing of symptoms as well as other background information.

Initial intake variables, which will be the primary focus of this report, include a spontaneous language sample with both parents and a clinician (used to derive Mean Length of Utterance (MLU), type-token ratio (TTR), error analysis, fluency analysis, rate, and Developmental Sentence Score (DSS), among the primary variables, conversational Adult-Child patterns as secondary variables), a battery of standardized tests for in-depth analysis of the child's lexicon, both receptively and expressively (receptive: *Peabody Picture Vocabulary Test- Revised* (PPVT; Dunn & Dunn, 1981), *Expressive One-Word Vocabulary Test* (EOWVT; Gardner, 1979), standardized assessment of grammatical understanding and production (*Clinical Evaluation of Language Fundamentals - Preschool* (CELF-P; Semel et al., 1987) subtests), a standardized phonetic inventory assessment (*Goldman-Fristoe Test of Articulation* (GFTA)), and oral-motor examination. Parents individually and separately complete case history information, a genetic history for communication disorders, and two scales meant to measure parental knowledge of the child's communicative development and opinions regarding the child's communicative adequacy (*MacArthur Communicative Development Inventory* (CDI), experimental extension, Dale, in press; *Speech and Language Assessment Scale* (SLAS), Hadley & Rice, 1993). Finally, one experimental measure is used to assess the child's auditory self-monitoring skills.

In our preliminary analyses to be reported here, we sought to evaluate the Demands and Capacities Model in a number of ways, posing alternative hypotheses about the nature of demand on the child's evolving communicative system. We have developed three operationally-defined levels of demand on the child's language system. The first *(1)* is that discrepancies in level of development among the child's capacity for particular components of language functioning could unduly stress the child's ability to produce speech fluently. That is, a child who has well-developed receptive language skills, but poorly developed articulation or expressive language skills may find it difficult to produce fluent speech. This hypothetical situation should produce "gaps" in the child's test performance on various tasks. The second hypothesis *(2)* is that fluency may be stressed when the child attempts to produce structures which are developmentally advanced according to published expectations. Thus, elevated MLU should reflect more ambitious sentence construction; elevated TTR should reflect higher levels of lexical demand. Finally, the third operational definition of demand *(3)* is defined by the child's own performance. We hypothesize that utterances produced without grammatical errors reflect lower level of demand on the child's language production system than those which are produced with grammatical errors, indicating lower levels of competence with this particular structure.

In the section below, we evaluate the degree to which stuttering reflects these operational levels of demand in our pilot group of children. Although this study is designed to be longitudinal, and to evaluate which factors eventually map to chronic, as opposed to transient stuttering (following the philosophy of Yairi, Ambrose et al., 1995), only cross-sectional data are available for report at this time.

First, this very small cohort (N = 8) consists of 6 boys and 2 girls. The average age of onset was 2;7, with a range of 2;3 to 3;1, consistent with earlier reports (Yairi, et al.). Our identification post onset was 1-3 months, average 2.5.

RESULTS

Our first hypothesis *(1)* was that there might be cross-domain instability within these children's systems. This is a popular notion, and both anecdotally and at conferences, one can see descriptions of children described as having "gaps" between comprehension and production, between phonology and syntax, etc. We looked for such gapping patterns. Within the limitations of comparing standardized scores across diverse tests, with a small population, the following was observed:

With the exception of one child's articulation skills, there was no evidence of clinically relevant language or speech "fragility." The sole exception was one child with a significant (1st percentile) deficit in articulation skills. All other children achieved scores well above the average on most instruments, and even those scores below average were well within the normal range of function. There was a trend for receptive lexicon (PPVT) to lead expressive lexicon (EOWVT) in this group, when analyzed both as a group and individual phenomenon (Figure 1).

As I have noted elsewhere (Bernstein Ratner, 1997), lexical factors have been ignored for the most part in psycholinguistic analyses of stuttering, but play an increasingly important role in accounts of the normal sentence generation process. There was no trend for receptive and expressive grammatical skills to be gapped, at least on the instruments we used (Figure 2). There was no trend, despite a large literature we respect, for children to demonstrate articulation delay or disorder (Figure 3).

We next *(2)* turned from defining demand as instability across linguistic domains such as grammar, lexicon and phonology, to measures of productive complexity, such as Mean Length of Utterance and Type-Token Ratio. Prior work with older children strongly suggests an effect of utterance length and complexity on the frequency of stutter behaviors. Particularly with children of this age level, MLU is an especially sensitive index of grammatical com-

VOCABULARY SCORES

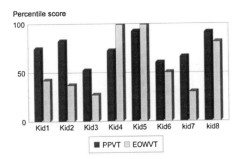

Figure 1. Standardized expressive (EOWVT) and receptive (PPVT) vocabulary scores.

CELF-P Expressive and Receptive Scores: Morphology

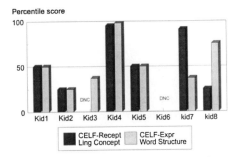

Figure 2. CELF-P expressive and receptive grammar scores.

Standardized Articulation Scores

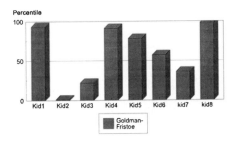

Figure 3. Goldman-Fristoe Test of Articulation (GFTA) scores.

plexity, although its utility falls as children generate longer utterances. In the following sections, data from only the first six subjects are reported.

When data from these six subjects are grouped, stuttered utterances were found to have higher MLU values (Figure 4), suggesting that as utterances become morphologically complex, they attract more stutter incidents. However, when viewed within subjects, it quickly became apparent that only two children evidenced such an association within their output (Figure 5). For the other four, no association between utterance length/complexity in morphemes and fluency could be discerned.

As part of this second definition of utterance complexity, we next examined Type-token Ratios, a measure of lexical variety and therefore, lexical complexity, within a spoken language sample. Five of six subjects showed a tendency to have stuttered utterances with higher type-token ratios than their fluent utterances (Figure 6). In previous work, we have noted that lexical analysis of stuttering has probably attracted less investigation than is warranted by current psycholinguistic theory, and we hope to follow up on this interesting finding.

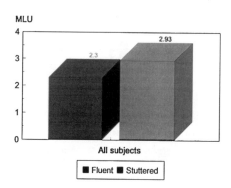

Figure 4. MLU of stuttered and fluent utterances (grouped data).

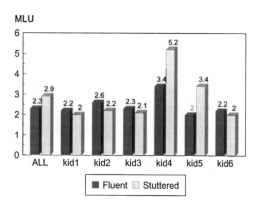

Figure 5. MLU of stuttered and fluent utterances (individual data).

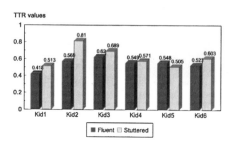

Figure 6. Type-Token Ratios of stuttered and fluent utterances (individual data).

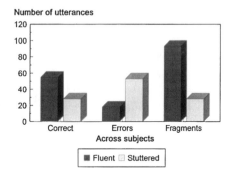

Figure 7. Relationship between fluency and grammatical correctness.

We also note that the children for whom this TTR gap was widest showed the largest discrepancies between their standardized expressive and receptive vocabulary scores.

Finally, we moved from what we might call "externally-defined" measures of utterance complexity (grammatical stage or length, lexical diversity), to "internally-defined" measures. We operationally defined demand by hypothesizing that utterances containing grammatical errors had placed more of a demand on the child's system than those which were produced correctly. A cross-tabulation of stuttered/fluent utterances by grammatical adequacy produced an interesting trend: (Figure 7)

There was an inverse pattern between the frequency of grammatically correct, fluent utterances, and errored, stuttered utterances. A chi-square analysis of the distribution of correct and errored utterances yields a highly significant value (chi-square = 29.14, df(1), $p < .001$).

Again, we believe that such an operational definition of communicative demand has relevance for further research, particularly at the earliest stages of stuttering, when children are still formulating grammar, and producing a variety of sentences, many of which show evolving and imperfect mastery of grammar. Unlike the case of lexical demand, however, we noted that neither scores on standardized tests of grammar nor MLU/fluency relationships tended to predict the degree to which ungrammatical utterances attracted stutters for a particular child.

Our experimental procedure examined auditory self-monitoring patterns in the children. Children who stutter appear to be different from other speech-language impaired children in important ways other than onset profile. The majority of children with grammatical or phonological disorders appear quite oblivious to their inadequacies in output, a feature conspicuously absent in stuttering, even at a young age. The literature on children's phonological development has historically used Delayed Auditory Feedback (DAF) to assess whether children are responsive to their own auditory output. The aging literature on this topic (cf. Yeni-Komshian et al., 1968; Chase et al., 1961) suggests that it is between 2-3 years that the first consistent effects of DAF are found with children, indicating that self-monitoring of auditory output is occurring.

The development of self-monitoring ability would appear interesting for a theory of stuttering onset because it potentially explains both observed struggle in stuttering toddlers, as well as predicts that stutters might not resemble normal nonfluencies. Specifically, if a child had some level of linguistic fragility, or gapping among components of the speech/language generating system, and was relatively hyper-attentive (for language age) to his own output, an increased incidence of planning failures (normal nonfluencies) could potentially be responded to with tension and concern, leading to the types of behaviors characteristic of early stuttering. In examining the DAF responses of this group of children and a control group, we are interested in the possibility that stuttering children, particularly those who show struggle behaviors, are more sensitive to their own feedback than are other children, and that this "strength", when coupled with deficits in either linguistic or motor planning, can lead to tension and struggle in speech output.

Our preliminary data show that the speech of four of the six children was greatly disrupted when single word naming tasks were switched from normal sidetone to a delay of 250 msec. Although we are currently pursuing ways of objectively qualifying and quantifying these data these children were also the four children who showed the greatest "struggle" during stuttered events. The two children who presented with "easy" multiple sound-syllable repetitions and blocks unaccompanied by secondary behaviors talked normally during DAF exposure, whereas the other four children greatly changed speech output, primarily by stretching the duration of segments by as much as 80%.

DISCUSSION

Inasmuch as one can interpret data from so few children, a number of observations are possible. First, one could probably justify a Demands and Capacities model for each of these children, using aspects of their standardized and spontaneous performance. An important issue is what to measure, when and how. Some measures were better suited to projecting when speech output was likely to be stuttered than others. Standardized tests scores appeared least interesting in this respect. We were able to find partial support for the first operational definition of demand, discrepancy among areas of functioning. A majority of our children demonstrated receptive vocabulary skills well in excess of expressive lexical performance. This finding was amplified by analysis of our second definition of demand, use of advanced linguistic structures. While MLU did not predict fluency well for this group of children, the same children who showed expressive-receptive lexical "gapping" showed a tendency for stuttered utterances to have higher TTR values, indicative of higher lexical demand. Finally, there was strong support, even in this small sample, for our third operational definition of demand, the child's own level of grammatical performance. There was a statistically significant relationship between the grammaticality of the child's output, and fluency. Stuttered utterances were highly likely to contain grammatical formulation errors.

Future directions

These data are pilot data, and we are using them primarily to refine the nature of future questions. In particular, it appears that if stuttering research is to seriously consider the role of language development and possible linguistic fragility on fluency, it needs to keep up with evolving research considerations in the language disorders literature. In particular, this field has moved beyond cataloguing what children do, to asking why it is that they do what they do. They have moved from what is often called "static" assessment (what does this child or group of children know when compared with other children) to "dynamic" assessment (how does this child learn or make use of learning opportunities). In this regard, research such as Ludlow, et al.'s (this volume), targeting nonsense word acquisition, is a valuable direction, as is the work being carried out by Smith et al. (this volume), and others. In taking a more dynamic approach, particularly at the onset of stuttering symptoms, we may better distinguish between the notion that stuttering children have reduced linguistic competence, and the possibility that stuttering children seem to have a competence for language which is poorly recognized in their performance. We may begin to recognize patterns of less efficient lexical or syntactic mapping, storage, or retrieval. This would be entirely consistent with newer views of specific language impairment (SLI) in children, whose limited language output has been shown to reflect slower processing (decoding) of incoming auditory input, and less efficient mapping of lexical representations, among other things (Bernstein Ratner, 1997). Thus, it would not be surprising to find that SLI children had inverse clinical "peers", children for whom the *encoding* of linguistic representations was slower or mismatched to the capacity of the child's speech motor system. But it also would not be surprising to find that the language encoding abilities of stuttering children were quite adequate, but poorly served by their motor systems. In this case, the well-documented effects of language tasks on fluency would be the unfortunate by-product of speech motor impairment exacerbated by excessive demand elsewhere in the system. The fact is, that until we better understand the typical developmental profile of a child at the onset of stuttering, before learned responses set in, we are not in a position to choose between these options.

REFERENCES

Bates, E., Dale, P., & Thal, D. (1995). Individual differences and their implications for theories of language development. In P. Fletcher, & B. MacWhinney (Eds.). *The handbook of child language.* Oxford: Basil Blackwell.

Bernstein Ratner, Nan (1997). Stuttering: a psycholinguistic perspective. In R. Curlee, & R. Siegel (Eds). *Nature and treatment of stuttering: New directions.* Boston: Allyn & Bacon.

Bernstein Ratner, Nan (in press). Atypical speech and language development. In J. Berko Gleason (Ed.) *The development of language (4th edition).* Boston: Allyn & Bacon.

Caruso, A., Max, L., & McClowry, M. (1997). Applications of motor learning theory to stuttering research. This volume.

Chase, R., Sutton, S., First, D., & Zubin, N. (1961). Developmental study of changes in behavior under delayed auditory feedback. *Journal of Genetic Psychology, 99* 101-112.

Colburn, N., & Mysak, E. (1982a). Developmental disfluency and emerging grammar I. Disfluency characteristics in early syntactic utterances. *Journal of Speech and Hearing Research, 25,* 414-420.

Colburn, N., & Mysak, E. (1982b). Developmental disfluency and emerging grammar II. Co-occurrence of disfluency with specified semantic-syntactic structures. *Journal of Speech and Hearing Research, 25,* 421-427.

Kent, R. (this volume). Speech motor models and developments in neurophysiological science: new perspectives. In W. Hulstijn, H.F.M. Peters, & P.H.H.M. Van Lieshout (Eds.), *Speech production: motor control, brain research and fluency disorders.* Amsterdam: Elsevier Science.

Locke, J. (1993). *The child's path to spoken language.* Cambridge, MA: Harvard University Press.

Ludlow, C., Siren, K., & Zikria, M. (1997). Speech production learning in adults with chronic developmental stuttering. This volume.

Neilson, M., & Neilson, P. (1987). Speech motor control and stuttering: a computational model of adaptive sensory-motor processing. *Speech Communication, 6,* 325-333.

Prins, D., Main, V., & Waupler, S. (1997). Lexicalization processes in adults who stutter. This volume.

Radford, A. (1995). Phrase structure and functional categories. In P. Fletcher & B. MacWhinney (eds.) *The handbook of child language.* Oxford: Basil Blackwell.

Silverman, S., & Bernstein Ratner, N. (in press). Fluency and sentence imitation abilities of adolescents who stutter. *Journal of Speech and Hearing Research.*

Smith, A. (1997). A multi-leveled, dynamic approach to stuttering. This volume.

Starkweather, C.W. (1987). *Fluency and stuttering.* Englewood Cliffs, NJ: Prentice-Hall.

Yairi, E., Paden, E., Ambrose, N., & Throneburg, R. (1996). Pathways of chronicity and recovery: longitudinal studies of early stuttering. *Journal of Communication Disorders, 29,* 51-77.

Yeni-Komshian, G., Chase, R., & Mobley, R. (1968). The development of auditory feedback monitoring II. Delayed auditory feedback studies on the speech of children between two and three years of age. *Journal of Speech and Hearing Research, 11,* 301-306.

Speech Production: Motor Control, Brain Research and Fluency Disorders
W. Hulstijn, H.F.M. Peters and P.H.H.M. Van Lieshout, editors

Chapter 58

COGNITIVE AND LINGUISTIC ABILITIES OF STUTTERING CHILDREN

Andrea Häge, Dieter Rommel, Helge S. Johannsen, Hartmut Schulze

In this study 94 stuttering children with a mean age of 5 years and 5 months (range 2:8 - 9:7) were assessed with psychometric tests measuring the basic performance level and possible partial deficits in specific cognitive or linguistic areas. These tests included the KABC (Kaufman Assessment Battery for Children), a test series for intellectual abilities and acquired skills, and two language development tests: The HSET (Heidelberger Sprachentwicklungstest) and the AWST 3-6 (Aktiver Wortschatztest für 3-6jährige Kinder). From videotaped playing situations we calculated the mean length of utterances (MLU), which is considered to be an indicator for language development. Additionally, these intellectual and cognitive abilities were recorded by a clinical screening procedure and by ratings of the children's parents. We compared the different methods for assessing cognitive and linguistic abilities and their relations to stuttering in children.

INTRODUCTION

This study is one part of a long term research project, supported by the DFG (Deutsche Forschungsgemeinschaft). Our purpose is to find out which linguistic or cognitive abilities provide prognostic validity for the development of childhood stuttering.

The focus of the research plan is to gather data about the onset and development of stuttering in 94 children over a period of five years per child. Follow-ups are carried out in six-months-intervals, provided that the stutter symptoms persist. If the children become permanently fluent, they are withdrawn from further follow-ups.

The theoretical framework of our study reflects a multifactorial view on the onset and development of the stuttering phenomenon published by Schulze and Johannsen (1986, 1990, 1993). This view holds that stuttering is etiologically not homogeneous and that every stutterer acquires his/her individual disorder on the basis of an interaction between physiological, psychosocial and psycholinguistic factors (see also the component model of Riley & Riley, 1984).

METHOD

When entering the longitudinal study, the children were examined with standardized psychometric tests and clinical screening procedures to assess the linguistic and cognitive stage of development. Language development data were recorded with the "Heidelberger Sprachentwicklunsgtest" (abbreviated HSET; Grimm & Schöler, 1991), a battery of 13 subtests assessing both receptive and expressive syntactic, semantic and pragmatic abilities. Additionally, the "Aktiver Wortschatztest" (AWST 3-6; Kiese & Kozielski, 1979) was applied for preschoolers, a vocabulary test requiring the naming of noncoloured drawings from every day objects and activities.

By means of the German version of the "Kaufman Assessment Battery for Children" (KABC; Kaufman & Kaufman, 1983, German version: Melchers & Preuß, 1991) we assessed cognitive abilities and possible partial deficits. This test series measures intellectual abilities as well as acquired skills. Additional measures are the clinical screening of the linguistic and cognitive stage by an experienced phoniatrician and the parents' ratings with the help of a scale divided into four steps (e.g.: above/ on/ below average/ seriously impaired). From videotaped and transcribed playing situations we got linguistic data as the mean length of utterances (MLU; McWhinney, 1992), which we compared with the other measures of linguistic ability. The paper by Rommel et al. (chapter 59) gives more linguistic data about the speech of the stuttering children in this sample.

RESULTS

Sample and stuttering

Data were derived from 94 children with a mean age of 5 years and 5 months, ranging from 2:8 to 9:7 years (see Table 1), brought to the phoniatrics department because of stuttering. The sample group consists of 71 boys and 23 girls and was not selected in any way.

Table 1. Description of the sample

		Boys	Girls	Total
number n (%)		71 (76%)	23 (24%)	94 (100%)
age: years;months	M (SD)	5;6 (1;7)	5;3 (1;4)	5;5 (1;6)
stuttering:				
in % of syllables	M (SD)	5,02 (3,59)	4,47 (3,45)	4,89 (3,55)
in % of words	M (SD)	6,34 (4,46)	5,53 (4,19)	6,14 (4,39)
age of onset	M (SD)	3;4 (1;0)	3;8 (0;11)	3;5 (0;10)

Table 2. Developmental problems of certain functions

rated by	cognitive development in %	language development in %	articulation in %	motor skills in %	oral motor skills in %	psychosocial development in %
examiner:						
below average	20,2	31,9	54,3	25,5	35,1	30,9
seriously impaired	2,1	17,0	7,5	2,1	16,0	1,1
parents:						
below average	7,5	31,9	40,4	20,2	--*	26,6

* Parents were not asked for their rating of oral motor function.

The distribution of boys and girls reflects the sex specification of the disorder, which is reported to have a ratio of 3:1 in recent literature (see, for example Bloodstein, 1995). The sex differences concerning age, stuttering and age of onset, as shown in Table 1, are statistically insignificant. The average stuttering frequency is about 5% stuttered syllables (about 6% stuttered words, respectively), which can be classified as moderate stuttering. Therefore, this could be considered to be a relatively representative sample of this age group of stuttering children.

Developmental stage

Table 2 gives a survey of developmental problems of the children, on the one hand rated by the examiner based on clinical experiences and on the other hand rated by the children's parents based on personal impressions. The expert's rating "below average" marks children with a mild impairment who need no therapy, while a rating of "seriously impaired" is considered to be an indication for therapy.

Of course, these estimations do not allow to draw conclusions about statistically relevant deviations from the standard population, because there are no comparable data from a non-stuttering control-group.

Asked for delayed or disordered development, the parents listed in 40% of the cases articulation, in 32% language, in 27% psychosocial development and in 20% motor skills. The cognitive development was rated most rarely as being delayed or disordered (7%). To the examiner, the children appeared more impaired than to their parents.

Cognitive abilities

By means of the psychometric test series KABC we found a perfect normal situation in the field of cognitive performances (see Table 3): The stuttering children show average values of their age group on all scales of the KABC. (The average of the IQ-scale covers the range from 85 to 115 with the mean of 100 and the standard deviation of 15 IQ-scores.)

Table 3. Cognitive Performance as measured by

KABC Global intellectual scale	KABC Achievement scale	KABC Nonverbal scale	KABC Sequential processing scale	KABC Simultaneous processing scale
n = 87 IQ-score	n = 87 IQ-score	n = 87 IQ-score	n = 87 IQ-score	n = 87 IQ-score
M SD	M SD	M SD	M SD	M SD
99 9	97* 13	98 11	99 12	99 11

* differs significantly from population standard (p<0,05)

The different subtests of the KABC are combined to two scales: First the sequential processing scale which includes serial processes in the visual and auditive perception field, secondly the simultaneous processing scale which includes spacial integrative perception and problem solving abilities. Both scales are condensed to the global intellectual scale (KABC-GS). The nonverbal scale includes those subtests which to a large extent can be used without spoken instructions; the achievement scale (KABC-AS) combines those subtests, which examine acquired skills and mainly verbally acquired knowledge as, for example, vocabulary, reading, arithmetics.

Only the mean of 97 in the achievement scale differs significantly from the population average 100 at the 5% level. We tested the significance by using a one-sample T-test (SAS System, Release 6.11, 1995).

Linguistic abilities

Assessed with psychometric methods, the sample shows no deficiencies in linguistic performances. The mean results of HSET with a T-score of 51 (standard deviation of 6) and AWST3-6 with a percentile rank of 46 confirm an appropriate state of the stuttering children's linguistic abilities in comparison with their non-stuttering age-group. The test scores' deviations from the population standard (T-score=50, percentile rank=50) are proved to be statistically not significant.

In sum, our sample of stuttering children shows no general linguistic or cognitive deficits at all. This result contributes to the discussion in specialist literature based on inconsistent results of different research groups concerning stuttering and cognitive or linguistic abilities (cf., Rommel, 1993).

Cognitive and linguistic measures in comparison

Possible relationships between the collected measures of cognitive and linguistic abilities are examined using correlation coefficients.

Table 4. Correlations between measures of cognitive and linguistic abilities

Correlations	HSET	AWST	MLU	parents' rating of language state	examiners' rating of language state	KABC-GS
HSET	-.-					* p < 0.05
AWST	.59**	-.-				** p < 0.01
MLU	.14	.37**	-.-			
parents' rating of language state	.37**	.27*	.25*	-.-		
examiners' rating of language state	.27*	.53**	.19	.33**	-.-	
KABC-GS	.48**	.46**	.00	.16	.38**	-.-
KABC-AS	.60**	.70**	.23**	.53**	.50**	.58**

Table 4 presents the correlation coefficients between the global test scores of KABC, HSET and AWST3-6, the examiners' and parents' ratings of language development and MLU. First, we can see that there are significant correlations between almost all cognitive and language state measures for the sample on hand. One may conclude that cognitive and linguistic abilities develop in close relationship to each other and that it is almost impossible to measure them independently by psychometric tests. Only the mean length of utterances (MLU) seems to measure a different dimension of linguistic abilities, totally independent from cognitive abilities as represented in the global scale of the KABC.

It seems that a relatively simple language development measure as MLU can cover different aspects of language development than a complex battery with several subtests. Possibly, we find these difference because MLU is derived from spontaneous speech whereas psychometric tests require answers within a given formal scheme. Spontaneous speech includes not only developmental aspects of grammar and vocabulary, but also situational aspects and personal characteristics of the speaking child.

Cognitive and linguistic abilities in relation to stuttering

Table 5 shows the correlation coefficients between the cognitive and linguistic measures and the single stutter symptoms as well as the total stuttering score. According to Riley and Riley (1984), the symptoms are divided into sound-, syllable-, and word-repetitions, blocks and prolongations.

There is no significant correlation except for the relationship between prolongations and the K-ABC global intellectual scale.

Table 5. Cognitive and linguistic abilities in relation to stuttering

Correlations	total stuttering	blocks	prolongations	word repetitions	syllable repetitions	sound repetitions
HSET	.04	.12	.02	-.04	.03	-.16
AWST	-.05	.03	.08	-.09	-.20	-.10
MLU	-.18	-.06	-.18	-.02	-.18	-.12
parents' rating of language state	.08	.02	.11	.05	.01	.10
examiners' rating of language state	-.06	-.07	-.07	.05	-.08	.06
KABC-GS	.12	-.04	.26*	.00	-.02	-.09
KABC-AS	-.14	-.10	-.05	-.08	-.11	-.10
age	-.31**	-.01	-.17	-.32**	-.29**	-.09

* $p < 0.05$
** $p < 0.01$

Interesting findings are the highly significant correlations between age and stuttering. Children show higher stuttering frequencies the younger they are at their entry in this study. Their main symptoms are word and syllable repetitions which are much more frequent as in the older children. Other symptoms show no correlations with age. There were no significant sex differences in comparing the cognitive and linguistic abilities and their relationship to stuttering. In making a distinction between stuttering children with less and more frequent stuttering, the MLU score was found to be lower for the latter group.

CONCLUSIONS

It should be noticed that in general there are no differences between the group of stuttering children and their fluent peers concerning cognitive and linguistic stages. Also the division into several subgroups according to sex, duration of stuttering and frequency of stuttering, did not reveal any differences, except the connection between MLU and subgroups of stuttering children mentioned above.

We can summarize our data by saying that up to now they provide no evidence for a prognostic validity of cognitive or linguistic factors in childhood stuttering. Possibly the longitudinal observation of small subgroups will provide more significant differences with regard to specific areas of cognitive or linguistic processing.

REFERENCES

Bloodstein, O (1995). *A handbook on stuttering.* London: Chapman & Hall.

Grimm, H., & Schöler, H. (1990). *HSET, Heidelberger Sprachentwicklungstest.* Göttingen, Germany: Hogrefe.

Johannsen, H.S., & Schulze, H. (1993). *Praxis der Beratung und Therapie bei kindlichem Stottern. - Werkstattbericht -.* Ulm, Germany: Phoniatrische Ambulanz der Universität Ulm.

Kaufman, A.S., & Kaufman, N.L. (1983). *Kaufman Assessment Battery for Children.* Minnesota: Circle Pines (German Version by Melchers, P. & Preuß, U., 1991. Amsterdam: Swets & Zeitlinger).

Kiese, C., & Kozielski, P.-M. (1979). *AWST 3-6, Aktiver Wortschatztest für drei- bis sechsjährige Kinder.* Weinheim, Germany: Beltz Testgesellschaft.

Riley, G.D., & Riley, J.A (1984). Component model for treating stuttering in children. In M. Prins (Ed.), *Contemporary approaches in stuttering therapy* (pp. 123-172). Boston, MA: Little, Brown & Co.

Rommel, D. (1993). Psycholinguistische Aspekte des Stotterns. In DBL und DGPP (Hrsg.) *Stottern. Münster 1993 Tagungsbericht* (pp. 59-73). Ulm, Germany: Phoniatrische Ambulanz der Universität Ulm.

Rommel, D., Häge, A., Johannsen, H.S., & Schulze, H. (this volume). Linguistic aspects of stuttering in childhood. In W. Hulstijn, H.F.M. Peters, & P.H.H.M. Van Lieshout (Eds.), *Speech production: motor control, brain research and fluency disorders.* Amsterdam: Elsevier Science.

Schulze, H., & Johannsen, H.S. (1986). *Stottern bei Kindern im Vorschulalter. Theorie, Diagnostik, Therapie.* Ulm, Germany: Phoniatrische Ambulanz der Universität Ulm.

Speech Production: Motor Control, Brain Research and Fluency Disorders
W. Hulstijn, H.F.M. Peters and P.H.H.M. Van Lieshout, editors

Chapter 59

LINGUISTIC ASPECTS OF STUTTERING IN CHILDHOOD

Dieter Rommel, Andrea Häge, Helge S. Johannsen, Hartmut Schulze

The verbal interactional behaviors of 94 stuttering children (mean age = 5;5) and their mothers were videotaped in a playing situation. The utterances were transcribed. The children's fluent and dysfluent utterances were analyzed separately. On the basis of the so-called speech-act theory and recent research results some selected psycholinguistic characteristics of the locutive and illocutive speech act have been analyzed concerning their significance for dysfluencies. Besides traditional characteristics (loci-variables) as the phonetic factor (consonants vs. vowels; sound transitions), syntactic structure (length of sentences, word length, position in the word or sentence) and propositional content (function words vs. content words) we took a look at the significance of the illocutive and perlocutive act for dysfluencies.

Results indicate that stuttering predominantly occurs on longer utterances, on vowels and before consonants, mainly on loci where vowel-consonant transitions take place, predominantly in the middle of the sentences and words. In the pragmalinguistic field we find less stuttering on expressiva and more stuttering on constativa and regulativa. The illocution of the parents' utterances has no effect.

Furthermore we found that the loci-variables do not depend upon the severity of stuttering, the linguistic or cognitive state of development and the motor and oral-motor skills of the children.

INTRODUCTION

An important approach in addition to the study of linguistic abilities (see Häge et al., chapter 58) towards an understanding of the language factor for the onset and development of stuttering, is to study the linguistic demands - through loci variables - of stuttering (Rommel, 1995). This tradition of research, which dates back to Brown (1945), tries to examine relationships between the occurence of dysfluencies and linguistic loci through a precise analysis. For this, studies have been made until today primarily with adult stutterers, which came up with quite homogeneous results (see Wingate, 1988), as follows:

- Phonetic field: stuttering most likely on consonants and on consonant-vowel transitions, and increased stuttering on stressed syllables;
- Syntactic field: increased stuttering on longer and/or grammatically more complex sentences, on longer words, more frequently at the beginning of sentences and most likely at the beginning of a word;

- Semantic field: increased stuttering on content words.

Within the last 20 years the need to examine children in the same way as adults, has become quite obvious. The results with adult speakers cannot simply be transferred to the situation of children - which unfortunately still happens quite frequently (see for review Bloodstein, 1995).

The few existing loci-studies on children - contradictory and in part questionable (few participants, insufficient or no description of the stuttering, insufficient or no clearing up of further problems of the child) - leave many questions open and point to the necessity of further studies, especially within the German-speaking area (Rommel, 1993).

METHOD

In this study the spontaneous linguistic behavior of 94 stuttering children was videotaped in a 30 minute standardized playing situation together with the mother. The utterances of the children and their partners were transcribed according to the guidelines of MacWhinney (1995); the utterances were analyzed by means of the CLAN-system described there. The raw transcripts of our study group are open to inspection in the CHILDES - database (see MacWhinney, 1995).

In examining the effects of the linguistic characteristics, we compared fluent with dysfluent utterances. All statistical comparisons where calculated as 'paired-difference t-Test' (SAS, v. 6.10).

Subjects

The participants - 94 stuttering children - are described in detail concerning their stuttering, their linguistic and cognitive abilities as well as their motor and oral-motor skills by Häge et al., (chapter 58).

Analyzed variables

On the basis of the Speech Act theory (Austin, 1962) we differentiate between the three levels of illocution, locution and perlocution (figure 1).

The *illocutionary act* denotes the communicative function of an utterance directed to a listener. To categorize the illocutions we went back to Habermas' (1982) classification of these speech acts into regulativa, expressiva and constativa. Regulativa are utterances that refer to a common social world. They regulate the interpersonal relationships (Examples: May I have your attention, please!; Mum, look!). Expressiva are utterances that express the speaker's and/or listener's feelings and attitudes. The speaker makes statements about his inner, subjective world or his partner's subjective world (Examples: I am worried; I like you). Constativa are utterances that refer to the objective world (Examples: This is a yellow cloth; The world is round).

speech act classification with reference to Austin	analyzed variables
I. illocutionary act ☞ communicative force (intention) of the utterance	taxonomy of communicative forces via Habermas: regulativa, expressiva and constativa
II. locutionary act ☞ actual utterance 1. *phonetic act* ☞ articulation of a complex sound structure 2. *phatic act* ☞ use of a grammatical construction 3. *rhetic act* ☞ use of words in a certain meaning	consonants vs. vowels; phonetic transitions sentence length; word length; position in the word / sentence function words vs. content words; word class
III. perlocutionary act ☞ consequent effect of the utterance	illocutionary force of the parents' utterance preceding the stutter event

Figure 1. Speech act classification of psycholinguistic variables in stuttering

The *locutionary act* denotes the actual act of utterance; the traditional loci variables can be assigned easily to the locutionary act:
- the phonetic act is attributed to the phonetic factor: the examination asks whether the stutter occurs on or before a vowel or consonant; furthermore it is of interest whether there is a relationship with certain sound transitions;
- the syntactic factor, i.e., the length of sentences, the length of words and the position in the sentence and word can be attributed to the phatic act;
- the semantic factor can be attributed to the rhetic act.

The *perlocutionary act* denotes the consequent effect of the utterance, i.e., the effect of a certain speech act on the partner. For example, the realization or the failure of the speaker's intention. This research examined the effects of the speech act of the mother preceding the child's stuttering.

Reliability

The interrater reliability in the allocation to the categories of the evaluation system, as defined in the pilot studies (Rommel et al., 1996), is high (96 - 100 %) regarding psycholinguistic characteristics. Only the categorization of illocutions of the children's utterances proved to be difficult, showing an interrater agreement of 75 %.

Table 1. Influence of phonetic factor on dysfluencies

Variables	Stuttering (frequencies in %)		Fluent (frequencies in %)		T-score	p (df=93)
	M	SD	M	SD		
Vowel (ss)	53.2	18	40.2	3.2	- 6.9	.0001
Consonant (ss)	46.8	18	59.8	3.2	6.9	.0001
Vowel (sfs)	22.9	12	40.2	3.2	13.1	.0001
Consonant (sfs)	77.1	12	59.8	3.2	-13.1	.0001
V-C	49	17	31.2	2.3	-10.2	.0001
C-V	17	12	32.9	2.1	10.6	.0001
C-C	29	16	27	4.3	- 1.6	.11
V-V	5	6	9	2.8	4.6	.0001

ss = stuttered sound   sfs = sound following stuttering
V-C = Vowel-consonant-transition C-C = Consonant-Consonant-transition

RESULTS

Phonetic act

In our sample stuttering occurs significantly more often on vowels and before consonants, and significantly more often at vowel-consonant transitions. Significantly less stuttering occurs on vowel-vowel and consonant-vowel transitions. Consonant-consonant transitions are irrelevant (see table 1).

Phatic act

Table 2 shows that stuttered utterances are significantly longer than fluent passages. Regarding word length it can be said that dysfluencies are more likely to occur on longer words. The position effect, however, predicting that a stutter is more likely at the beginning of a word or sentence can not be confirmed. On the contrary we usually observe dysfluencies in the middle of a word or sentence.

Rhetic act

As shown in table 3 we find less stuttering on conjunctions, adverbs and adjectives compared to prepositions, interjections and pronouns. The content words 'nouns' and 'verbs' showed no effects. With respect to the comparison between 'content' and 'function words', no other effects were found.

Illocutionary and perlocutionary act

We observed more frequent stuttering on the children's constativa and regulativa and less stuttering on expressiva. The relevance of the illocutionary effect of the mother's utterances preceding the act of stuttering was not confirmed (see table 4).

Table 2. Influence of sentence lenght and word length on dysfluencies

Variables	Stuttering		Fluent		T-score	p
	M	SD	M	SD		
Sentence lenght (in words)	7	2	3.7	.98	-21.6	.0001
Word lenght (in letters)	4.1	.7	3.8	.21	-5	.0001

Table 3. Influence of 'word categories' on the dysluencies

Variables	Stuttering (frequencies in %)		Fluent (frequencies in %)		T-score	p (df=93)
	M	SD	M	SD		
Nouns	12.9	10.4	13.1	5.6	.2	.85
Adjectives	2.3	3.5	3.6	2.4	3.1	.002
Adverbs	22.8	12.8	28.6	5.4	4.3	.0001
Verbs	19.9	10.1	19.2	4.3	- .7	.5
Interjections	10.3	10.6	6.2	4.9	-3.5	.001
Content words	68.2	14.4	70.7	5.5	1.5	.13
Pronouns	21.2	12.2	17.1	5.2	-3.1	.003
Conjunctions	1.0	2.3	3.5	2.6	7.0	.0001
Prepositions	3.3	4.9	1.7	1.6	-3.4	.001
Articles	6.3	6.9	7.0	3.4	1.3	.21
Function words	31.8	14.5	29.3	5.5	-1.4	.17

Subgroups

Subgroup analyses, e.g., a division according to stuttering severity, linguistic, articulatory and oral-motor abilities, showed identical results in the fields of phonetic, syntactic, semantic and pragmatic requirements (loci-variables).

Summary

These results seem to indicate that linguistic demands, required by the daily use of language, have the same effect for all stuttering children; this is true regardless additional problems (e.g., retarded language development, or oral-motor deficits). This means that the dysfluencies of young stuttering children occur - regardless of other characteristics of the sample - predominantly at the following linguistic loci: in longer sentences, in longer words,

Table 4. Influence of the child's illocutions and the preceding speech act of the mother on the dysfluencies

Variables	Person	Stuttering (frequencies in %)		Fluent (frequencies in %)		T-score	p (df=93)
		M	SD	M	SD		
Regulativa	Mother	49.5	19.8	48.7	12.7	- .4	.7
	Child	32.4	16.4	29.2	8.9	- 2	.05
Constativa	Mother	16.2	14.2	16.5	8.1	.2	.8
	Child	35.1	18.8	26.8	12.3	-4.4	.0001
Expressiva	Mother	34.2	19.6	34.8	14	.41	.7
	Child	32.4	15.2	44	11.5	6.3	.0001

in the middle of sentences or words, on vowels at vowel-consonant transitions and predominantly in constativa and regulativa.

The 'information load' of words (content vs. function words) has no effect, nor does the illocution of parents' utterances preceding the stutter.

DISCUSSION

Phonetic act

Our results contradict results of studies that have been carried out exclusively with adults. We assume that the core of the problem of stuttering lies in the area of the vowels or the vowel-consonant transitions. This corresponds to the results of our pilot studies (Rommel et al., 1996). Wingate (1998, p. 156) points in his extensive linguistic analysis of stuttering at the same direction. He thinks that the true core of stuttering lies possibly in the vowels and not in the physiologically and oral-motorically more difficult consonants. Further hints for this assumption can be found in studies that examine the symptoms of stuttering with the help of a computer-aided acoustic analysis. Stromsta's results (1986, p.111 ff) can be looked upon as pioneering. According to his studies a disturbed transition (coarticulation) from a vowel to the following consonant points at a chronic stutter. Furthermore, there are indications that stuttering children have problems forming vowels in consonant- vowel-consonant combinations adequately (cf., Howell et al., 1991). Other confirmations can be derived from the studies by Throneburg et al. (1994) and Howell and Au-Yeung (1995). Phonetically difficult words have no 'trigger' effect for a stutter, the difficulty of a word being defined via the consonants.

Phatic act

Our results concerning the length of the sentences correspond with other results (for review see Bernstein Ratner, 1995). This means that our examined children are dysfluent in longer and linguistically more complex utterances. However, an interpretation is quite difficult because both, psychological, linguistic and physiological explanations could be used here (Rommel et al., 1996). Some, if not most of the stutter-relevant variables correspond with the sentence length in the sense that all linguistic, physiological, cognitive and emotional demands become bigger in longer and more complex sentences (Starkweather, 1987, 1991).

As to the *position effect*, however, we find results contrary to the present state of research. Our results from the phonetic field indicate that stuttering occurs predominantly in the middle of words. German as well as - according to Wingate (1988) - English words have mainly a consonant-vowel-consonant structure. Our results showing that a stutter occurs predominantly in the middle of utterances needs further explanation or discussion. The effect may have its origin in the language itself and related grammatical regularities. But a precise analysis of studies in this area makes us doubtful whether until now really stuttering or merely normal disfluent children have been examined. Repetitions of whole sentences and parts of sentences prevail in the category 'stutter symptoms' of the examined 5 children in Bloodstein and Grossman (1981). Bernstein (1981, p. 348) also points to the fact that her examined 'stuttering' children can hardly be distinguished from fluent children concerning the stutter symptoms. We therefore assume at present that dysfluencies are not tied to the beginning of sentences or words; they occur mostly in the middle of sentences or words.

Rhetic act

If we observe only the main categories 'content vs. function words', we find no effect in the semantic field. This means that occurring dysfluencies of young stuttering children must be looked upon as independent from the word's information load. Significant effects can merely be observed in some word classes, but these effects are very contradictory as regards the results of other study groups and our own pilot studies (Bloodstein & Gantwerk, 1967; Bloodstein & Grossman, 1981; Rommel et al., 1996). We assume at present that the semantic factor is irrelevant for young stuttering children, although we recognize the need for further research.

Illocutionary and perlocutionary act

Here our results show that even pragmatic aspects, which go beyond the traditional loci-variables, add to the onset of dysfluencies. To our knowledge, there are no other results reported in the literature to compare our data with, except for a single case study report by Pollack et al. (1986). Further research in this area is clearly needed. Due to the presently very unsatisfactory state of research we will refrain from further speculations at this point.

REFERENCES

Austin, J. (1962). *How to do things with words*. Oxford: Oxford University Press.
Bernstein, N. (1981). Are there constraints on childhood disfluency? *Journal of Fluency Disorders, 6*, 341-350.

Bernstein Ratner, N. (1995). Language complexity and stuttering in children. *Topics in Language Disorders, 15*, 32-47.

Bloodstein, O.(1995). *A handbook on stuttering*. London: Chapman & Hall.

Bloodstein, O., & Gantwerk, B.F. (1967). Grammatical function in relation to stuttering in young children. *Journal of Speech and Hearing Research, 10*, 786-789.

Bloodstein, O., & Grossman, M. (1981). Early stutterings: Some aspects of their form and distribution. *Journal of Speech and Hearing Research, 20*, 148-155.

Brown, S.F. (1945). The loci of stutterings in the speech sequence. *Journal of Speech Disorders, 10*, 181-192.

Habermas, J. (1982). *Theorie des kommunikativen Handelns. Bd. I: Handlungsrationalität und gesellschaftliche Rationalisierung*. Frankfurt: Suhrkamp.

Häge, A., Rommel, D., Johannsen, H.S., & Schulze, H. (this volume). Cognitive and linguistic abilities of stuttering children. In W. Hulstijn, H.F.M. Peters, & P.H.H.M. Van Lieshout (Eds.), *Speech production: motor control, brain research and fluency disorders*. Amsterdam: Elsevier Science.

Howell, P., Williams, M., & Young, K. (1991). Production of vowels by stuttering children and teenagers. In H. F. M. Peters, W. Hulstijn, & C. W. Starkweather (Eds.), *Speech motor control and stuttering* (pp. 409-414). Amsterdam: Elsevier.

Howell, P., & Au-Yeung, J. (1995). The association between stuttering, Brown's factors, and phonological categories in child stutterers ranging in age between 2 and 12 years. *Journal of Fluency Disorders, 20*, 331-344.

MacWhinney, B. (1995). *The CHILDES project. Tools for analyzing talk*. Hillsdale, New Jersey: Lawrence Erlbaum.

Pollack, J., Lubinski, R., & Weitzner-Lin, B. (1986). A pragmatic study of child dysfluency. *Journal of Fluency Disorders, 11*, 231-239.

Rommel, D. (1993). Psycholinguistische Aspekte des Stotterns. In H.S. Johannsen (DGPP), & L. Springer (DBL) (Hrsg.), *Stottern, Tagungsbericht, Münster 19.-22.5.1993* (S. 59-73). Ulm : Phoniatrische Ambulanz der Universität Ulm.,

Rommel, D. (1995). Psycholinguistic Aspects of Stuttering in Childhood. Cross-sectional results with 50 pre-school stuttering children. In C.W. Starkweather, & H.F.M. Peters (Eds.), *Stuttering: Proceedings of the first world congress on fluency disorders* (pp. 168-174). The International Fluency Association: Nijmegen University Press.

Rommel, D., Johannsen, H. S., Schulze, H., Moldaschel, S., & Müller, M. (1996). Psycholinguistische Merkmale des Sprechverhaltens stotternder Kinder unterschiedlicher Altersstufen in verschiedenen Sprechsituationen. *Sprache - Stimme - Gehör, 20*, 72-79.

Starkweather, C.W. (1987). *Fluency and stuttering*. Englewood Cliffs, NJ: Prentice-Hall.

Starkweather, C.W. (1991). The language-motor interface in children. In H.F.M. Peters, W. Hulstijn, & C.W. Starkweather (Eds.), *Speech Motor Control and Stuttering* (pp. 385-391). Amsterdam: Elsevier.

Stromsta, C. (1986). *Elements of stuttering*. Oshtemo: Atsmorts Publishing.

Throneburg, R. N., Yairi, E., & Paden, E. P. (1994). Relation between phonologic difficulty and the occurrence of disfluences in the early stage of stuttering. *Journal of Speech and Hearing Research, 37*, 504-509.

Wingate, M.E. (1988). *The structure of stuttering. A psycholinguistic analysis*. New York: Springer.

Speech Production: Motor Control, Brain Research and Fluency Disorders
W. Hulstijn, H.F.M. Peters and P.H.H.M. Van Lieshout, editors

Chapter 60

QUANTITATIVE ASSESSMENT OF DYSARTHRIA AND DEVELOPMENTAL APRAXIA OF SPEECH

Ben Maassen, Geert Thoonen, Inge Boers

For a particular child, a multiplicity of factors may underlie defective articulation. In order to assess the degree of involvement of neuromotor, phonological and developmental factors, procedures to obtain quantitative measures of motoric and phonemic involvement in dysarthria and developmenal apraxia of speech (DAS) are presented. The test procedures used were Maximum Performance Tasks (MPTs), and Word- and Nonword imitation tasks. The analysis techniques consisted of acoustic analyses, and broad phonetic transcription followed by automatic analyses of error types. The results showed, that dysarthria is mainly characterized by slowness and by a high proportion of distortions. DAS is characterized by a high error rate, sequencing problems, and many errors of place-of-articulation; there are striking qualitative correspondences with speech errors ('slips of the tongue') in the speech of normally speaking children. Comparison of these disorders suggests that children with defective articulatory development show individual degrees of dysarthric and dyspraxic involvement.

INTRODUCTION

The present paper is the result of a series of studies that started one conference ago; aim and methods, and preliminary results were then presented (Maassen et al., 1991). The studies were motivated by the lack of an articulation test that yields a differential diagnosis of speech disorders in children. Although tests are available to assess aspects of articulation and speech motor capacities in children, to date, no tests exist that yield quantitative measures for "dysarthria", "apraxia of speech" or speech delay. In current clinical practice the speech pathologist not only must rely on evaluations of articulo-motoric aspects by means of perceptual judgements, but also must interpret scores and judgements on diverse aspects of speech to come up with a differential diagnosis.

Motivated by this state of affairs two research goals were formulated: (1) To quantify and objectify the assessment of aspects of speech that can be considered relevant symptoms for the diagnosis of articulation disorders; and (2) To obtain *speech profiles* which allow for a differential diagnosis, that is speech profiles that can be classified as being primarily related to *Developmental Apraxia of Speech* (DAS), to *(Spastic) Dysarthria (SDys)*, or to the broader category *Speech-Language Delay* (SLD).

When starting this series of studies, the first issue that came across, was that it is hard to find children with 'pure' DAS, 'pure' SDys or 'pure' SLD. Instead, for most children the underlying deficit is not so much an all-or-none matter but a matter of degree of involvement. So the second aim of the study should be read as to obtain a speech profile which gives quantitative measures of apraxic, dysarthric and/or phonological involvement (see also Dodd, 1995; Shriberg, 1994).

METHODS

Two studies are presented. In the first study performances of carefully selected children with DAS and SDys were compared with those of normally speaking children. In the second study the tasks that contributed most to diagnostic differentiation in the first study were administered to larger groups of subjects, as well as a group of children with SLD.

Subjects

For the selection of children with DAS and SDys, the following criteria were employed. The criteria for DAS were derived from Hall et al. (1993), and previously used in Thoonen et al. (1994). The most important criteria for DAS were: persistent speech difficulty and unintelligibility; deviant rather than immature articulation; quality of articulation strongly dependent on length of utterance; seemingly inconsistent error patterns; and groping. The criteria for SDys were derived from Darley et al. (1975), and previously used in Wit et al. (1993). The most important criteria for SDys were: quadriplegia due to cerebral palsy; slow speech rate; imprecise consonant production; hypernasality; and low and monotonous pitch.

Particularly in Study 2 it became obvious that DAS is a rare disorder in isolation. Sixty-four children were referred by speech pathologists with the diagnosis DAS. By means of anamnestic information (questionnaire filled out by teacher and parents) and a pre-test (articulation test plus MRR and word- and pseudo-word repetition) evaluated by independent judges, 28 of these children were assessed as DAS. These children were administered an articulation test, a language comprehension test, and a neuropsychological examination. It turned out that 7 children showed a delay of more than 1 standard deviation in language comprehension or intelligence, 1 child showed hearing loss, 1 child showed fluency problems, and 1 child rather severe concentration problems, such that of the originally referred 64 children, 18 could be classified as pure DAS.

This is not to say that the remaining children were not dyspraxic; however, they did not pass the criteria that are commonly used to make the clinical diagnosis DAS.

Tasks and Materials

Children were requested to produce words and nonwords. The words were first elicited by means of picture-naming, immediately followed by imitation (experimenter

Table 1. Characteristics of children participating in each of the three studies.

Diagnosis:	Study 1		Study 2	
	n	age	n	age
DAS	11	6;3- 7;9	18	4;11-6;10
			10#	similar
SDys	9	6;4-10;3		
SLD			23	4;6- 7;0
NS	11	6;0- 8;3	29	4;9- 6;10

Notes: DAS: Dev. apraxia of speech; SDys: (Spastic) dysarthria, due to cerebral palsy; SLD: Speech-language delay; NS: Normally speaking; n: number of children; age: age range, expressed in years;months; # Children in this group were diagnosed and referred as DAS, but obtained low language comprehension or intelligence scores.

speaks the word - child imitates). Only the imitations were analyzed because the spontaneous picture naming procedure gave too many responses with a different word than intended. Nonwords were also elicited by imitation. The use of an imitation task is motivated by the requirement of standardization; the ultimate aim is to come up with an articulation test.

For the *maximum performance tasks* (MPTs) children were requested to imitate the mono-syllabic sequences "papa..", "tata..", and "kaka.." and the multi-syllabic sequence "patakapataka..". After instruction and practice trials, at least 3 attempts were elicited. Because some children had difficulty with the task (particularly the multi-syllabic sequence) the number of extra trials was an additional assessment parameter (Thoonen et al., 1996). Also, the task maximum sound prolongation was administered (sustain the sounds /a/, /s/, and /z/ for as long as possible). Results are reported elsewhere (Thoonen et al., 1996). MPTs are generally considered to yield valid data for dysarthria or more generally motor speech involvement (Netsell, 1982).

Analysis procedure

The word and nonword imitations were broadly phonetically transcribed, followed by a quantitative analysis by means of the LIPP-program (Oller, 1991). The advantage of transcription analysis with LIPP is that once data have been typed in, frequency counts can be easily obtained, features can be isolated, and also analyses related to context (anticipations, perseverations, transpositions) can be performed.

The utterances from the MPTs were analyzed with help of Kay-CSL. Onsets of all syllables were marked by interactive inspection of the acoustic signal and a semi-automatic procedure that calculated from these marks syllable durations, standard deviations and also the scanning index. The scanning index is an index of regularity between 0.0 and 1.0, which is independent of the unit of measurement, and which is defined as the product of all syllable durations divided by the mean syllable duration to-the-power-of the number of syllables (Kent et al., 1994). The formula to calculate the scanning index is: *(S1 * S2 * ... * Sn) / (mean S) ** n*. In this formula *S1, S2 ... Sn* represent the syllable durations of the utterance; *n* represents the number of syllables in the utterance; *mean S* the mean syllable duration; and ** represents to-the-power-of.

RESULTS

Word and Nonword Imitation

In Table 2 main error types are compared for children with SDys and DAS, and normally speaking (NS) children (Study 1). Children with DAS produce the highest error frequencies, followed by children with SDys and NS. SDys children produce the highest proportions of distortions after correction for error rate. In Table 3 consonant substitutions are divided into substitutions by place-of-articulation, manner-of-articulation and voicing. Children with SDys produce relatively many voicing errors; DAS children relatively many place substitutions.

Because the diagnosis DAS is particularly controversial, the next step in the analysis comprised a search for 'typical' apraxic symptoms, that are often reported in literature. First, an in-depth comparison was made between the DAS and NS children of Study 1. Percentages retention were calculated by dividing the number of substitutions that are correct with respect to a particular feature or feature-value (but incorrect with respect to another feature or feature-value) by the total number substitutions (Thoonen et al., 1994).

Table 2. Main error types produced by children with SDys and DAS as compared to normally speaking children, expressed in percentages relative to the number of consonants in the material (**Study 1**); for each error type between brackets its proportion (relative to the sum of error types) is given.

Error Type	NS	SDys	DAS
Substitutions	11.8 (.67)	29.1 (.48)	57.2 (.58)
Omissions	3.8 (.21)	13.6 (.22)	24.3 (.24)
Distortions	2.2 (.12)	17.9 (.30)	18.2 (.18)

Table 3. Substitutions by feature: place-of-articulation, manner-of-articulation and voicing, as percentages of the total number of consonant substitutions (*Study 1*)

Feature	SDys	DAS
place	33 %	58 %
manner	27 %	43 %
voicing	60 %	41 %
TOTAL	120 %	132 %

Table 4. Confusion matrices of place-of-articulation substitutions in Study 1 (*Table 4a*) and Study 2 (*Table 4b*).

Table 4a

Group: DAS (Study 1)

	labial	alveolar	dorsal	retention	mean retention
labial	**82**	31	16	64 %	
alveolar	36	**116**	40	60 %	54 %
dorsal	17	32	**6**	11 %	

Group: NS (Study 1)

	labial	alveolar	dorsal	retention	mean retention
labial	**43**	13	3	73 %	
alveolar	6	**28**	8	67 %	59 %
dorsal	2	8	**1**	9 %	

Table 4b

Group: DAS (Study 2)

	labial	alveolar	dorsal	retention	mean retention
labial	**113**	62	38	53 %	
alveolar	104	**91**	55	36 %	38 %
dorsal	37	72	**22**	16 %	

Group: SLD (Study 2)

	labial	alveolar	dorsal	retention	mean retention
labial	**118**	26	19	72 %	
alveolar	32	**75**	52	47 %	57 %
dorsal	10	19	**18**	38 %	

Note: The Tables present confusion matrices of place-of-articulation substitutions. Only substitutions are presented, which are either correct (labial-labial, etc. on the diagonal) or incorrect (off-diagonal) with respect to place-of-articulation. For each particular place, dividing the correct cell by the number of targets yields a percentage of retention of that place.

The DAS and NS children, presented in Table 4a, show striking similarities with respect to the feature place-of-articulation, as well as the distinct feature-values (labial, alveolar, dorsal). The slightly lower percentage place-retention of the DAS children as compared to the NS children, might turn out a genuine effect, however, because a similar but larger difference was found between the SLD children and the DAS children of Study 2, presented in Table 4b. (Differences in percentages can be the result of differences in speech material.) The similarities across subject groups for manner-of-articulation (feature values: plosive, fricative, nasal, semivowel), and voicing (voice, voiceless) were even more striking in both studies.

The substitutions of Study 1 were also analyzed with respect to context. It turned out that de percentage of syntagmatic (as compared to paradigmatic) substitutions was similar -not significantly different- for DAS (64%) and NS children (59%).

Finally, similar distributions of substitutions and omissions over syllable-initial and syllable-final position were found across the DAS, SLD and NS children of Study 2. The results are presented in Figure 1. All 3 groups produce more substitutions in syllable-initial position, and more omissions in syllable-final position.

Conclusions Imitation Task

In this extensive comparison of error profiles of DAS, SLD, SDys and NS children, we first found large *quantitative* differences between groups: DAS children producing the highest error frequencies, followed by SLD and SDys, and NS children. SDys children can be distinguished on the basis of the high proportion of distortions. There is a tendency for DAS children to produce a relatively high number of place-of-articulation errors. The remaining comparisons, particularly with respect to context, syllable position and feature value, revealed striking similarities between groups.

Maximum Performance Tasks (MPT)

In Figure 2 maximum repetition rates of DAS, SDys and NS children are presented (Study 1).

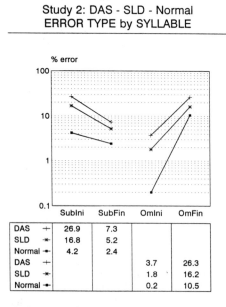

Figure 1. Percentages of substitutions and omissions in syllable-initial (SubIni resp. OmIni) and syllable-final (SubFin resp. OmFin) position for each of the 3 groups of children in Study 2; profiles are similar.

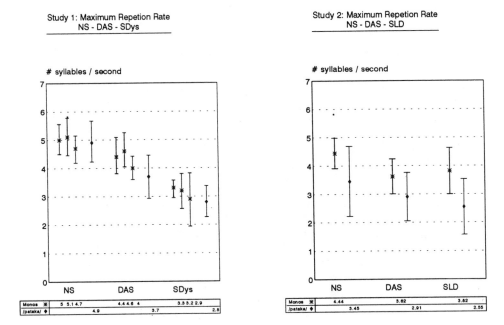

Figure 2. Maximum repetition rates of normally speaking (NS), developmental dyspraxic (DAS), spastic dysarthric (SDys) and speech-language delayed (SLD) children: Mean number of syllables per second for the mono-syllabic and multi-syllabic ("pataka..") sequences. (For Study 1 "papa.., tata.., kaka.." are presented separately; for Study 2 means of monosyllabic sequences are presented.)

Children with SDys produce overall the slowest repetition rates. DAS children are similar to NS children with respect to the mono-syllabic sequences, but have difficulty producing the multi-syllabic sequence (4 out of 11 children failed) and, if they are able to produce these, they produce them slower. In Study 2, with younger age groups, all children produce the multi-syllabic sequences slower than the mono-syllabic. The differentiation between pathological groups and control group can be based on overall syllable repetition rate (DAS and SLD are slower than NS) and the relative numbers of children that are able to produce the multi-syllabic sequences (NS: 22 out of 25 ; DAS: 9 / 25 ; SLD: 11 / 23).

Subgroups of SLD
    The similarities in relative error frequencies and repetition rates between DAS and SLD children suggest similarities in underlying deficit. Perhaps some SLD children also have speech problems which are of a dyspraxic nature. In an attempt to answer this question, the SLD children were divided into 2 groups: (1) SLD children who could produce "pataka.." 5 times in succession (SLD+ children: n=11); and (2) SLD children who could not produce "pataka.." 5 times in succession (SLD- children: n=12).

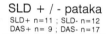

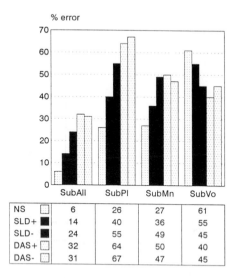

Figure 3. Comparison of error percentages for SLD and DAS children, both groups divided into those able to produce "pataka.." (SLD+ and DAS+) and those not able to produce "pataka.." (SLD- and DAS-). The error profile of SLD- children is more similar to that of DAS children than the SLD+ profile; much smaller differences are observed for both DAS groups. Normally speaking (NS) children are shown as reference. *Note. SubAll: Overall percentage substitutions (relative to number of consonants); SubPl, SubMn, SubVo: Percentage substitutions by place-of-articulation, manner-of-articulation and voicing (relative to number of substitutions).*

Results, which are presented in Figure 3, show that error percentages for the SLD-children, those who were not able to produce "pataka..", are much more similar to the DAS profile than the errors percentages produced by the SLD+ group.

From these results it can provisionally be concluded that among the SLD children about 50% shows clear dyspraxic characteristics.

SUMMARY AND CONCLUSION

To summarize the results, it was found that children with spastic dysarthria (SDys) produce slower speech, with relatively many distortions and voicing errors. Children with developmental apraxia of speech (DAS) have difficulty producing alternating sequences of syllables, and produce the highest error rates with relatively many errors of place-of-articulation. A striking result was the similarities in error profile between DAS and normally speaking (NS) children. Performance of children with speech-language delay

(SLD) were in between those of the NS and DAS groups. The division of SLD children in 2 groups on the basis of their multi-syllabic maximum repetition rate performance, showed that those SLD children who are not able to produce rapid sequences of "pataka.." produce similar error profiles as the DAS children.

In clinical practice, most children with articulation disorders show a mixture of problems. Assessing the degree of involvement of dysarthria, apraxia or just delay yields guidelines for an individualized, goal-directed speech therapy program.

REFERENCES

Darley, F.L., Aronson, A.E., & Brown, J.R. (1975). *Motor speech disorders.* Philadelphia/London/Toronto: W.B. Saunders.

Dodd, B. (1995). *Differential diagnosis & treatment of children with speech disorders.* London: Whurr Publishers.

Hall, P.K., Jordan, L.S., & Robin, D.A. (1993). *Developmental Apraxia of Speech.* Austin, TX: Pro-ed.

Kent, R.D., Kent, J.F., Weismer, G., & Rosenbek, J.C. (1994). Evidence of speech timing errors in cerebellar disease. *ASHA Convention program* (p. 59), oct.1994.

Maassen, B., Thoonen, G., & Wit, J. (1991). Toward assessment of articulo-motoric processing capacities in children. In H.F.M. Peters, W. Hulstijn, & C.W. Starkweather (Eds.), *Speech Motor Control and Stuttering* (pp. 461-469). Amsterdam: Excerpta Medica.

Netsell, R. (1982). Speech Motor Control and Selected Neurologic Disorders. In S. Grillner et al. (Eds.) *Speech Motor Control* (pp. 247-261). Pergamon Press.

Oller, D. Kimbrough (1991). *Logical International Phonetics Program V 1.40 (LIPP).* Miami, FL: Intelligent Hearing Systems.

Shriberg, L.D. (1994). Five subtypes of developmental phonological disorders. *Clinical Communication Disorders, 4(1)*, 38-52.

Thoonen, G., Maassen, B., Gabreëls, F., & Schreuder, R. (1994). Feature analysis of singleton consonant errors in developmental verbal dyspraxia (DVD). *Journal of Speech and Hearing Research, 37*, 1424-1440.

Thoonen, G., Maassen, B., Wit, J., Gabreëls, F., & Schreuder, R. (1996). The integrated use of maximum performance tasks in differential diagnostic evaluations among children with motor speech disorders. *Clinical Linguistics & Phonetics, 10*, 311-336.

Thoonen, G., Maassen, B., Wit, J., Gabreëls, F., Schreuder, R., & de Swart, B. (1996). Developmental verbal dyspraxia: Criteria for subject selection and quantitative assessment of speech. *European Journal of Communication Disorders*, in press.

Wit, J., Maassen, B., Gabreëls, G., & Thoonen, G. (1993). Maximum Performance Tests in Children With Developmental Spastic Dysarthria. *Journal of Speech and Hearing Research, 36*, 452-460.

Wit, J., Maassen, B., Gabreëls, F., Thoonen, G., & de Swart, B. (1994). Traumatic versus perinatally acquired dysarthria: Assessment by means of speech-like maximum performance tasks. *Developmental Medicine and Child Neurology, 36*, 221-229.

Speech Production: Motor Control, Brain Research and Fluency Disorders
W. Hulstijn, H.F.M. Peters and P.H.H.M. Van Lieshout, editors

Chapter 61

CLINICAL APPLICATION OF SPEECH SCIENCE INSTRUMENTATION IN THE DETERMINATION OF TREATMENT PRIORITIES IN ACQUIRED AND CONGENITAL CHILDHOOD DYSARTHRIA

Bruce E. Murdoch, Susan K. Horton, Deborah G. Theodoros, Elizabeth C. Thompson

Comprehensive studies of the physiological functioning of the speech production apparatus in children with either acquired or congenital dysarthria have not been previously reported. In this paper, profiles of the functioning of the major components of the speech production mechanisms of 3 children with acquired dysarthria of varying etiologies (including closed head injury, cerebrovascular accident and intracerebral tumour) and 1 child with congenital dysarthria associated with Moebius syndrome are presented. Each subject was administered a battery of physiological assessments which included: spirometric and kinematic assessments of respiratory function; aerodynamic and electroglottographic evaluations of laryngeal function; pressure and strain gauge transducer evaluations of articulatory function; and nasal accelerometric assessments of nasality. In addition, perceptual profiles of each subject were compiled using perceptual ratings of deviant speech parameters, intelligibility ratings from the Assessment of Intelligibility of Dysarthric Speech and perceptual judgements of subsystem function determined from the Frenchay Dysarthria Assessment. The clinical implications of the findings of the physiological and perceptual analyses are discussed with regard to determination of specific treatment priorities for each of the 4 cases. It was therefore concluded that physiological instrumentation has the potential to play an important role in the clinical assessment and treatment of dysarthria in children.

INTRODUCTION

Instrumental investigations of the functioning of the speech production mechanism in children with dysarthria subsequent to acquired or congenital damage to the central nervous system have been rarely reported (Bak et al., 1983; Murdoch & Hudson-Tennent, 1993, 1994; van Dongen et al., 1994). It is now widely recognised that a knowledge of the underlying pathophysiology of the speech production mechanism is necessary for the development of optimal treatments for motor speech disorders (Abbs & dePaul, 1989). To date, however, no study has reported the findings of a comprehensive physiological analysis of the functioning of the major components of the speech production apparatus of a child with acquired or congenital dysarthria.

The purpose of the present study, therefore, was to develop a comprehensive perceptual and physiological profile of the functioning of the major motor subsystems of the speech mechanisms (i.e. respiratory, laryngeal, velopharyngeal and articulatory subsystems) of 4 children with dysarthria of varying etiologies with a view to demonstrating the potential importance of speech science instrumentation in defining treatment priorities for children with dysarthria.

METHODOLOGY

Subjects

The 4 subjects included 1 child with acquired dysarthria subsequent to severe closed head injury (Subject 1), one child with acquired dysarthria following a basilar artery cerebrovascular accident (Subject 2), one child with acquired dysarthria subsequent to treatment for a posterior cranial fossa tumour (Subject 3), and one child with congenital dysarthria associated with Moebius syndrome (Subject 4).

Procedure for Perceptual Assessment

A perceptual profile of each subject's speech was compiled through administration of 3 different perceptual assessments. These included: The Assessment of Intelligibility of Dysarthric Speech (ASSIDS) (Yorkston & Beukelman, 1981), which provides an index of severity of dysarthric speech by quantifying both single-word and sentence intelligibility as well as the speaking rate of dysarthric speakers; the Frenchay Dysarthria Assessment (Enderby, 1983), which provides a standardised assessment of speech neuromuscular activity; and a perceptual analysis of a speech sample (FitzGerald et al., 1987) based on a rating scale involving 32 deviant speech dimensions encompassing prosody, respiration, phonation, resonance and articulation.

Procedure for Physiological Assessment

The respiratory, laryngeal, velopharyngeal and articulatory function of each of the 4 subjects was assessed instrumentally using a battery of physiological techniques. For the purpose of establishing whether or not the scores achieved by each subject on the various physiological tests were within normal limits, their data were compared to values achieved by non-neurologically impaired control subjects matched for age and sex. Respiratory function was assessed, using both spirometric and kinematic techniques, as described by Murdoch and Hudson-Tennent (1993) and included such measures as vital capacity, forced expiratory volume per second, percentage of relative contribution of the rib cage, lung volume initiation and termination levels during production of a range of speech tasks, mean syllables per breath, speaking rate and the incidence of slope changes and paradoxical chest wall movements. One other important indicator of respiratory function for speech, namely subglottal pressure, was estimated using an Aerophone II (Kay Elemetrics) airflow measurement system consistent with the methods used by Theodoros and Murdoch (1994).

Vocal fold vibration and laryngeal aerodynamics were assessed in each subject using electroglottography (Kay Elemetrics laryngograph with waveform display system - Model 6091) and an airflow measurement system (Aerophone II - Kay Elemetrics Model 6800) respectively. The parameters measured in these assessments included fundamental frequency (Fo), duty cycle, closing time, ab/adduction rate, sound pressure level, glottal resistance and phonatory flow rate. Velopharyngeal function was assessed using the acclerometric technique described by Theodoros et al. (1993) which provides a nasality index (the Horii Oral Nasal Coupling Index). In addition, velopharyngeal function was also assessed using the Nasometer (Kay Elemetrics Model 6200-2) yielding a 'nasalance' score comprised of a ratio of nasal to oral plus nasal acoustic energy calculated as a percentage. The assessment of articulatory function involved measurement of lip and tongue strength, endurance and rate of repetitive movements using strain-gauge and pressure transduction systems. The transducer used for assessing tongue function was identical to the rubber-bulb pressure transducer described by Murdoch et al. (1995). A miniaturised pressure transducer based on semi-conductor strain-gauge technology similar to that described by Hinton and Luschei (1992) was used to estimate lip strength and endurance. In addition, changes in the dimensions of the lips during performance of speech and non-speech tasks were monitored by a quantifiable video assessment procedure.

CASE REPORTS

A summary of the deviant perceptual features and physiological profile of each of the 4 subjects is shown in Figure 1.

Subject 1
Subject 1 was a 14-year-old, right-handed male who sustained a severe closed head injury (Glasgow Coma Score=5) when hit by a motor vehicle. A computed tomographic scan performed on the day of admission revealed a large soft tissue haematoma present over the right temporal region and left zygomatic region of his left cerebral hemisphere. A small, high attenuation area was also identified in the left lentiform nucleus. Further small, high attenuation foci were scattered over the peripheral grey/white region anteriorly and superiorly. No significant mass effect was noted. Subject 1 was mute for 2-5 months post-injury. Although from that time speech did begin to return, Subject 1 remained moderately dysarthric until referred to the Motor Speech Research Unit at 8 months post-injury.

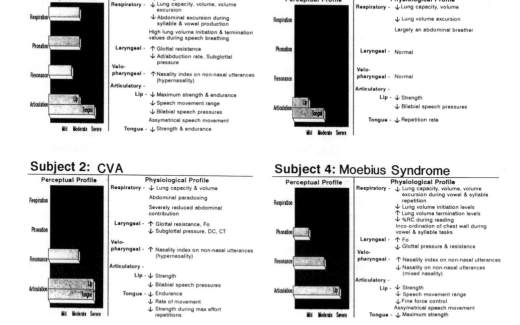

Figure 1. Perceptual and physiological profiles of the four children with dysarthria.
Mild = mild level of impairment; Moderate = moderate level of impairment; Severe = severe level of impairment.

↑ = increased compared to age and sex matched controls
↓ = decreased compared to age and sex matched controle

Perceptual analysis of speech

The perceptual analyses revealed the presence of deficits in all five aspects of the speech production process (prosody, respiration, articulation, resonance and phonation). In particular, the perceptual analyses revealed a profile of speech impairments which included: A severe degree of tongue dysfunction; a moderate level of impairment in the areas of lip function, respiratory support for speech and phonation; and a mild-moderate degree of hypernasality.

Physiological analysis of speech

The instrumental assessment confirmed the presence of a number of deficiencies in Subject 1's respiratory function that could have contributed to the reduction in his respiratory support for speech evidenced by the perceptual analyses. These included reduced lung volumes and capacities, reduced abdominal excursions during vowel and syllable production and high lung volume initiation and termination levels during speech production. Assessment of laryngeal function using electroglottography and aerodynamic examination identified the presence of a number of features suggestive of laryngeal hyperfunction. These features included increased glottal resistance and decreased ad/abduction rate suggestive of laryngeal spasticity. The findings of the aerodynamic assessment using the Aerophone II also indicated the presence of decreased subglottal pressure. This reduction in subglottal pressure could have been the outcome of two independent factors. Firstly, it could have resulted from the observed reduction in respiratory support for speech. Secondly, and more likely, however, the noted reduction in subglottal pressure may be an artifact of the instrumental procedure used in its estimation. The Aerophone II estimates subglottal pressure indirectly on the basis of a recording of oral pressure during production of the voiceless stop /p/. In those subjects where there is a leakage of air from the oral cavity due to either an inadequate bilabial seal or due to velopharyngeal incompetence, estimation of subglottal pressure using this technique will lead to an underestimation of subglottal pressure. As Subject 1 demonstrated both inadequate lip closure for bilabial consonants and velopharyngeal incompetence, such underestimation of subglottal pressure may well have occurred here.

The findings of both the nasal accelerometry technique and the nasometer confirmed the presence of hypernasality, most likely as a consequence of velopharyngeal incompetence. Likewise the pressure and strain-gauge transducer systems confirmed problems in both lip and tongue function. Specifically, the musculature of both the lips and tongue was impaired with respect to strength and endurance with the tongue being severely affected and the lips moderately affected. Further, the video lip movement analysis revealed that lip movement was reduced, especially during performance of speech tasks and that Subject 1 exhibited asymmetric lip movement, the right side of his lips being weaker than the left.

Overall the findings of the physiological assessments confirmed the presence of impairments at all levels of the speech production apparatus in Subject 1, but went further than the perceptual analysis in defining the physiological nature of the impairments in each of the speech motor subsystems, thereby providing more accurate directions for treatment.

Treatment priorities

On the basis of the perceptual and physiological assessments, the major features contributing to the dysarthria exhibited by Subject 1 included severely reduced tongue function and moderately reduced lip, velopharyngeal and laryngeal function and a mild-moderately reduced respiratory function. His speech was moderately unintelligible with decreased rate of speech, reduced variability of pitch and imprecision of consonants. The single greatest contributor to Subject 1's unintelligibility appeared to be the dysfunction in the articulatory system, especially the impaired tongue function. The recommended treatment priorities for Subject 1 would include: Firstly, simultaneous treatment of tongue and lip function aimed at increasing tongue and lip strength and endurance, and increasing the range of movement of the lips. This should be followed by treatment for the laryngeal dysfunction, with therapy specifically aimed at reducing glottal resistance and improving the ad/abduction rate. Treatment should then focus on reducing velopharyngeal incompetence and improve the respiratory support for speech by targeting improvement in the excursion of the abdominal muscles and increasing various lung volumes and capacities.

Subject 2

Subject 2, a 9-year-old, right-handed male, suffered a brainstem infarct following basilar artery occlusion secondary to arteritis when he was 5 years old. An MRI scan performed 10 days post-CVA revealed the presence of multiple infarcts in the cerebellum with no mass effects. Infarcts were also identified in the thalami and in the deep white matter medial to the posterior horn of the left lateral ventricle. Later scans showed the infarcts to be persistent and also indicated the presence of global cerebellar atrophy. Subject 2 was mute for 2 months post-CVA and remained moderately to severely dysarthric when referred to our research clinic approximately 4 years later on.

Perceptual analysis of speech

Tongue function was the most deviant dimension identified by the perceptual analysis, with severe impairment of the elevation and moderate impairment of the lateral movements of the tongue being observed. Loudness, lip seal and palatal function during maintenance tasks were severely impaired. Hypernasality was obvious during speech to a moderate level. Perceptually respiration appeared adequate for speech and phonatory function was within normal limits.

Physiological analysis of speech

In contrast to the findings of the perceptual assessment, the physiological assessments of respiration showed that Subject 2 had an abnormal speech breathing pattern. Expiration during production of various speech tasks was produced with virtually no contribution from the diaphragm/abdomen, his breathing resulting almost 100% from ribcage activity. On all tasks, Subject 2 displayed a significant component of abdominal paradoxing indicating that during expiration his abdominal circumference actually expanded to a degree rather than decreased and was indicative of flaccid paralysis of the abdominal wall. To compensate for the lack of abdominal contribution, Subject 2 utilised the secondary muscles of respiration (e.g. the scalenus muscles, sternocleidomastoid etc) to raise the ribcage during deep inspirations.

Also in contrast to the findings of the perceptual evaluations, the instrumental assessments revealed the presence of features indicative of laryngeal hyperfunction, including elevated Fo, increased glottal resistance and reduced duty cycle. Estimated subglottal pressures were also low, but as in Subject 1, the low values recorded may have been associated with reduced oral pressure caused by velopharyngeal incompetence and impaired lip function. Both the nasal accelerometric technique and the nasometer confirmed the presence of velopharyngeal incompetence. Likewise the various pressure and strain-gauge transducers confirmed the perceived articulatory deficits. Although the instruments identified that Subject 2 had good tongue strength on maximum tongue strength tasks, his tongue muscles showed reduced endurance. In addition, tasks requiring repetitive tongue movements were performed slowly and with reduced pressure. Lip pressures recorded during production of bilabial consonants as well as on tasks requiring maximum lip strength were reduced.

Treatment priorities

It is suggested that the first targets for treatment of the speech disorder exhibited by Subject 2 should be his impaired speech breathing, reduced lip strength and velopharyngeal incompetence. According to Rosenbek and LaPointe (1985), impaired speech breathing often requires remediation prior to other areas being targeted. Hayden and Square (1994) also place the correction of breathing patterns and the achievement of adequate breath support for sequenced speech early on their motor speech treatment hierarchy. Subsequent to treatment of the above-listed areas, treatment should then focus on improvement of tongue muscle endurance and eventually to reduction of laryngeal hyperfunction.

Subject 3

Subject 3 was an 8-year-old, right-handed female who had a large cerebellar astrocytoma surgically removed when aged 6 years. During the operation, the left cerebellar hemisphere was completely removed along with a large portion of the right cerebellar hemisphere. Neither radiotherapy nor chemotherapy were administered as part of the treatment regimen. Subject 3 was mildly dysarthric when referred to the Motor Speech Research Unit approximately 2 years post-surgery.

Perceptual analysis of speech

The perceptual assessments indicated that Subject 3 had a mild dysarthria, characterised primarily by a slow rate of speech and an equal and even stress pattern. Some impairment in articulation was noted, with lip function being mildly affected and tongue function moderately impaired. There was no evidence of impairments in the processes of respiration, phonation or velopharyngeal function and intelligibility was only mildly affected.

Physiological analysis of speech

Although not evidenced by the perceptual evaluations, instrumental analysis revealed that Subject 3 had below normal lung volumes and capacities. In addition she was primarily an abdominal breather and demonstrated an overall reduction in chest wall excursion during performance of a range of different speech tasks. Instrumental investigation of laryngeal and velopharyngeal function confirmed that these subsystems were performing within normal limits. As suggested by the perceptual assessments, some evidence of articulatory dysfunction was detected by the strain-gauge and pressure transducers. Maximum lip pressure on non-speech tasks was reduced as was the lip pressures achieved by Subject 3 when producing bilabial consonants. However, this did not lead to noticeable distortion of bilabial consonants. Tongue pressure and endurance levels were within normal limits although repetitive tongue movements were slow. It is suggested that in the latter task, Subject 3 reduced the number of repetitions to preserve strength and accuracy of the tongue movements.

Treatment priorities

Subject 3 presented with a mild dysarthria characterised primarily by prosodic disorders, in particular a slow rate of speech and poor intonation. The physiological assessments also revealed some respiratory and articulatory problems which may well contribute to the prosodic disorders. For instance, it is possible that Subject 3 may have reduced her rate of speech in order to conserve expiratory output and to ensure accuracy and strength of articulatory movements. Owing to the nature of the subsystem impairments observed and their possible inter-relatedness with the prosodic disturbances, it is recommended that the treatment framework be more concurrent than hierarchical in this case. Therefore treatment should concurrently focus on the following: Treatment of the prosodic aspects of the speech disturbance aimed at increasing speech rate and improving intonation; treatment of respiratory dysfunction aimed at increasing the excursion of the chest wall during speech breathing; and treatment of the articulatory disorder.

Subject 4

Subject 4 was a right-handed female, who presented with congenital hypoplasia of the muscles supplied by the facial (VII) and glossopharyngeal (IX) cranial nerves consistent with Moebius syndrome. Neurological examination soon after birth revealed an absence of facial expression, ptotic eyelids, no discernible palatal movement and head lag. Subject 4 was mildly dysarthric when referred to the Motor Speech Research Unit at age 12 years.

Perceptual analysis of speech

The perceptual analyses revealed a moderate reduction in intelligibility with deficits in the articulatory, resonatory and phonatory aspects of the speech production process. The most frequently occurring deviant speech dimensions related to disturbances of articulation and resonance, as would be expected given the neuropathological basis of Moebius syndrome.

Physiological analysis of speech

Although not detected by the perceptual evaluations, instrumental analysis revealed the presence of a number of problems with the speech breathing abilities of Subject 4. These included depressed lung volumes and capacities, inco-ordination of the chest wall, elevated lung volume termination levels and depressed lung volume initiation levels during performance of various speech tasks, and depressed ribcage contribution to breathing when reading. While the perceptual analysis indicated that Subject 4 demonstrated mild, intermittent breathiness and difficulty maintaining phonation for an extended period of time, the instrumental assessments of laryngeal function further identified decreased sound pressure levels, reduced glottal resistance and subglottal pressure and a reduction in vocal fold closing time. As indicated for Subject 1, however, the value for sublottal pressure may have been an underestimation due to concomitant problems with bilabial seal and velopharyngeal incompetence. Both the nasal accelerometric method and the nasometer confirmed the presence of velopharyngeal incompetence, Subject 4 demonstrating hyponasality when producing nasal sounds and hypernasality when producing non-nasal sounds indicative of mixed nasality due to improper functioning of the velopharyngeal valve.

The tongue transducer analysis demonstrated reduced lingual strength on all tasks. Subject 4 did, however, exhibit normal ability to maintain and repeat maximal contractions of the tongue muscles on sustained pressure and repetition tasks. It is suggested that rather than her reduced performance on maximum tongue strength tasks being associated with weakness in the tongue muscles, her reduced pressures were the result of the presence of a high arched palate which may have reduced Subject 4's ability to compress the tongue bulb transducer. As expected, Subject 4 demonstrated reduced lip pressure, an inconsistent ability to maintain lip pressure and poor fine motor control of the lips. In addition, Subject 4 also showed impairment in the range of movement of the upper and lower lips laterally and vertically.

Treatment priorities

It is evident that Subject 4 demonstrated impairments in all 4 major subsystems of the speech production apparatus. Undoubtedly, however, those subsystems having the greatest influence on her associated dysarthria were the articulatory and velopharyngeal valves. The recommended treatment should focus on improving articulation, especially with reference to improving the strength and fine motor control of the lips; treatment of velopharyngeal dysfunction aimed at improving valving at the velopharyngeal port; and finally treatment aimed at improving laryngeal and respiratory dysfunction.

CONCLUSIONS

The results demonstrated that speech science instrumentation has the potential to play an important role in the clinical assessment and treatment of both acquired and congenital dysarthria in children. In particular, in the 4 cases presented, the physiological instruments were able to identify dysfunction at various levels of the speech production mechanism not evidenced by the perceptual assessments. Further, the physiological instruments were better able to identify the nature and severity of the motor disturbances underlying the deficits in the various speech motor subsystems. The advantage of instrumental analysis over perceptual assessments in defining treatment goals for children with dysarthria is therefore highlighted.

The results also indicate that dysarthria in children varies from case to case with respect to perceptual and physiological characteristics, thereby necessitating the development of individually designed treatment programs. It is recommended that such programs be based on a combination of perceptual and physiological measures.

REFERENCES

Abbs, J., & DePaul, R. (1989). Assessment of dysarthria: The critical prerequisite to treatment. In M.M. Leahy (Ed.), *Disorders of communication: The science of intervention* (pp.206-227). London: Taylor & Francis.

Bak, E., van Dongen, H.R., & Arts, W.F.M. (1983). The analysis of acquired dysarthria in children. *Developmental Medicine & Child Neurology*, *25*, 81-94.

Enderby, P. (1983). *Frenchay dysarthria assessment*. San Diego: College-Hill Press.

FitzGerald, F., Murdoch, B.E., & Chenery, H.J. (1987). Multiple sclerosis: Associated speech and language disorders. *Australian Journal of Human Communication Disorders*, *15*, 15-33.

Hayden, D.A., & Square, P.A. (1994). Motor speech treatment hierarchy: A systems approach. *Clinics in Communication Disorders*, *4*(3), 162-174.

Hinton, V.A., & Luschei, E.S. (1992). Validation of a modern miniature transducer for measurement of interlabial contact pressure during speech. *Journal of Speech and Hearing Research*, *35*, 245-251.

Murdoch, B.E., Attard, M., & Ozanne, A.E. (1995). Impaired tongue strength and endurance in developmental verbal dyspraxia: A physiological analysis. *European Journal of Communication Disorders*, *30*, 51-64.

Murdoch, B.E., & Hudson-Tennent, L.J. (1993). Speech breathing anomalies in children with dysarthria following treatment for posterior fossa tumours. *Journal of Medical Speech-Language Pathology*, *1*, 107-119.

Murdoch, B.E., & Hudson-Tennent, L.J. (1994). Speech disorders in children treated for posterior fossa tumours: Ataxic and developmental features. *European Journal of Disorders of Communication*, *29*, 379-397.

Rosenbek, J.D., & LaPointe, L.L. (1985). The dysarthrias: Description, diagnosis and treatment. In D.F. Johns (Ed.), *Clinical management of neurogenic communicative disorders* (2nd ed.)(pp.251-310). Boston: Little Brown & Co.

Theodoros, D.G., & Murdoch, B.E. (1994). Laryngeal dysfunction in dysarthric speakers following severe closed head injury. *Brain Injury*, *8*, 667-684.

Theodoros, D.G., Murdoch, B.E., & Stokes, P.D. (1993). Hypernasality in dysarthric speakers following severe closed head injury: A perceptual and instrumental analysis. *Brain Injury*, *7*, 59-69.

Van Dongen, H.R., Catsman-Berrevoets, C.E., & van Mourik, M. (1994). The syndrome of cerebellar mutism and subsequent dysarthria. *Neurology*, *44*, 2040-2046.

Yorkston, K., & Beukelman, D. (1981). *Assessment of intelligibility of dysarthric speech*. Austin: Pro-Ed.

Index of authors